UNDERSTANDING NUTRITION

WEST PUBLISHING COMPANY · St. Paul · New York · Los Angeles · San Francisco

UNDERSTANDING NUTRITION

Eleanor Noss Whitney
Eva May Nunnelley Hamilton

Library of Congress Cataloging in Publication Data

Whitney, Eleanor N.
Understanding nutrition.
    Includes index
    1. Nutrition. 2. Metabolism. I. Hamilton, Eva May, joint author. II. Title.

QP141.W46   641.1   77–23252

ISBN 0–8299–0052–7

6th Reprint—1979

To the memory of Sam G. Harrison, Jr., who encouraged me to begin, and with love and gratitude to my children, Lynn, Russell, and Kara Lee, who saw me through.

Ellie Whitney

To my husband, Marshall W. Hamilton, who throughout our marriage has supported me in my academic ventures; and to our daughters, Gayle, Nancy, and Bonnie, who have sustained me with their joy in my varied activities.

May Hamilton

Acknowledgements

We have many people to thank for their contributions to this book: Margaret A. Sitton, Dean of the College of Home Economics, Lucille M. Wakefield, Chairman of the Department of Food and Nutrition, and Nancy R. Green, Professor of Nutrition — our colleagues at The Florida State University, for their moral support; Jean Zibrida for her painstaking detective work in the library; Brian Shelley for his cheerful emergency assistance on obtaining permissions; and Ann Bass for her heroic and sustained typing efforts. Our gratitude goes also to those who read and criticized the manuscript: author Whitney's parents, Henry and Edith Tyler Noss; Simon D. Silver, Jean A. T. Pennington, H. Ira Fritz, Marsha Read, Howard Appledorf, Joan Howe, Mary K. Korslund, Olivia Bennett, Gideon E. Nelson, Joan E. Herr, Isabelle M. Koehler, Gladys Jennings, Bertha M. Bresina, and Val Hillers.

Many others have helped us in many ways and we would like to thank them all. Any errors in style or content which remain are our own.

Contents

Note to the Student

You may have some questions in mind as you approach the study of nutrition. In getting to know students over the years, we have some idea of what your concerns may be, and are anticipating a few here.

I keep hearing exciting news about nutrition. How can I tell what to believe? This is the commonest complaint we hear from students in the classroom today. Because of it, we have designed this book not to be just a book of facts, but a book of principles that you can use to assess the nutrition information you encounter elsewhere. Today's nutrition science stands firmly on the principles of chemistry and molecular biology. This book is based on those principles.

Even with the principles clearly in mind, however, it is sometimes hard to tell whether a statement made in the market place is a valid fact or a myth. Some major controversies are currently raging in our field over sugar, cholesterol, vitamin C and the common cold, the roles of vitamin E, and many other issues. It would not be fair to present these issues to you in textbook fashion as if they were settled, but it makes the study of our lively science needlessly dull to omit them. Our decision has been to reserve the **CHAPTERS** mostly for solid information, on which the experts in our field largely agree, and to present separate **HIGHLIGHTS** on the current issues, where more speculative material appears. The Highlights alternate with the

Chapters and are printed on beige pages to remind you that they convey more tentative information.

The fact is that even though we are scientists, in some cases we have no facts. Researchers in nutrition are earnestly endeavoring to learn more, but in the meantime there are many areas where we are still in the dark. Students can be infuriated when a teacher seems to weasel. "I want the facts, and you are hedging. Give me the answer, straight and simple." It is frustrating when you ask "Why?" and a cautious scientist replies, "Well, we know this, and this, and . . . " — but your question is left dangling. It is insulting to be told, "It's too complicated to understand," and sounds suspiciously like what mother used to say: "Wait until you are older, dear." But the truth of the matter is that there are a great many things we do not understand. One of the most exciting, as well as frustrating, of students' experiences can be the dawning realization that they are approaching the outer bounds of human knowledge. The answers are simply not all in yet; no one knows what they all are; no one ever has. In nutrition, this is true in many areas. Nutrition is a growing, young science. While its questions are immensely important and fascinating, that is all they are: questions. We have tried to be honest in this respect: to show you what we *do* know (with a high probability) and to admit what we don't.

In attempting to present a fair picture of current nutrition research in the Highlight sections, we have found ourselves at times confused, frustrated, angered, and amused. If you too respond this way in reading the *maybe's* and *probably's* of today's nutrition issues, then be assured that you are close to the reality of our science. Any book that claims at this time to present absolute answers to all questions is actually only presenting one person's prejudices. The writer may be proved right in years to come, but some of the winners have not yet been declared. If you wish to be informed on the current issues, you will have to accept the ambiguities and contradictions in the evidence and the disagreements among the experts as an intrinsic part of scientific research in progress.

But then how can I choose what to believe? In the absence of all the facts, we still have to live and make decisions. Should I eat polyunsaturated fats? Avoid tunafish? Beef? Sugar? It would not be fair to answer simply, "We don't know," to all these questions. Where the answers are uncertain today, we owe it to you to help in developing the skill to evaluate new information as it appears tomorrow. Our field is beset with claims and appeals, and all of us as consumers need to be equipped to deal with them.

There are some guidelines that help us to discriminate between reliable information and false advertising. It seems to us that a separate chapter devoted to this subject would not serve the purpose. You need continuous, repeated exposure to the kinds of claims made to consumers, and you need practice in assessing them. We offer frequent opportunities, by way of **DIGRESSIONS** throughout the text, for you to examine such sources of nutrition information and to assess their reliability against the criteria of accurate scientific reporting.

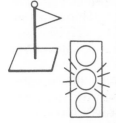 In these digressions we have identified the most common characteristics of fraudulent advertising with **FLAG SIGNS** that will help you to recognize spurious claims, and the most common misunderstandings that arise from reading about nutrition research with **CAUTION** signs, to help you interpret them correctly.

The Digressions are set off with color; if they prove too distracting you can skip them and possibly come back to them later. But they constitute a theme that runs throughout the book. In nutrition as in any other science, every "fact" in which we have confidence is based on scientific evidence and experimentation. To appreciate the value and weight of these facts, one must have a sense of how they emerged from research. If the research was well controlled, its findings will stand up to further testing. **SUGGESTED ACTIVITIES** throughout the book invite you to practice evaluating nutrition information using these guidelines.

In some cases, we have clear-cut evidence that a claim being made on the market place is fraudulent. In these cases, we feel obligated to explain and elaborate. It is not enough to say, "That's a myth," and provide nothing to replace it. But there is another problem: it seems to us that it is also not enough to say "That is a myth and this is a fact." After all, aren't "they" saying their myth is a fact? The student, confronted with a choice between what "they" say and what "we" (in a nutrition text) say is in the bind of having to choose whom to believe, with nothing further to go on. We hope, by providing relevant information, to show you that what we say is more probably true than the myth you might otherwise believe. You will understand why the low-carbohydrate diet is ill-advised when you know that carbohydrate is needed to metabolize fat in the body and how the body may be damaged when carbohydrate is not available (Chapter 7). You will understand why taking large doses of vitamin C may be harmful when you know what might happen to the child born of a mother who indulges in that practice (Highlight 10).

In using some of our space to deal with current issues, consumer questions, and health food myths, we have elected not to present an encyclopedic book of all the important knowledge that has been accumulated in our rapidly expanding field. Instead, we have stressed concepts, using selected facts to illustrate the principles on which they are based. The larger number of facts available in other texts are listed in the **APPENDICES**. We hope you will explore them and find them useful. Rather than simply becoming knowledgeable, we believe it is important to gain an acquaintance with the general principles of nutrition, as well as to develop the incentive and ability to identify reliable nutrition information on your own. Armed with this skill, you can continually gather and apply the information that is relevant to your own particular concerns.

I have heard some very scary rumors about foods. Am I right to worry about what I may be doing to myself with my diet? Under a wide range of conditions, the body cares beautifully for itself. To indicate this, we have emphasized physiology more heavily than most texts do. Only when people *understand* and *appreciate* natural health can they use their knowledge to enhance it. Still, there are circumstances in which physiology becomes abnormal and diseases arise. Cardiovascular disease, cancer, diabetes, and alcoholism are among the major diseases in the United States. Nutritional factors and carcinogens found in foods have an influence on the incidence and severity of all these diseases. While the relation of nutrition to disease does not traditionally fall within the province of a beginning text, we feel that it is important to show how nutritional status and food choices may affect susceptibility to these diseases and so have devoted a few pages to each of them.

We invite you to study your own diet and compare its characteristics with recommendations of nutrition authorities. The first one or two activities at the end of every chapter suggest informative comparisons you may wish to make. Highlight 14 suggests summing up all you have learned about your diet and considering appropriate changes.

But your science scares me. Do I have to learn chemistry to understand nutrition? Yes, this is the hard part, and the most rewarding. We make no apologies: this is a science book, a book that presents the realities as they are understood, as they really are. We are not privileged to change those realities for your convenience or our own. Our approach is biochemical. However, we believe that it is not necessary to have studied chemistry and biology extensively before embarking on the study of nutrition. We have assumed only a high school background in these sciences. The background chemistry is reviewed and explained in Appendix B to provide a refresher course. Further concepts that underlie nutrition are presented gradually in a logical sequence as they are needed; they are fully explained. Inclusion of detailed biochemical structures in Appendix C provides the option for further study of this aspect of nutrition.

In mastering the chemical concepts you may find it helpful first to read each chapter for the general ideas involved and then to study the marginal **DEFINITIONS**, which explain the chemistry in words. We have also employed verbal analogies wherever possible to assist you, comparing enzymes to machines, the process of digestion to a disassembly line, and nutrient molecules to tinker toys whose sticks are the electrons. These are not intended to insult you; if they seem too simpleminded for you (and they may, especially if you have studied chemistry before), please be patient and allow us to indulge in what for us is the enjoyable and harmless practice of playing with words and ideas.

The rewards of understanding nutrition at the molecular level are as great as the effort needed to gain that understanding. When you have struggled with an unfamiliar system, picked it apart, looked at it from every angle, and finally put it back together again, you'll find that suddenly everything falls into place. The experience of grasping a whole new concept in chemistry is an "Aha!" experience that can generate tremendous excitement and pleasure. Once understood, these concepts will not slip away. When you learned to read (through effort), to play the piano (with practice), to ride a bicycle (with painful falls), these skills stayed with you. So will nutritional chemistry once you learn it. It too will stay with you, giving you a skill and a new dimension of understanding that can be used again and again to see deeper into things.

In our introduction, we have stated that human beings are a collection of molecules that move. The biologists who have provided us with this atomic view have made great strides in recent years towards understanding what we are and how we work. They are proud of their progress, but they are humble too: proud, because their tools and analyses have given the world deeper insights into the workings of nature—and humble, because with all of the new discoveries their probings among molecules have yielded, they know even better than before how *little* they know. They know that as you read this page, the light reflecting from it is entering your eye. They know the pattern strikes your retina, where it hits molecules in your nerve cells that respond by changing their shape, and these in turn move other molecules in other nerve cells deeper in your brain. But they cannot account for what happens next—when in a fraction of a second, you process what you see into information and meaning. At this point, these scientists lose track of their molecules and are struck with wonder.

Human beings are remarkable creatures. As your eyes scan these lines you are extracting meanings from it that we who wrote this book encoded for you at another time and place. We are the only animals in nature that can do this: we can communicate our experience through symbols, bridging the gaps of time and space. And through symbols—words and pictures—we can think, remember, imagine, plan, compose poetry and music, and express our feelings for one another. How we do all these things, no one really knows.

Do not be affronted, then, at what may seem to be a mechanistic view of humankind. We are sharing with you our way of seeing things, not because it is "the" reality, but because it is a part of reality, a way of seeing that can deepen and enhance your understanding of yourself. We realize that many readers of this book will not choose to devote their lives to the study of atoms and molecules but will return to the world of people, society, and other ways of seeing reality. It is our hope that if you accept our invitation to take a tour through our world, you will return to yours better equipped to pursue your own goals, whatever they may be. We too dwell in the world of people and society, and find the chief reward of our study of nutrition to be that it enhances our lives, our understanding, and our effectiveness as human beings.

Keeping in mind that we do not pretend to account for all of human experience, let us gain what we can from the molecular nutrition point of view.

Introduction
Molecules,
the Unseen Actors

*All things are in process
and nothing stays still ...
you would not step twice
into the same river.*
—HERACLITUS

You are a collection of molecules that move. All these moving parts are arranged into patterns of extraordinary complexity and order—cells, tissues, and organs. The arrangement is constant, but its parts are continuously being replaced. Your skin, which has reliably covered you from the time you were born, is not the same skin that covered you seven years ago; it is made entirely of new cells. The fat beneath your skin is not the same fat that was there a year ago. Your oldest red blood cell is only six weeks old, while the entire lining of your digestive tract is renewed every three days. To maintain your "self," you must continually replace the pieces you lose.

All of these pieces have come from your food: you are made

food: nutritive material taken into the body to keep it alive and to enable it to grow (**nutritive:** containing nutrients).

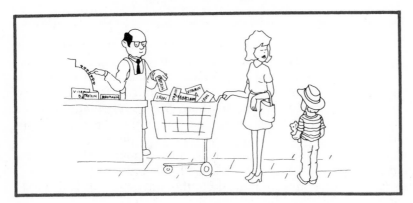

"Darling, would you go back to aisle 6 and get us another 40 milligrams of iron?"

1

nutrient: a substance obtained from food and used in the body to promote growth, maintenance, or repair.

adequate diet: a diet providing all the needed nutrients in the right total amounts. Such a diet is ideally also **balanced**, that is, it provides nutrients in the proportion that best meets the body's needs.

science of nutrition: the study of nutrients and of their digestion, absorption, metabolism, interaction, storage, and excretion. A broader definition includes the study of the environment and of human behavior as it relates to nutrition.

atoms, molecules, compounds: Appendix B summarizes basic chemistry facts and definitions.

organic: see following pages.

entirely of what you have eaten. This is not meant to imply, of course, that if you ate spaghetti last night, you are made of spaghetti now! Some complex events take place between your eating of food and its becoming "you." A bowl of spaghetti or a piece of apple pie must be entirely taken apart and rearranged before its pieces can be used to make the structures of your eye, brain, or skin. You eat *foods*, but what you obtain from them is *nutrients*, and these undergo many transformations and rearrangements in your body. If the spaghetti or the apple pie you choose to eat does not contain the nutrients you need, you lose a little: for optimum nutrition you need an adequate diet.

The science of nutrition is the study, not of foods, but of the nutrients they contain and the body's handling of these nutrients.

The Nutrients

Almost any food you eat is composed of dozens or even hundreds of different kinds of materials, tinier by far than the smallest things that can be seen with the highest power microscope; they are atoms and molecules. The complete chemical analysis of a food such as spinach shows that it is composed mostly of water (95 percent) and that most of the solid materials are organic compounds: carbohydrate, fat, and protein. If you could remove these materials, you would find a tiny residue remaining, consisting of minerals and of vitamins and other organic materials. Water, carbohydrate, fat, protein, vitamins, and some of the minerals are nutrients. Some of the other organic materials and minerals are not.

The six classes of nutrients:	
carbohydrate	vitamins
fat	minerals
protein	water

A complete chemical analysis of your body would show that it is made of very similar materials. If you weigh 150 pounds, your body contains about 90 pounds of water, and (if 150 pounds is the proper weight for you) about 30 pounds of fat. The other 30 pounds are mostly protein, carbohydrate, and related organic compounds made from them, and the major minerals of your bones: calcium and phosphorus. Vitamins, other minerals, and incidental extras constitute a fraction of a pound. Thus you too, like spinach, are composed mostly of nutrients.

(This book is devoted mostly to the nutrients, but you should be aware that there are other constituents found in foods and in

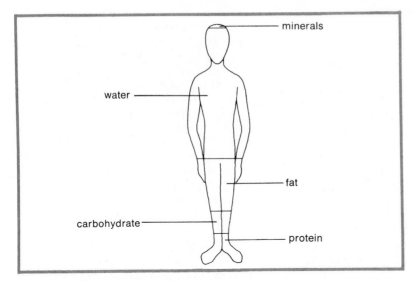

minerals

water

fat

carbohydrate

protein

Chemical composition
of the human body.

your body—organic additives, both intentional and incidental, and trace minerals—of no recognized positive value to humans. Some may even be harmful. Later sections of the book focus on these and their significance.)

If you burn a food, such as spinach, in air, it disappears. The water evaporates, and all of the organic compounds are oxidized to gas (carbon dioxide) and water vapor, leaving only a residue of ash. This leads us to a definition of the word *organic.*

The meaning of organic. An organic compound is one which contains carbon atoms. The first such compounds known were natural products synthesized by plants or animals; indeed, it used to be thought that only living things contributed organic compounds to our world. The term has since been expanded to include all carbon compounds, whatever their origin. Actually, in a sense, all organic compounds are produced by living things. Some of them, like petroleum (which comes from the remains of trees that grew in prehistoric times), began life millions of years ago. Others are produced by plants and animals alive today. Still others come from the laboratories where chemists (who are also "living things") produce them in the test tube.

Additives, including the pesticides and possible carcinogens, are the subject of Highlight 13.

ash: the minerals that remain after a food is completely burned.

organic: containing carbon or, more strictly, containing carbon and hydrogen or carbon-carbon bonds. This definition excludes coal (in which there are no defined bonds); a few carbon-containing compounds, such as carbon dioxide (which contains only a single carbon and no hydrogen); and salts such as calcium carbonate ($CaCO_3$), magnesium carbonate ($MgCO_3$), and sodium cyanide ($NaCN$).

Throughout this book digressions from the main topic will be made to develop your skill in evaluating what you read about nutrition. Labels on food products sometimes make the claim that the product is *organic,* and imply that it is therefore somehow superior to a chemically fertilized food. By the definition given above, any carbon compound is organic, even a synthetic vitamin preparation from the laboratory of a pharmaceutical

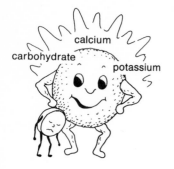

company. Is there any reason to believe that *organic* or *natural* foods or nutrient preparations sold in "health food" stores are superior to grocery store foods or synthetic vitamins? Let us take vitamin C as an example.

Vitamin C, or ascorbic acid, is an organic compound with a certain chemical structure (see Chapter 10). Regardless of its source, it always has the same structure. One carbon atom (or hydrogen atom or oxygen atom) is exactly like all the others. They have no individuality; all molecules with this structure are identical. When a molecule of vitamin C enters your bloodstream, your body cannot tell where it came from. Hence the vitamin C from a chemist's lab is no different from the vitamin C in an orange fresh from a Florida citrus grove. An important point made by the American Dietetic Association in 1975 is:

> All foods are "organic" because they are composed of organic compounds containing carbon.[1]

On the other hand, the orange may be better for you, not because its ascorbic acid is qualitatively superior to the ascorbic acid in the vitamin pill, but because the orange also contains carbohydrate, calcium, potassium, and other nutrients, as well as beneficial nonnutrient fiber, while the pill contains only vitamin C—nothing more. In other words:

> There is no advantage to eating an organic *nutrient* from one source as opposed to another, but there may be fringe benefits to eating that nutrient in a natural *food* as opposed to a purified nutrient preparation.

To interpret what you read on food labels you need two kinds of information. First, of course, you need to know the meanings of the terms that are used (an acquaintance with the definitions given throughout this book will help). Secondly—and this is especially important with *health food* products—you must be aware that a term may be used to imply a meaning different from the officially accepted one. The word *organic* is an example. As used on health food labels it is intended to imply superiority to ordinary foods. The product labeled organic has merely been organically grown; that is, in soil to which no "chemical fertilizer" has been added (only "natural fertilizer" such as manure and compost),

[1]Position paper on food and nutrition misinformation on selected topics. *Journal of The American Dietetic Association* 66:277-279, 1975.

and without the use of any insecticide sprays such as DDT. The term "health food" is another example, implying that the food has extraordinary power to promote health. Actually, a food promotes health depending solely on the amounts and balance of nutrients it contains and on the response to it of the person who eats it.

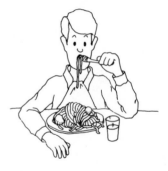

Your choice of what foods to buy is a personal choice. Insofar as it is based on your knowledge of the nutritional value of the foods, the information in this book may help you to choose wisely. The subject is a big one, and different aspects of it will be taken up in the series of digressions that follow. For the present, let us content ourselves with one additional important point—about fertilizers.

Plants take up minerals from the soil (including those from fertilizers) depending not on what is present in the soil but on what the plant needs. A tomato grown on synthetic fertilizer achieves the same chemical composition as one grown on decomposed organic material, such as compost. To put it most simply, the composition of a plant depends on the plant, not on the soil. Nutritionally, therefore, an "organically grown" plant is not superior to a "chemically fertilized" one, and a label which implies otherwise is misleading. All fertilizers are composed of chemicals.

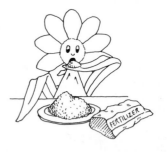

A flag sign of a spurious claim is the use of the words:

> organic
> health food

spurious: false, fraudulent.

Pending legislation proposes forbidding the use of these words on labels. See Highlight 13.

Of course if a needed element is absolutely lacking in the soil, the plant cannot select it. Any poorly- (inadequately) fertilized soil is inferior to well- (adequately) fertilized soil. There are good and poor "organic" fertilizers, as well as good and poor "chemical" fertilizers. By the same token, there may be fringe benefits from the use of natural fertilizers, such as compost. For example, such a fertilizer has a beneficial effect on the structure (*tilth*) of the soil which most chemical fertilizers do not. This is not a nutritional but a mechanical advantage to the plant.

An adequate diet for a plant might be defined as any plant food (fertilizer) that supplies all the needed nutrients for the plant.

The only unequivocal statement about the nutritive quality of a fertilizer is a statement of the specific chemicals it contains, and the amount of each; their source is irrelevant. The only unequivocal statement about the nutritive quality of a food is a statement of the specific nutrients it contains and the amount of each; their source is irrelevant.

unequivocal: clear, unambiguous, leaving no doubt.

The Principal Actors: The Energy Nutrients

> **The organic nutrients:**
>
> carbohydrate   protein
> fat   vitamins

The distinction between the organic and inorganic nutrients is important for several reasons. For one thing, in cooking foods you need to be aware that some organic nutrients are sensitive to and can be altered or destroyed by chemical and physical agents, such as acids, heat, and light. This is especially important with respect to the vitamins. The minerals, on the other hand, are simple elements whose nature cannot be changed physically or chemically.

metabolism: the processes by which nutrients are re-arranged into body structures or broken down to yield energy (precise definition, page 202.

oxidation: a reaction in which atoms from a molecule are combined with oxygen, usually with the release of energy. Chemical oxidation of nutrients differs from oxidative combustion (burning) in that the energy released is largely chemical and mechanical, rather than heat and light energy. A further explanation is given in Appendix B.

Moreover, when organic nutrients are metabolized, waste materials (such as carbon dioxide) are produced. Everything has to go somewhere, and the metabolism of certain organic nutrients taxes the body, which has the burden of excreting these wastes.

Furthermore, organic nutrients can release heat or other kinds of energy. When oxidized, they break down; that is, their carbon atoms and others come apart and are combined with oxygen. If you burn a potful of food on the range, the same thing happens. Heat is released together with carbon dioxide and water vapor, and you are left with a ruined pot, blackened with the carbon and mineral residue from the food. But when you oxidize food in your body, the energy is not all released as heat. Some is transferred into other compounds (including fat) that compose the *structures* of your body cells, and some of the energy which holds the atoms of the energy nutrients together is used to power your activities, enabling you to *move*.

At the outset it was stated that you are a collection of molecules that move. Now you can see a little more clearly what this means. Human beings *are* atoms taken from the molecules of food and rearranged into the molecules of their bodies. We *move* thanks to the energy released when these food molecules are taken apart.

You can metabolize all four classes of organic nutrients, but only three yield energy for the body's use. These three are the energy nutrients.

> **The energy nutrients:**
>
> carbohydrate
> fat
> protein

The amount of energy they release can be measured in "calories," (or more properly, kilocalories), which no doubt are familiar to you as those things that make foods "fattening." The energy content of a food thus depends on how much carbohydrate, fat, and protein it contains. If not used immediately, these nutrients and the energy contained in them are rearranged mostly into body fat and then stored. Thus an excess intake of any of the three energy nutrients can lead to overweight. Too much meat (a protein-rich food) is just as fattening as too many potatoes (a carbohydrate-rich food).

It is important not to forget the organic compound found in alcoholic beverages: alcohol. This compound is not properly called a nutrient by the definition given on page 2, but it shares several characteristics with the energy nutrients. Like them, it is metabolized in the body to yield energy. When taken in excess of energy need, it too is converted to body fat and stored. But when alcohol contributes a substantial portion of the energy in a person's diet, its effects are damaging. Highlight 9 is devoted to this compound.

Practically all foods contain mixtures of all three energy nutrients, although they are sometimes classed by the predominant nutrient. A protein-rich food such as beef actually contains a lot of fat as well as protein; a carbohydrate-rich food such as corn also contains fat and protein. Only a few foods are exceptions to this rule, the common ones being sugar (which is pure carbohydrate) and oil (which is almost pure fat).

kilocalories: the units in which the energy in food is measured. These are often mistakenly called calories. Definitions of both are given on pages 235-236.

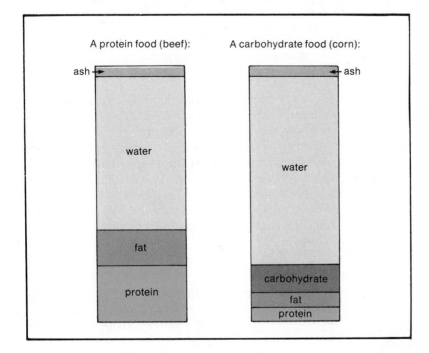

A protein food (beef):

A carbohydrate food (corn):

ash

ash

water

water

fat

carbohydrate

protein

fat

protein

The energy nutrients are the principal actors in the drama of nutrition and are the subject of Part One of this book. The vitamins and the inorganic nutrients—minerals and water—serve functions other than providing energy and the direct building of body compounds; they are the subject of Part Two. The figure in the summary below outlines very simply the flow of the energy nutrients into and through the body, a recurring theme throughout Part One.

Summing Up

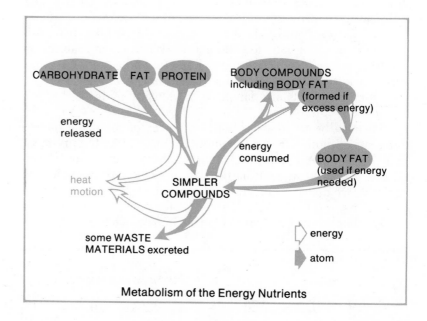

Metabolism of the Energy Nutrients

The six classes of nutrients found in foods are carbohydrate, fat, protein, vitamins, minerals, and water. The first four are organic compounds, the last two inorganic. The first three of these are the energy nutrients and are the subject of Part One of this book. After entering the body, these nutrients are metabolized to simpler compounds which can be oxidized, releasing energy. The simple compounds may then be excreted, or reassembled into body compounds, while the energy they release may be used to construct body compounds, to move body parts, or to generate heat.

To Explore Further—

This article develops further the ideas presented in the Digression in this introduction:

Jukes, T. H.: The organic food myth. *Journal of the American Medical Association* 230(2):276-277, 1974.

Suggested readings and resource materials follow each Chapter and Highlight. A few excellent *general references which would be useful throughout the study of nutrition* are the following.

A short, clear explanation of cell biology, recommended for the student who is unfamiliar with cells:
Loewy, A. G. and Siekevitz, P.: *Cell Structure and Function.* 2nd ed. Holt, Rinehart and Winston, Inc., New York, 1969.

A biology textbook, an unusually clear and beautiful presentation of the biological principles on which the science of nutrition is based:
Curtis, H.: *Invitation to Biology.* Worth Publishers, Inc., New York, 1972.

An advanced textbook including detailed treatments of the nutrients, digestion and absorption, the cell and cell types, growth, and other topics:
Pike, R. L. and Brown, M. L.: *Nutrition: An Integrated Approach.* 2nd ed. John Wiley and Sons, Inc., New York, 1975.

"The" reference book for nutrition facts: encyclopedic articles on major topics:
Goodhart, R. S. and Shils, M. E., editors: *Modern Nutrition in Health and Disease.* 5th ed. Lea and Febiger, Philadelphia, 1973.

A journal for the interested layman, with easily readable articles of current interest: *Nutrition Today. Scientific American* often also has excellent articles on foods and nutrition.

A more technical journal, which includes a very useful section of abstracts of recent articles from many other journals of nutrition and related areas is: *Journal of the American Dietetic Association.*

A journal which does much of the work for the library researcher, compiling recent evidence on current topics and presenting extensive bibliographies, is: *Nutrition Reviews.*

Three more technical reputable (see page 76) journals in the field: *Journal of Nutrition, American Journal of Clinical Nutrition, Journal of the American Medical Association.*

PART ONE

THE ENERGY NUTRIENTS: CARBOHYDRATE, FAT, PROTEIN

1

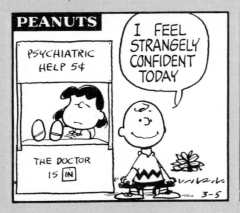
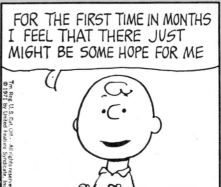
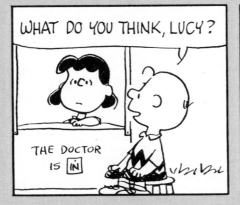
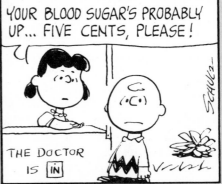

The Carbohydrates ▬

The Universe is not only queerer than we imagine —it is queerer than we can imagine.
—J. B. S. HALDANE

Feeling Good

Most of us would like to feel good all the time. The enjoyment available in a day, no matter what the day may bring, can be tremendous if your body and mind are tuned for it. The feeling of well-being that comes from being full of energy, alert, clear-thinking and confident, is so rewarding that if you know how to produce it, you will probably make the effort required.

It would be an exaggeration to say that good eating habits alone produce the feeling of well-being that we find so desirable. If you try to think of what makes you feel good, you can come up with any of several answers. Being in love, for example, is certainly one! Facing and solving a personal problem is another. Being well rested helps too; when you wake up after a good night's sleep, you may feel bright eyed and bushy tailed, ready to take on the world, without having eaten a thing for twelve hours or more. Exercise helps too; the feeling of being physically tired after climbing a mountain or running a mile is a "good tired." Being clean is still another; a cold shower after heavy work or exercise can be bracing and exhilarating. Sparkling weather, clean air, beautiful scenery, pleasant company— all these play a part.

Even among the best of these pleasures, however, some limits are set by your nutritional state. You can feel really good only when your blood sugar (glucose) level is right. If that con-

glucose: a simple sugar, often known as "blood sugar" because it is the principal carbohydrate found in mammalian blood (see also page 25).

13

But see page 207.

oxidation: see page 6.

dition isn't met, neither the most beautiful mountaintop nor the most stimulating companion can compensate.

The health and functioning of every cell in your body depend on blood sugar to a greater or lesser extent. Ordinarily the cells of your brain and nervous system depend solely on this sugar for their energy. Since the brain cells are continually active, even while you're asleep, they are continually drawing upon the supply of sugar in the fluid surrounding them. They oxidize it for the energy they need to perform their functions. To maintain the supply, a continuous flow of blood moves past these cells, replenishing the sugar as the cells use it up.

Because your brain and other nerves ordinarily cannot make use of any other energy source, they are especially vulnerable to a temporary deficit in the blood sugar supply. This is why sugar is sometimes known as *brain food*. When your brain is deprived of energy, your mental processes are affected. You may be unable to think clearly. Your brain controls your muscles, so you may feel weak and shaky. You are likely to miscalculate—either to make an error in balancing your checkbook, or to trip while walking downstairs. And since the mind resides in the brain, your attitude toward life, the world, and other people may also be distorted. You may become anxious, easily upset, depressed, or irritable. Your head may ache; you may feel dizzy or even nauseated. These are the symptoms of hypoglycemia: too little glucose in the blood.

hypoglycemia (HIGH-po-gligh-SEEM-ee-uh): an abnormally low blood glucose concentration.

hypo = too little
glyce = glucose
emia = in the blood

The hypoglycemia being described here is a temporary state known as **functional hypoglycemia** that may be experienced briefly by any normal person. **Spontaneous hypoglycemia**, a condition experienced by certain individuals with abnormal carbohydrate metabolism, requires diagnosis and medical treatment.

Hypoglycemia became a fad some years ago with the publication of several popular and not entirely reliable books on the subject. Since then, people suffering from the symptoms listed above have tended to self-diagnose their conditions as hypoglycemia when in fact, of course, there are many other possible causes for such symptoms. A position paper by the American Dietetic Association warns of the risks of self-diagnosis of this condition;[1] a later digression (page 285) develops this theme more fully.

The body has an amazing ability to adapt to changing conditions by altering its own chemistry to maintain an internal balance. For example, when you get too hot, your blood circulation is routed closer to the skin surface so that the blood can be cooled; you perspire, and the evaporation of the secreted moisture cools you still further. When you are too cold, your circulation is rerouted inwards, so that heat will not be lost by expo-

[1] _____ : Position paper on food and nutrition misinformation on selected topics. *Journal of the American Dietetic Association* 66:277-279, 1975.

sure of the blood to the outside air. In the same way, when your blood sugar concentration rises too high or falls too low, your body makes internal adjustments to bring it back to normal. Still, human folly can defeat the body's best efforts to keep in balance. An awareness and understanding of how blood sugar is regulated can enable you to cooperate with your body in the best interest of both of you.

The following paragraphs show how the body maintains its blood glucose level, and what can be done to help. There follow descriptions of how energy is contained in glucose, and finally where glucose is found in foods.

The Constancy of the Blood Glucose Level

When you wake up in the morning, your blood probably contains between 80 and 120 milligrams (mg) of glucose in each 100 milliliters (ml) of blood (about one-half cup). This range, which is known as the *fasting blood glucose* concentration, is normal and is accompanied by a feeling of alertness and well-being (provided that nothing else is wrong, of course—that you don't have the flu, for example). If you don't eat, the blood glucose level will gradually fall as your cells draw upon the supply. At 70 mg/100 ml, the low end of the normal range is reached. Often at this point a feeling of hunger is experienced. The normal response to this sensation is to eat, and provided that the meal includes some carbohydrate, or an alternative source of glucose, your blood sugar level soon rises again above this threshold.

If your meal has been unusually high in carbohydrate, and especially if it has consisted mostly of simple carbohydrate (ordinary, granulated sugar or syrup), your blood sugar concentration may threaten to rise too high. This too is an undesirable condition, known as hyperglycemia. A simple way for the body to contend with this imbalance would be to excrete the excess sugar in the urine. But the body is conservative; it stores the excess against a possible future need. The first organ to respond is the pancreas, which detects the excess and puts out a message about it; then liver, muscle, and fat cells receive the message, remove the sugar from the blood, and store it.

The beta cells of the pancreas are sensitive to the blood glucose concentration. When it rises, they respond by secreting more of the hormone insulin into the blood. As the circulating insulin bathes the liver cells, they in turn respond by taking up sugar from the blood, just as all cells in the body do. Within the liver cells, the small glucose units are assembled into long

normoglycemia (NOR-mo-gligh-SEEM-ee-uh): a normal blood glucose concentration: 80-120 mg/100 ml.

normo = normal

milligrams, milliliters: metric measures of weight and volume. For definitions of these terms see Appendix D.

hyperglycemia (HIGH-per-gligh-SEEM-ee-uh): an abnormally high blood glucose concentration.

hyper = too much

pancreas, liver: Chapter 5 describes some of the functions of these organs. Their anatomical relation to the digestive system is shown in Figure C5.1.

beta cells: one of the four types of cells in the pancreas. The beta cells secrete insulin in response to increased blood glucose concentration.

hormone: see page 157.

insulin (IN-suh-lin): a hormone secreted by the pancreas in response to increased blood glucose concentration.

glycogen (GLIGH-co-gen): a storage form of glucose in liver and muscle (see also page 23).

glyco = glucose
gen = gives rise to

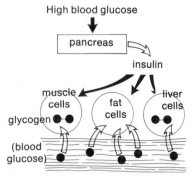

Insulin brings blood glucose down by stimulating its removal into the cells and its storage as liver and muscle glycogen and as fat.

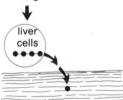

Low blood glucose is raised by the return of liver glycogen to glucose and its release into the blood. (Other hormones are involved: not shown.)

maladaptive behavior: behavior intended to help an organism meet its needs, but which is not actually in its best interest.

simple carbohydrate: see page 22.

diabetes: see page 43.

chains of glycogen and stored in this form. These can later be dismantled if the need arises. The sugar units can then be returned to the circulating blood.

Muscle and fat cells also participate in bringing blood glucose down to normal. In muscle, as in the liver, the glucose is stored as glycogen, but this glycogen cannot be converted back directly to blood glucose. (It converts to an intermediate substance, lactate, and is released into the blood, from which it is taken up by the liver and converted to glucose.) In fat cells, the glucose is converted to fat and stored as such. Very little can be reconverted to glucose. Thus, liver glycogen is the only ready reserve of blood glucose.

The maintenance of a normal blood glucose level thus depends on two types of safeguards. When the level gets too low, it can be replenished quickly either by drawing upon liver glycogen stores or by eating a meal that includes a food source of glucose—normally carbohydrate. When it gets too high, insulin will be secreted to siphon off the excess into storage. (There is more to this story. Insulin performs other roles than the one described here; this description is only intended to give a sense of how the body maintains balance.)

If your blood glucose level reaches 70 mg/100 ml, and you don't eat, the level may fall further still as the glycogen reserves are used up. Then you will feel the undesirable symptoms associated with hypoglycemia. In addition to those already described above (weakness, mental confusion, dizziness), you may experience a craving for sweets. At this point, some people succumb to the craving and eat a quick energy food, such as a coke or a candy bar—thus beginning what could be called *maladaptive behavior*. The blood glucose level shoots up rapidly in response to pure simple carbohydrate of this type, and an insulin overreaction may occur. Then blood glucose rebounds to a too-low level, and hypoglycemia once again sets in. This alternation between the extremes upsets the system, destroying the normal state of well-being.

One of the many theories about the cause of diabetes is that frequent flooding of the circulation with simple carbohydrate can overstrain the pancreas by placing repeated sudden demands on it to secrete large quantities of insulin. Finally, after years of such abuse, the beta cells can no longer produce insulin at all. This, however, is only a theory. The evidence for it is largely circumstantial. Experts disagree on the subject. Some of the evidence relating to sugar and diabetes is discussed in the Highlight following this chapter.

For maximum well-being, you need to eat in such a way as to avoid either extreme. This primarily means doing two things. First, when you are approaching hypoglycemia, you should probably eat, without waiting until you are famished. For most people, hunger is a reliable indicator of the appropriate time to eat (although in some—notably the intractably obese and diabetics—hunger is not necessarily a sign of physiological need for food). Secondly, when you do eat, you should eat a balanced meal, including some protein and fat as well as complex carbohydrate. The fat slows down the digestion and absorption of carbohydrate, so that it trickles gradually into the blood, rather than flooding the system all at once. The protein provides a more slowly digested alternative source of blood glucose for use in case the glycogen reserves are exhausted.

hunger, appetite: see pages 238-239.

How fat slows down digestion and absorption of carbohydrate: see Chapter 5.

Carbohydrates: The Chemist's View

Those who work with atoms and molecules—chemists, physicists, and other scientists—are people whose curiosity has impelled them to ask questions about everything. The answers they seek are explanations of substances in terms of the next smaller units of which they are made. These scientists also explain *you* in this way; that is, you are a bundle of a great many atoms (perhaps 3,000,000,000,000,000,000,000,000,000, give or take 1,000,000,000,000,000,000,000,000,000), held together and moved about by virtue of their associated energy.

If your mind boggles at such a thought, don't be dismayed. It staggers anyone's imagination to contemplate the ultimate realities of our universe. If we willingly go along with the chemists, all the way down to the atoms of which the carbohydrates are made, we may feel a little bit out of our depth, but we stand to gain much. An understanding of how energy is contained in glucose molecules and of how it is released when these molecules are metabolized in the body will help us achieve some desirable ends—to acquire the energy we need from our food at a minimum dollar cost, for example, or to balance our food energy sources for maximum health and efficiency without weight gain.

To promote an understanding of the carbohydrates, the following two sections are devoted to (1) the structure of glucose, and (2) the reactions by which glucose and similar molecules are put together to make the larger carbohydrates. The release of energy from glucose and the ways the body uses this energy are the subjects of Highlight 7.

(1) Glucose. A chemist views a glucose molecule as a compound composed of 24 atoms: six carbon, six oxygen, and twelve hydrogen atoms. These atoms are symbolized by the letters C,

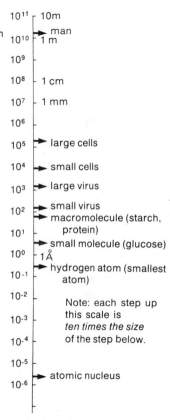

From *Cell Structure and Function* by Ariel G. Loewy and Phillip Siekevitz. Copyright © 1963 by Holt, Rinehart & Winston, Inc. Adapted by permission of Holt, Rinehart & Winston.

compound, chemical formula: for basic chemistry, see Appendix B.

O, and H. Thus, the chemical formula for glucose, which reflects the number of atoms it contains, is $C_6H_{12}O_6$.

Each type of atom has a characteristic amount of energy available for forming chemical bonds with other atoms. A carbon atom can form four such bonds; an oxygen atom, two; and a hydrogen atom, only one. One way to represent the number of bonds associated with each type of atom is to use lines radiating from the letters. The bonds of a carbon atom are represented by showing four lines radiating from each C, while the bonds of an oxygen atom are represented by two such lines, and that of a hydrogen atom by one, like this:

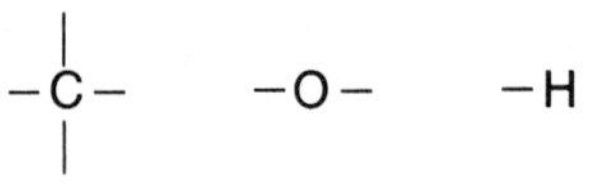

$$-\overset{\displaystyle |}{\underset{\displaystyle |}{C}}- \qquad -O- \qquad -H$$

Now, C, H, and O atoms may be put together in any way that satisfies their bonding requirements. The drawing of the active ingredient of alcoholic beverages (below) shows that each atom's bonding capabilities are fully used in its structure:

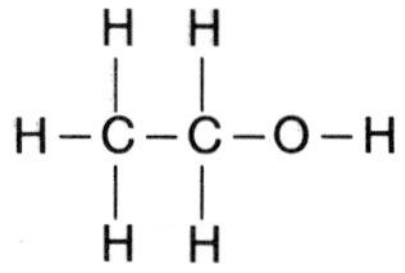

$$H-\overset{\displaystyle \overset{H}{|}}{\underset{\displaystyle \underset{H}{|}}{C}}-\overset{\displaystyle \overset{H}{|}}{\underset{\displaystyle \underset{H}{|}}{C}}-O-H$$

Chemical structure of ethyl alcohol

The carbons both have four lines (bonds), the oxygen has two, and the hydrogens each have one that connect them to other atoms. In any drawing of a chemical structure these conditions must be met, not because a fussy scientist made up these rules, but because this represents the way nature demands it.

Glucose is a larger and more complicated molecule than alcohol, but it obeys the same rules—as do all chemical compounds. The complete structure of a glucose molecule is shown below:

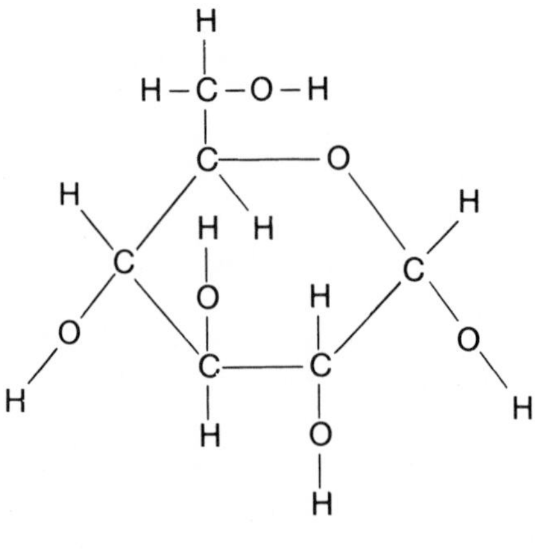

Chemical structure of glucose

Again, each carbon atom has four, each oxygen two, and each hydrogen one bond connecting it to other atoms.

This diagram may look formidable, but it does show all the relationships between the parts and proves simple on examination. Since we will be viewing other complex structures (not necessarily to memorize them, but rather to understand certain things about them), let us adopt a simpler way to depict them—one which shows fewer details. In the drawing shown below, each corner, where lines intersect, represents a carbon atom, and many of the bonds are not shown. Wherever a carbon atom needs H's to complete its four bonds, the H's are assumed to be present. From such a picture, knowing the rules of chemical structure, it is possible to reconstruct the complete structure with all its details:

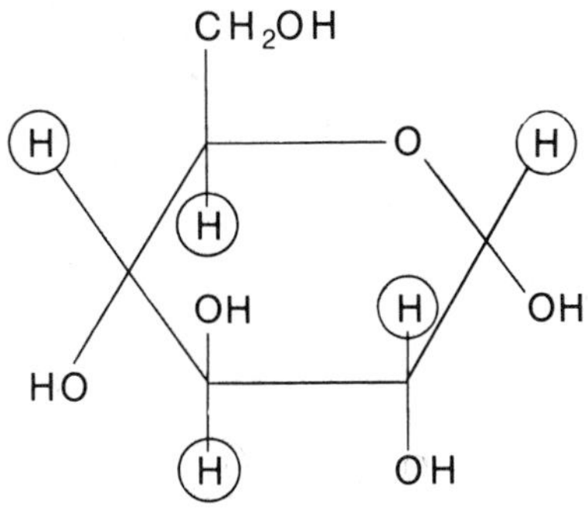

Chemical
structure of
glucose (simplified)

In future drawings of the glucose structure, the circled hydrogens will be omitted

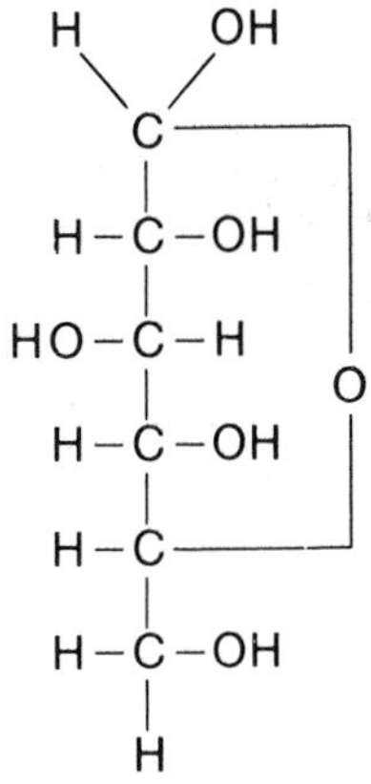

Another way to depict the structure of glucose. Note that both the first and the fifth carbons are bonded to oxygen. Hydroxyl (—OH) groups, which are shown on the right of the "line" structure are placed below the carbon in the "ring" structure. Similarly, note that the lone —OH group shown on the left of the line structure is placed above the carbon in the ring structure.

All carbohydrates are composed of glucose and other C—H—O compounds very much like glucose in structure. They come in three main sizes: single molecules like glucose itself; pairs (for example, two glucose molecules bonded together); and chains (for example, 300 glucose molecules strung in a line). The chemist's terms for these three types of carbohydrates are mono-, di-, and polysaccharides.

With this information, the chemist's terms defining the carbohydrates are understandable, and the common terms we use to describe them—*sugars* and *starches*—can be understood

carbohydrate: a compound composed of carbon, hydrogen, and oxygen, arranged as monosaccharides or multiples of monosaccharides.

carbo = carbon (C)
hydrate = water (H_2O)

monosaccharide (mon-oh-SACK-uh-ride): a carbohydrate of the general formula $C_nH_{2n}O_n$; n may be any number, but the monosaccharides important in nutrition are all **hexoses** (monosaccharides containing 6 carbon atoms—$C_6H_{12}O_6$).

> mono = one
> saccharide, -ose = sugar
> hex = six

disaccharide: a pair of monosaccharides bonded together.

> di = two

polysaccharide: many monosaccharides bonded together.

> poly = many

chemical reaction: see Appendix B.

condensation: a chemical reaction in which two reactants combine to yield a major product with the elimination of water or a similar small molecule.

more precisely. The sugars are the mono- and disaccharides; the starches are the polysaccharides. Store-bought cane or beet sugar is one of the disaccharides.

It remains to be seen how these units are put together and taken apart in the continuous flow of matter and energy through living things.

(2) *Making pairs: chemical reactions.* When a disaccharide is formed from two monosaccharides, a chemical reaction takes place, known as a condensation reaction.

In a condensation reaction, a hydrogen atom is removed from one monosaccharide, and an oxygen-hydrogen (OH group) from the other, leaving the two molecules bonded by a single —O—:

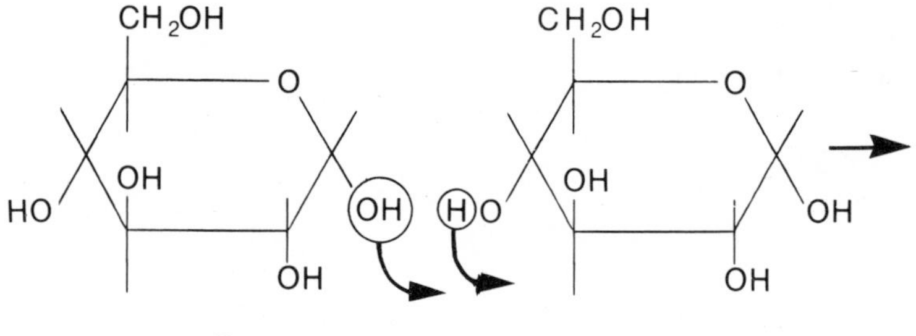

Two glucoses, water being removed.

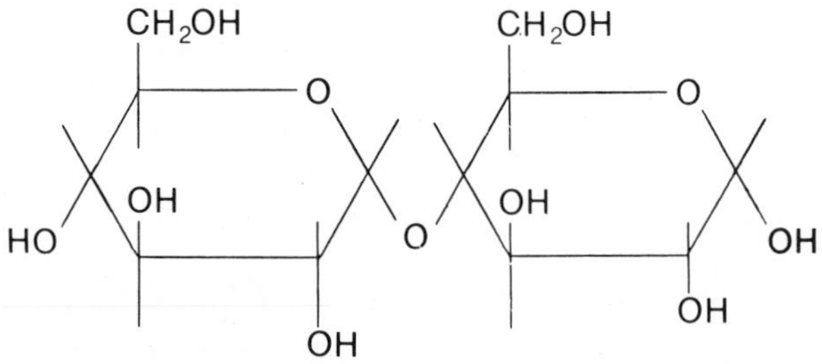

The disaccharide maltose (new bond between two glucoses).

The H— and —O—H which were removed from the monosaccharides in this reaction also bond to each other and form a molecule of H—O—H, or water (H_2O):

$$H- + -O-H \rightarrow H-O-H$$

hydrolysis (high-DROL-uh-sis): a chemical reaction in which a major reactant is split into two products with the addition of H— to one and —OH to the other, from water.

> hydro = water
> lysis = breaking

When a disaccharide is taken apart to form two monosaccharides again, as for example during digestion in the human body, a molecule of water participates in the reaction, with the H— being added to one, and the —O—H to the other monosaccharide, to reform the original structures. This reaction is called a hydrolysis reaction:

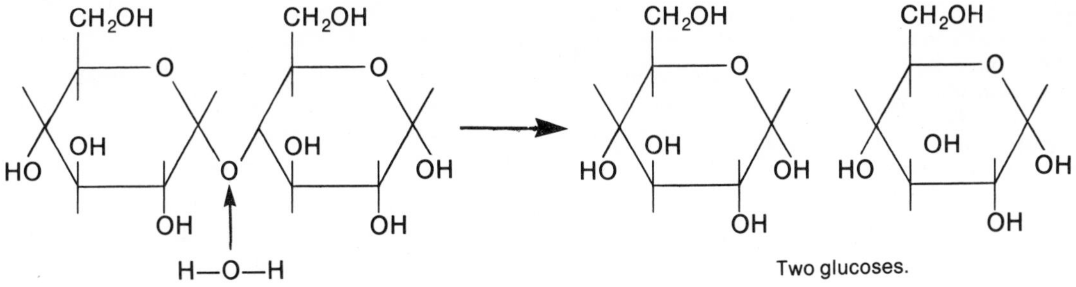

Disaccharide maltose
water enters

Two glucoses.

It is by these two types of reactions, condensation and hydrolysis, that all of the carbohydrates are put together and taken apart. For this reason, among many others, *water* is of tremendous importance to living things such as ourselves; without it, literally nothing would happen. Chapter 14 is devoted to this extraordinary substance. Meanwhile, as you read, notice that water is involved in every process that is described in this book.

The facilitators of the above reactions, the enzymes, are also of great importance. They are described fully in Chapter 3. For the moment, however, let us adopt a simple definition. An enzyme is a giant molecule (about the same size as a molecule of starch) which provides a surface on which other molecules (such as glucose) may come together and react with each other. Since the making and breaking of chemical bonds tells the whole story of growth, maintenance, and change in living creatures, the enzymes which facilitate these reactions are indispensable to life.

enzyme: see also page 89.

But enough of chemistry. We know now that glucose is the predominant energy source for all the body's cells and can appreciate the importance of having a constant energy supply if we are to feel well. So let's return to the more familiar chemicals called foods, which are the sources of glucose in the diet.

Starches and Sugars in Foods

Virtually all our energy comes from the food we eat, about half from carbohydrate and half from fat and protein. In fact, one of the principal roles of carbohydrate in the diet is to supply energy in the form of blood glucose. A look at the carbohydrates found in foods and the way they are put together will show why this is so.

The carbohydrates are conveniently divided into two classes: the complex carbohydrates, of which starch is the most familiar example, and the simple carbohydrates, exemplified

complex carbohydrates: the polysaccharides (starch, glycogen and cellulose).

simple carbohydrates: the monosaccharides (glucose, fructose, and galactose) and the disaccharides (sucrose, lactose, and maltose). Also called the sugars.

by ordinary table sugar. All are composed of monosaccharides, as you have seen. By far the most common monosaccharide in these compounds is glucose. Since starch itself is the most significant contributor of glucose to most people's diets, it will be considered first.

Starch. You know what foods are starchy by their reputation: bread, rice, macaroni and other pastas, potatoes. Possibly these are the foods you and your friends or relatives avoid when you are on a diet since they are believed to be high in calories. Actually, all foods contain calories because they contain energy nutrients—protein, fat, and carbohydrate—and the hundred calories from a 3½−ounce baked potato are no more and no less fattening than the 100 calories from a 2-ounce slice of roast beef, although they are a lot less expensive. Starchy foods supply calories at the rate of approximately 20 calories per teaspoon of pure starch they contain. But what is starch?

● = glucose

etc.   etc.

etc. ●—●—●—●—●—● etc.

Portion of a starch molecule.

Starch, as the chemist sees it, is a branched chain of dozens of glucose units connected together. These units would have to be magnified more than ten million times to appear at the size shown on this page. A single starch molecule may contain from 300 to 1,000 or more glucose units linked together in this way. These giant molecules are packed side by side in the rice grain or potato root—as many as a million in a cubic inch of the food.

In the plant, starch serves a function similar to that of the glycogen in your liver. It is a storage form of glucose that will be needed for the plant's first growth. (When you eat the plant, of course, you get the glucose to use for your own purposes.)

starch: a plant polysaccharide composed of glucose, digestible by humans.

Notice that all starchy foods are in fact plant foods. Seeds

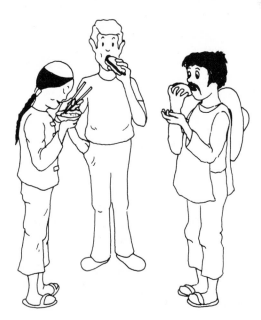

are the richest food source of starch; 70 percent of their weight is starch. Many human societies have a staple grain, from which 50 to 80 percent of their food energy is derived. Rice is the staple grain of the Orient. In much of America and Europe the staple grain is wheat. If you consider all the food products made from wheat in our country—bread and other baked goods made from wheat flour, cereals, and pasta—you will realize how all-pervasive this grain is in our food supply. The Italians use wheat to make their pasta, while the Mexicans use corn in their tacos and tortillas. Corn is the staple grain of much of South America and in the American South. The staple grains of other peoples include millet, rye, barley, oats, and others. In each society a bread, meal, or flour is made from the grain, which is then used for many purposes.

A second important source of starch is the bean and pea family, including such *dry beans* found in the supermarket as lima beans, kidney beans, "baked" beans, blackeyed peas (cowpeas), chickpeas, garbanzo beans, soybeans, and many others. These vegetables are about 40 percent starch by weight, and contain a significant amount of protein also. A third major source of starch is the tubers, such as the potato, yam, cassava, and others. For many non-Western societies, one of these may serve as the primary starch source.

When you eat any of these foods, the starch molecules are taken apart by enzymes in your mouth and intestine. The enzymes hydrolyze the starch molecules to yield glucose units, which are absorbed across the intestinal wall into the blood. One to four hours after a meal, all the starch has been digested and is circulating to the cells as glucose.

Glycogen. Glycogen is not found in plants and is stored in animal meats only to a limited extent. It is not, therefore, of major importance as a nutrient, although it performs an important role in the metabolism of carbohydrates in the body, as already described. Glycogen is more complex and more highly branched in structure than starch.

glycogen (GLIGH-co-gen): an animal polysaccharide composed of glucose, manufactured in the body and stored in liver and muscle.

Cellulose. The third polysaccharide of importance in nutrition is cellulose. Cellulose, like starch, is found abundantly in plants. Cellulose, again like starch, is composed of glucose units connected in long chains. It differs from starch because the bonds holding its glucose units together are different. The difference is of major importance for humans because each type of bond requires a different enzyme to hydrolyze it. The human digestive tract is supplied with abundant enzymes to hydrolyze the bonds in starch but has none that can attack the bonds in cellulose. As a result, starch is digestible for humans and cellulose is not. Cellulose instead passes through the digestive tract largely unchanged—which explains the different roles of these two major plant polysaccharides: starch is the most abundant

cellulose (CELL-yoo-lose): a plant polysaccharide composed of glucose, indigestible by humans.

Glycogen in a liver cell. The black "rosettes" are aggregates of glycogen granules. The circular membrane-bound bodies such as the one in the upper left corner, are subcellular energy-producing organelles known as mitochondria. This cell was photographed under an electron microscope at a magnification of 65,000x.

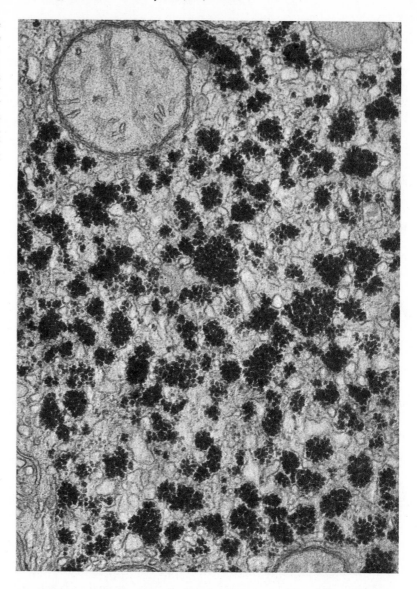

From Fawcett, D.W.: *An Atlas of Fine Structure.* W. B. Saunders Company, Philadelphia and London, 1966, Figure 161. Courtesy of the author and publisher.

Other carbohydrates providing indigestible residue are **pectin** and **hemicellulose**; **lignin** is a noncarbohydrate fiber that occurs in foods.

constipation: see also Highlight 5.

energy source in the staple foods of the world, while cellulose provides no energy for humans at all.

The fact that cellulose is indigestible, however, and widely distributed in plant foods, gives it a role of unique importance in human digestion. It is a *fiber* which provides *roughage* in the human diet, supplying the bulk against which the muscles of the digestive tract can push. The presence of fiber in the stomach and intestines stimulates the action of these muscles, facilitating the passage of all the nutrients which accompany it through the tract. A lack of fiber in the diet is a common cause of constipation, in which the contents of the digestive tract become compacted and their passage slowed. Constipation problems are most commonly found in elderly people who eat too few of the fruits, vegetables, and whole-grain breads and cereals in which the cellulose content is high.

 The sugars. There are actually six common sugars found in foods, of which the monosaccharide glucose is but one. Glucose is not especially sweet tasting; a pinch of the purified sugar on your tongue gives only the faintest taste sensation. On the other hand, it is absorbed with extraordinary rapidity into the bloodstream; if a diabetic has gone into a hypoglycemic coma (as for example from an overdose of insulin), a quick way to supply the needed blood glucose is to tip his/her head to one side and drip a water solution of glucose into his/her cheek pocket. The glucose will be absorbed directly into his/her bloodstream.

 When you bite into a ripe peach or plum and savor the natural sweetness of its juice, the sugar you are enjoying is fructose. Curiously, fructose has exactly the same chemical formula as glucose—$C_6H_{12}O_6$—but its structure is very slightly different:

● = glucose

glucose: a monosaccharide. Sometimes known as blood sugar, sometimes as grape sugar. Also called **dextrose**.

▲ = fructose

fructose: a monosaccharide. Sometimes known as fruit sugar.

Glucose   Fructose

The different arrangements of the atoms in these two sugars stimulate the taste buds on your tongue in different ways. The next time you sit down to a plate of pancakes dripping with pure Vermont maple syrup, give thanks to the way nature has ordered the carbon, hydrogen, and oxygen atoms in fructose to make it the sweetest of the sugars.

 Fructose can be absorbed directly into your blood stream. When the blood circulates past the liver, the fructose is taken up into the liver cells, where enzymes rearrange the C, H, and O atoms to make glucose. The glucose may be released into the blood or stored as glycogen. Thus this sugar is as good a source of blood glucose as glucose itself.

 Food chemists have studied the exact arrangement of the atoms in sweet-tasting substances, such as fructose, and have identified the structures in them that stimulate your sweetness taste buds. They have developed a number of artificial, non-nutritive sweeteners, such as saccharin, cyclamates, and aspartame, which taste sweet because they stimulate your taste receptors in the same way but which cannot be oxidized by the body to yield energy. Thus they are noncaloric.

Liver cell

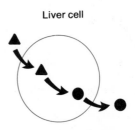

Fructose → glucose

For the advantages and disadvantages of these additives, see Highlight 13.

■ = galactose

galactose: a monosaccharide. Part of the disaccharide lactose.

Glucose and fructose are the only two monosaccharides of importance in foods; a third, galactose, is seldom found free in nature but is instead found as part of the dissacharide lactose. Galactose is also a hexose with the formula $C_6H_{12}O_6$, but has a slightly different structure from glucose and fructose:

$$CH_2OH$$

Galactose

(Can you see the difference?)

The other three common sugars are dissacharides—pairs of monosaccharides linked together. Glucose is found in all three; the second member of the pair is either fructose, galactose, or another glucose.

Sucrose (*sucro* means sugar) is the most familiar of these three common sugars: table sugar. It is the sugar found in sugar cane and sugar beets; it is purified and granulated to various extents to provide the brown, white, and powdered sugars available in the supermarket. Since it is the disaccharide in which fructose is paired with glucose, it is the sweetest of the common sugars.

●——▲ = sucrose

sucrose: a disaccharide composed of glucose and fructose. Commonly known as table sugar, beet sugar, or cane sugar.

> Next time you buy white sugar, look at the label and notice whether it comes from sugar cane or sugar beets. The label may imply that sugar from one source is better than sugar from the other. Because you know that the chemical structures of the two are identical, you can let the price be the sole factor in determining which you buy.

(DIGESTION)

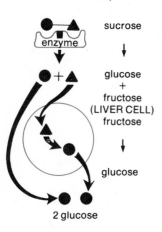

sucrose

glucose
+
fructose
(LIVER CELL)
fructose

glucose

2 glucose

●——■ = lactose

When a food containing sucrose has been eaten, enzymes in the digestive tract hydrolyze the sucrose to yield glucose and fructose. These monosaccharides are absorbed, and the fructose is converted to glucose in the liver. Thus, one molecule of sucrose ultimately yields two of glucose.

Sucrose is the principal nutrient ingredient of carbonated beverages, candy, cakes, frostings, cookies, and other concentrated sweets. A special section at the end of this chapter highlights the questions whether sucrose is necessary in the diet at all and whether it may be, in fact, a threat to our health.

Lactose is the principal carbohydrate found in milk, comprising about 5 percent of its weight. A human baby is born with the digestive enzymes necessary to hydrolyze lactose into its component monosaccharides, which can then be absorbed. Since the galactose is converted to glucose in the liver, each molecule of lactose yields two molecules of glucose to supply energy for the baby's growth and activity. On the other hand, babies don't develop the ability to digest starch until they are several months old. This is one of the many reasons why milk is such a good food for babies; it provides a simple, easily digested carbohydrate in the right amount to provide energy to meet their needs.

Some individuals lose the ability to digest lactose as early as the age of four, becoming *lactose-intolerant.* They react badly to milk, feeling nauseated and sometimes having diarrhea when they drink it. Lactose intolerance is especially common among the Black races, American Indians and Orientals; it is less frequently found in Caucasians. It is not the same as the commonly observed milk allergy, which is caused by certain babies' hypersensitivity to the protein in cow's milk, and sometimes to that in other milks.[2]

Maltose is found at only one stage in the life of a plant. When the seed is formed, it is packed with starch—stored glucose—to be used as fuel for the germination process. When the seed begins to sprout, an enzyme cleaves the starch into maltose units. Another enzyme splits the maltose units into glucose units. Other enzymes degrade the units still further, releasing energy for the sprouting of the shoot and root of the plant. By the time the young plant is established and growing, all the starch in the seed has been used up, and the plant is able to capture the sun's light in its leaves. The plant uses this light energy to put new molecules of glucose together and to elaborate chains of starch, cellulose, and other plant constituents from them. Thus the sugar maltose is present briefly during the early germination process, as the starch is being broken down. The malt found in beer contains maltose formed as the grains germinate (the alcohol is produced by yeast in a process known as fermentation).

As you might predict, when you eat or drink a food source of maltose, your digestive enzymes hydrolyze the maltose into two glucose units, which are then absorbed into the blood.

How Much Carbohydrate?

Most authorities agree that a dietary source of glucose is essential. We must have some every day—but how much? A recent estimate[3] sets the amount of carbohydrate needed in a

lactose: a disaccharide composed of glucose and galactose. Commonly known as milk sugar.

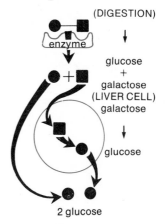

lactose intolerance: inherited or acquired inability to digest lactose, due to failure to produce the enzyme lactase. Lactose intolerance is prevalent in the majority of adult human population groups.[2]

maltose: a disaccharide composed of two glucose units. Sometimes known as malt sugar.

fermentation: breakdown of sugar in the absence of oxygen, yielding alcohol.

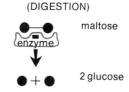

[2]Kretchmer, N.: Lactose and lactase. *Scientific American* 227:70-78, 1972.
[3]Fineberg, S. K.: Diet, the realities of obesity and fad diets. *Nutrition Today,* July/August: 23-26, 1972.

Energy value of carbohydrate: 1 gram supplies 4 kilocalories.

person's daily diet at "not less than 500 calories." Since each gram of pure carbohydrate supplies about 4 kilocalories of energy, we need at least 125 grams of carbohydrate a day. How can we be sure we get at least that amount?

The number and variety of different foods commonly eaten by Americans is staggering. Appendix H lists 615 of the most common ones, and no two are alike. Must we memorize the nutrient composition of all these foods in order to plan and assess our diets properly? This would be a formidable task.

To avoid such a tedious undertaking, dietetic experts have devised a variety of systems by which similar foods can be grouped together. None is satisfactory for all purposes, yet there are many advantages of using some such system. The most widely used system in current use is the Food Exchange System originally developed by the American Diabetes Association and the American Dietetic Association in 1950 and revised in 1976. At first intended only for use in diet planning for diabetics, this system has since been adapted to a wide variety of uses by doctors, dietitians, nutritionists, and other health professionals —as well as by weight reduction groups, such as Weight Watchers. It is presently in use, with modifications, all over the world.

ADA Food Exchange System

In the Exchange System there are six groups of foods: milk, vegetables, fruit, bread, meat, and fat. Almost every food commonly used by Americans has a place in one of these groups. The only exceptions are foods containing large amounts of sucrose (cakes, candies, cola beverages, and the like) and alcoholic beverages; these are omitted because they are forbidden to diabetics. Within each group all foods are similar in their content of carbohydrate, fat, and protein. A look at the lists of foods on pages 33-38 will familiarize you with these groups.

The Exchange System will be referred to in every chapter of this book and repeated opportunities to study it will be offered. At present we are concerned only with the carbohydrate content of foods. The following table highlights the four groups which contain carbohydrate. Knowing what foods are in these groups and the amount of carbohydrate in each will provide you with a shortcut for estimating the total carbohydrate in a meal or a day's diet.

Exchange Group	Carbohydrate (g)	Protein (g)	Fat (g)	Energy (kcal)
(1) **Skim milk**	12	8	0	80
(2) **Vegetables**	5	2	0	25
(3) **Fruit**	10	0	0	40
(4) **Bread**	15	2	0	70
(5) Lean meat	0	7	3	55
(6) Fat	0	0	5	45

As you can see, carbohydrate is found in four of the six types of foods listed.

(1). The milk list (see page 33) itemizes the servings of food which are equivalent to skim milk in their energy nutrient content. As you can see, all of these are milk and milk products. A one cup serving of any of these foods supplies 12 grams of carbohydrate.

Foods Containing Carbohydrate:

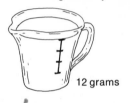

12 grams

1 milk exchange = 12 grams carbohydrate
(serving size: 1 CUP)

The variable amounts of *fat* in milk exchanges will be explained fully in Chapter 2.

(2). The vegetable list (see pages 33-34) shows the low-starch vegetables. A ½ cup serving of any of these supplies 5 grams of a carbohydrate.

1 vegetable exchange = 5 grams carbohydrate
(serving size: ½ CUP)

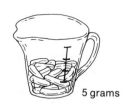

5 grams

(3). The fruit list (see page 34) shows the fruits, with serving sizes adjusted so that each serving supplies 10 grams of carbohydrate.

1 fruit exchange = 10 grams carbohydrate
(serving size: VARIES)

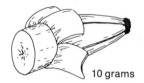

10 grams

(4). The bread list (see page 35) includes the breads, cereals, and starchy vegetables. These foods are grouped together because they contain similar amounts of carbohydrate and protein. For example, ½ cup of lima beans or green peas contains as many grams of carbohydrate as a slice of bread. The same is true of 1/3 cup of corn. Dried peas and beans are also included in this group. One serving of any of these foods supplies 15 grams of carbohydrate.

1 bread exchange = 15 grams carbohydrate
(serving size: 1 SLICE BREAD or VARIES)

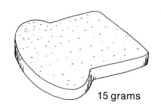

15 grams

(5). One food is not included in the ADA Exchange System but does, at least in America, contribute a substantial amount of carbohydrate to the diet. This food is sugar.

To make the Exchange System useful for the present purpose, we need a means of estimating the amount of carbohydrate sugar contributes to the diet. The fact to remember is that one teaspoon of white sugar supplies 5 grams of carbohydrate.

One teaspoon of any of the following can be considered equivalent in sucrose content to one teaspoon of white sugar:

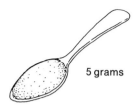

5 grams

1 tsp brown sugar	1 tsp honey
1 tsp molasses	1 tsp jam
1 tsp corn syrup	1 tsp jelly
1 tsp maple syrup	1 tsp candy

Other useful numbers:

1 tbsp catsup = 1 tsp sugar
1 8-ounce can cola beverage
= 6 tsp sugar

For a person who uses catsup (ketchup) liberally, it may help to remember that one tablespoon of catsup supplies about one teaspoon of sugar. For the soft drink user, an 8-ounce can of a cola beverage contains about 6 teaspoons of sugar, or 30 carbohydrate grams.

A familiarity with these five groups of foods provides a way to estimate the carbohydrate in your diet. For example, suppose that one day's meals included a fried egg and a piece of toast with margarine for breakfast; a peanut butter and jelly sandwich with a cup of milk for lunch; a 6-ounce steak, green beans, and mashed potato with margarine for dinner; and strawberry shortcake and whipped cream for an evening snack. That day's meals contained the following carbohydrate exchanges:

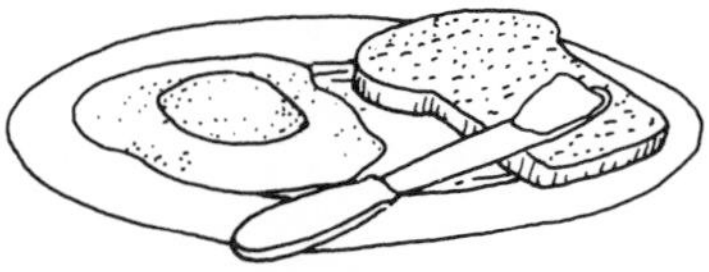

Breakfast: 1 bread exchange

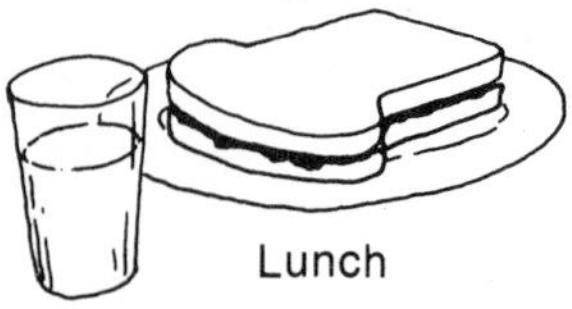

Lunch: 2 bread exchanges
           2 tsp sugar[4]
           1 milk exchange

Dinner: 2 bread exchanges[5]
           1 vegetable exchange[6]

Snack:[7] 1 bread exchange
           1 fruit exchange
           6 tsp sugar

Breakfast

Lunch

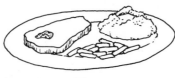

Dinner

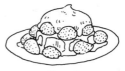

Snack

Thus your total carbohydrate consumption for the day was:

6 bread exchanges   = 90 grams carbohydrate
8 teaspoons sugar   = 40   ''   ''
1 milk exchange   = 12   ''   ''
1 vegetable exchange   = 5   ''   ''
1 fruit exchange   = 10   ''   ''
           TOTAL: 157 grams carbohydrate

This is more than the necessary 125 grams and so is adequate.

This kind of calculation provides only an estimate but is close enough for most purposes. A more accurate way to determine the carbohydrate composition of foods is to refer to Ap-

[4]The sandwich contained 2 teaspoons jelly.
[5]This was a one-cup serving of mashed potato.
[6]This was a ½-cup serving of green beans.
[7]This was a 2'' diameter biscuit with ¾ cup strawberries, one tbsp heavy cream, and 6 tsp sugar added in preparation.

pendix H, which lists individual foods rather than food groups. Adding the carbohydrate values obtained from Appendix H yields 138 grams of carbohydrate.

The difference between the 157 gram estimate and the 138 gram amount obtained by the more accurate calculation may be disconcerting. Rough estimates are often more valuable than close calculations, however, because of the time saved and because often only a "ball park" figure is needed. In this example, we know that 50 grams of carbohydrate would be too little, while 260 grams would be more than twice the recommended number. The numbers 157 and 138 both fall between these extremes; the difference between them becomes insignificant from this perspective.

Most estimates of the nutrient contents of foods are rough but serviceable approximations. In this book we refer repeatedly to a "90 kcalorie potato;" the reader should understand this to mean "90 plus-or-minus about 20 percent," which makes it not significantly different from a "100 kcalorie potato." In general, for our purposes, a variation of about 20 percent is tolerable.

It takes only one or two calculations of this kind to get a feel for the carbohydrate content of the diet. Once aware of the major carbohydrate-contributing foods you eat, you can return to thinking in terms of these foods alone, developing a sense of how much of each is enough.

This chapter began by stating that, while all three energy nutrients—protein, fat, and carbohydrate—fuel body processes, carbohydrate is the only one which ordinarily supplies fuel in a form the brain can use, that is, as glucose. The discussion of carbohydrates has explained this. Of the three polysaccharides, starch is our principal energy food, and starch is glucose—long chains of it strung together. As for the three disaccharides, each of them yields two molecules of glucose after they are taken into the body. The three monosaccharides, too, provide glucose after absorption.

Armed with this information, you can explode some of the myths perpetrated by television commercials advertising sweets. Sugar is brain food? True, but which sugar are we talking about? Not sucrose! When you need quick energy, what is the best source? A candy bar? A coke? For efficient functioning of all your cells you must keep glucose available to them at all times, but to supply glucose for your blood, must you eat table sugar? No, starch is a better choice, for many reasons.

Summing Up

The world's people derive 50 to 80 percent of their food energy from carbohydrate, most of it from starch, although sugar (sucrose) makes a large contribution to the American diet. The carbohydrates can be grouped into complex carbohydrates—the polysaccharides—and simple carbohydrates—the mono- and disaccharides. Of the polysaccharides, starch and cellulose are found in plants, starch is found predominantly in grains, and cellulose is found in grains, fruits, and vegetables. Cellulose, being an indigestible carbohydrate, provides the diet with fiber. Glycogen, or animal starch, is the polysaccharide synthesized in animal liver and muscle from temporary excess glucose.

All three polysaccharides are chains of glucose units strung together; cellulose differs from the other two in the character of the bonds holding the glucose units together.

Of the monosaccharides, fructose, or fruit sugar, is the sweetest; it gives honey, syrup, and many fruits their sweet flavor. Both fructose and glucose are found free in these and other plant foods. All three monosaccharides—glucose, fructose, and galactose—share the chemical formula $C_6H_{12}O_6$, but differ from one another in the arrangement of their atoms. This difference in arrangement gives each its particular character.

Each of the three disaccharides contains a molecule of glucose paired with another monosaccharide. The two of importance in nutrition are lactose and sucrose. Lactose is the simple carbohydrate of milk. It is very digestible except for those who lack the digestive enzyme to hydrolyze lactose and thus are lactose-intolerant. Sucrose, or table sugar, is the sugar of candies, sweets, and confections. It is highlighted in the following section. Nutritionists are attempting to decide whether sucrose is innocent or guilty-as-charged with causing a rise in diabetes and heart disease.

The Food Exchange System, which groups foods according to their carbohydrate, fat, and protein content, includes four groups of food which contain carbohydrate: milk (12 grams per cup), vegetable (5 grams per ½ cup serving), fruit (10 grams per serving), and bread (15 grams per serving). In addition to these four groups, a category which might be called the sugar group contributes five grams of carbohydrate per teaspoon; an 8-ounce cola type beverage contains six teaspoons.

These five groups of food constitute a complete list of the carbohydrate-containing foods in the diet.

ADA Food Exchange Lists

(1) The Milk List

Nonfat Fortified Milk

1 cup	skim or nonfat milk
1 cup	buttermilk made from skim milk
1 cup	yogurt made from skim milk (plain, unflavored)
1/3 cup	powdered, nonfat dry milk, before adding liquid
½ cup	canned evaporated skim milk, before adding liquid

Lowfat Fortified Milk

1 cup	1% fat fortified milk (add ½ fat exchange)*
1 cup	2% fat fortified milk (add 1 fat exchange)*
1 cup	yogurt made from 2% fortified milk (plain, unflavored) (add 1 fat exchange*)

Whole Milk (add 2 fat exchanges)*

1 cup	whole milk
1 cup	buttermilk made from whole milk
1 cup	yogurt made from whole milk (plain, unflavored)
½ cup	canned, evaporated whole milk, before adding liquid

A MILK EXCHANGE is a serving of food which is equivalent to one cup of skim milk in its energy nutrient content. One milk exchange contains substantial amounts of carbohydrate and protein and about 80 kcalories.

(12 grams carbohydrate, 8 grams protein)

*These foods contain more fat than skim milk. When calculating fat values, add fat exchanges as indicated. (1 fat exchange=5 grams fat.)

(2) The Vegetable List

½ cup asparagus
½ cup bean sprouts
½ cup beets
½ cup broccoli
½ cup Brussels sprouts
½ cup cabbage
½ cup carrots
½ cup cauliflower
½ cup celery
½ cup cucumbers
½ cup eggplant
½ cup green pepper

Greens:

  ½ cup beet greens
  ½ cup chards
  ½ cup collard greens
  ½ cup dandelion greens

Greens continued:

  ½ cup kale
  ½ cup mustard greens
  ½ cup spinach
  ½ cup turnip greens
½ cup mushrooms
½ cup okra
½ cup onions
½ cup rhubarb
½ cup rutabaga
½ cup sauerkraut
½ cup string beans, green or yellow
½ cup summer squash
½ cup tomatoes
½ cup tomato juice
½ cup turnips
½ cup vegetable juice cocktail
½ cup zucchini

ADA Food Exchange Lists

(2) The Vegetable List (continued)

A VEGETABLE EXCHANGE is a serving of any vegetable that contains a moderate amount of carbohydrate, a small but significant amount of protein, and about 25 kcalories.

(5 grams carbohydrate, 2 grams protein)

The following vegetables may be assumed to have negligible carbohydrate, protein, and calories:

chicory   lettuce
Chinese cabbage   parsley
endive   radishes
escarole   watercress

Starchy vegetables are found on the Bread Exchange List.

(3) The Fruit List

1 small	apple	⅛ medium	honeydew melon
1/3 cup	apple juice	½ small	mango
½ cup	applesauce (unsweetened)	1 small	nectarine
		1 small	orange
2 medium	apricots, fresh	½ cup	orange juice
4 halves	apricots, dried	¾ cup	papaya
½ small	banana	1 medium	peach
½ cup	blackberries	1 small	pear
½ cup	blueberries	1 medium	persimmon
¼ small	cantaloupe melon	½ cup	pineapple
10 large	cherries	1/3 cup	pineapple juice
1/3 cup	cider	2 medium	plums
2	dates	2 medium	prunes
1	fig, fresh	¼ cup	prune juice
1	fig, dried	½ cup	raspberries
1 half	grapefruit	2 tbsp	raisins
½ cup	grapefruit juice	¾ cup	strawberries
12	grapes	1 medium	tangerine
¼ cup	grape juice	1 cup	watermelon

A FRUIT EXCHANGE is a serving of fruit which contains about 10 grams of carbohydrate and 40 kcalories. The protein and fat content of fruit is negligible.

(10 grams carbohydrate)

Cranberries may be assumed to have negligible carbohydrate and calories if used without sugar.

ADA Food Exchange Lists

**(4) The Bread List
(includes bread, cereals, and starchy vegetables)**

Bread

1 slice	white (including French and Italian)
1 slice	whole wheat
1 slice	rye or pumpernickel
1 slice	raisin
1 half	small bagel
1 half	small English muffin
1	plain roll, bread
1 half	frankfurter roll
1 half	hamburger bun
3 tbsp	dried bread crumbs
1 6-inch	tortilla

Cereal

½ cup	bran flakes
¾ cup	other ready-to-eat cereal, unsweetened
1 cup	puffed cereal (unfrosted)
½ cup	cereal (cooked)
½ cup	grits (cooked)
½ cup	rice or barley (cooked)
½ cup	pasta (cooked): spaghetti, noodles, or macaroni
3 cups	popcorn (popped, no fat added)
2 tbsp	cornmeal (dry)
2½ tbsp	flour
¼ cup	wheat germ

Crackers

3	arrowroot
2	graham, 2½" square
1 half	matzoth, 4" x 6"
20	oyster
25	pretzels, 3⅛" long x ⅛" diam.
3	rye wafers, 2" x 3½"
6	saltines
4	soda, 2½" square

Dried Beans, Peas, and Lentils

½ cup	beans, peas, lentils (dried and cooked)
¼ cup	baked beans, no pork (canned)

Starchy Vegetables

1/3 cup	corn
1 small	corn on cob
½ cup	lima beans
2/3 cup	parsnips
½ cup	peas, green (canned or frozen)
1 small	potato, white
½ cup	potato (mashed)
¾ cup	pumpkin
½ cup	squash: winter, acorn, or butternut
¼ cup	yam or sweet potato

Prepared Foods*

1 biscuit, 2" diameter (add 1 fat exchange)
1 corn bread, 2" x 2" x 1" (add 1 fat exchange)
1 corn muffin, 2" diameter (add 1 fat exchange)
5 crackers, round butter type (add 1 fat exchange)
1 muffin, plain, small (add 1 fat exchange)
8 potatoes, French fried, length 2" by 3½" (add 1 fat exchange)
15 potato chips or corn chips (add 2 fat exchanges)
1 pancake, 5" x ½" (add 1 fat exchange)
1 waffle, 5" x ½" (add 1 fat exchange)

A BREAD EXCHANGE is a serving of bread, cereal, or starchy vegetable which contains appreciable carbohydrate and a small but significant amount of protein, totaling about 70 kcalories.

(15 grams carbohydrate, 2 grams protein)

*These foods contain more fat than bread. When calculating fat values, add fat exchanges as indicated. (1 fat exchange = 5 grams fat.)

ADA Food Exchange Lists

---

(5) The Meat List

Low-fat Meat

1 ounce beef:	baby beef (very lean), chipped beef, chuck, flank steak, tenderloin, plateribs, plate skirt steak, round (bottom, top), all cuts rump, spare ribs, tripe
1 ounce lamb:	leg, rib, sirloin, loin (roast and chops), shank, shoulder
1 ounce pork:	leg (whole rump, center shank), ham, smoked (center slices)
1 ounce veal:	leg, loin, rib, shank, shoulder, cutlets
1 ounce poultry:	meat-without-skin of chicken, turkey, cornish hen, guinea hen, pheasant
1 ounce fish:	any fresh or frozen
¼ cup fish:	canned salmon, tuna, mackerel, crab, and lobster
5 (or 1 ounce):	clams, oysters, scallops, shrimp
3	sardines, drained
1 ounce cheese:	containing less than 5% butterfat
¼ cup	cottage cheese, dry and 2% butterfat
½ cup	dried beans and peas (add 1 bread exchange*)

Medium-fat Meat (add ½ fat exchange)*

1 ounce beef:	ground (15% fat), corned beef (canned), rib eye, round (ground commercial)
1 ounce pork:	loin (all cuts tenderloin), shoulder arm (picnic), shoulder blade, Boston butt, Canadian bacon, boiled ham
1 ounce	liver, heart, kidney, and sweetbreads (these are high in cholesterol)
¼ cup	cottage cheese, creamed
1 ounce cheese:	mozzarella, ricotta, farmer's cheese, Neufchatel
3 tbsp	Parmesan cheese
1	egg (high in cholesterol)

High-fat Meat (add 1 fat exchange)*

1 ounce beef:	brisket, corned beef (brisket), ground beef (more than 20% fat), hamburger (commercial), chuck (ground commercial), roasts (rib), steaks (club and rib)
1 ounce lamb:	breast
1 ounce pork:	spare ribs, loin (back ribs), pork (ground), country style ham, deviled ham
1 ounce veal:	breast
1 ounce poultry:	capon, duck (domestic), goose

---

*These foods contain more carbohydrate or fat than lean meat. When calculating carbohydrate or fat values, add bread or fat exchanges as indicated.

ADA Food Exchange List

(5) The Meat List (continued)

1 ounce cheese:	cheddar types
1 slice	cold cuts, 4½" x ⅛" slice
1 small	frankfurter

Peanut Butter

2 tbsp	peanut butter (add 2 fat exchanges*)

A MEAT EXCHANGE is a serving of protein-rich food which contains negligible carbohydrate, but a significant amount of protein and fat, roughly equivalent to the amounts in one ounce of lean meat; contains about 55 kcalories.

(7 grams protein, 3 grams fat)

*These foods contain more carbohydrate or fat than lean meat. When calculating carbohydrate or fat values, add bread or fat exchanges as indicated.

(6) The Fat List

Polyunsaturated Fat

1 tsp	margarine, soft, tub, or stick*
1 eighth	avocado (4" in diameter)†
1 tsp	oil, corn, cottonseed, safflower, soy, sunflower
1 tsp	oil, olive†
1 tsp	oil, peanut†
5 small	olives†
10 whole	almonds†
2 large whole	pecans†
20 whole	peanuts, Spanish†
10 whole	peanuts, Virginia†
6 small	walnuts
6 small	nuts, other†

Saturated Fat

1 tsp	margarine, regular stick	1 tbsp	cream cheese
1 tsp	butter	1 tbsp	French dressing‡
1 tsp	bacon fat	1 tbsp	Italian dressing‡
1 strip	bacon, crisp	1 tsp	lard
2 tbsp	cream, light	1 tsp	mayonnaise‡
2 tbsp	cream, sour	2 tsp	salad dressing, mayonnaise type‡
1 tbsp	cream, heavy	¾ inch cube	salt pork

*Made with corn, cottonseed, safflower, soy, or sunflower oil only.
†Fat content is primarily monounsaturated.
‡If made with corn, cottonseed, safflower, soy, or sunflower oil, can be assumed to contain polyunsaturated fat.

ADA Food Exchange Lists

(6) The Fat List (continued)

A FAT EXCHANGE is a serving of any food which contains negligible carbohydrate and protein, but appreciable fat, totaling about 45 kcalories.

(5 grams fat)

Unlimited Foods

These are *free foods*, which contain negligible carbohydrate, protein, and fat, and therefore negligible calories.

Diet calorie free beverage	Salt and Pepper	Mustard
Coffee	Red pepper	Chili powder
Tea	Paprika	Onion salt or powder
Bouillon without fat	Garlic	Horseradish
Unsweetened gelatin	Celery salt	Vinegar
Unsweetened pickles	Parsley	Mint
	Nutmeg	Cinnamon
	Lemon	Lime

The exchange lists in this book are based on material in EXCHANGE LISTS FOR MEAL PLANNING prepared by Committees of the American Diabetes Association and the American Dietetic Association in cooperation with The National Institute of Arthritis, Metabolism, and Digestive Diseases and the National Heart and Lung Institute, National Institutes of Health, Public Health Service, U.S. Department of Health, Education, and Welfare.

To Explore Further—

A programmed instruction book for the student who wishes to understand chemical bonding better:

Eichinger, J. W., Jr.: *Chemical Bonds—Introduction and Fundamentals.* Lyons and Carnahan, Inc., Chicago, 1968.

Highlight One ━━━━━━
Sugar: Is It Bad for You?

Rabbit said, "Honey
or condensed milk with
your bread?" (Pooh) was
so excited that he said,
"Both," and then, so as
not to seem greedy, he
added, "But don't bother
about the bread, please."
—A. A. MILNE,
Winnie the Pooh

A heated argument over sugar is presently in progress in the nutrition literature. The questions being debated are (1) how much sugar do Americans consume? (2) is the consumption of sugar a causative factor in the rising incidence of diabetes and cardiovascular diseases? (3) is sugar a physiologically worthless substance, a contributor of empty calories? Not only opinions but also evidence will be cited to support contradictory answers to these questions.

It is important that we understand the term *sugar* in the context of this discussion. Sugar in the normal household usage refers to the disaccharide sucrose. It may appear in various forms: white, granulated table sugar, brown sugar, honey, molasses, syrups, or sugar used in the preparation of food products, such as cakes, pies, cookies, candy, cola beverages, or alcohol.

Some areas of agreement appear in the literature. For one thing, it is known that obesity correlates with both diabetes and cardiovascular diseases. Obesity has become a prime health problem in this country largely because we are exercising less than previous generations. Excess energy intake from any energy source, including sugar, can only exacerbate this problem. One 12-ounce fruit flavored carbonated drink, for instance, contributes about 170 kcalories (Appendix N). Anytime a person consumes about 3500 kcalories in excess of need, a pound of fat is produced.[1] In other words, if we drink one 12-ounce orange

[1]Krause, M. V. and Hunscher, M. A.: *Food, Nutrition and Diet Therapy.* W. B. Saunders Company, Philadelphia, 1972, p. 427.

soda a day *in excess of our energy need*, we will gain one pound about every 20 days.

Another concern about which nutritionists are agreed is that in some individuals calories from sugar may be replacing calories from other carbohydrate sources which would contribute *vitamins, minerals, protein, complex carbohydrates, and fiber* in addition to the calories. How often someone says, "I can't eat that baked potato because I have to count my calories." Then that same person may drink a cola beverage without giving a thought to its caloric content. Yet a baked potato of medium size has only about 90 kcalories and gives the body at the same time 3 grams protein, 21 grams complex carbohydrates, 9 milligrams calcium, and 20 milligrams vitamin C. (Notice that nothing has been said about the calories from the butter or sour cream that may be on that potato.) Table H1.1 compares the contribution of nutrients made by 100 kcalorie portions of several supposedly "high calorie" foods with 100 kcalorie portions of table sugar and cola beverage.

Another thing nutritionists agree on is the role of sugar in the development of *dental caries*. Of all the carbohydrates we eat, sucrose is the one most readily used by mouth bacteria for acid production and is the most consistently damaging to the teeth. The longer the acid is allowed to remain in contact with

dental caries (CARE-eez): tooth decay, cavities.

Table H1.1. Nutrient composition of 100 kcalorie portions of selected common foods, expressed as percent* of U.S. Recommended Daily Dietary Allowance (RDA) for adults.

Item Number in Appendix H	Food	Size of 100 Kcal Portion	Protein	Calcium	Iron	Vitamin A	Thiamin	Riboflavin	Niacin	Vitamin C
369	Bread, whole wheat	1½ slices	7%	4%	7%	—	9%	3%	6%	—
338	Cereal, enriched 40% bran	1 cup	6%	3%	68%	0%	9%	4%	11%	0%
2	Milk, partly skim, 2% fat	¾ cup	17%	26%	—	3%	5%	23%	—	3%
550	Sugar, white	2½ tbsp	0%	0%	0%	0%	0%	0%	0%	0%
562	cola beverage	1 cup	0%	0%	0%	0%	0%	0%	0%	0%
167	Vegetables, lima beans	½ cup	10%	4%	12%	5%	10%	5%	6%	25%
236	sweet potatoes	2/3 potato (5" x 2")	2%	3%	4%	118%	4%	3%	2%	26%

*Percentages are rounded to nearest whole number. A dash means the percentage has not been determined, but is insignificant.

the enamel, the greater the damage. Eventually the enamel will be broken down and a cavity will form. The American Dental Association recommends that foods and snacks be selected which are lower in sucrose content, for example, milk rather than chocolate milk, fresh fruits as opposed to dried fruits, popcorn or toast as opposed to sweet rolls or cookies, or sugar-free soft drinks rather than drinks flavored with caloric sweeteners.[2]

While these three areas—obesity, displacement of foods that contribute a variety of nutrients, and dental caries—may be related to excess sugar consumption, the questions outlined at the beginning of this Highlight remain. Let us examine each of these.

How Much Sugar Do Americans Consume?

During the last 60 years, the pattern of carbohydrate consumption has shifted, with potato and cereal consumption dropping about 50 percent, vegetable (other than the potato) and fruit consumption remaining about the same, and with sugar consumption rising about 20 percent. The effect is shown in Figure H1.1. The rise in sugar consumption does not include the

[2]*Diet and Dental Health*. Pamphlet: American Dental Association. Chicago, Illinois.

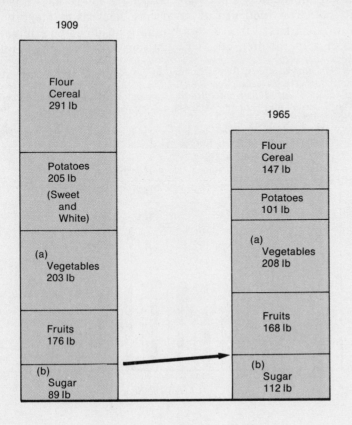

Figure HI.1. Trends in Carbohydrate Consumption* in Pounds per Person Per Year

a—Excluding white and sweet potatoes
b—Excluding beverages (alcoholic and carbonated)
* —Retail Weight Equivalent
Adapted from Friend, Berta.: Nutrients in U.S. Food Supply. *American Journal of Clinical Nutrition* 20:8, 1967.

sugar used in the manufacture of alcoholic and carbonated beverages. Dr. John Yudkin, of the Department of Nutrition, London University, has estimated that if these are included, the consumption of sugar per American in 1973 averaged about 126 pounds.[3]

You may be able to say truthfully that you have not eaten 126 pounds of sugar in a year, that you drink your coffee black, that you don't eat much cake or pie, and that you never drink cola or alcoholic beverages. However, if Dr. Yudkin's estimate is correct, this means that for every person like you there is another who consumes enormous amounts of sugar, thereby bringing the average up to 126 pounds. It has been estimated that some teenaged boys consume about 400 pounds of sugar a year, mostly in the form of carbonated beverages and snack foods.[4] Figure H1.2 shows the average consumption of soft drinks by individuals of different ages on one day in spring 1965; you will note that older teenage boys had the highest consumption.

Other scientists disagree with these data. Notable among them is Dr. Frederick J. Stare, Department of Nutrition, Harvard School of Public Health. Dr. Stare agrees that sugar consumption rose markedly prior to 1925, but he believes it has not increased appreciably since then.[5] Dr. Stare states that "it is true that industrial food use of sugar has been rising steadily for many years, but at the same time there has been an equivalent decrease in the household use of sugar." Food consumption

[3]*Nutrition and Diseases.* Select Committee on Nutrition and Human Needs, 93rd Congress (Washington: G.P.O., 1973), p. 147.
[4]Yudkin, J.: *Dietary Sugar and Disease.* Hearings before the Select Committee on Nutrition and Human Needs, 93rd Congress (Washington: G.P.O., 1973), pp. 233-236.
[5]Stare, F. J.: Sugar in the diet of man. In *World Review of Nutrition and Dietetics.* Bourne, G. F., editor. S. Karger AG, Basel, 1975.

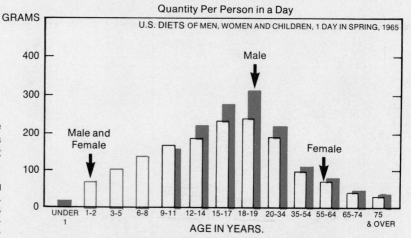

Figure HI.2. Average consumption of soft drinks by individuals of different ages.

From Page, L. and Friend, B.: Level of use of sugars in the United States. Ch. 7 in *Sugars in Nutrition.* Sipple, H. L. and McNutt, K. W., editors. Academic Press, N.Y., 1974.

tables of the Department of Agriculture really concern disappearance of the food from the market, he points out, and do not accurately reflect the food consumed by people. Dr. Stare estimates that the average per capita intake of sugar is about 80 pounds per year.

Dr. Louise Page and Dr. Berta Friend, nutrition analysts with the Consumer and Food Economics Institute of the U.S. Department of Agriculture, state that there has been a one-third increase in the per capita quantity of refined sugar used in this century, while the consumption of *all* carbohydrates has dropped by about one-fourth. At the present time, beverages account for the largest industrial use of sugar, about one-fifth; cereal and bakery goods account for about one-sixth of the total used.[6]

It seems, then, that there is agreement that the home use of sugar is declining and that food industrial use is rising. (See Figure H1.3.) The disagreement among the experts seems to be over the size of the increase and its significance—which makes it difficult to answer the next question.

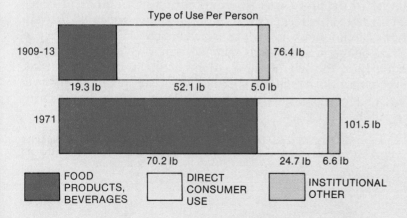

Figure HI.3. Per capita per year use of refined sugar in industrially prepared food products and beverages, direct consumer use, and use by institutional and other users, selected periods.

From Page, L. and Friend, B.: Level of use of sugars in the United States. Ch. 7 in *Sugars in Nutrition*. Sipple, H. L. and McNutt, K. W., Editors. Academic Press, New York, 1974.

cardiovascular disease: a disease affecting the heart or circulatory system. (See the description of atherosclerosis in Highlight 2.)

diabetes (dye-uh-BEET-eez): a hereditary metabolic disease characterized by an inadequate supply of effective insulin, which renders an individual unable to regulate blood glucose level normally. Diabetes affects carbohydrate, fat, and protein metabolism and gives rise to pathological changes in nerves and blood vessels. Properly called *diabetes mellitus*.

Is Increased Consumption of Sugar Causing a Rising Incidence of Diabetes and Cardiovascular Disease?

According to the Vital Statistics of the United States,[7] deaths due to all causes increased by 13 percent in the decade 1961-1971. During that time deaths due to cardiovascular diseases increased by 10 percent while deaths due to diabetes increased by a whopping 27 percent. In 1971 more than half of all the people who died in the United States died of heart disease.

[6]Page, L. and Friend, B.: Level of use of sugars in the United States. In *Sugars in Nutrition*. Sipple, H. L. and McNutt, K. W., editors. Academic Press, New York, 1974.

[7]*Vital Statistics of the United States*. 1971 Vol. II Part B. United States Department of Health, Education and Welfare. Public Health Service.

It is very likely that diabetes contributed to a number of these deaths but did not appear on the death certificate as the primary cause.

The concern over the rising deaths due to these two diseases and the rising consumption of sugar prompted the United States Senate in 1973 to form a Select Committee to conduct hearings on "Sugar in Diet, Diabetes, and Heart Disease." Scientists from various parts of the world who had been studying the relationship of sugar to these diseases were invited to appear before the committee. Among the many interesting testimonies presented was one by Dr. Aharon M. Cohen of the Hebrew University, Hadassah Medical College of Jerusalem, Israel.[8]

Dr. Cohen had had the opportunity to study in his homeland the changes in diseases which occur when a group of people emigrate to a new culture. He studied the flow of immigrants from Yemen and from the Western World into Jerusalem. Over a period of ten years, he tested 16,000 immigrants for diabetes. None of the 5,000 newly-arrived Yemenites he tested had diabetes, while there was a remarkably high number of cases among the settled Yemenites. A dietary study revealed that the Yemen immigrants had not consumed sucrose before coming to Israel but soon afterwards adopted a more Western diet, particularly in the use of sugar. Many of them, he found, drank large quantities of coffee, stirring five or six spoonsful of sugar into each cup; moreover, they ate little other food in the early part of the day.

[8]Cohen, A. M.: *High Sucrose Intake as a Factor in the Development of Diabetes and its Vascular Complications.* Hearings before the Select Committee on Nutrition and Human Needs, 93rd Congress (Washington: G.P.O., 1973), pp. 167-198.

A **variable** is a factor which may vary (increase or decrease). One variable may depend on another; for example, the height of the average child depends on his age. One variable may be independent of another; for example, the intelligence of a child is independent of his height.

This digression is intended to help you learn to evaluate what you read about nutrition from experimental results. A long-term study has just been described in which two variables increased at the same time: sugar consumption and diabetes.

Noting a correlation between two variables does not necessarily mean that there is a cause and effect relationship between them. For example, you may have noticed that the sun always rises shortly after the milkman has made his delivery to your doorstep. This does not mean that the milkman causes the sun to rise! Further investigation will show that the milkman's coming and the sun's rising are independent events; either can happen without the other, though both tend to correlate with a third variable, the time of day. In the same manner, noting that a rise in sugar consumption correlates with a rise in the incidence of diabetes does not prove that the sugar has caused the diabetes.

correlation: the simultaneous increase, decrease, or change of two variables.

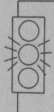

CAUTION WHEN YOU READ!

If A increases as B increases, or if A decreases as B decreases, it does not follow that A causes B. When you note such an association, ask yourself, are there other variables with which both A and B may correlate?

There are many factors in the etiology of diabetes. One of these is age, another is heredity. Diabetes is usually an adult-onset disease. It may be that the cause of the diabetes in those Yemenites who immigrated to Israel was simply that they had become older; perhaps if they had remained in Yemen they would have developed diabetes with the same incidence. This possibility was studied; it was found that diabetes developed uniquely in the immigrants and not in those of the same age who remained in Yemen.

etiology (ee-tee-OLL-uh-gee): causation, the study of all of the causes. The term is used especially with respect to disease.

The factor of heredity was also considered. Those who developed diabetes and those who did not had a common racial background; but if they had come from varying racial groups the fact that one group (consuming sucrose) had become diabetic while the other group (consuming no sucrose) had not might reflect differences in their genetic makeup and be unrelated to the differences in their diets.

When epidemiological studies are made on human beings, many variables are present which will not be identified. Dr. Cohen could not expect that the 5,000 Yemenites he tested had lived lives in every respect identical to those of their countrymen who had stayed in Yemen. It might be that some other unidentified factor in their new environment was responsible for their becoming diabetic after living some years in Jerusalem.

epidemiology (ep-uh-deem-ee-OLL-uh-gee): study of the incidence and distribution of disease in a population.

CAUTION WHEN YOU READ!

When epidemiological studies are made, many variables are present which will not be identified. Ask yourself, did the researcher consider the many possible variables which might have had an effect on the results when he *interpreted* his results?

One way to test theories resulting from an epidemiological study on human beings is to design an experiment using animals, in which all variables other than the one in question (in this case, sugar in the diet) can be kept constant. Animals with physiological systems similar to the human system under study are excellent subjects for examining a human disease theory. Such animals can share a common heredity, their life span is short compared to that of human beings, and they can be maintained in laboratory conditions where most variables can be controlled.

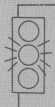

CAUTION WHEN YOU READ!

When animals are used as experimental subjects most variables can be controlled. Ask yourself, did the researcher design the experiment so that the variables critical to this study were controlled?

To test the theory that diabetes is more likely to result when sucrose replaces complex carbohydrates in a diet, Dr. Cohen designed an experiment using rats. He controlled the genetic factor that operates in human diabetes by breeding a single, uniform strain of rats which was particularly sensitive to sucrose feeding. He divided this new strain into two groups, one group being fed a high starch diet, and the other group being fed an identical diet except that sugar, providing the same number of calories, replaced the starch.

In the animals fed the starch diet, the tissues of the kidney and the retina of the eye remained normal. However, in the animals which were fed a high sucrose diet, these tissues showed a type of damage similar to that which is seen in the diabetic human; that is, the blood vessels were constricted and there were deformities in the tissues of the kidneys and the retina.

Cohen came to the conclusion that this experiment offered hope to potential diabetics; if from birth they consume a low sucrose diet, they may never become diabetic.

Has it then been firmly established that rising intake of sugar has precipitated the rise in the incidence of diabetes? No. Certainly Cohen's studies suggest as much and point toward the use of complex carbohydrates instead of refined sugar in the diet. However, it is not clear that sugar consumption in the United States has risen in parallel with the rise in diabetes.

Even if it has, what has been observed in the United States and Israel is a correlation, not a cause and effect relationship. Perhaps both diabetes and cardiovascular diseases are on the rise because they are more often correctly diagnosed than formerly or because the incidence of other diseases such as tuberculosis and diphtheria has fallen. Perhaps early diagnosis and treatment of diabetics is allowing them to live long enough to produce offspring who carry the genes for the disease, thus adding to the number of potential diabetics in the population.

Dr. E. L. Bierman and Dr. R. Nelson, of the University of Washington School of Medicine and the Mayo Clinic, disagree with the view that there may be a causal relationship between the consumption of sugar and the development of diabetes. They state that "the cause of primary diabetes mellitus in man remains unknown; there is no evidence that excessive consumption of sugar causes diabetes."[9]

Moreover, Dr. F. Grande, School of Public Health, University of Minnesota, does not attribute significance to the correlation between rising sugar consumption and rising deaths from coronary heart disease. He states that the true rate of individuals' consumption of sugar is unknown and that the rise in coronary heart disease deaths may be due to changes in medical diagnosis of the causes of death.[10] The whole question of cardiovascular disease is so complex that further discussion of it has been reserved for the second Highlight. Meanwhile, the third question concerning the value of sugar in the diet needs to be discussed.

Is Sugar "Physiologically Worthless" and a Contributor of "Empty Calories"?

Sucrose, in the process of metabolism, eventually becomes two molecules of glucose. Glucose is used for energy to power the body, an excess is stored as glycogen in the liver, ready to be later reconverted to glucose. If glucose is needed, then sucrose is not "physiologically worthless." The condemnation of sucrose probably came about because of nutritionists' concern over obesity and the replacement of vegetables and grains by refined sugar in the U.S. diet. Sugar may be a worthless addition to the diet of a person who is already overfed.

The term *empty calories* is often used to denote calories **empty calories** from foods which contribute no nutrients such as amino acids, vitamins, and minerals. Some nutritionists object to the use of the term, since a large portion of the world's population is

[9]Bierman, E. L. and Nelson, R.: Carbohydrates, diabetes, and blood lipids. In *World Review of Nutrition and Dietetics.* Bourne, G. F., editor. S. Karger AG, Basel, 1975.

[10]Grande, F.: Sugar and cardiovascular disease. In *World Review of Nutrition and Dietetics.* Bourne, G. F., editor. S. Karger AG, Basel, 1975.

junk food

calorie poor. Still it is widely used. Soft drinks made of sugar and water are often referred to as *junk foods*. (See Table H1.1.) Meanwhile, the original question in the title of this Highlight remains.

Is Sugar Bad for You?

There is no reason to believe that sugar is in any way poisonous to the normal, healthy human being. Clearly, however, it may be associated with other factors that are harmful: obesity, the displacement of needed nutrients and fiber, and dental decay. If on these grounds you conclude that sugar is indeed to be avoided, it is important to recognize that other caloric sweeteners, such as honey, are no better (see Activity 5). Notice should also be taken of the sugar that is hidden in many supposedly healthful products.

Labeling laws are described in Highlight 13.

The advertising industry would have us believe that some products provide an excellent replacement for a balanced meal. One such product, advertised as a substitute for breakfast, contains more sugar than any other single ingredient. Labeling laws require that food product ingredients be listed on the container in the order of their weight, with the ingredient in the largest amount listed first. In the breakfast substitute just mentioned, the order of the first three ingredients is sugar, vegetable shortening, water. The recommended serving contains 370 kcalories. For only 335 kcalories, a person could have ½ cup orange juice (60), a poached egg on toast (150), a pat of margarine (35), and a cup of skim milk (90). This breakfast has the added advantage of being high in protein, which would help to keep the blood glucose elevated for a longer period of time.

On the other hand, as is stressed heavily in Highlight 4 and in Chapters 7 and 8, energy is the prime nutritional need of humans. Many countries of the world suffer severe malnutrition from an energy deficit. If sugar is available to make up this deficit, it may be a life-saving resource. If nutrients are otherwise adequate and the teeth are healthy, what harm can there be in getting needed energy from sugar?

To Explore Further—

This book shows the role sugar has played in history:
Aykroyd, W. R.: *The Story of Sugar.* Quadrangle Books, Chicago, 1967.

This is a highly technical book but excellently written; chapters are by experts in the field:
Sipple, H. L. and McNutt, K. W., editors: *Sugars in Nutrition.* Academic Press, New York, 1974.

Suggested Activities

(1) Study your own diet.

This is the first of a series of suggested activities that will appear at the end of each chapter. They will invite you to study your own diet as one nutrient after another is discussed throughout the following chapters. At present the focus is on carbohydrate. To study your carbohydrate consumption, make a record of all the foods you eat for a twenty-four hour period, a three-day period, or a week. If you choose a single day, pick a typical one in order to get as accurate a picture as possible of your typical nutrient intakes. If you choose three days, it would be a good idea to use two weekdays and one weekend day, to get a still more accurate reflection of your average consumption. If you record for a week, you can select from your record the three days you consider most typical.

For each food, record the type of food, the way prepared (for example, boiled, fried, or scrambled eggs), and the amount (for example, cups or half-cups for vegetables, teaspoons for butter or sugar). For mixed dishes such as casseroles and salads, record each major ingredient separately with an estimate of its amount.

Look up each food in Appendix H and record the amount of carbohydrate it contained. (You may wish to prepare for all the exercises that follow by recording now the amounts of *all* nutrients these foods contained. If so, you will find it convenient to follow the form of the table on page 445. Note that if the size of the serving you ate was different from that listed in Appendix H you must correct all values. If, for example, you ate a 4-ounce hamburger and the nutrient contents of a 3-ounce hamburger are listed in the Appendix, you must multiply all nutrient amounts listed by 4/3. (Appendix D, example 3, gives help with this kind of calculation.)

Total your carbohydrate grams for each day. How many grams of carbohydrate do you consume per day, on the average? How many kilocalories a day do you consume from carbohydrate?

(2) Take a closer look at your carbohydrate consumption.

Now select all of the food items you ate that contained more than 3 grams of carbohydrate. Sort these into three groups: (1) foods containing complex carbohydrate (these would be foods found on the Bread and Vegetable Lists in the Exchange System, pages 33-35), (2) nutritious foods containing simple carbohydrate (these would be foods on the Milk and Fruit lists), and (3) foods containing carbohydrate mostly as sucrose: candy, cakes, honey, cola beverages, etc. How many grams of carbohydrate did you consume in each of these three categories? What *percent* of your carbohydrate calories comes from sweets? (See Appendix D, example 4, for help in calculating percent.) How many *pounds* of sugar do you eat in a year? (See Appendix D, Conversion Tables.)

(Note: The last Highlight in the book invites you to survey your entire diet for adequacy, balance, and economy. You may wish to save these two activities until you have read that Highlight, or you may wish to read the Highlight now for a sense of perspective.)

(3)   Find the hidden sugar in the processed foods you buy.

Examine the packages of processed foods you buy—canned, frozen, or dried—and make a list of the ones which contain sugar. Note the position of sugar in the list of ingredients. The next time you are purchasing these same foods, determine if you can buy the same item without sugar. For example, frozen strawberries can be bought with or without sugar.

(4)   Find the hidden sugar in the cereals.

The cereal section of a supermarket is a good place to go in pursuit of hidden sugar. Make a list of all the brand names of cereals and indicate if there is sugar in the list of ingredients, and where in the list it is positioned. (Be certain you count honey, brown sugar, and corn syrup as sugar.) It will be interesting to see how many cereals are primarily a sugar product, not a grain product, and how many contain no sugar.

(5)   Is honey better for you than sugar?

The following table compares for you some of the nutrients supplied by white sugar and by honey, and shows you how much of each of these nutrients might be needed in your diet in

Vitamins and Minerals Supplied by One Tablespoon

	Calcium (mg)	Iron (mg)	Vitamin A (IU)	Thiamin (mg)	Riboflavin (mg)	Vitamin C (mg)
Sugar (white granulated	0	trace*	0	0	0	0
Honey (strained or extracted)	1	0.1	0	trace*	0.01	trace*
Possible daily nutrient need†	1000	18	5000	1.5	1.7	60

*A *trace* is an amount large enough to be detectable in chemical analysis, but too small to be significant in comparison to the amounts recorded in these tables.

†These are U.S. RDA amounts (see page 419). Not all the vitamins and minerals are listed.

a day. What *percent* of your daily need for these nutrients is supplied by honey? (See Appendix D, example 4, for help in calculating percent.) Does this justify your including honey in your diet as an important source of essential nutrients?

(6) Notice your own serving sizes.

Many people think that the spoon with which they help themselves to sugar is a teaspoon, but when it is heaped high with sugar it may be more nearly two. Using your sugar spoon as you usually do, spoon ten helpings of sugar into a bowl. Now measure this sugar with a measuring spoon, using level spoonsful. How many teaspoons is a spoonful of sugar as you use it?

2

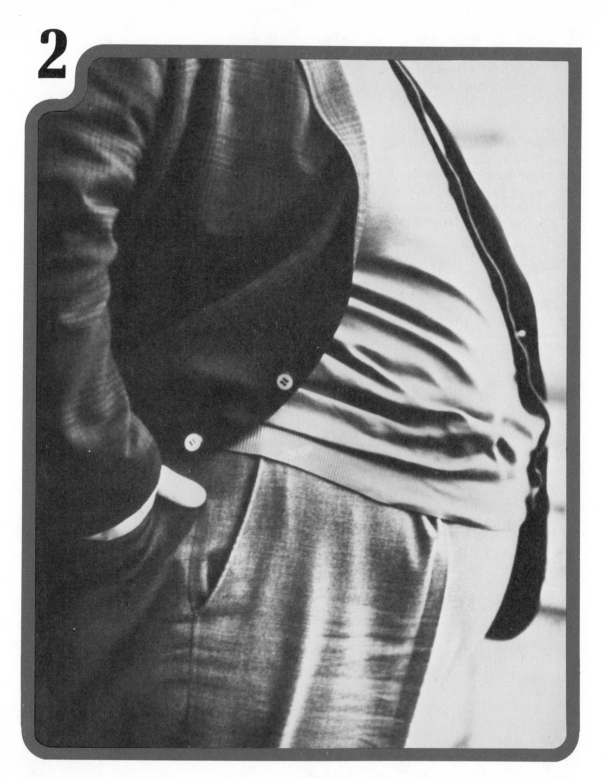

Joe Baker—Medical World News

The Lipids

The notion that matter is something inert and uninteresting is surely the veriest nonsense. If there is anything more wonderful than matter in the sheer versatility of its behavior, I have yet to hear tell of it.
—FRED HOYLE

Pros and Cons of Body Fat

We Americans have been conditioned to believe that slim is beautiful. The less fat you carry on your frame, the lovelier (sexier, healthier) you are. One-third of the world's population is underfed, while one-third of the United States' population is overfed. And indeed, overweight is a major health problem in our country, contributing as it does to the incidence of heart disease, diabetes, and many other ills.

On the other hand, there are things your body fat does for you that you would be sorry to do without. If you carry neither too much nor too little body fat, you will enjoy the benefits nature intended in providing stores of this very important nutrient.

The fats—more properly called the lipids—are actually a family of compounds which include both fats and oils. There are both in your body, and both help to keep it healthy. Natural oils in the skin provide a radiant complexion, while in the scalp they help nourish the hair and make it glossy. The layer of fat beneath the skin, being a poor conductor of heat, protects the body from extremes of temperature. A pad of hard fat beneath each kidney protects it from being jarred and damaged, even during a motorcycle ride on a bumpy road. The soft fat in the breasts of a woman protects her mammary glands from heat and cold and

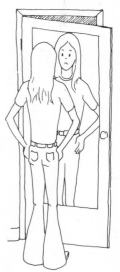

"I have got to go on a diet."

53

cushions them against shock. The fat that lards the muscles provides a ready supply of usable energy for their action.

An uninterrupted flow of energy is so vital to life that in a pinch any other function will be sacrificed to maintain it. If a growing child is fed too little food, for example, the food he does consume will be used for energy to keep his heart and lungs going, while his growth comes to a standstill. The urgency of the need for energy has ensured, over the course of evolution, that all creatures have built-in reserves to protect themselves from ever being deprived of it. To go totally without an energy supply, even for a few minutes, would be to die. One provision against this has already been described: the stores of glycogen —chains of sugar (glucose) units—in the liver which can be returned to circulation whenever the blood glucose supply runs short.

However, the cells can only store a limited amount of energy as glycogen; once this is depleted, the body must receive new food or turn to its backup reserve, the body fat. Unlike liver cells, fat cells have an unlimited storage capacity. Depending on how much fat has been stored (in other words how fat a person is), an individual can keep going without energy nutrients for days or even weeks or months.

The average twenty-year-old American woman needs about 2,000 kcalories a day to fuel her body's maintenance and activities. If she fasts (drinking only water to flush out her metabolic wastes), she will oxidize her own body fat to meet this need. One pound of body fat provides 3,500 kcalories, or enough for almost two days of her energy need. Obviously, in conditions of enforced starvation, for example during a siege or famine, the fatter person will survive longer. Fifty pounds of excess body fat will provide about three months' worth of energy.

For the dangers of fasting, see Highlight 8.

1 pound "body fat"=3,500 kcal (but see page 241).

If you happen to be acquainted with a polar bear, you will be aware that the same thing is true for him. As he lumbers about on his iceberg, great masses of fat ripple beneath his thick fur coat. When he hibernates, he oxidizes that fat, extracting tens of thousands of kcalories from it to maintain his body temperature and to fuel other metabolic processes while he sleeps. Come spring, he is several hundred pounds thinner than when he went to sleep.

On the other hand, since we do not yet anticipate facing a famine in America, the thinner person actually has most of the advantages. To lose 50 pounds, you would have to deprive yourself of food totally for at least three months—and for much longer if you didn't elect total starvation. No one acquainted with the risks of this course would undertake such a program except under close medical supervision.

Living on body fat has other disadvantages too. Fat can provide energy, true, but not as glucose, the form from which brain and nerve cells can best extract energy. After a long period of glucose deprivation, those cells do develop the ability to metabolize fat for energy and so continue to function; but under these conditions the body is in a state of *ketosis*, with headaches and other undesirable symptoms.

To sum up what's good about body fat: it helps maintain the health of the skin and hair, protects body organs from temperature extremes and mechanical shock, and provides a reserve fuel supply for use whenever body carbohydrate is depleted. As for what is bad about body fat: there can simply be too much of it. When fat is being oxidized for energy in the absence of glucose, ketosis results.

ketosis (kee-TOE-sis): excess ketones in the blood (see pages 210-211).

Fat in Foods

Many of the compounds that give foods their flavor and aroma are found in fats and oils; they are fat-soluble. Four vitamins—A, D, E, and K—are also soluble in fat. Understanding this fact provides insight into many different areas in nutrition, so let us spend a moment here considering the phenomenon of "fat solubility." As you know, fats and oils tend to separate from water and watery substances. The oil floats to the top when salad dressing stands. As hot meat drippings cool, the fat separates and hardens on top of the other juices. You can probably think of many other examples of this phenomenon.

Whenever a mixture of a fatty liquid and a watery liquid separates in this manner, other compounds in the mixture must go either with the fat or with the water. The significance of this is evident if you think what happens when the fat is removed from a food.

If you skin chicken meat before cooking it, the layer of fat is removed with the skin. The result is a tasteless, odorless meat. Chicken meat without its fat is almost indistinguishable from defatted veal, lamb, or water-pack tuna; many of the compounds that give the meat its flavor are removed with the fat.

The aromatic nature of many fat-soluble compounds becomes obvious in the house when foods are cooking. Meat fat, especially bacon, ham, pork, and fatty beef (hamburgers), and the fat added to vegetables—onions smothered in butter, French fries—all contribute to a good "food" smell. Milk when skimmed loses much of its buttery flavor too, and more importantly it loses all of the vitamins A and D the cow secreted into the milk. To make skimmed milk equivalent to whole milk nutritionally, these vitamins must be mixed in; hence the "vitamin A & D fortified" label you see on skimmed milk. In general, foods from which the fat or oil has been removed lack much of their original flavor, aroma, and fat-soluble vitamins.

fat solubility

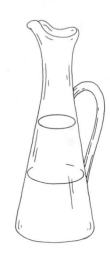

Fortification actually involves adding back more vitamin D than was in the whole milk originally. See Highlight 13.

Reminder: the calorie of everyday speech is properly called a *kilocalorie* (kcal).

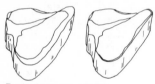

Pork chop with ½" fat
(260 kcal)
Pork chop with fat trimmed off
(130 kcal)

Potato with butter and sour cream
(1 tbsp each) (260 kcal)

Energy value of fat: 1 gram supplies 9 kilocalories

ADA Food Exchange Lists, pages 33-38.

exchange: see definitions on Exchange Lists.

One additional feature is lost when fat is removed: calories. A medium pork chop with the fat trimmed to within one-half inch of the lean meat contains 260 kcalories; with the fat trimmed off completely it contains 130 kcalories. A baked potato with butter and sour cream (one tablespoon each) is 260 kcalories; plain, it is 100 kcalories. So it goes. The most effective single measure you can take to reduce the energy (caloric) value of a food is to eat it without the fat.

Plain potato (100 kcal)

Whole milk 1 cup (170 kcal)

Skim milk 1 cup (80 kcal)

How Much Fat?

Removing the fat from a food reduces the energy value to a far greater extent than removing the carbohydrate or protein because fat is a concentrated energy source. A gram of fat supplies about 9 kcalories, while a gram of carbohydrate supplies only 4. Knowing where fats are found provides a powerful way to control the energy content of the diet.

Three of the lists in the Food Exchange System include foods containing appreciable amounts of fat: the milk list, the meat list, and the fat list. The three lists differ in that milk exchanges also contain protein and carbohydrate, and meat exchanges contain protein, while fat exchanges contain only fat. It will be helpful to look at the fat list first (see page 37). In addition to the obvious items (butter, margarine, and oil) this list includes bacon, olives, and avocados. These foods are classed as fat exchanges because the amount of lipid they contain makes them essentially pure fat contributors. One-eighth of an avocado or one slice of bacon contains as much fat as a pat of butter, and, like butter, they contain negligible protein and carbohydrate. Hence, when you eat bacon, you are not eating a protein food; you are eating a food which is equivalent to butter in the energy nutrients it contributes to your diet.

1 fat exchange = 5 grams fat
(serving size: VARIES)

The foods on the milk list (see page 33) contain variable amounts of fat. A cup of skim milk has negligible fat, a cup of 2 percent fortified milk has 5 grams of fat, and a cup of whole milk has 10 grams. In calculating the amount of fat present in a food, it is convenient to think in terms of fat exchanges: thus, a cup of 2 percent milk contains one fat exchange, while a cup of whole milk contains two.

1 skim milk exchange = 0 grams fat
1 2% milk exchange = 5 grams fat
1 whole milk exchange = 10 grams fat

Serving size: 1 CUP

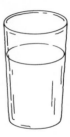

10 grams

The foods on the meat lists (see pages 36-37) also contain varying amounts of fat. An ounce of lean meat has 3 grams of fat, an ounce of medium-fat meat has about 2½ grams more, or 5½ grams, while an ounce of high-fat meat has 8 grams of fat. Peanut butter, which is a protein-rich food grouped with meat, has 13 grams of fat per two-tablespoon serving.

1 lean meat exchange = 3 grams fat
1 medium-fat meat exchange = 5½ grams fat
1 high-fat meat exchange = 8 grams fat
1 exchange of peanut butter = 13 grams fat

Serving size: 1 OUNCE or VARIES

A person studying the meat list for the first time may be surprised to note how many fat calories there are in meat. An ounce of lean meat supplies 28 kcalories from protein and 27 kcalories from its fat. An ounce of high-fat meat supplies the same number—28 kcalories—from protein, but 72 kcalories from fat. Two tablespoons of peanut butter, also with 28 kcalories from protein, supply 117 kcalories from fat! Thus meat, which is often thought of as a protein food, actually contains more fat energy than protein energy, and is an unexpectedly fattening food, often accounting for the excess weight that meat eaters tend to gain.

1 ounce=28.4 grams (Appendix D). Nutritionists usually use either 28 or 30.

3 grams

Note that one exchange of meat is only one ounce. To make the exchange system work for you it is important not only to be familiar with the foods on each list, but also to be aware of the number of exchanges that constitutes a serving. For most foods, the normal serving size is one exchange. For meat, one serving may be one exchange (an egg), two or three exchanges (a hamburger), or even eight exchanges (a dinner steak).

The following table shows the fat content of some foods in the context of their overall energy nutrient composition:

Exchange Group	Carbohydrate (g)	Protein (g)	Fat (g)	Energy (kcal)
(1) Skim milk*	12	8	0	80
(2) Vegetables	5	2	0	25
(3) Fruit	10	0	0	40
(4) Bread*	15	2	0	70
(5) **Lean meat***	0	7	3	55
(6) **Fat**	0	0	5	45

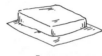

5 grams

*For exchanges containing more fat, add fat exchanges as indicated (see Exchange Lists, pages 33, 35-37.

These values provide an easy way to estimate the amount of fat eaten at a meal or in a day. Two reminders are needed. Fat is often hidden in cooked vegetables. As a rule of thumb, vegetables served with butter or margarine can be assumed to contain one fat exchange (one teaspoon) per half-cup serving. Some baked goods also contain appreciable fat: these are listed on the bread list.

Using these values, let us see how much fat was provided by the day's meals described on page 30. Adding up the meat exchanges for the egg, peanut butter, and steak, taking into account the extra fat in these meats, the whole milk, and the short-cake biscuit, adding the fat used in frying the egg and flavoring the beans and potato, and finally adding a fat exchange for the heavy cream, we reach a total of 106½ grams of fat for the day:

Breakfast	# Exchanges	# Grams Fat
1 egg fried in	1 meat	3
1 tsp fat	1 fat	5
1 piece toast		
1 tsp margarine	1 fat	5
Lunch		
2 slices bread		
2 tbsp peanut butter	1 meat + 2½ fat	15½
2 tsp jelly		
1 cup milk	+ 2 fat	10
Dinner		
6-ounce steak	6 meat + 6 fat	48
½ cup green beans served with		
1 tsp margarine	1 fat	5
1 cup mashed potato served with		
1 tsp margarine	1 fat	5
Dessert		
2" diameter biscuit	1 fat	5
¾ cup strawberries		
1 tbsp heavy cream	1 fat	5
6 tsp sugar		
	TOTAL	106½ grams fat

The day's meals thus supplied (9 x 106½) or about 960 kcalories from fat.

In addition to facilitating calculations of this kind, the Exchange System divides fats into two classes—saturated and polyunsaturated—to aid in meal planning for the diabetic. The importance of being aware of the quality of dietary fat as well as of its quantity, will be evident in the next section.

Triglycerides and Cholesterol: A Closer Look at the Fats in Foods

"Your blood triglycerides are up." If a doctor says this, the patient may, perhaps rightly, be alarmed. Most of us are aware nowadays that there is a close relation between the fats found in the blood and the state of health of the heart. A closer look at the fats in foods will lay the foundation for an understanding of this relation, which is treated in detail in the Highlight at the end of this chapter.

Almost all (95 percent) of the lipids in the diet are triglycerides; the other two classes of dietary lipid are the phospholipids and sterols, which amount to 5 percent. (Cholesterol is a member of the latter group.) Let us look at these groups as they are found in foods.

A word of warning: cholesterol has been much maligned as being "the" cause of cardiovascular disease. Compared with the triglycerides, however, cholesterol may be less important than we have been led to believe. Other factors such as smoking, hypertension, and obesity are also of great importance. Since the triglycerides predominate in the diet, the following section focuses on them.

The Triglycerides. Triglycerides come in many sizes and several varieties, but they all share a common structure; they all have a "backbone" of *glycerol*, to which three *fatty acids* are attached. All glycerol molecules are alike:

$$
\begin{array}{c}
H \\
| \\
H-C-O-H \\
| \\
H-C-O-H \qquad \text{Glycerol} \\
| \\
H-C-O-H \\
| \\
H
\end{array}
$$

But the fatty acids may vary in two ways: length and degree of saturation.

Understanding the fats, and the beneficial and harmful effects they have on your body, means descending to the level of their molecular structure. It is not as complicated as it may seem at first. If you follow the few steps of reasoning presented here, you can reap the reward of an appreciation for the whole subject—and of its beauty—that you may never otherwise enjoy. Let us examine the fatty acids to see how they differ in (1) length and (2) saturation, and to see how they are attached to glycerol to make triglycerides.

A fatty acid is a chain of carbon atoms with hydrogens at-

triglycerides: the major class of dietary lipids (precise definition, page 60).

phospholipids: a minor class of dietary lipids (precise definition, page 69).
sterols, including cholesterol: other dietary lipids (precise definition, page 69).

glycerol (GLIS-er-ol): an organic alcohol, composed of a 3-carbon chain, each with an alcohol group attached. An alcohol is a comound containing an —OH group.

—ol=alcohol

acid: a compound which tends to ionize in water solution, releasing H⁺ions. The more H⁺ions are free in the water, the stronger the acid. See Appendix B.

acid group: the —COOH group of an organic acid. This can also be represented

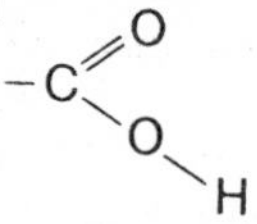

tached and with an *acid group* (—COOH) at one end. The one shown below is acetic acid, the compound that gives vinegar its sour taste:

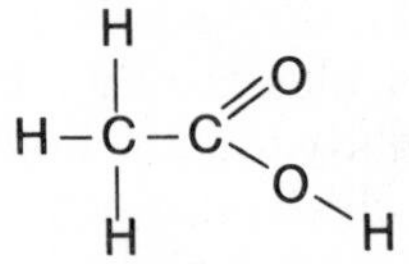

Acetic Acid

This is the simplest of the fatty acids; the chain is only two carbon atoms long. A longer fatty acid may have four, six, eight (they do mostly come in even numbers) or more carbon atoms. Among those common in dairy products are fatty acids 6-10 carbons long; butyric acid, which is present in butter, is a 4-carbon fatty acid. Fatty acids that predominate in meat and fish are 16 or more carbon atoms long.

fatty acid: an organic compound composed of a carbon chain with hydrogens attached and an acid group at one end.

To illustrate the characteristics of these fatty acids, let us look at the 18-carbon series. Stearic acid is one of these:

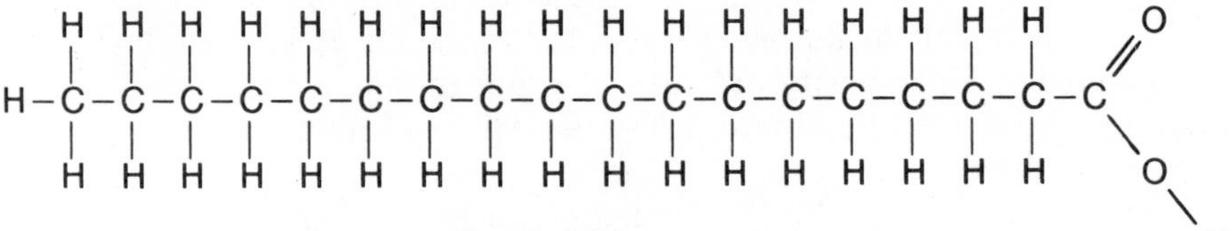

Stearic Acid

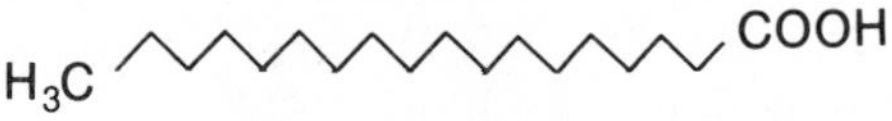

Stearic Acid (simplified)

(see rules for simplified structure, page 19)

triglyceride (try-GLIS-uh-ride): a compound composed of carbon, hydrogen, and oxygen arranged as a molecule of glycerol with three fatty acids attached to it.

    tri=three (fatty acids)
glyceride=a compound of glycerol

To make a triglyceride, we would attach three of these to a molecule of glycerol. A triglyceride composed of glycerol and three molecules of stearic acid is shown below:

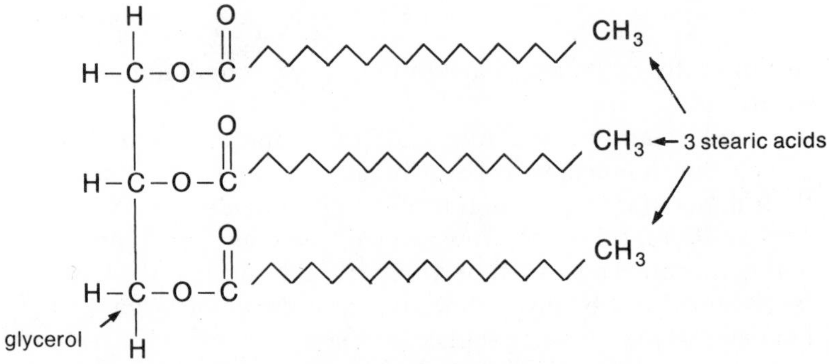

3 stearic acids

glycerol

A fat (triglyceride) found in butter.

(Note that the fatty acids are connected to glycerol by their acid ends; that is, they are reversed compared to the drawing of stearic acid alone. You might also notice that two H's and an O are lost when a fatty acid is attached to glycerol: water—H$_2$O— is formed.)

People under the threat of heart trouble may be told to reduce their intake of saturated fats and increase their intake of polyunsaturated fats. Cutting out butter, and using soft margarine in its place, is one way to do this. The triglyceride shown above is a saturated fat: one which is loaded, or saturated, with all the hydrogen (H) atoms it can carry. Some (soft) margarines are rich in polyunsaturated fats: triglycerides in which the fatty acids are carrying less than their full complement of hydrogens. To understand them, let us consider stearic acid once more. If we remove two H's from the middle of the carbon chain, we are left with a compound that looks like this:

saturated fatty acid: a fatty acid carrying the maximum possible number of hydrogen atoms. Example: stearic acid. Thus a **saturated fat** is a triglyceride composed of glycerol and 3 saturated fatty acids.

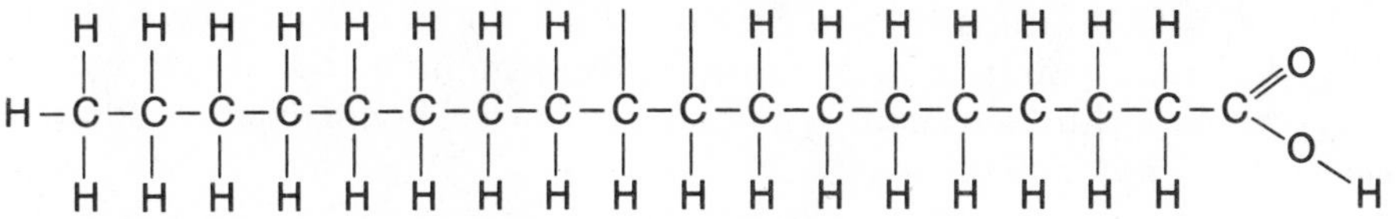

impossible structure

The two carbon atoms which formerly held the H's are, in a sense, empty-handed. Each has an available bond which is going unused. Such a compound cannot exist in nature. But an extra bond can be formed between the two carbons to satisfy nature's requirement that every carbon must have four bonds connecting it to other atoms. There is then a "double bond" between them:

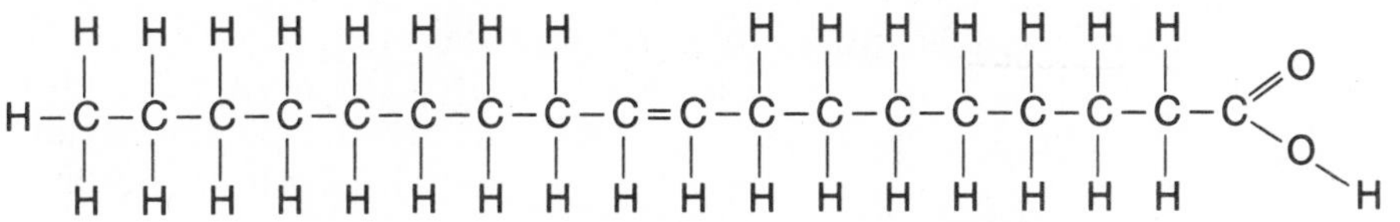

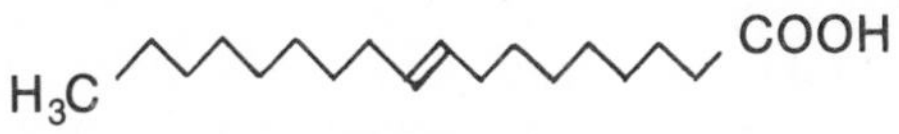

Oleic Acid

(The same situation exists in the acid group at the end of the chain, where an O is double-bonded to the terminal C. That carbon has its full four bonds, while the oxygen meets its requirement of having two.) The resulting structure is that of the unsaturated (in this case *monounsaturated*) fatty acid, oleic acid, which is found abundantly in the triglycerides in olive oil (example below):

monounsaturated fatty acid: a fatty acid that lacks two hydrogen atoms and has one double bond between carbons. Example: oleic acid.

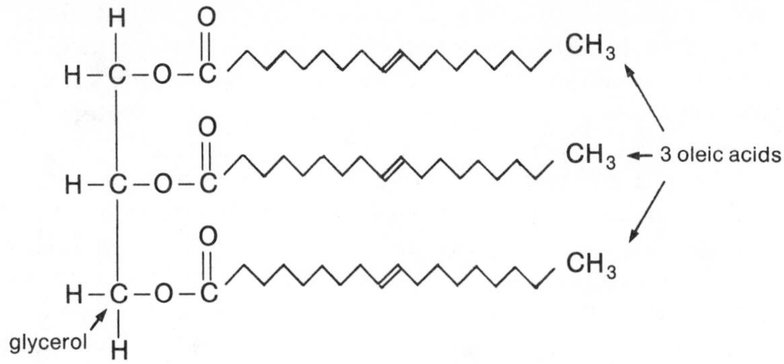

A triglyceride found in olive oil.

polyunsaturated fatty acid:
a fatty acid that lacks four or more hydrogen atoms and has two or more double bonds between carbons, often abbreviated PUFA. Examples: linoleic acid (2 double bonds), linolenic acid (3 double bonds). Thus a **polyunsaturated fat** is a triglyceride containing PUFA.

The heart patient, however, is advised to eat *polyunsaturated* fats, for reasons explained in Highlight 2. A polyunsaturated fat is a triglyceride in which the fatty acids have *two* or more points of unsaturation. An example is the one shown below, linoleic acid, which lacks four H's and has two double bonds:

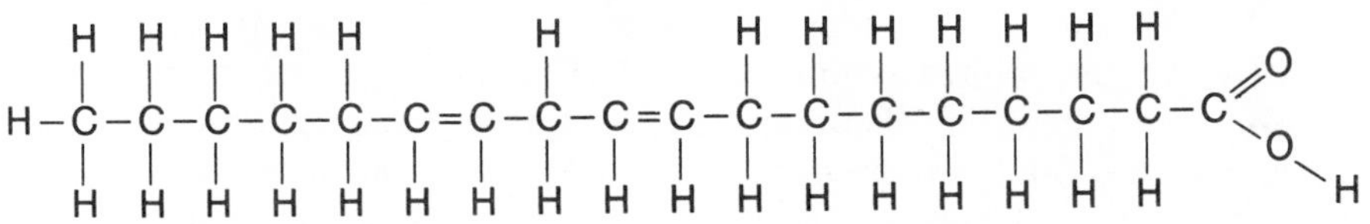

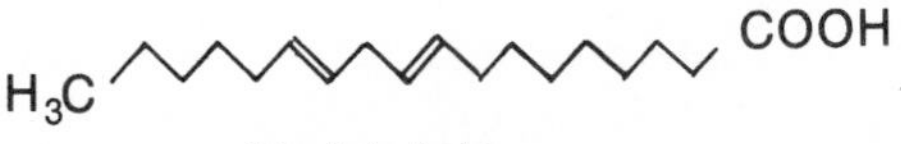

Linoleic Acid

Linoleic acid is found in the triglycerides of most vegetable oils: corn oil, safflower oil, and the like. It is the most common of the polyunsaturated fatty acids in foods and the most important. In fact it is an *essential* nutrient. We will discuss it further after the end of this section.

Having looked at three of the most common fatty acids in foods, you can probably anticipate what the others look like. There is a fourth member of the family of "18-carbon fatty acids": linolenic acid, which has three double bonds. A similar series of 20-carbon fatty acids exists as well as another series of 22-carbon fatty acids. These are the long-chain fatty acids. In lesser amounts, medium-chain (14-16 C) and short-chain (8-12 C) fatty acids are also present in foods.

Note: lino*leic* acid (18C, 2 double bonds) should not be confused with lino*lenic* acid (18C, 3 double bonds).

For these series, names, and structures, see Appendix C.

To repeat, the fats and oils in foods are mostly (95 percent) triglycerides: glycerol backbones with fatty acids attached. To complete the picture, it only remains to say that any combination of fatty acids is possible. A mixed triglyceride, one which contains more than one type of fatty acid, is shown below:

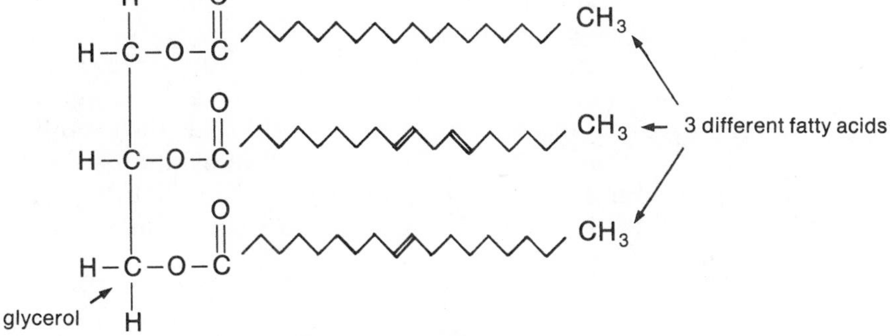

A mixed triglyceride.

The essential nutrient, linoleic acid. Since the concept of essential nutrients pervades much of nutrition science, let us devote our attention to it for a moment. Why is this fatty acid essential for health, while a lack of any of the others would produce no ill effects?

When polyunsaturated fatty acids are missing from an infant's diet, the skin reddens and becomes irritated and the liver develops abnormalities. Addition of the fatty acids back to the diet clears up these symptoms. It turns out that what the body cells need is arachidonic acid (20C, 4 double bonds) and that infants can make this compound for themselves if linoleic acid is supplied in their diets.

The body's cells are equipped with many enzymes which can convert one compound to another. To make body fat or oil—triglycerides—all the enzymes need is a usable food source of the atoms triglycerides contain: carbon, hydrogen, and oxygen. Glucose will do perfectly well. In fact, given an excess of blood glucose (and a filled glycogen storage space), this is precisely what the enzymes do: they cleave the glucose to make the two-carbon compound acetic acid and then combine many of these molecules with the appropriate alterations to make long-chain fatty acids. (This is why the fatty acid carbon chains come in even numbers: they are multiples of two.) But the cells do not possess an enzyme which can arrange the double bonding of linoleic acid.

The conversion of compound A into B and of B into C by enzymes in the body can be represented as follows:

$$A \rightarrow B \rightarrow C$$

with the arrows representing enzyme action. The problem described above can be stated:

essential nutrient: a compound which cannot be synthesized in the body in amounts sufficient to meet physiological needs. Many nutrients are needed by the body, but the word "essential" refers only to those which must be supplied by eating food.

The irritation of the skin is known as **dermatitis** (derm-uh-TIGHT-us): infection or inflammation of the skin evidenced by itching, redness, and various skin lesions.

derma = skin
itis = infection or inflammation

Acetic acid, or acetyl CoA, is formed from glucose. (See Chapter 7 and Highlight 7.)

The **precursor** of a compound, B, is a compound, A, that can be converted into B.

A (a precursor of linoleic acid) —✗→ B (linoleic acid) → C (arachidonic acid: needed in cells)

The "X" means that the enzyme that can manufacture linoleic acid is missing in human beings.

As you can see, the needed compound, C, can be supplied by either B or C. Supplying B will remedy a deficiency of both. Linoleic acid has thus come to be considered "the essential fatty acid,"[1] although arachidonic acid will alleviate the dermatitis, and to a limited extent linolenic acid will also help. By including corn oil (or any other linoleic acid source) in your diet, you obtain this fatty acid ready made.

[handwritten: three polyunsaturated fatty acids →]

allergen (AL-er-gen): an agent which provokes an allergic reaction.

symptom: the outward manifestation of a disease condition. A **disease** is the impairment or failure of a vital function, due to viral or bacterial infection, lack of an essential nutrient, genetic abnormality, or other causes.

diagnosis: identification.

The relief of dermatitis by linoleic acid might suggest to the unwary observer that all cases of dermatitis indicate a deficiency of this nutrient. Not so! Dermatitis is, by definition, a skin condition; the word does not imply a single cause. Actually, there are more than a hundred body compounds—including other oils, vitamins, minerals, and hormones—that are needed in certain proportions to one another to ensure the health of the skin. A deficiency or imbalance of any of these, caused either by a dietary lack or by failure of the body to produce necessary compounds in the normal way, may create a dermatitis condition. Bacterial and viral infections, allergens, physical agents such as radiation, and chemical irritants also cause dermatitis. There may also be a "psychosomatic" cause, as when excessive nervous activity in the brain (mind) generates a hormone imbalance that affects the skin (body). (See Highlight 6.) For these reasons, when you notice a symptom, never conclude that the cause is necessarily one with which you are familiar.

A distinction must be made between a symptom and a disease. A symptom can be alleviated (soothing oils can be applied to the skin to make it feel better, for example), but until you know the cause, you cannot achieve a cure. With dermatitis, the rule is that if a certain nutrient clears up the symptom, then a deficiency of that nutrient may have been the cause.

A symptom is not a disease. Prescription of a cure depends on correct diagnosis of the of the disease.

[1]Alfin-Slater, R. B. and Aftergood, L.: Fats and other lipids. In *Modern Nutrition in Health and Disease.* Goodhart, R. S. and Shils, M. E., editors. Lea and Febiger, Philadelphia, 1973.

You can also be fooled into thinking that a particular *food*—safflower oil, for example—is essential for healthy skin. Health food stores make millions of dollars a year promoting misconceptions like this. Actually, of course, safflower oil is not essential at all; you need never taste a drop of it all your life. All you need, to avoid essential fatty acid deficiency, is to include polyunsaturated fat in your diet from any of several hundred different possible food sources. The chance that you will then lack an essential fatty acid is virtually nil, since they are found in almost all oils (Appendix H).

The distinction between foods and nutrients has been emphasized once before (page 2). The implication that any specific food has magical, miraculous or curative powers is false.

A flag sign of a spurious claim is the use of:

the implication that any specific *food* is needed for any reason.

Each culture has its own favorite food sources of fats and oils. The peoples of the Mediterranean (Greeks, Italians, and Spaniards) rely heavily on olive oil, which is high in monounsaturates, while the Orientals use the polyunsaturated oil of soybeans. Jewish cookery traditionally employs chicken fat, while southern Americans rely heavily on pork fat—lard and bacon. The saturated fat consumption of Blacks is cause for concern among health authorities who note a high incidence of

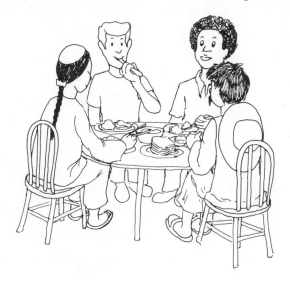

hypertension: high blood pressure. This problem may also be related to salt consumption.[2]

hypertensive heart disease among these people. This high rate of heart disease may be diet-related, genetically caused, or both.

Polyunsaturated fats: the "good guys" in the lipid family. Ever since researchers first began to conclude that saturated fats were linked to heart disease while polyunsaturated fats were preventive, advertisers have been touting the value of their margarines and oils as "high in polyunsaturates." If we agree (and Highlight 2 gives reasons why we might) that it is advisable to make a habit of selecting foods rich in polyunsaturated and low in saturated fat for our daily consumption, we need to know which foods are which.

> Generally speaking, vegetable and fish oils are rich in polyunsaturates while the harder fats—animal fats—are more saturated. But once again, beware. Not all vegetable fats are polyunsaturated. If you are looking for a substitute for cream, you may well use a non-dairy creamer in its place. Many non-dairy creamers substitute coconut oil for butterfat. But coconut oil is also saturated and hence no "better" for you than cream!

saturated fats: high melting point; solid at room or body temperature.
polyunsaturated fats: low melting point; liquid at room or body temperature.

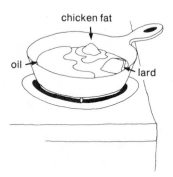

chicken fat

oil

lard

A rule of thumb in determining the degree of saturation is to observe how hard a lipid is at room temperature. Chicken fat is softer than pork fat, which is softer than lard. Of the three, lard is the most, and chicken fat the least saturated. The double bonds in polyunsaturated fats make them melt more readily.

Unfortunately, what we gain in health from polyunsaturated fats we lose in keeping quality. The more double bonds there are in a fatty acid, the more easily oxygen can destroy it. The oxidation of a fatty acid is shown below: an oxygen molecule attacks the double bond and combines with the carbons at that site to yield two aldehydes:

$$O = O$$

$$-\overset{\overset{\displaystyle H}{|}}{\underset{\underset{\displaystyle H}{|}}{C}}-\overset{}{\underset{\underset{\displaystyle H}{|}}{C}}=\overset{}{\underset{\underset{\displaystyle H}{|}}{C}}-\overset{\overset{\displaystyle H}{|}}{\underset{\underset{\displaystyle H}{|}}{C}}-$$

Fatty acid and oxygen.

$$-\overset{\overset{\displaystyle H}{|}}{\underset{\underset{\displaystyle H}{|}}{C}}-C\overset{\displaystyle O}{\underset{\displaystyle H}{\big\langle}} \quad + \quad \overset{\displaystyle O}{\underset{\displaystyle H}{\big\rangle}}C-\overset{\overset{\displaystyle H}{|}}{\underset{\underset{\displaystyle H}{|}}{C}}-$$

Two aldehydes.

aldehyde (AL-duh-hide): an organic compound containing a —CHO group:
$$-C\overset{\displaystyle H}{\underset{\displaystyle O}{\big\langle}}.$$

Aldehydes smell bad; the product has spoiled. Other types of spoilage, due to bacterial or mold growth, can, of course, occur

[2]Seedat, Y. K. and Reddy, J.: A study of 1000 South African nonwhite hypertensive patients. *South African Medical Journal* 48(19):816-820, 1974.

too. In general, unsaturated fatty acids are less stable than their saturated counterparts.

Marketers of fat-containing products have three alternatives, none perfect. They may keep the product tightly sealed and under refrigeration—an expensive storage system. The consumer will have to do the same, and most people prefer not to buy a product that spoils readily. Marketers may protect the fat by adding preservatives and antioxidants, but there are disadvantages to this course also. Finally, they may increase the product's stability by extracting the unsaturated fat and replacing it with a more saturated one, or by hydrogenating it. This also makes it more solid, which is often desirable. Margarine made from vegetable oils is solid at room temperature because the oils have been partially hydrogenated. Hydrogenation, however, diminishes its polyunsaturated fat content and possibly, therefore, its health value. You pay your money and you take your choice!

Digestion of triglycerides. If milk is spilled, it will spatter and splash all over the floor, some drops bouncing almost as high as the table top. Not so with oil. A spilled cup of oil runs over the countertop, flows in a single stream to the floor, and spreads in a pool. If it separates into droplets, they will tend to merge again. A child observing this once said, "They love each other." The molecular structures of the triglycerides shown earlier reveal a reason for this behavior. Fatty acid chains tend to stick together: they are lipophilic (fat-loving) and hydrophobic (water-fearing). In the stomach and intestines, as well as on the countertop, they tend to adhere to one another in droplets.

The enzymes which digest them, on the other hand, are hydrophilic (water-loving). Water molecules tend to ionize: to separate into positively charged H^+ and negatively charged $-OH^-$ ions, both of which attract their opposites. Enzymes also have positively and negatively charged groups on their surfaces and so mix comfortably among the ions in water. To be digested, the triglycerides must first be brought into closer association with the enzymes in the watery medium of the intestines; that is, they must be emulsified. The liver manufactures emulsifiers for this purpose: the bile acids. Not surprisingly they are made from lipids themselves. The system seems to have been designed for maximum efficiency and balance—the more fat you eat, the more is available to manufacture the bile acids needed for the emulsification of fat.

The bile acids, like all emulsifiers, have the structure that best suits their purpose (bringing hydrophilic and lipophilic molecules together). Each molecule of bile acid has at one end an ionized group which is attracted to water, and at the other end a fatty acid chain which has an affinity for fat. As a skilled hostess takes your hand, draws you away from the company of

For the disadvantages of these additives, see Highlight 13.

hydrogenation (high-dro-gen-AY-shun): a chemical process by which hydrogens are added to unsaturated or polyunsaturated fats to make them more solid and more resistant to oxidation.

For the effects of hydrogenation on the oils in peanut butter, see Activity 6 at the end of this chapter.

ionize: see Appendix B.

emulsify (ee-MULL-suh-fye): to disperse and stabilize fat droplets in a watery solution.

bile: see also page 153.

1. Fat and water separate:

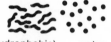

fat (hydrophobic)   water

2. Emulsifier has affinity for both:

emulsifier

3. Emulsifier helps distribute fat into water:

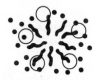

emulsified fat

your friends, and leaves you shaking hands with a new acquaintance, so a molecule of bile acid will attach itself to a lipid molecule in a droplet and draw it out into the surrounding water solution where the lipid can come into contact with an enzyme. Detergents work the same way (they are also emulsifiers), which is why they are so effective in removing grease from clothes and dishes. Molecule by molecule, the grease is dissolved out of the spot and suspended in the water, where it can be rinsed away. (You can guess where the manufacturers of "detergents with enzymes" got their idea.)

After emulsification, a triglyceride is hydrolyzed by enzymes which remove two or three of the fatty acids, leaving a monoglyceride or glycerol. In this form, as monoglycerides, glycerol, and fatty acids, most of the products of lipid digestion are absorbed into the intestinal wall cells. As with the hydrolysis of carbohydrates, that of lipids requires the participation of water, as shown below:

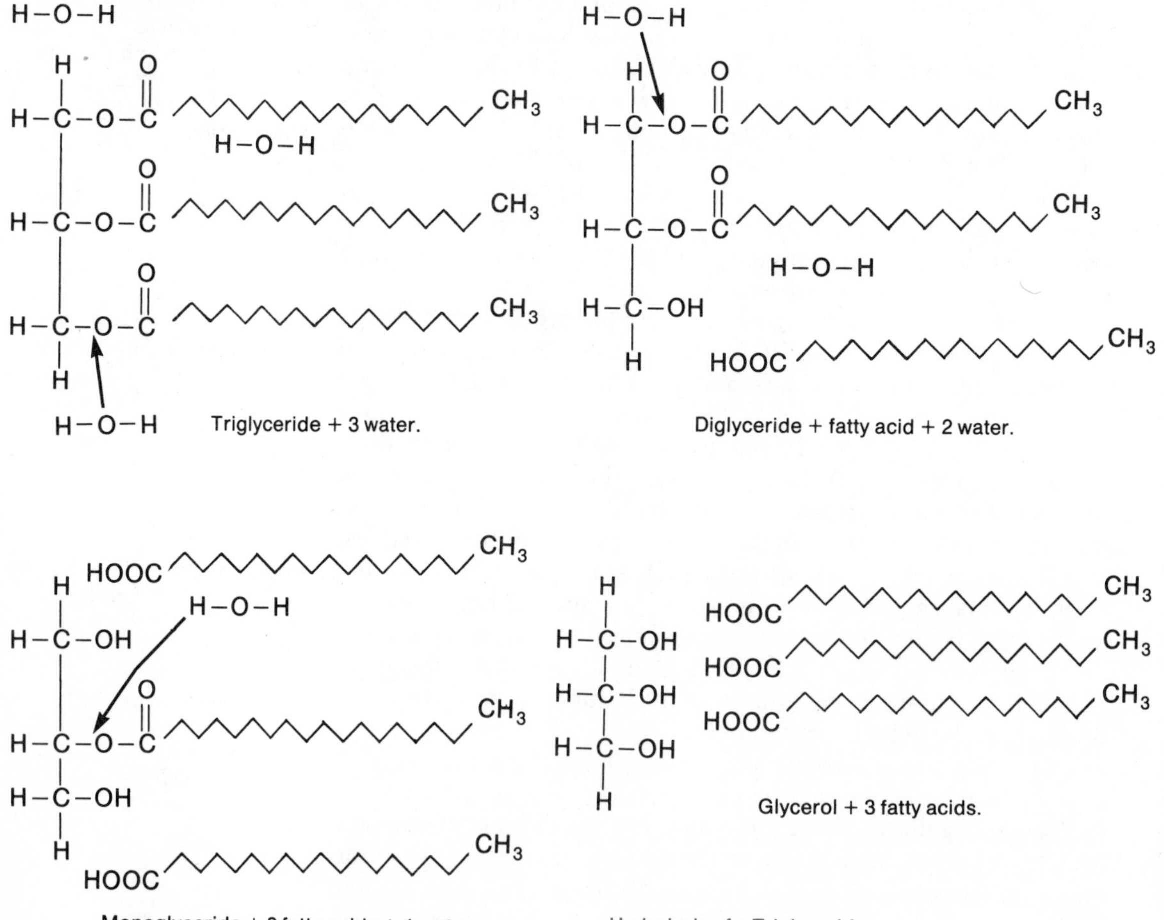

Triglyceride + 3 water.

Diglyceride + fatty acid + 2 water.

Monoglyceride + 2 fatty acids + 1 water.

Glycerol + 3 fatty acids.

Hydrolysis of a Triglyceride.

The *phospholipids*. The preceding pages have been devoted to one of the three classes of lipids, the triglycerides. The other two classes, the phospholipids and sterols, comprise only 5 percent of the lipids in the diet. They will be discussed briefly, partly for the sake of completeness, but also because they are interesting.

One of the magical nutrients, so called, that is presently receiving much attention, is *lecithin*. We are told that this nutrient is a major constituent of cell membranes (true), that the functioning of all cells depends on the integrity of their membranes (true, and on a great many other structures), and that we must therefore include large quantities of lecithin in our daily meals (false). The lecithins are not essential nutrients; the liver manufactures all that are needed for cell membrane building and other functions. One might as well believe that in order to grow healthy hair, or maintain the brain, we must eat hair or brains!

The lecithins and the other phospholipids are compounds similar to the triglycerides because they have a backbone of glycerol; they are different because they have only two fatty acids attached to them. In place of the third fatty acid is a molecule of choline or a similar compound containing phosphorus (P) and nitrogen (N) atoms. A lecithin is shown below (others differ in the nature of the attached fatty acids):

lecithin

phospholipid: a compound similar to a triglyceride, but having choline or another P-containing acid in place of one of the fatty acids.

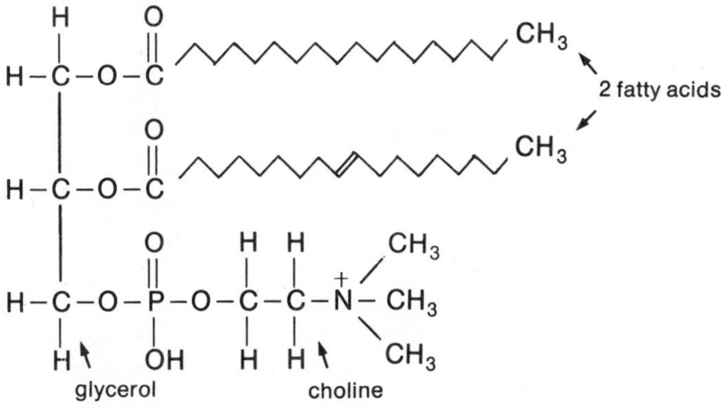

Lecithin.

The sterols: *cholesterol*. A student observing the chemical structure of cholesterol for the first time once remarked, "Would you believe dimethyl dihydroxy chicken wire?" He was not far wrong; chemists do remarkable "terminologizing." According to them, cholesterol is a member of the cyclopentanoperhydrophenanthrene family, whose particular designation is 3-hydroxy-5, 6-cholestene! Never mind. It is not necessary to memorize a structure as complex as this one. But once having viewed it, you *can* say "I have seen the structure of cholesterol."

sterol: a compound composed of C, H, and O atoms arranged in rings like those of cholesterol, with any of a variety of side chains attached.

Cholesterol.

cholesterol

This is not at all an unusual type of molecule. With minor differences there are dozens of similar ones in the body; all are interesting and important. Among them are the bile acids, the sex hormones (such as testosterone), the adrenocortical hormones (such as cortisone), and vitamin D.

Like lecithins, cholesterol is needed metabolically but is not an essential nutrient. Your liver is manufacturing it now, as you read, at the rate of perhaps 50,000,000,000,000,000 molecules per second. It is vital to life. Yet cholesterol in foods has come to be viewed as something to be avoided, even if we have to give up eggs and beef to do it. The following Highlight puts cholesterol in perspective as a possible cause of heart disease.

Summing Up

Lipids in the body serve as a major energy reserve and also provide nourishment and structural material for many tissues; in specific locations body fat protects organs from heat, cold, and mechanical shock. The oxidation of one pound of human adipose tissue supplies 3,500 kcalories usable to meet energy needs.

In the Exchange System, the foods which contribute fat to the diet are found mainly on the milk list, the meat list, and the fat list. The size of a milk exchange is one cup; an exchange of 2 percent milk contains 5 grams, and an exchange of whole milk contains 10 grams of fat. For meat, the size of an exchange is one ounce or the equivalent; an exchange of lean meat contains 3 grams, of medium-fat meat 5½ grams, and of high-fat meat 8 grams of fat. An exchange (2 tablespoons) of peanut butter contains 13 grams of fat. For fat itself, the exchange size is one teaspoon or the equivalent, and one fat exchange contains 5 grams of fat. When fat is added to vegetables, the amount is usually 5 grams per half-cup serving. Some baked goods also contain fat. (See Bread List, page 35.)

In the diet, 95 percent of the lipids are triglycerides: compounds composed of glycerol with three fatty acids attached. The fatty acids may be saturated, in which case the triglycerides are known as saturated fats; or mono- or polyunsaturated, in which case the triglycerides are known as unsaturated or polyunsaturated fats. Known familiarly as the fats and oils, these compounds are not soluble in water, but serve as a solvent themselves for the fat-soluble vitamins and for the aromatic compounds that give foods their flavor and aroma. During digestion, the triglycerides must be emulsified (dispersed in water) by bile, before they can be hydrolyzed by enzymes to di- and then to monoglycerides and fatty acids, which are absorbed into the body fluids.

Essential fatty acid deficiency manifests itself in human infants as a dermatitis and associated liver abnormality. The symptoms can be cleared up by administering linoleic acid, which has therefore come to be called "the" essential fatty acid.

The other 5 percent of dietary lipids are the phospholipids and sterols, cholesterol being a member of the latter group.

The single most important approach to alleviating almost any disease is the reduction of stress ... Better still is the elimination of constant worry about your heart, plus the restoration of relaxation and pleasure to your mealtimes. Enjoy food rather than fear it.
—EDWARD R. AND CATHEY PINCKNEY

Highlight Two
Cholesterol and Atherosclerosis

atherosclerosis (ath-er-oh-scler-OH-sis): a type of arteriosclerosis characterized by patchy, nodular thickenings of the intima of the arteries especially at branch points.
arteriosclerosis (ar-TEER-ee-oh-scler-OH-sis): hardening of the arteries (a broader term which includes atherosclerosis).
intima (IN-tuh-muh): the inner layer of the arterial wall.

plaques

More than half the deaths in the United States are due to heart disease.[1] The underlying condition which contributes to a large proportion of these deaths is *atherosclerosis*. This disease, which takes its heaviest toll among males in the most productive period of their lives, actually begins in adolescence or even earlier, as revealed in the autopsies performed on young American soldiers killed in the Vietnam War.[2]

Atherosclerosis is the term which denotes the soft, lipid accumulation, called *plaques*, on the inner wall of the arteries. If these plaques are allowed to continue enlarging, the artery walls will lose their elasticity and the passages will become narrower.

The arterial walls, to remain healthy, must be elastic so that when the heart pumps blood outward, the arteries can expand to accommodate the increased volume; and when the heart is resting, they can contract again. If the arteries lost their elasticity, they wouldn't be able to hold the large volume of blood being pumped out by the

[1] *Vital Statistics of the United States*. 1971 Vol. II part B. United States Department of Health, Education and Welfare. Public Health Service.
[2] Corey, J. E.: Dietary factors and atherosclerosis prevention should begin early. The Journal of School Health XLIV: 511-513, 1974.

heart, thus building up the blood pressure. The increased pressure could damage the walls.

If the plaques continue to accumulate on the inner walls, they protrude into the lumen of the artery, narrowing the size of the bore. This, too, causes a rise in the blood pressure, as the heart strives to push the blood through the narrowed passages.

In addition to being elastic, the inner walls of the arteries must be glass-smooth so that the blood can move over the surface with as little friction as possible. Blood clotting is an intricate series of events triggered by blood platelets moving against a rough surface, such as the edge of a cut. As long as the inner wall remains smooth, clotting will not occur inside the vessel, but if the plaques should encroach upon the lumen of the artery, their roughness could cause clotting reactions to begin. A clot thus formed might travel along the system until it reached an artery too small to allow its passage. With the clot lodged in the artery, the tissues fed by this particular vessel would be robbed of oxygen and nutrients and would die. Should such a clot lodge in an artery of the heart, a kind of heart attack will occur; if the clot should lodge in an artery in the brain, a stroke will follow.

lumen (LOO-men): interior space.

platelet (PLATE-let): cell fragment in the blood.

The kind of heart attack described here is a **coronary thrombosis.**

> coronary = crowning
> (the heart)
> thrombo = clot

A stroke is a **cerebral thrombosis.**

> cerebrum = part of the brain.

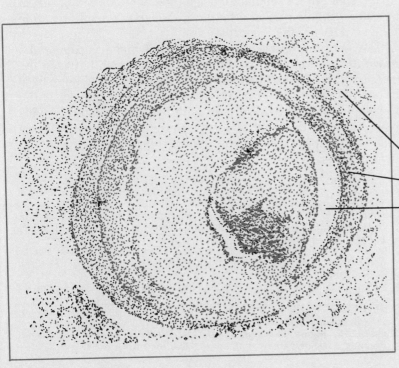

Outer mantel of blood vessel wall

Middle layer of blood vessel wall

Inner layer (intima), invaded by lipid accumulation: a plaque

The diameter of this coronary artery has been reduced to half its normal dimensions by the formation of an atherosclerotic plaque. This same section is shown 14 times actual size. Courtesy of Yearbook Medical Publishers.

serum: the watery portion of the blood that remains after the cells and clot-forming materials have been removed. (Unclotted blood with the cells removed is **plasma**.)

The breakdown of the energy nutrients to 2-carbon fragments and the use of these fragments to meet the body's energy needs is described in Highlight 7.

mg = milligrams/ml = milliliters: see Appendix D.

etiology: see page 45.

In the early research on atherosclerosis it was determined by chemical analyses that the composition of plaques was largely lipid, particularly cholesterol. The conclusion was drawn that *dietary cholesterol* was the villain. Patients who had high serum cholesterol levels or who had suffered a heart attack were advised to limit severely their intake of foods containing cholesterol. However, further research revealed that dietary cholesterol was not the only source of serum cholesterol; the body synthesizes as much as 2,000 mg per day from any 2-carbon fragment.

Food sources of 2-carbon fragments are those containing nutrients which during their metabolism become the 2-carbon compound, acetate. Thus glucose and amino acids, as well as fatty acids, contribute to the synthesis of cholesterol. For example, saturated fats are excellent sources of 2-carbon fragments and it has now been shown that diets high in saturated fats will raise the serum cholesterol as much as 40 to 50 mg per 100 ml serum, whereas dietary cholesterol will increase the serum cholesterol by only a few mg per 100 ml.[3]

As research continued, it was found that elevated serum triglycerides were involved, in addition to high serum cholesterol,[4] and that sodium may be implicated.[5] Evidence was accumulated, too, suggesting that diets high in refined sugar[6] and/or low in fiber[7] might be causative. There was much conflicting evidence in the literature over the roles played by the various nutrients, but there seemed to be general agreement that serum cholesterol levels played a major, although not a solitary, role in the etiology of atherosclerosis.

Dawber and his associates in a study which has come to be known as the Framingham Study[8] found that men between the ages of 30 and 59 who had serum cholesterol levels below 200 mg per 100 ml of serum had half as many heart attacks as the total population. For those men with serum cholesterol levels above 260 mg per 100 ml of serum, there were almost twice as many heart attacks as in the general population. Evidently, lower is better.

[3]Krause, M. V. and Hunscher, M. A.: *Food, Nutrition and Diet Therapy*. W. B. Saunders Company, Philadelphia, 1972, p. 60.

[4]Friedman, G. J.: Nutrition in relation to atherosclerosis. In *Modern Nutrition in Health and Disease*. Wohl, M. G. and Goodhart, R. S., editors. Lea and Febiger, Philadelphia, 1968.

[5]Leiter, L.: Nutrition in cardiovascular disease. In *Modern Nutrition in Health and Disease*. Wohl, M. G. and Goodhart, R. S., editors. Lea and Febiger, Philadelphia, 1968.

[6]Ahrens, R. A.: Sucrose, hypertension, and heart disease: an historical perspective. *American Journal of Clinical Nutrition* 27: 403-422, 1974.

[7]Kritchevsky, D. and Story, J. A.: Binding of biosalts in vitro by nonnutritive fiber. *Journal of Nutrition* 104:458-462, 1974.

[8]Dawber, T. R., Moore, F. E. and Mann, G. V.: Coronary heart disease in the Framingham study. *American Journal of Public Health* 4:23, 1957.

Blood lipids are not the only factors related to heart disease. As a result of studies of populations, such as the Framingham Study, it has been shown that *risk factors* include: high blood pressure, heavy cigarette smoking, obesity, and physical inactivity, in addition to an elevation in plasma lipids. Nevertheless, all evidence points to the fact that high serum cholesterol levels (above 220 mg per 100 ml serum) do correlate with the risk of coronary heart disease independently of the presence of the other risk factors.[8] It remains to be shown that lowering serum cholesterol levels actually reduces the incidence of heart attacks; one study[9] suggests that it does.

In the continuing effort to discover if there were dietary measures that would lower the serum cholesterol, it came to light that polyunsaturated fatty acids had a lowering effect. Keys[10] advanced the idea that these fatty acids *decrease* serum cholesterol levels half as much per gram as saturated fatty acids *raise* these levels.

In a joint policy statement of the American Medical Association (AMA) and the Foods and Nutrition Board of the NAS-NRC, it was stated that lowering of the serum cholesterol "can be achieved most practically by partial replacement of the dietary source of saturated fat with sources of unsaturated fat, especially those rich in polyunsaturated fatty acids, and by a reduction in the consumption of foods rich in cholesterol."[11]

risk factors: the factors in a person's life which increase his chances of having a heart attack, such as smoking, hypertension, heredity, diabetes, maleness, advancing age, etc.

Different dietary measures may be needed to correct different abnormal blood lipid profiles. See suggested readings.

NAS-NRC: National Academy of Sciences-National Research Council.

Don't be misled into accepting the excerpt above (from the NAS-NRC policy statement concerning dietary measures for lowering serum cholesterol) as a final statement of ultimate truth. When controversy and conflicting evidence appear in the literature on a theory, it is customary for an organization such as the AMA or the ADA to issue a policy statement. This statement results from a committee's sifting through evidence and reaching an agreement on the fairest statement that can be made *at present*. Before this text can be printed and into your hands, new evidence may have outdated that policy statement.

ADA: American Dietetic Association.

Meanwhile, the controversy continues and there is mounting evidence that simple carbohydrates—refined sugars—have

[9]Miettinen, M., Karvonen, M. J., Turpeinen, O., Elosuo, R. and Paavilainen, E.: Effect of cholesterol lowering diet on mortality from coronary heart disease and other causes. *Lancet* ii:836-837, 1972.

[10]Keys, A., Anderson, J. and Grande, F.: Serum cholesterol response to dietary fat. *Lancet* i:787, 1957.

[11]Council on Foods and Nutrition: Diet and coronary heart disease. *Journal of the American Medical Association* 222 (13), 1972. Reprint.

a cholesterol and triglyceride-raising effect.[6] This theory is not accepted by the proponents of the saturated fat theory and it is being heatedly discussed in the literature.[12] [13] [14] If nutritionists can't agree, how is the layman to decide what or whom to believe?

reputable journal: a periodical which enjoys the reputation of being accurate and reliable. See Digression, Highlight 8.

In order to assess opposing views expressed by well-known scientists in reputable journals, the layman needs to understand how and why such articles appear. In addition, when these articles are reviewed in the popular press, the layman should understand how the article was chosen for publication and how much faith he can put in its conclusions.

A report of a study in a scientific journal is written by the people responsible for the research. They will receive the criticism of the work done; thus their reputations as scientists stand or fall on the accuracy of the reporting. Articles submitted for publication to a professional journal are scrutinized by a committee of the authors' peers (scientists in the same or allied fields). Acceptance for publication signifies that the committee judges it a valid piece of research. The written report includes all information necessary for other scientists to replicate the work or further test its validity. Thus, on a continuing basis, the research is judged by the authors' peers. Both these judgments, before and after publication, act as restraints on the publication of inaccurate reports or of poorly designed research.

A report in a scientific journal is intended for reading by other scientists who would recognize that the authors are recording the results of one piece of research and not attempting to report viewpoints other than their own.

The general public, however, is also interested in scientific research and would like to know about new discoveries, such as possible cures for cancer. Because of this interest, science writers of another breed have appeared. Seeking a newsworthy piece, they search the professional journals for unusual or controversial reports coming out of the nation's laboratories. When they find one that is exciting, they translate it into layman's language and enlarge it into a salable article. (The reports in the journals are usually written in a rather dull,

[12]Grande, F.: Sugar and cardiovascular disease. In *World Review of Nutrition and Dietetics.* Bourne, G. H., editor. S. Karger AG, Basel, 1975.

[13]Reiser, R.: Saturated fat in the diet and serum cholesterol concentration: a critical examination of the literature. *American Journal of Clinical Nutrition* 26:524-555, 1973.

[14]Keys, A., Grande, F. and Anderson, J.: Bias and misrepresentation revisited: perspective on saturated fat. *American Journal of Clinical Nutrition* 27: 188-212, 1974.

scholarly style). These science writers may not note that there are opposing results coming from other, equally well-known laboratories; in addition, they may be interested in promoting a particular viewpoint because of their own biases, because it is newsworthy, or because they have an alliance with an organization which stands to profit by the promotion of a viewpoint. For instance, a writer may be employed by a tobacco grower's association which would be interested in widespread publication of any research that suggests cigarette smoking does not cause cancer.

By no means are all science-article writers motivated by greed above all else. There are many who render a valuable service to the public by their honest reports. Nor are all scientists above the profit motive. Laymen, then, should learn to discriminate among the myriad reports available to them.

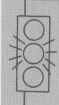

CAUTION WHEN YOU READ!
To weigh the reliability of nutrition information, ask yourself,
 who wrote it?
 who published it?
 why was it published?

The informed layman learns to judge scientific reporting on the basis of:

(1) The media in which it is published. (Was the article judged by other scientists before it was published? Does the magazine have a vested interest in the viewpoint expressed in the article?)

(2) The author of the written article. (Was the author the person responsible for the research? What are the qualifications of the author of the article?)

(3) The purpose for which the article is written. (Is the author promoting a viewpoint because he will profit from the acceptance of that view? Is he a writer who will make a profit from the sale of the article to a publication? Is he a scientist who is putting the results of his research into print so that it may be judged by other scientists in his field?)

When theories arising out of epidemiologic studies into the causes of heart disease had been examined in the laboratories and argued on the pages of the scientific journals,[13] [14] the crucial question remained: What can be done to prevent heart disease? Obviously, any project undertaken to answer that question must involve large numbers of subjects and continue for many years.

One such project attempted to discover the specific effect of diet modification on the probability of developing coronary heart disease.[4]

The Anti-Coronary Club Study Project was begun in 1957 by the late Dr. Norman Jolliffe of the Bureau of Nutrition, New York City Department of Health. The diet for the experimental group was designed to lower total calories, saturated fat, cholesterol, and refined sugar but to remain as nearly as possible a typical American eating plan. It was found that the "Prudent Diet" resulted in a significant decrease in three of the high risk factors: obesity, cholesterol levels, and blood pressure. It also resulted in a significant decrease in the incidence of coronary heart disease in the experimental group as compared with the control group.[4]

The purpose of this Highlight was to present the role of one dietary component, cholesterol, in the development of atherosclerosis and, at the same time, to give a sense of the divergence of opinions among scientists; as well as to suggest ways the layman can sift the truth out of the voluminous writings on the subject. One question remains to be dealt with here: in the light of present knowledge, what measures should be taken to prevent atherosclerosis and thus heart disease?

The American Heart Foundation has issued a Position Statement on Diet and Coronary Heart Disease which offers a comprehensive review of the various programs for prevention of heart disease and offers the following recommendations.[15] Beginning in childhood:

(1) Caloric content of the diet should be controlled and physical activity should be increased so that obesity will be prevented.
(2) The amount and type of fat eaten should be controlled to avoid elevated serum cholesterol and serum triglycerides.
(3) Carbohydrates eaten should be predominantly of the complex type.
(4) Salt content should be controlled to avoid predisposition to high blood pressure.

Until all the results are in, it would seem prudent to follow the above diet modifications, recognizing also the importance of smoking, high blood pressure, physical inactivity, and stress to the development of coronary heart disease.

To Explore Further—

Rosenthal's recipes are based on the Prudent Diet, which is described in Bennett's book and in Livingston's article:

[15]Board of Scientific Consultants of the American Heart Foundation: Position statement on diet and coronary heart disease. *Preventive Medicine* 1: 255-286, 1972.

Bennett, I.: *The Prudent Diet.* David White Publishers, New York, 1973.

Livingston, C. E.: The prudent diet: what? why? how? *Preventive Medicine* 2:321-328, 1973.

Rosenthal, S.: *Live High on Low Fat.* Lippincott, Philadelphia, 1962.

These excellent cookbooks are helpful to calorie watchers and to persons needing low-saturated fat recipes:

Eshelman, R. and Winston, M.: *The American Heart Association Cookbook.* David McKay Company, Inc., New York, 1973.

Keys, A. and Keys, M.: *How to Eat Well and Stay Well the Mediterranean Way.* Doubleday and Co., Inc., Garden City, New York, 1974.

Schoenberg, H.: *Good Housekeeping Cookbook for Calorie Watchers.* Good Housekeeping, New York, 1971.

A sampling of some of the very fine work being done to determine ways of reducing mortality from heart disease:

Bodber, G. E.: Diet and coronary heart disease. *Nutrition Today,* January/February, 1975.

Dawber, T. R.: Risk factors in young adults. *Journal of the American College Health Association* 22:85-95, 1973.

Glueck, C. J., Fallat, R. W. and Tsang, R.: Hypercholesterolemia and hypertriglyceridemia in children. *American Journal of Diseases of Children* 128:569-577, 1974. (A review article)

Podell, R. N.: Current status of the cholesterol hypothesis. *American Family Physician* 9(1):145-148, 1974.

Schaefer, O.: Relative roles of diet and physical activity on blood lipids and obesity. *American Heart Journal* 88(5):673-674, 1974.

Trowell, H.: Dietary fibre, ischaemic heart disease and diabetes mellitus. *Proceedings of the Nutrition Society* 32:151-157, 1973.

Chapters on cardiovascular disease and atherosclerosis give abundant information on distinguishing among abnormal blood lipid profiles and appropriate dietary treatments:

Goodhart, R. S. and Shils, M. E., editors: *Modern Nutrition in Health and Disease.* Lea and Febiger, Philadelphia, 1973.

Reprints: *Council Statement on Diet and Heart Disease,* and *The Healthy Way to Weigh Less* can be ordered from:
The Department of Foods and Nutrition
American Medical Association
535 North Dearborn
Chicago, Illinois 60610

Suggested Activities

(1) Study your own diet.

Review the record you made in Activity 1 of Chapter 1. If you haven't already done so, look up each food in Appendix H and record the amount of fat it contained. How many grams of fat do you consume per day, on the average? How many kilocalories a day do you consume from fat?

(2) Take a closer look at your fat consumption.

Now select all of the food items you ate that contained more than 3 grams of fat. Sort these into two groups: animal foods and plant foods. How many of your fat grams come from each group?

Look up these foods in Appendix H and record the number of grams of linoleic acid and of saturated fat they contain. Calculate the P:S ratio of your diet. (Appendix D offers help with this calculation.)

It is recommended that 2 percent of your total calories come from linoleic acid. Is your diet in accord with this recommendation?

(Note: The last Highlight in the book invites you to survey your entire diet for adequacy, balance, and economy. You may wish to postpone these activities until you have read that Highlight, or you may wish to read it now for a sense of perspective.)

(3) Discover the effect of the hamburger-stand habit of Americans.

Plan a typical 3000 calorie diet for an adolescent boy using his (supposedly) favorite foods: hamburgers, French fries, etc. What is the P:S ratio of his diet?

Make substitutions in the above diet which you think would raise the P:S ratio. Recalculate the ratio to see if it actually increased with your substitutions.

How many milligrams of cholesterol does this boy's diet contain before and after the substitutions you made (Appendix G)? Can you conclude that cholesterol and saturated fat are usually found in the same foods?

(4) Practice preventive medicine.

Select five items from the list below and suggest ways in which they could be selected and/or prepared that would be detrimental to a heart patient and ways of preparation that would be helpful in lowering the patient's cholesterol. (Hint: ask a friend who is a member of Weight-Watchers, Inc., to lend you some recipes.)

hamburger	creamed carrots
spaghetti	steak

turnip greens
mashed potatoes
eggs
buttered toast
green beans

chicken
fried chicken served in a
    restaurant
dry cereal with milk

(5) Be alert for flag signs.

Vitamin A deficiency sometimes causes a skin condition that resembles acne. Criticize this statement: "Vitamin A should be used in the treatment of acne."

(6) Debate the peanut butter issue.

Mashed whole peanuts can be used as peanut butter without further processing. However, the highly polyunsaturated peanut oil rises to the top of the mash when the peanut butter is left standing. For easy spreading, the oil has to be remixed with the mash at every use. Hydrogenation of the oil renders it more solid so that the product does not separate. Most consumers prefer the more spreadable product. Argue the case from both sides: why should food processors hydrogenate the oils in their peanut butter? Why should they not? What are the consequences of each choice?

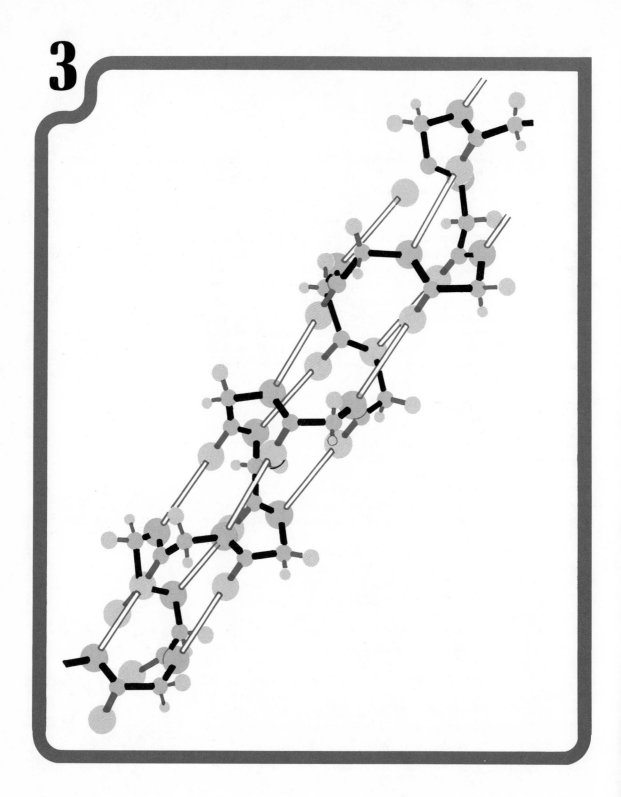

Proteins (A) Structure and Need

Everybody knows that protein is important. It is advertised on every cereal box; it is said to "build strong bodies" and provide "super go power." In fact, as you will see, protein has been so overemphasized that most Americans eat more than enough, sometimes at the expense of other nutrients that are equally important. An understanding of the quantity and quality of protein will help put it in its proper place—as only one of the many essential nutrients needed in correct proportions to achieve a balanced diet.

To put your protein intake in perspective, see Activity 2 at the end of this chapter.

The preceding two chapters on carbohydrates and lipids both began with sections describing the roles of these nutrients in the body, then moved on to a consideration of their structure. This chapter, on the contrary, describes the structure of protein first, because the structure makes clear how protein is able to play so many more roles than carbohydrate and lipid. All three nutrients are important, and all three share the common function of providing energy, but protein is far more versatile.

Energy value of protein: 1 gram provides 4 kilocalories.

Protein structure is also far more interesting than that of carbohydrate or lipid. The regularity and simplicity of protein structure have yielded only recently to human investigation. Those who have worked on elucidating the structure of proteins have been rewarded with a rare insight into the elegance of nature's designs.

83

Protein as the Chemist Sees It

protein: a compound composed of C, H, O, and N, arranged into amino acids linked in a chain. Proteins also contain some S (sulfur).

Atomic composition. A protein is a chemical compound composed of the same atoms as carbohydrate and lipid—that is to say carbon, hydrogen, and oxygen—but in addition, protein contains nitrogen atoms. These C, H, O, and N atoms are arranged into amino acids, which are linked into chains to form proteins. It is easy to construct a protein once we know what an amino acid looks like, and the unit structure of an amino acid is far simpler than that of either carbohydrates (the monosaccharides) or lipids (glycerol and fatty acids).

Amino acid structure. An amino acid has a backbone of one nitrogen and two carbon atoms linked together. You will recall that carbons must form four bonds with other atoms, oxygens two, and hydrogens one. Nitrogens must form three bonds with other atoms: $>$N—. The structure which all amino acids have in common fulfills these requirements as shown below:

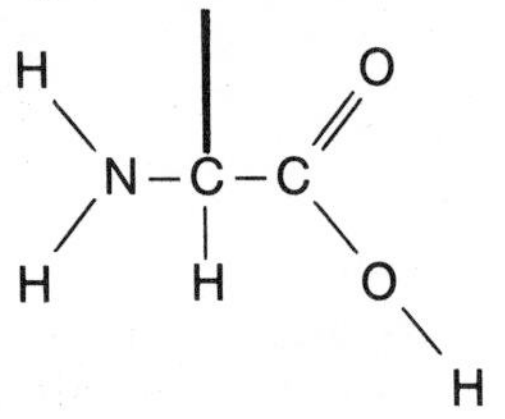

amino (uh-MEEN-oh) **acid** (incomplete structure)

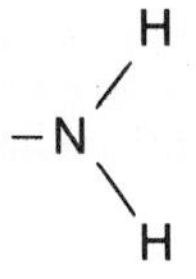

Amino group

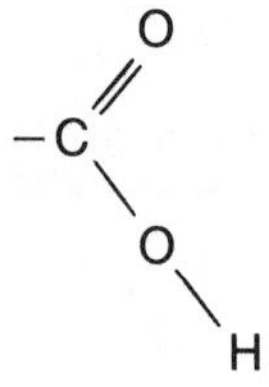

Acid group

At one end is an amino group (—NH₂), at the other is an acid group (—COOH). Both are attached to a central carbon which also carries a hydrogen (—H). As you can see, there is one position left unfilled: the central carbon atom must have another atom or group of atoms attached to it to make a complete structure.

This central carbon atom and the attached structures are what make proteins so different from either carbohydrates or lipids. A polysaccharide (starch, for example) is composed of glucose units one after the other. It may be a hundred or two hundred units long, but every unit in the chain is a glucose molecule just like all the others. In a protein, on the other hand, 22 different possible amino acids are commonly found. Each differs from the others in the nature of the side group that it carries on the central carbon. The simplest amino acid, glycine, has a hydrogen atom in that position:

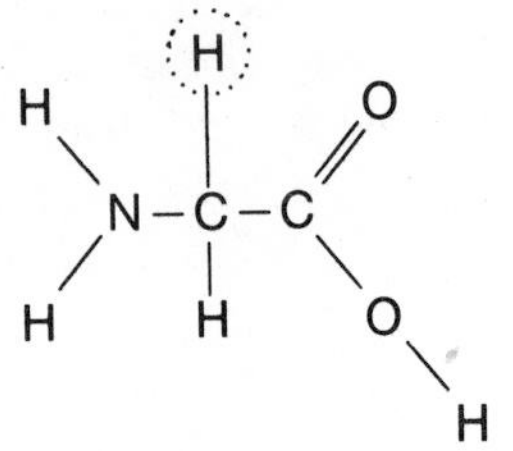

Glycine

Examples of Amino Acids

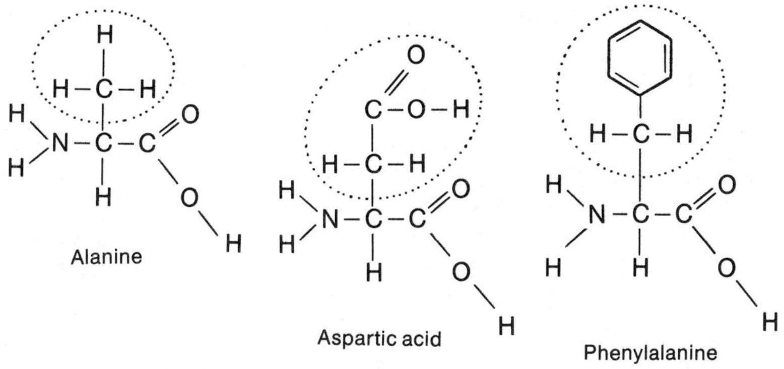

Alanine

Aspartic acid

Phenylalanine

A slightly more complex amino acid, alanine, has an additional carbon, which carries three H's, attached to the central carbon. Other amino acids have still more complex side groups. For example, one amino acid may have an acid group attached to the central carbon, another may have an amino group. Still others may have aromatic structures similar to the "rings" of cholesterol. Thus while the basic structure of an amino acid is simple, the side groups may be quite elaborate.

Amino acid sequence. The 22 different common amino acids may be linked together in a great variety of ways to form proteins, by means of a condensation reaction similar to that which joins two glucoses to form maltose (page 20). An —OH is removed from the acid end of one, and an —H from the amino group of another amino acid. A bond is formed between the two amino acids, while the H— and —OH join to form a molecule of water. The resulting structure is called a dipeptide:

dipeptide: two amino acids bonded together. The bond between two amino acids is a **peptide bond**.

di = two
peptide = amino acid

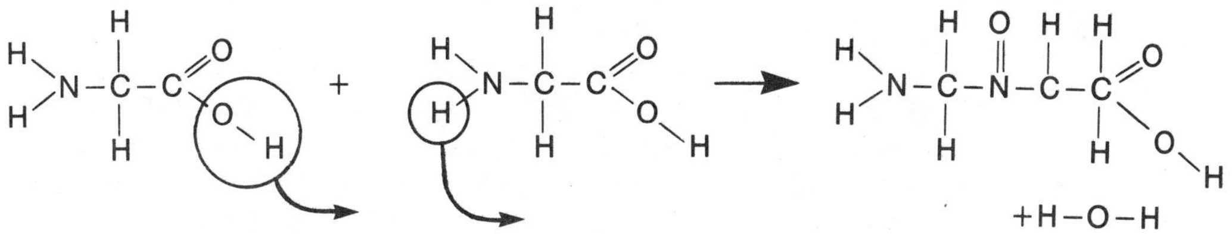

Formation of a dipeptide by condensation of two amino acids.

By an exactly similar reaction, the —OH can be removed from the acid end of the second amino acid, and an —H from the amino group of a third, to form a tripeptide. As additional amino acids are added to the chain, a polypeptide is formed. Most proteins are polypeptides, 100 to 300 amino acids long.

It would be misleading, however, to leave the picture of proteins this way, because in showing the structures on a piece

tripeptide: three amino acids bonded together by peptide bonds.

tri = three

polypeptide: many amino acids bonded together by peptide bonds. "Many" refers to ten or more. An intermediate length of between four and ten amino acids is an **oligopeptide**.

poly = many
oligo = few

The description given here is of the **primary structure of proteins**: the sequence of amino acids.

The folding of the chain gives a protein its **secondary structure**. This structure may be stabilized by covalent bonding (Appendix B) between —SH side groups on certain amino acids, giving protein a further structural complexity known as **tertiary structure**.

Two folded polypeptides may associate closely by hydrogen bonding (Appendix B), giving protein a **quaternary structure**.

The change in shape of a protein brought about by heat, acid, or other conditions is known as **denaturation**.

tryptophan (TRIP-toe-fane) **serine** (SEAR-een): amino acids. A complete list of the amino acids with their structures appears in Appendix C.

of paper we have drawn a straight, flat chain. Actually, polypeptide chains fold and tangle so that they look not like rods but like crazy jungle gyms or tangled balls of yarn. The sequence of amino acids in a protein will determine which specific way the chain will fold.

Folding of the chain. The chain structure can best be visualized by keeping in mind that each side group on the amino acids has special characteristics that attract it to other groups. Some side groups are negatively charged, others are positively charged, and the aromatic rings are attracted to other aromatic rings. As amino acids are added to a polypeptide chain to make a protein and the chain lengthens, those acids which are negatively charged fold back on the chain in order to be positioned as closely as possible to those that are positively charged. Since the molecule is in a watery solution, these charged groups, being hydrophilic (page 67), tend to expose themselves on the outer surface of the completed protein, while the aromatic groups, being hydrophobic (page 67), tend to tuck themselves into the inside. The shape the polypeptide finally assumes is usually globular, giving it the maximum stability possible in water solution. Finally, two or more of these giant molecules may associate together to form a still larger working aggregate. Thus, the completed picture of a protein is of one or more very complex tangled chains of amino acids, bristling on its surface with positive and negative charges.

When a protein molecule is subjected to heat, acid, or other conditions which disturb its stability, it will uncoil or change its shape, thus losing its function to some extent. That is what happens to an egg when it is cooked; alterations of the egg proteins occur during cooking that largely account for the observable changes in the egg white and yolk.

The completed protein. If you could step onto a *carbohydrate* molecule like starch and walk along it, the first stepping stone would be a glucose. Your next stepping stone would be glucose again, and then glucose, and then glucose, and then glucose. On the other hand, if you were to step onto one end of a *polypeptide* chain your first stepping stone might be a glycine. Your second might be an alanine. The third might be a glycine again, and the fourth a tryptophan, then a serine, and so on. In other words, the variety of both the nature and the sequence of the units in a protein is far greater than it is in a carbohydrate molecule.

By another analogy, if you were to try to make a sentence using only the letter G, you could only speak gibberish: G-G-G-G-G-G-G. But with 22 different letters available, you could say "To be or not to be, that is the question"—or on a different plane, "The way to a man's heart is through his stomach." The Greek alphabet contains only 24 letters, and all of Homer can be written

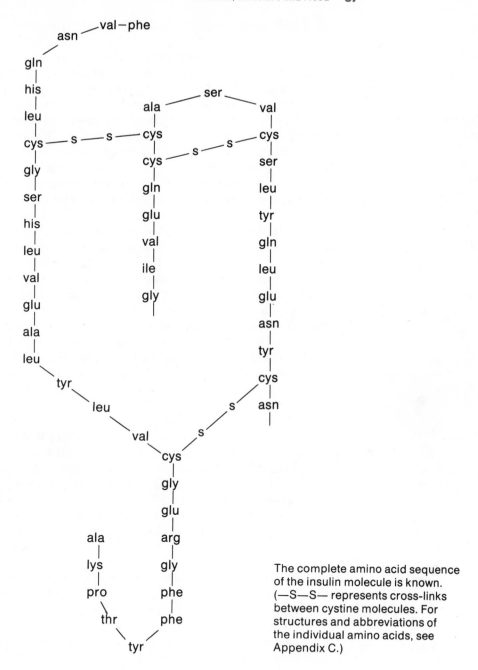

The complete amino acid sequence of the insulin molecule is known. (—S—S— represents cross-links between cystine molecules. For structures and abbreviations of the individual amino acids, see Appendix C.)

with it. The variety of sequences in which the amino acids can be linked together is even greater than that possible for letters in a sentence because proteins do not have to be pronounced. This gives them a tremendous range of possible surface structures, and this in turn enables them to perform very distinct, individual and specialized functions.

A Function of Proteins: Enzymes

In Chapter 1 the enzymes were mentioned for the first time and a promise was made that when protein structure had been explained, we would look at these magnificent molecules more closely. Let us start by looking at the enzyme maltase.

A typical protein, maltase is a tangled ball-shaped polypeptide chain, a hundred or so amino acids long. The little molecule maltose, on the other hand, is a disaccharide perhaps a hundred times smaller. If you were one of the glucoses in this maltose, you would be joined to the other like a Siamese twin, incomplete and unable to stand alone for lack of an H— or an —OH. Suppose you were swallowed by a person: you would travel down his esophagus, and after spending some time in his stomach would presently find yourself floating around in the watery medium of his small intestine. Looking about, you would see many giant enzymes working on, breaking down, and putting together a variety of other compounds like yourself. Sooner or later you would find yourself snapping into position on the surface of a maltase: an enzyme custom-designed to fit your contours. On this surface you would encounter a molecule of water, and as you split away from your glucose twin the water would also split apart, its H— being added to one of you, and its —OH to your twin. Released as a free glucose, you might turn around to see other pairs being attracted into that same position and being hydrolyzed just as you were.

Since enzymes and what they do are so fundamental to all life processes, it may be worthwhile to introduce a somewhat fanciful analogy in order to clarify two important characteristics they all share. Enzymes could be compared to the ministers and judges who respectively make and dissolve human matrimonial bonds. When two individuals come to a minister to be married, the minister performs the ceremony and the couple leaves with a new bond between them. They are joined together. The minister is only momentarily involved in this process, and remains unchanged and available to perform other ceremonies between other pairs of people. One minister can perform thousands of marriage ceremonies. In a divorce court, the judge plays a similar but opposite role. A couple enters the court, the judge performs the dissolution, and the couple leaves as two separate individuals. Like the minister, the judge may decree many divorces before he dies or retires.

The minister represents those enzymes which synthesize larger compounds from smaller ones, that is, the synthetases, which build body structures. The judge represents those enzymes which hydrolyze larger compounds to smaller ones— the proteases, lipases, carbohydrases, disaccharidases and others. Maltase is a disaccharidase.

---

maltase: the enzyme which hydrolyzes maltose to 2 glucose units.

maltose: the disaccharide composed of 2 glucose units (see page 20).

-ase = enzyme. The prefix usually identifies the compound worked on. Thus malt-ase is "the enzyme which works on maltose."

Apology for the use of fanciful descriptions appears in Note to the Student.

Model of Enzyme Action

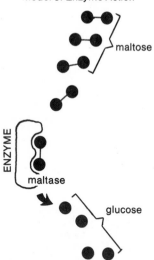

The roles of coenzymes in processes like this are shown in Chapter 9.

synthetase (SIN-the-tase): an enzyme which synthesizes compounds.

protease (PRO-tee-ase): an enzyme which hydrolyzes proteins.

The first point to be learned is that some enzymes put compounds together, while others take them apart. Since you yourself are a very "put-together" kind of organism, superbly organized out of billions of molecules that have been bonded together to make muscle, bone, skin, eyes, and blood cells, you can imagine that in your body those enzymes which put things together are numerous and very active.

The second point to be learned is that the enzymes, which facilitate chemical reactions, are not themselves affected in the process: they are catalysts. The technical definition of an enzyme, which biologists and chemists use, is *a protein catalyst.*

What makes you yourself unique and distinct from any other human being is minute differences between your body proteins (enzymes, antibodies, and others) and those of any other person. These differences are determined by the amino acid sequences of your proteins. It is these sequences that are written into the genetic code of the DNA you inherit from your parents and ancestors. Each of us receives at conception a unique combination of DNA codes for these sequences. A description of the genetic basis of human individuality is beyond our scope, but suffice it to say that the exciting scientific discoveries of the last few decades have led to a profound understanding of molecular biology. The references at the end of this chapter will lead you further along this path, if you like.

Perhaps you have realized by now that the protein story moves in a circle. All enzymes are proteins. All proteins are made of amino acids. Amino acids have to be put together to make proteins. Enzymes put together the amino acids. No other system in the universe works with such self-renewal. A broken toaster cannot be fixed by another toaster. A car cannot make another car. Only living creatures and those parts that they are composed of, the cells, can duplicate themselves and make the parts of which they are made. To follow the circle in nutrition, start with a person eating proteins. The proteins are broken down by proteins (enzymes) into amino acids. The amino acids enter the cells of the body, where proteins (enzymes) put them together in long chains with sequences specified by DNA. The chains fold and what are they? They are enzymes themselves. These enzymes may then be used to break apart other compounds or to put other compounds together. Day by day, billion reactions by billion reactions, these processes repeat themselves and life goes on.

A Closer Look at Enzyme Action

If we look closely at the details of the reaction sequences governed by enzymes, some additional important facts emerge.

lipase (LYE-pase): an enzyme which hydrolyzes lipids.

carbohydrase, disaccharidase, sucrase, lactase, phospholipase: definitions self-evident.

catalyst (CAT-uh-list): a compound which facilitates chemical reactions without itself being destroyed in the process.

enzyme: a protein catalyst.

The following description is an example of the way enzymes work to alter the structure of a compound. It is the only example given in this book of biochemistry at the level at which biochemists actually think about it. The object is to give you an insight into the kinds of processes that account for human nutritional needs.

Let us take a biochemical pathway at a point partway along its length and see how each enzyme alters the structure of a compound until one thing has been converted into another, quite different, thing. Beginning with glucose, a 6-carbon compound, enzymes add a phosphate group, altering and breaking this structure until a 3-carbon compound results—which looks like this:

$$
\begin{array}{c}
H \\
| \\
H-C-O-PO_3H \\
| \\
H-C-OH \\
| \\
COOH
\end{array}
$$

An intermediate in glucose metabolism.

This compound floats around until it encounters an enzyme which has the specialized function of removing hydrogen atoms (from these compounds). The encounter results in the altered compound, like this:

$$
\begin{array}{c}
H \\
| \\
H-C-O-PO_3H \\
| \\
C=O \\
| \\
COOH
\end{array}
$$

Removal of hydrogen from this intermediate by a dehydrogenase.

This compound is released from the enzyme, and later encounters another enzyme, which removes oxygens and substitutes amino groups. What results is the following:

$$
\begin{array}{c}
H \\
| \\
H-C-O-PO_3H \\
| \\
H-C-NH_2 \\
| \\
COOH
\end{array}
$$

Removal of oxygen and substitution of NH_2 by a transaminase.

The next enzyme removes the phosphate group from the top carbon:

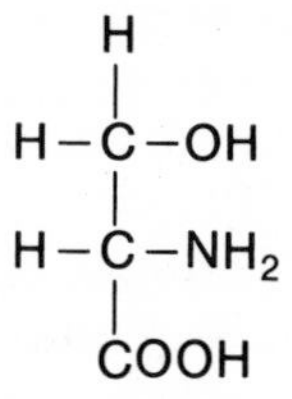

$$
\begin{array}{c}
H \\
| \\
H-C-OH \\
| \\
H-C-NH_2 \\
| \\
COOH
\end{array}
$$

Removal of phosphate by a phosphatase.

If you look closely at this picture, you may recognize its characteristics and not be surprised by the statements that follow. But first let us take the process one more step. Another enzyme, whose function is to remove CH_2OH groups from these molecules, forms the compound shown below:

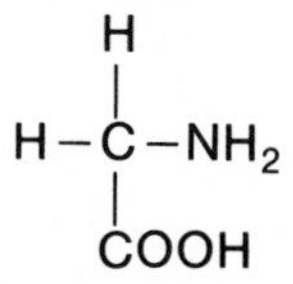

$$
\begin{array}{c}
H \\
| \\
H-C-NH_2 \\
| \\
COOH
\end{array}
$$

Look at this product closely. It is one that you may recognize, for you have seen it before, but from a different angle. It has an amino group at one end, an acid group at the other, and a central carbon carrying two H's. It is the amino acid, glycine (page 84).

Well, how about that! We started with a molecule of glucose, a derivative of dietary carbohydrate, and by making one minute change after another we transformed it into an amino acid, a member of the protein family.

The lesson to be learned from this sequence of events is that the body can make, from glucose and nitrogen-containing compounds, many of the amino acids needed to build body proteins. Glycine is one of those. The compound which precedes it on the pathway outlined above is the amino acid serine (which has a CH_2OH on its central carbon). This too is an amino acid the body can make.

The Essential Amino Acids

It should now be clear that the role of protein in the *diet* is not to provide body proteins directly but to supply the amino acids from which the body can make its own proteins. Since the body can make glycine and serine for itself, the proteins in the diet need not contain these two amino acids in order to supply

essential amino acid: an amino acid that the body cannot synthesize in amounts sufficient to meet physiological need. Eight amino acids known to be essential for human adults are:

methionine (meh-THIGH-o-neen)
threonine (THREE-o-neen)
tryptophan (TRIP-toe-fane)
isoleucine (eye-so-LOO-seen)
leucine (LOO-seen)
lysine (LYE-seen)
valine (VAY-leen)
phenylalanine (fee-nul-AL-uh-neen)

Children and possibly adults also require:

histidine (HISS-tuh-deen)

Infants also require:

arginine (ARJ-uh-neen).

complete protein: a protein containing all of the amino acids essential for humans.

amino acid balance: the proportion in which each amino acid occurs in a protein, relative to the others.

EFT TURN ON Y

limiting amino acid: the amino acid found in the shortest supply relative to the amounts needed for protein synthesis in the body.

Measures of protein quality (PER, BV, NPU) are explained in Appendix E.

the body with the necessary amounts. But there are some amino acids that the body cannot make (because it does not possess the genetic code for making the enzymes necessary to synthesize these amino acids). These amino acids are referred to as *essential amino acids*; it is essential that they be included in the diet.

In Chapter 2, one *fatty* acid was singled out as a dietary essential for the same reason: because it cannot be synthesized in the body. All compounds in your body are needed for your health, but those that you cannot make for yourself are needed in your *diet*, and these are called *essential nutrients*. With the addition of the eight essential amino acids, your list of these nutrients has now expanded to nine.

To make body protein, a cell must have all 22 amino acids available simultaneously. A first important characteristic of dietary protein is therefore that it should supply at least the eight essential amino acids, plus enough of the nonessential ones to provide a source of nitrogen for the synthesis of the others.

Protein Quality

A complete protein is defined as a protein which contains all of the eight (or nine) essential amino acids; it may or may not contain all of the others. Complete proteins are far more commonly found in animal sources (meat, milk, cheese, and eggs) than in vegetable sources.

A second characteristic of dietary proteins that affects their quality as human amino acid sources is the ratio of the amino acids to each other, or the amino acid balance. Ideally, dietary protein will supply each amino acid in the amount needed for protein synthesis in the body. If one amino acid is supplied in an amount smaller than that needed, it will limit the total amount of protein that can be synthesized from the others. By analogy, suppose that a signmaker plans to make 100 identical signs, each saying LEFT TURN ONLY. He needs 200 L's, 200 N's, 200 T's, and 100 of each of the other letters. If he has only 20 L's, he can only make 10 signs, even if all the other letters are available in unlimited quantities. The L's *limit* the number of signs that can be made.

The quality of dietary protein depends first on whether or not the protein supplies all the essential amino acids, and second on the extent to which it supplies them in the relative proportions needed. A protein of high quality is one in which the amino acid proportions most nearly approximate those needed by human beings. The most perfect protein by this standard is egg protein. Egg has been designated the *reference protein*, against which other proteins are measured as good sources of amino acids in human nutrition. Other high quality proteins include those of milk, cheese, meat, poultry, and fish.

Proteins from plants are of lower quality. Some are inadequate to meet human needs by themselves because they are low in one or more of the essential amino acids. Only when they are supplemented with the limiting amino acids do they approach the quality of animal protein. For example, soy protein, which is used for making the TVP products sometimes substituted for meat, must be supplemented with methionine.

Since the highest quality proteins are found in animal meats and animal products and those from vegetables are generally of lower quality, those who follow vegetarian diets must be somewhat better informed about nutrition than the average person, in order to meet their nutritional needs. Milk, cheese, and eggs, as mentioned above, are excellent sources of high quality protein, so lacto-ovo-vegetarians are unlikely to suffer any amino acid deficiencies. Strict vegetarians, on the other hand, must be aware of the lacks in their plant protein sources in order to balance their diets. For example, wheat is low in lysine, while corn is low in tryptophan. Combining the two to supply the protein at a meal, the strict vegetarian can obtain the needed lysine from the corn, and the tryptophan from the wheat. Similarly, peanut butter and whole wheat bread, or rice and beans make complete protein combinations.

Geneticists have developed new varieties of plants that contain proteins with a better amino acid balance, such as high-lysine wheat and opaque-2 corn, in the effort to help solve the world's malnutrition problem. The complex story of this effort to bring about a "green revolution" is a story of technological triumphs and frustrating obstacles. References at the end of Highlight 4 describe its history.

How Much Protein?

Nitrogen balance studies. Quality is not the only factor of importance in the selection of protein for your diet. The amount of protein that you need depends upon the amount of lean tissue in your body. Fat tissue requires relatively little protein to maintain itself, but the muscle and blood and other metabolically active tissues must be maintained by a continuous supply of essential amino acids. To determine how much protein a person needs, the laboratory scientist can perform a nitrogen balance study.

Since protein is the only one of the three energy nutrients which contains nitrogen, it is possible to follow its path through the body simply by following the nitrogen. Furthermore, the amount of nitrogen in a mixture of substances can easily be

reference protein: egg protein, used by WHO (World Health Organization) as a standard against which to measure the quality of other proteins.

TVP: textured vegetable protein, a plant product used as a meat substitute.

lacto-ovo-vegetarian: a vegetarian who eats no animal flesh, but does eat animal products such as milk, cheese, and eggs.

lacto = milk
ovo = egg

strict vegetarian: a vegetarian who eats neither animal flesh nor animal products. Such a vegetarian is also called a **vegan**.

nitrogen balance: the amount of nitrogen consumed (N in) as compared with the amount of nitrogen excreted (N out) in a given period of time.

Activity 3 at the end of this chapter helps clarify the concept of nitrogen balance.

nitrogen equilibrium (zero nitrogen balance): the condition in which

N in = N out.

positive nitrogen balance:

N in > N out.

negative nitrogen balance:

N in < N out.

measured. When we measure the amount of nitrogen in a meal we are indirectly also measuring the amount of protein in the meal. When we measure the nitrogen excreted by a person in his feces and urine (and to a lesser extent in his hair, fingernails, and perspiration), we are indirectly measuring the amount of protein that is being lost from the body.

Under normal circumstances healthy adults are in nitrogen equilibrium or *zero nitrogen balance*—that is to say they have at all times the same amount of total protein in their bodies. When nitrogen-in exceeds nitrogen-out, they are said to be in *positive nitrogen balance*; this means that somewhere in their bodies more proteins must be being built than are being broken down and lost. When nitrogen-in is less than nitrogen-out, they are said to be in *negative nitrogen balance*. Let us consider some of the circumstances in which these nonzero balances occur.

Growing children add to their bodies new blood, bone, and muscle cells every day. Since these cells contain protein, children must have in their bodies more protein (and therefore more nitrogen) at the end of each day than they had at the beginning. A growing child is therefore in positive nitrogen balance. Similarly, when a woman is pregnant she is, in essence, growing a new organism; she too must be in positive nitrogen balance (although on the day she gives birth she loses a tremendous amount of the protein she has accumulated at one fell swoop!). When she is lactating, she may be in equilibrium again, but it is a sort of enhanced equilibrium. She is eating more protein than before to make her milk and is excreting it whenever the baby nurses.

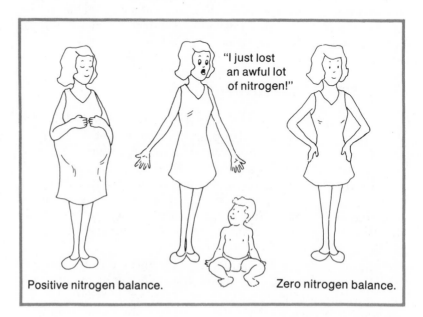

Positive nitrogen balance.   Zero nitrogen balance.

Negative nitrogen balance occurs when muscle or other protein tissue is broken down and lost. Consider the situation in which people have to rest in bed for a period of time. Their muscles are atrophying, and they suffer a net loss of protein. One of several problems faced by nutritionists responsible for the welfare of the astronauts is that of the negative nitrogen balance that occurs when they lie down for days in the space capsule; their muscles then fail to receive enough exercise to maintain themselves.

atrophy (AT-ro-fee): to decrease in size or waste away.

The protein RDA. On the basis of nitrogen-balance studies, the Food and Nutrition Board of the NAS-NRC published its most recent estimate of adult protein needs in 1973 (see Box, pages 96-99). It stated that a healthy adult needs about 0.8 grams of high quality protein per kilogram of ideal body weight per day. They use the ideal weight for this calculation because that weight is proportional to the lean body mass of average persons (if they get fat, their adipose tissue increases in mass; but adipose tissue is composed largely of fat—C, H, and O—and does not require much protein for maintenance). To figure how much protein is recommended for you per day, then, you would need to know your ideal body weight in kilograms. Suppose that you are a person who ideally weighs 50 kilograms. You would then need 0.8 times 50, or 40 grams of protein each day.

RDA = Recommended Dietary Allowances.

NAS = National Academy of Sciences.

NRC = National Research Council.

ideal weight: definition, page 239. Tables of ideal weights: Appendix F.

1 kilogram = 2.2 pounds (Appendix D).

Sample calculation of protein needs: Appendix D, example 2.

Amounts of protein in foods. In the Exchange System, the foods which supply protein in abundance are those in the milk and meat lists. One milk exchange provides 8 grams of protein; one meat exchange provides 7 grams, as shown in the following table:

ADA Food Exchange Lists, pages 33-38.

1 milk exchange = 8 grams protein (serving size = 1 CUP)

Exchange Group	Carbohydrate (g)	Protein (g)	Fat (g)	Energy (kcal)
(1) **Skim milk**	12	8	0	80
(2) Vegetables	5	2	0	25
(3) Fruit	10	0	0	40
(4) Bread	15	2	0	70
(5) **Lean meat**	0	7	3	55
(6) Fat	0	0	5	45

1 meat exchange=7 grams protein (size=1 OUNCE).
1 SERVING of 4 ounces of meat therefore=28 grams protein.

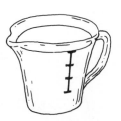

8 grams

7 grams

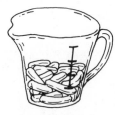

2 grams

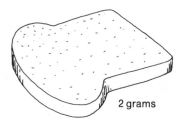

2 grams

As you can see, the foods in the vegetable and bread lists also contribute small but significant amounts of protein to the diet.

The ADA Exchange System provides an easy way to estimate the amount of protein a person consumes in a day. The day's meals described on page 30, for example, supplied:

Breakfast

1 egg (= 1 meat exchange)	7 grams protein
1 slice toast (= 1 bread exchange)	2

Lunch

2 tablespoons peanut butter (= 1 meat)	7
2 slices bread (= 2 bread)	4
1 cup milk (= 1 milk)	8

Dinner

6-oz steak (= 6 meat)	42
½ cup beans (= 1 vegetable)	2
1 cup mashed potato	4

Dessert

shortcake (= 1 bread)		2
	TOTAL	78 grams protein

This totals more than enough protein for the day. You will notice from the discussion of the RDA below that 2/3 RDA is a sufficient intake of protein for most people. If your RDA is 40 grams, then very possibly you can get by with as little as 27 grams. Assuming that you choose to eat one-third of this amount at each meal, you will need only 9 grams of protein at each meal—provided, of course, that the protein is of high quality. From the Food Exchange lists, it is clear that one cup of milk or one ounce of meat along with the incidental additional protein provided by a serving of vegetable, bread, or cereal, will provide this amount. This means that two cups of milk and a very small serving of meat would suffice for a day.

Needless to say, most Americans consume a great deal more high quality protein than that. Further considerations relating to the consumption of protein by Americans and to the special needs and problems of vegetarians are offered in the Highlight at the end of this chapter.

The Recommended Dietary Allowances (RDA)

The Food and Nutrition Board (FNB) of the National Academy of Sciences—National Research Council (NAS-NRC) has established recommendations for the daily consumption of many nutrients by the American population (protein, seven vitamins, and six minerals, as well as calories). Every five years, the FNB meets to reexamine and revise these recommendations on the basis of new evidence regarding people's nutrient needs. The Board then publishes a new set of Recommended Dietary Allowances.

The RDA have many uses. One use is to provide a yardstick against which the nutrient intakes of *segments of our population* can be measured. If, for example, virtually all the children in a community are consuming over 100 percent of the RDA for vitamin C, we can assume we have no need to worry about their diets with respect to this nutrient. If on the other hand half the children are consuming less than 50 percent of the RDA for vitamin C, we have cause for alarm. Another use of the RDA is to set a standard for diet planning. In feeding large groups of people, a planner is well advised to aim at providing 100 percent of the RDA for each nutrient to each person each day.

Before applying these numbers to *individuals*, however, it is important to understand that this application has the limitations inherent in any logic which applies statistical norms to individuals. The RDA have been so widely misinterpreted, misunderstood, and misused, that the American Dietetic Association (ADA) has published a paper entitled "The RDA's Are Not for Amateurs."[1] It cannot be said, for example, that if an individual consumes 100 percent of the adult protein RDA, he/she is certainly getting enough protein. This amount may be too little, or more than enough, for any particular individual.

At the end of each chapter in this book that is devoted to a nutrient with a published RDA we have included a boxed section like this one presenting additional cautions about the interpretation and use of the RDA numbers. The protein RDA illustrates especially well the way in which the FNB arrived at its recommendations, and will be used here to illustrate the reasoning process.

To use the U.S. RDA for interpreting labels, see Highlight 13.

The Protein RDA for Adults: 0.8g/kg body weight

The protein needs of hundreds of healthy people were established by nitrogen-balance and other studies. It was found that people do indeed vary in their protein needs with an approximately normal distribution—some need more, some less, protein to maintain nitrogen

normal distribution: a distribution in which the majority of points cluster at the mean. The graph of such a distribution is symmetrical and bell-shaped.

[1]Leverton, R. M.: The RDA's are not for amateurs. *Journal of the American Dietetic Association* 66:9-11, 1975.

The **standard deviation** describes the spread of the distribution: if small, the curve is narrow, if large the curve is broad. One standard deviation each side of the mean includes 68 percent of the sample; two include 95 percent. To determine the standard deviation of a particular distribution, the statistician adds up the squares of all the deviations from the mean, divides that total by the number of cases minus one, and finds the square root of the resulting number. The square root figure equals the standard deviation.

The Minimum Daily Requirements (MDR), formerly used for purposes similar to the RDA, have been discontinued.

equilibrium. A protein deficit is harmful, however, while a slight excess is not. A deficit cannot be made up from any other source, but an excess can easily be excreted. Suppose the RDA for protein were set at the average amount needed. The danger then would be that everyone would take this number literally and consume exactly (or close to) this amount. Approximately half the population (those who needed that amount or less) would then receive enough protein or a surplus, while half (those who needed more) would suffer a protein deficit.

If the RDA were set higher and all people consumed exactly this higher amount, only a few would suffer a deficit. The choice made by the authorities was to set it two standard deviations above the mean—high enough to cover the needs of 97.5 percent of the population. This choice sets the RDA so high that most people will meet their protein needs if they consume no more than 2/3 of the RDA. Then to allow for variation in protein quality, they set it higher still.

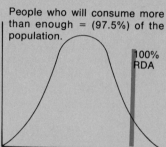

People who will consume more than enough = (97.5%) of the population.

100% RDA

Range of individual needs for protein.

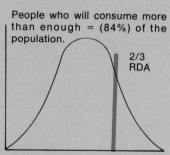

People who will consume more than enough = (84%) of the population.

2/3 RDA

Range of individual needs for protein.

As a result, a healthy person who consumes 2/3 of the RDA for protein can be assumed (with a high probability) to have enough protein.

There are thus two important cautions to apply when the RDA are used as a yardstick to measure individual intakes:

(1). The RDA are not minimum daily requirements. Most people do not have to consume 100 percent of their RDA for all nutrients in order to be adequately nourished.

CAUTION WHEN YOU READ!
A margin of safety is built into the RDA.

(2). The RDA apply only to healthy persons. Illness or malnutrition may greatly increase an individual's needs for certain nutrients.

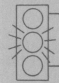

CAUTION WHEN YOU READ!
The RDA apply to healthy persons only.

Additional cautions regarding interpretation of the RDA are offered in Chapters 8, 9, 10, 11, 12, and 13.

Summing Up

Proteins are composed of carbon, hydrogen, oxygen, and nitrogen atoms arranged as amino acids, which are covalently linked in chains some 100 to 300 amino acids long. Each amino acid has an amino group and an acid group bonded to a central carbon which also carries a hydrogen and a side group. There are some 22 amino acids which differ from one another in the nature of the side groups they carry. The protein chain is constructed by linking the amino group of one amino acid to the acid group of the next simultaneously with the elimination of water. The bond formed is a peptide bond. The polypeptide thus formed has for each protein a distinctive sequence of amino acids and so has great specificity, as great as that of the different sentences that can be constructed from a 22 letter alphabet. The sequence of a protein's amino acids is known as its primary structure. Folding of the chain, usually into a globular tangle, gives the protein its secondary structure and establishes surface characteristics which enable the protein to act in specific ways: for example, as an enzyme which catalyzes a particular chemical reaction. In some proteins the chains are cross-linked (tertiary structure), and two or more folded chains can associate by hydrogen bonding (quaternary structure). Other roles of protein are described in Chapter 4.

The catalytic role of enzymes is exemplified by the sequence of reactions in which a derivative of glucose-phosphate is converted step by step to an amino acid. Each step is catalyzed by a different enzyme named for its function. Thus, a dehydrogenase removes hydrogens, a transaminase transfers an amino group into the structure; and a phosphatase removes a phosphate group.

Many amino acids can, thereby, be synthesized in the body from other energy nutrients and a nitrogen source. Eight (listed on page 92) cannot; these are the essential amino acids. An additional amino acid, histidine, is required by children and possibly by adults, and arginine is required by infants. The major role of dietary protein in human nutrition is therefore to supply amino acids for the synthesis of proteins needed in the body, although dietary protein can also serve as an energy source, providing 4 kcal per gram. A complete protein is defined as one which supplies all of the essential amino acids; a high quality protein is one which not only supplies them but also provides each in the appropriate amount relative to human physiological need. When one essential amino acid is in short supply relative to the others in a protein source, it is said to be a limiting amino acid; that is, it limits the total amount of protein that can be synthesized from that source. Egg protein is the World Health Organization's reference protein; it is a high quality protein used as a standard against which the quality of other proteins can be measured.

Animal protein sources are generally of higher quality than vegetable protein sources. The latter may have to be combined in pairs so that each supplements the other's limiting amino acids. Efforts to improve the quality of vegetable proteins are being made by plant geneticists who have been developing new strains of wheat, corn, and other food plants with amino acid balances tailored to meet human nutritional needs.

The amount of protein needed by human beings can be determined by nitrogen balance studies, since the element nitrogen is unique to protein among the energy nutrients. The healthy adult should be in nitrogen equilibrium (N in = N out), while a growing child requires a net increase in total body nitrogen per unit of time and so should be in positive nitrogen balance. Muscle wasting and other disease conditions cause negative nitrogen balance. The protein RDA (Recommended Dietary Allowance) for the healthy adult is 0.8 grams of protein per kilogram of ideal body weight. This is a generous allowance, published by the Food and Nutrition Board of the National Academy of Sciences-National Research Council and is set high enough to cover even people whose individual needs for protein (as determined by nitrogen balance and other studies) range as high as two standard deviations above the mean. Two-thirds of the RDA is probably an adequate intake for most members of the American population.

In the ADA Food Exchange System, the exchange groups which supply protein in abundance are those on the milk list (8 grams per exchange, or cup) and those on the meat list (7 grams per ounce and therefore 28 grams per 4-ounce serving). Vegetable and bread exchanges contribute 2 grams per exchange. The average consumption of protein by Americans is considerably higher than the RDA and is largely from high quality sources. The Highlight which follows this chapter deals with some aspects of American protein consumption and the special needs of vegetarians.

To Explore Further—

A clear picture of our new and profound understanding of how genes code for enzymes, which in turn determine the structure and function of cells, tissues, and whole organisms. Paperback:

Watson, J. D.: *Molecular Biology of the Gene.* 2nd ed. W. A. Benjamin, Inc., Menlo Park, California, 1970.

An amusing autobiographical account of Watson and Crick's discovery of the structure of DNA. Paperback:

Watson, J. D.: *The Double Helix.* Atheneum Publishers, New York, 1968.

Both of these articles present excellent discourses on how the RDA's are set and how they are revised. They both contribute to an understanding of the use that should be made of the RDA's:

Harper, A. E.: Those pesky RDA's. *Nutrition Today,* March/April: 15-28, 1974.

Leverton, R. M.: The RDA's are not for amateurs. *Journal of the American Dietetic Association* 66:9-11, 1975.

Cassette tape, *Recommended Dietary Allowances* (CAM 8-74) can be ordered from:

The American Dietetic Association
620 North Michigan Avenue
Chicago, Illinois 60611

Highlight Three
Meat Eaters vs Vegetarians

The middle-aged man who says with braggadocio that he is a
"meat and potatoes man" and the college age young person who,
almost defiantly, disdains any restaurant that will not serve
a meal of vegetables, fruit, and nuts have a lot more in com-

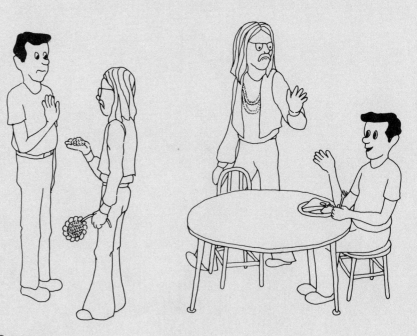

mon than either would like to believe. Both are extremists in their use of a valuable class of food—protein—and both could be suffering from malnutrition due to the rigidity of their daily food intake.

In today's world of contrasts between the affluent nations with their overconsumption of food and the poorer nations with their famines, there is a need for better understanding of protein nutrition by everyone, from policy maker to consumer.

In earlier times, recommendations on proper diet were made on the basis of observation only. A doctor might note, for instance, that persons who ate meat and eggs and drank milk were healthier, stronger, taller, or more resistant to infections. Therefore, he recommended to all his patients that they needed more protein and should include animal and dairy products in their diets. Later, when more sophisticated laboratory tests had been developed, it became clear that it was necessary to include certain amino acids in the diet and that animal and dairy products contained all of these essential amino acids. Vegetables, it was found, were lacking in one or more of these. Another observation made by many persons was that populations existing on cereal diets, either for reasons of meat taboos or of economic necessity, were malnourished, as revealed by their shorter stature, lower resistance to diseases, shorter life span, and higher infant mortality. All these observations and laboratory work underscored a common belief that animal and dairy products were good protein foods and that plants were poor protein foods. Present day clinical tests have shown that this earlier concept of animal proteins being better than plant proteins was not entirely justified.

essential amino acids: page 92.

It is true that animal and dairy foods contain complete proteins; it does seem to be true that milk-and-meat-eating populations are generally healthier than grain-eating populations. But it has been shown by clinical tests that if the vegetables, legumes, fruits, and grains are *wisely* chosen, growth in children will proceed as well on a diet devoid of animal protein as on one that includes milk and other animal proteins.[1]

complete protein: page 92.

clinical tests: see page 386.

In the United States, a love affair with meat has been flourishing for a century or more. No doubt the wide expanses of good grazing land in this country and the easy availability of wild animals to be had for the hunting (especially in our early history) contributed to our acquiring a taste for meat three times a day. In this century, as Americans have become more affluent and steak houses and hamburger chains have become more numerous, the amount of protein in the U.S. diet coming from animal sources has increased from 51.8 percent to 68.7 percent,

[1] Register, U. D. and Sonnenberg, L. M.: The vegetarian diet. *Journal of the American Dietetic Association* 62: 253-263, 1973.

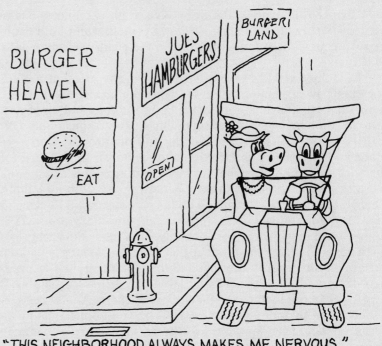

"THIS NEIGHBORHOOD ALWAYS MAKES ME NERVOUS."

while protein from plant sources has decreased from 48.2 percent to 31.3 percent.[2]

However, a counter trend has been developing among the young people who are turning from the "eggs-and-bacon, hamburger-and-French-fries, steak-and-potatoes" meals of their parents to vegetarian diets. There is a wide variation in the reasons given for this change by the "new" vegetarians:[3] some have been influenced by Eastern religions; some are eschewing meat on humanitarian grounds; some are expressing antiestablishment feelings; and some are merely caught up in a new fad. There is also a wide variation in the extent to which meat and dairy products are excluded from these diets, ranging from the highest Zen macrobiotic diet, made up exclusively of cereals, to those which, while eliminating animal meat, do include animal products such as eggs, milk, and cheese.

types of vegetarians: page 93.

In order to help us gain an understanding of the nutritional problems of these two groups, let us examine the calorie, protein, and fat content of meals consumed by a "meat and potatoes" man and by a "vegetables, fruits, and nuts" man to see *why* they both may be malnourished. (In order to make a valid comparison, we must use people of the same size, age and sex.)

[2]Friend, B. and Marston, R.: *Nutritional Review*, 1975. Bulletin of The Consumer and Food Economics Institute, U. S. Department of Agriculture, 1976.
[3]Dwyer, J. T., Kandel, R. F., Mayer, L. D. V. H. and Mayer, J.: The new vegetarians. *Journal of the American Dietetic Association* 64: 376-381, 1974.

If the ideal weight of each is 70 kilograms (154 pounds) and they are under 35 years of age, their daily calorie allowance would be 2,700 kcalories (see the RDA tables in Appendix I). One hundred percent of the RDA for protein would be 0.8 grams for each kilogram of ideal body weight, or 56 grams protein. If we assume that each eats one-third of his calorie and protein allowance at each meal, then the dinner calories should be 900 kcalories (1/3 x 2,700 = 900), and the dinner protein should be 19 grams (1/3 x 56 =18.6).

The Meat and Potato Man's Dinner

	Exchanges*	Kcalories	Grams Protein	Grams Fat
6 ounces boneless beefsteak	6 high-fat meat	330	42	18
	6 fat	270	—	30
1 large baked potato	2 bread	140	4	—
2 teaspoons margarine	2 fat	90	—	10
1 lettuce salad	vegetable (free)	—	—	—
2 tbsp French dressing	2 fat	90	—	10
1 slice (1/7) apple pie†		350	3	15
Totals		1,270‡	49**	83

*Food composition values are from the Food Exchange Lists (pages 33-38).
†Calculated by using the Table of Food Composition (Appendix H).
‡One-third of calories for the day (1/3 x 100% RDA) = 900 kcalories.
**One-third of grams protein for the day (1/3 x 100% RDA) = 19 grams.

By examining this man's consumption of one meal, what implications can we see for his future health? The first observation must concern excess calories. If we extrapolate from this one meal to estimate his total daily intake, he probably consumes in excess of 3,500 kcalories (3 x 1,270 = 3,810 kcalories). This is about 800 kcalories over his daily allowance and would cause a weight gain of about a pound every five days unless he is engaged in heavy physical labor. It is relatively easy to exceed the energy allowance when a large portion of the calories comes from animal meat, particularly beef and pork. Some fat can be trimmed from the meat, but much of it is in the marbling. Marbling deceives the eater who doesn't realize that he is consuming considerable invisible fat. The fat also contributes to palatability, which encourages larger servings.

The *protein* needs for the entire day may also have been exceeded in this one meal—49 grams when only 38 grams (2/3 the RDA) are needed by the average person. You will recall that protein is important in the diet because of its contribution of essential amino acids and nitrogen. The ease with which a per-

extrapolation (ex-trap-oh-LAY-shun): an educated guess, from a known series of numbers, as to what others may be. For example, knowing that ten dimes is one dollar and that twenty dimes is two dollars, we might extrapolate (in this case correctly) to conclude that fifty dimes must be five dollars.

marbling: a lacy network of fat embedded in meat, sometimes so fine as to be invisible. Sometimes called **invisible fat**, in contrast to the visible fats—butter, margarine, oil, and the fats removable from meat.

Removal of nitrogen from amino acids and use of the remaining 2-carbon fragments for energy is described in Chapter 6.

son can meet his essential amino acid needs with animal products is one of the advantages of including such products in the diet. But if more amino acids are present than are needed by the body for several hours after ingestion, these amino acids will be degraded to 2-carbon fragments which will be used for energy, and if not needed for energy will be used to build body *fat*. Thus, valuable, essential amino acids, eaten in excess of need, can lead to obesity.

If beef is being used for *calories*, it is costly, both in terms of money and in terms of land use. If a cut of beef costs $1.79 a pound, its cost is 15 cents for 100 kcalories; if an 18-ounce box of rolled oats costs $0.55, its cost is 2.3 cents for 100 kcalories. If it is energy rather than amino acids you are buying, it is obvious which of these is the better buy.

Plant calories also cost less land. A million kcalories in wheat can be produced on less than one acre of land; a million kcalories in beef require seventeen acres.[4] (These figures have some harsh implications for groups interested in solving the nutrition problems in the developing countries: introducing meat into a vegetarian economy may worsen the food balance. See Highlight 4. Even in the United States we may find that in the near future we will not be able to afford the luxury of using 17 times as much land as needed to produce an energy food.)

As for *fat*, 83 grams were consumed in this meal. Each gram of fat produces 9 kcalories, so about 750 kcalories are produced by this fat—more than 55 percent of the total kcalories in this meal. This amount makes this meal not only high in fat but also one that contains virtually all saturated fats and could, therefore, tend to lead to the development of atherosclerosis. Fat is a necessary nutrient in the diet for several reasons and useful for its high satiety value. However, satiety is not always desirable; the appetite can sometimes be satisfied before enough vegetables, fruits, and grains are consumed to ensure that all essential nutrients have been included.

atherosclerosis: page 72.

satiety (sat-EYE-uh-tee): the feeling of fullness or satisfaction after a meal. Fat provides satiety more than carbohydrate or protein because it slows gastric motility.

diverticulosis (DYE-ver-tick-yoo-LO-sis): a condition in which the walls of the intestines are weakened in spots and form "blowouts" or outpocketings. These may become inflamed or infected, a condition known as **diverticulitis** (DYE-ver-ti-cu-LI-tis) which is dangerous because the intestinal walls may rupture.

Finally, this is a low-fiber meal. Only the lettuce has appreciable fiber content. Fiber aids in digestion and may be important for the prevention of diverticulitis,[5] cancer of the colon,[5] and atherosclerosis.[6] People who are interested in prevention of these diseases of modern life would be wise to choose with care the foods they consume regularly.

We have seen that this meal contains more than enough protein. There is no need to be concerned that all essential amino

[4]Stare, F.: Sugar in the diet of man. In *World Review of Nutrition and Dietetics,* Vol. 22. Bourne, G. H., editor. S. Karger AG, Basel, 1975.
[5]Tunaley, A.: Constipation—the secret national problem. *Nutrition* 28(2): 91-96, 1974.
[6]Kritchevsky, D. and Story, J. A.: Binding of bile salts in vitro by nonnutritive fiber. *Journal of Nutrition* 104: 458-462, 1974.

acids are present, since the protein is predominantly of animal origin. There is, however, an excess of calories, largely from saturated fat, which leads us to be concerned about obesity and atherosclerosis. There may not be enough vegetables and fruits in the diet as a whole to ensure that all essential nutrients and fiber are present, but we cannot make this judgment without knowing the intake for the other meals of the day.

In the introduction we stated that the only unequivocal statement about the nutritive quality of a food is a statement of the specific nutrients it contains and the amount of each. In this Highlight, the nutritive quality of two *diets* is being examined, and the above statement can be amplified. In assessing these diets it is useful (1) to note the specific nutrients they contain and (2) to state the amount of each. We also undertake two additional means of evaluation: (3) to examine the quality of the nutrients (complete vs incomplete protein, saturated vs polyunsaturated fat), and (4) to compare the amounts of the nutrients with the RDA. Each of these two additional judgments deserves a comment.

Notice that in assessing the quality of the nutrients we are not concerned about their source but about their molecular characteristics. The food sources of amino acids need not be "organically grown," but they do need to contribute a complete and balanced spectrum of essential amino acids. The fat need not be "natural," but it does need to have a high percentage of polyunsaturated fatty acids. These observations reinforce the points made in the digression on pages 64-65.

In comparing the amounts of the nutrients with the RDA, we can make a meaningful statement about their contribution to a person's needs. Failing to use such a yardstick can cause serious misunderstanding on the part of a careless reader/consumer. For example, when you read that a vitamin-mineral supplement provides 10 milligrams of calcium, you may be hoodwinked into believing that a pill a day will meet your needs for this nutrient. Only when you compare this statement with the calcium RDA for an adult (800 milligrams) do you realize that you would have to take eighty of these pills a day to meet your RDA!

CAUTION WHEN YOU READ!

Make a habit of using a yardstick to measure quantities.

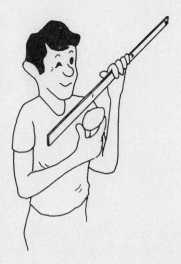

Many food companies make statements about their products that can be critically analyzed this way. A "high protein cereal" sounds like a cereal that provides a lot of protein for human needs, but on closer examination it turns out to be high in protein only when compared with other cereals. In small lettering on the side panel, the label of such a cereal may reveal that one serving *including the milk added to it* supplies only 10 percent of the RDA for protein!

If there is no statement of quantity on the label or in the advertisement, beware. The statement that a food contains a nutrient, without specifying how much, may be intended to mislead.

Labeling laws are discussed in Highlight 13.

A flag sign of a suspect claim is

the statement "contains X," with no amount specified.

Now let us look at the "vegetables, fruits, and nuts" man' meal.

The Vegetables, Fruits and Nuts Man's Dinner

	Exchanges*	Kcalories	Grams Protein	Grams Fat
1 cup cooked cabbage	2 vegetable	50	4	—
1 teaspoon safflower oil	1 fat	45	—	5
½ cup cooked carrots	1 vegetable	25	2	—
1 large baked potato	2 bread	140	4	—
1 tablespoon margarine	3 fat	135	—	15
fruit salad:				
1 small banana	2 fruit	80	—	—
1 small apple	1 fruit	40	—	—
½ cup pineapple	1 fruit	40	—	—
2 tablespoons raisins	1 fruit	40	—	—
6 nuts	1 fat	45	—	5
Totals		640†	10‡	25

*See Food Exchange Lists, pages 33-38.
†One-third of calories for the day (1/3 x 100% RDA) = 900 kcalories. (See page 105).
‡One-third of grams protein for the day (1/3 x 100% RDA) = 19 grams. (See page 105).

This one meal is not typical of a knowledgeable vegetarian's meal but it illustrates several of the difficulties an amateur vegan may encounter. You will notice there is a very large quantity of food in this meal yet the calories are deficient by about 250 kcalories. This deficiency, amounting to about 750 kcalories per day, could result in a loss of weight of about a pound every four to five days—unless, of course, it is corrected at the other meals. This is, as a matter fact, a common observation about vegans: they are usually underweight, and must eat huge amounts of food if they are to maintain their weight.

Another obstacle the vegetarian faces in planning his/her meals is in obtaining sufficient protein. In this vegetarian dinner, there is about one-half the recommended amount of protein. Furthermore, the protein present has a poor combination of essential amino acids. Vegetables must be carefully chosen if they are to be the only source of protein. Potatoes and carrots provide many important nutrients as well as adding to the fiber content of the diet, but a child would not grow properly on a diet in which the only sources of protein were potatoes and carrots.

protein quality: page 92.

If you examine the Vegetable Exchange List on pages 33-34, you will note that there are a few vegetables which provide such an insignificant amount of protein and calories that they are treated as having no protein or calories. Then there is a long list of vegetables that provide 2 grams of protein and 25 kcalories per half cup. Turn to the Bread Exchange List to find still other vegetables (legumes, tubers, and other starchy vegetables), which provide 2 grams of protein and 70 kcalories per exchange.

In selecting protein food sources for the diet, we must not only know the amount of protein in the source but also must be certain that the essential amino acids are present and are present in the correct proportions. Most of the vegetable or grain sources are low in some essential amino acids, such as lysine, methionine, threonine, or tryptophan; however, by eating specific combinations at the same meal, we can obtain the equivalent of a complete protein. Soybeans, which are rich in lysine, can supplement wheat or corn or rye, which are deficient in lysine; a mixture of soy and sesame proteins has a high nutritive value comparable to milk proteins;[1] peanut proteins can supplement wheat, corn, oats, and rice. A rule of thumb could be that mixtures of grains and legumes eaten at the same meal provide a fairly good proportion of the essential amino acids.

This strategy is called **mutual supplementation**: use of two different protein sources, each lacking a different amino acid, so that each provides the amino acid missing from the other. See suggested readings for further information.

Another point to consider in planning the protein for a meal is to be certain that there are sufficient calories so that the amino acids will not be degraded for energy. With a 250 kcalorie deficit, the 10 grams of protein in this vegetarian's meal will certainly be used for energy rather than for building and maintaining his body tissues.

linoleic (lin-oh-LAY-ic) **acid:** an essential polyunsaturated fatty acid (see pages 62-63).

There are about 25 grams of fat in this meal which supply 225 kcalories, or about 35 percent of the total calories. This is not a high fat diet. In addition, about a third of the fat is linoleic acid, whereas in the meat and potato diet only a sixth of the fat was linoleic acid. Also, there is no cholesterol in this meal. These are among the unique advantages of the vegetarian diet as compared to the meat and potato diet: plant sources contain no cholesterol and, except for coconuts, very little saturated fat.

We have seen that this one meal of vegetables, fruits, and nuts contains a large quantity of food but a deficit of calories. This deficit could lead, not only to loss of weight, but to poor utilization of the protein present. The protein is low in amount and has a poor amino acid spectrum, since the two protein sources are not mutually supplemental. The meal does contain a wide variety of fruits and vegetables which would ensure an ample supply of vitamins and minerals and a good fiber content.

For the pure vegetarian there are some problems with other nutrients which will be discussed later in this text but which should be recognized here. With the absence of milk and milk products, calcium, riboflavin, and vitamin B_{12} needs must be met in other ways. Occasional use of dark green leafy vegetables, legumes, and nuts will not supply enough calcium and riboflavin, but the use of two cups of soybean milk will protect against deficiencies of these two nutrients.[1] Soybean milk has been on the market for many years as a substitute milk for infants who are allergic to cow's milk. There is, however, no known plant source of vitamin B_{12}; therefore, all vegans should supplement their diets with this vitamin.[1]

empty calories: see Highlight 1.

Menu planning for the vegetarian is helped immensely by the new meat analogs on the market. These analogs have flavor and texture similar to various kinds of meat. However, it is not necessary to use these meat substitutes to obtain all the essential amino acids. One precaution should be taken by the vegan in menu planning: avoid the use of empty calorie foods. Vegans must eat large quantities of food to meet their protein needs. They are dependent on the accumulation of small amounts of amino acids from each of many items. Empty calorie foods would make no contribution of any nutrient except glucose.

The ideal diet for Americans lies somewhere between the two examples studied. The meat and potatoes eater should select smaller servings of meat and include a variety of vegetables, fruits, and cereals. By substituting meats which are lower in saturated fats (such as fish, chicken, and veal) for beef and pork, the fat and cholesterol content of this diet would be lowered substantially as would the total calories. If vegans would decide to become lacto-ovo-vegetarians, they could easily correct most of the deficiencies noted in the vegetarian menu shown. One egg and two cups of milk (2% fat) would provide 23 grams of complete protein and 305 kcalories, as well as other valuable nutrients. Activities at the end of this chapter suggest that you make the changes in these two menus.

If vegetarians insist on omitting all animal and dairy products, they should strive to meet 100 percent of the RDA for protein, should use a vitamin B_{12} supplement, and should meet 100 percent of the RDA for calories, without resorting to empty calorie foods. They must also be willing to become very well informed on nutrition and strict about including, at every meal, plant proteins which supplement each other.

From the above comparison, it seems that people get into trouble, nutritionally, when they select foods from just one or two categories, even if these are high quality protein foods. On the other hand, if they exclude one entire group of foods, as vegetarians sometimes do, they run the risk of malnourishment of another kind. The old maxim among nutritionists appears to be true: GOOD NUTRITION DEPENDS MOSTLY ON INCLUDING A WIDE VARIETY OF FOODS IN THE DIET.

To Explore Further—

Two easy reading books for the vegetarian. Lappe's book has an especially good discussion of complementarity of amino acids:

Deutsch, R.: *The Nuts among the Berries.* Ballantine Books, New York, 1962.

Lappe, F. M.: *Diet for a Small Planet.* Ballantine Books, New York, 1971.

Majumber's article has a good discussion of economic and ecological implications of vegetarianism while Shun's article is an account of a case study of one vegan who developed megaloblastic anemia:

Majumber, J. K.: Vegetarianism: fad, faith, fact? *American Scientist* 60 (2):175-179, 1974.

Shun, O. J. and Kabakow, B.: Nutritional megaloblastic anemia in vegan. *New York State Journal of Medicine,* pp. 2893-2894, 1972.

A good source of recipes for persons seeking help on modified fat diets or less expensive protein sources. Calculations are included for fat and calories in the recipes:

Keys, A. and Keys, M.: *The Benevolent Bean*. Farrar, Straus and Giroux Publishers, New York, 1972.

Cassette with syllabus can be ordered from the American Dietetic Association: *Animal Flesh Analogs from Vegetable Protein* (CAM 12-75).

A study kit which includes pre- and post-tests and information for planning vegetarian diets, also reprints of journal articles: *The Vegetarian Diet* by Register, U. D. and Zolber, K.

Both of these teaching aids can be ordered from:

The American Dietetic Association
430 North Michigan Avenue
Chicago, Illinois 60611

Suggested Activities

(1) Study your own diet.

Review the record you made (Chapter 1, Activity 1) of your food intake. Record from Appendix H the number of grams of protein in each item. Estimate your protein consumption from your milk, meat, vegetable, and bread exchanges. How many of your protein grams are from animal sources? From vegetable sources? How many calories a day do you consume from protein?

Calculate your protein RDA (see Appendix D, example 2 if you need help). How does your protein intake compare with your RDA?

(2) Put protein in its place as one part of a balanced diet.

Add up the kcalories you consumed from carbohydrate (Chapter 1, Activity 1), those from fat (Chapter 2, Activity 1), and those from protein (Activity 1 above). The USPHS (United States Public Health Service) suggests that a well-balanced diet should derive 10 to 15 percent of its kcalories from protein, not more than 35 percent from fat,[1] and the remainder from carbohydrate. Many Americans consume more protein and fat and less carbohydrate than this. How does your balance compare with this recommendation? (For aid in calculating percentages, turn to Appendix D, example 4.)

(Note: The last Highlight in the book invites you to survey your entire diet for adequacy, balance, and economy. You may wish to save these two activities until you have read that Highlight, or you may wish to read the Highlight now for a sense of perspective.)

(3) Think about the meaning of nitrogen balance.

(a) You have been physically inactive for more than a year and are now embarking on a strenuous body-building campaign, designed especially for muscle building. You are eating an adequate and well-balanced diet. During the body-building program would you be in positive, zero, or negative nitrogen balance? When you have reached your desired goal and are maintaining it with daily jogging, will you be in positive, zero, or negative balance?

Since most athletes are in top physical condition and are maintaining their muscles with daily exercise, do athletes need more protein than less active people?[2]

(b) Suppose you degrade 30 grams of tissue protein per day and excrete the nitrogen. Suppose you eat 70 grams of protein a day. You use 30 to replace your losses. What happens to the other 40 grams? Are you in positive, zero, or negative nitrogen balance?

(ANSWER: zero balance. The extra 40 grams are also degraded and the nitrogen excreted, never becoming a part of the body tissue proper. The amino acid residues follow the fate described in Chapter 6. Thus a person consuming a lot of protein excretes a lot of nitrogen and remains in zero balance.)

(4) Don't be an amateur in using the RDA.

A friend tells you "my roommate only ate . . . yesterday. I'm sure her diet is deficient in protein." You calculate the

---

[1]Livingston, G. E.: The prudent diet: what? why? how? *Preventive Medicine* 2:321-328, 1973.

[2]Position paper on food and nutrition misinformation on selected topics. *Journal of the American Dietetic Association* 66(3):277-279, 1975.

roommate's protein intake and find she consumed 40 grams of animal protein. The protein RDA for a woman that age, height, and weight is 46 grams. How do you advise your friend? Should she worry about her roommate?

(5) Be dollar-wise with protein.
You have been asked to advise a college student on ways to reduce the cost of his/her food. Since protein is one of the most costly items in the food budget, you will need to know the cost per gram of protein delivered by the foods. The following chart, when completed, will help you make a valid comparison of costs.

Food Item	Regular Hamburger	Low-fat Milk	Plain Corn-flakes	Peanut Butter	Eggs	Canned Pork and Beans
Brand, type, etc.						
G protein per measure of food	$\frac{23 \text{ g}}{3 \text{ oz}}$			$\frac{4 \text{ g}}{1 \text{ tbsp}}$		
Amount of food to provide 40 g protein						
Cost of unit amount of food						
Cost of amount of food to provide 40 g of protein						
Cost of 1 g protein						

(6) Consider changing your life style.
Prepare a day's menus for a lacto-ovo-vegetarian using your ideal weight. The day's intake must meet your RDA for protein and calories.
Now delete the eggs, milk, or cheese foods in the above menu and make substitutions so that it will continue to provide the RDA for calories and protein. In addition, this menu must show mutual supplementation of the amino acids.

(7) Caution when you read!
A "high protein supplement" advertises that it supplies "an unbelievable 690 milligrams of purified high quality protein in every tablet!" Using the RDA as a yardstick, what percent of a

person's daily need for protein does a tablet supply (check Appendix D to compare milligrams with grams)?

Make a collection of labels from foods in the grocery store, the health food store, and supplements in the drug store. Which labels convey accurate information about their products? Which are implying untrue things about their products? How can you tell?

4

Proteins (B) Roles and Deficiency

There is present in plants and in animals a substance which ... is without doubt the most important of all the known substances in living matter, and, without it, life would be impossible on our planet. This material has been named Protein.
—GERARD JOHANNES MULDER, 1838

Roles of Protein

The next twelve sections describing roles of protein do not represent an arbitrary selection, but rather a selection of those body functions for which other nutrients (vitamins and minerals) are also essential. The minerals sodium and potassium, for example, help proteins maintain the water balance, while vitamin C helps make the protein collagen, which is involved in scar formation. For the present, we suggest you read the following sections keeping in mind that "proteins do all these things." This thought will provide the background you need in order to appreciate the roles of the helper nutrients, details of which are given in Chapters 9-14. Then read those chapters keeping in mind that "these other nutrients *help* the proteins to do all these things." Margin references show where each of the helper nutrients is described.

Some proteins act as enzymes. Our earlier description of enzyme molecules and the way they are constructed depicted them as giant tangled chains of amino acids, bristling with positive and negative charges, and bouncing about in the fluids of the body. Because of the differing nature of their surface characteristics each enzyme is able to perform a different role. Each can work on a different compound, either to break it apart into smaller compounds, to add something to it and make it larger, or to change some part of it in order to change its chemical identity.

enzyme: see pages 88-91.

Helper nutrients: coenzymes (like the B vitamins) and cofactors (minerals). See Chapters 9, 12, 13.

117

There are many other proteins besides enzymes in the body. The roles of some of these are understandable at the molecular level if you keep this "bristling ball" picture in mind.

Proteins help maintain the water balance. In order to understand how this extremely important function is managed it is necessary to appreciate the fact that there are three principal compartments for fluids in the body: the intravascular space, the intracellular space, and the interstitial space. In normal and healthy people, there is a proper amount of fluid in each of these compartments. Fluid can flow back and forth across the boundaries between these systems, but whenever the volume of fluid deviates, it is rapidly brought back to normal. Protein (with certain minerals) helps to maintain the amount of water at the proper volume in each compartment.

water balance: distribution of body water among the body compartments.

intravascular space: the continuous space inside the circulatory system (heart, arteries, capillaries, veins).

> intra = inside (within)
> vascular = vein

intracellular space: the spaces inside the cells.

interstitial space (in-ter-STISH-ul): the spaces between the cells, outside the vascular system.

> interstice = space between

Helper nutrients: minerals. See pages 431-435.

Diagram of section of body tissue.

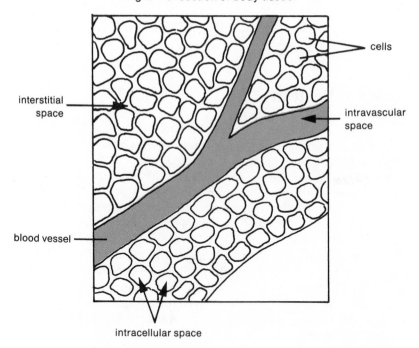

The way this works is neat and simple. Proteins are so large that they cannot pass across the walls or membranes which separate the compartments from one another. They are trapped where they are—and they are hydrophilic; that is, they are attractive to water molecules. The water molecules therefore stay with, or near, the proteins. Thus by regulating the amount of protein (and minerals) in each compartment, the body indirectly regulates the amount of water.

The flow of water across a membrane in the direction of a solute such as protein or minerals is due to osmotic pressure (see Chapter 14).

When something goes wrong with this sytem—when a person is suffering from a condition in which the blood protein concentration falls, for example—fluid may leak out of the vascular system and accumulate in the interstitial tissues, resulting in the symptom known as edema. This causes a visible swelling or puffiness in the tissue. In pregnant women, it is not uncommon to see a swelling of the ankles which reflects fluid leakage from the leg veins into the tissues. In other individuals, fluid may leak out of the veins in the abdomen, resulting in a swollen "pot belly." In others the hands may swell or the face may become puffy.

edema (uh-DEE-muh): accumulation of fluid in the interstitial spaces. In the special case where edema occurs in the abdomen, it is known as **ascites** (uh-SITE-eez).

The uninformed person may believe that the way to prevent this swelling is to drink less water or to increase excretion by taking a diuretic. Indeed if edema has become extreme, these measures, as well as salt restriction, may be a necessary part of treatment. Yet you can never *cause* edema by drinking too much water. The more you drink, the more you carry in your vascular system, and as the vascular fluid is circulated through your kidneys, the more you automatically excrete.

diuretic (dye-yoo-RET-ic): a drug that stimulates increased renal water excretion.

renal = kidney

kidneys: see illustration, page 182.

> This discussion illustrates a principle that pervades the study of health. Provided that you *are* healthy, your body will maintain its own health. No drug is known which renders the healthy body more capable of regulating its own functions than it is already. Drugs are needed to remedy situations in which body functions have become impaired. Diuretics may be needed only when excess fluid has already accumulated. They are not useful as preventive medicine.
>
> Since the taking of a diuretic increases water excretion, it causes a sudden weight loss. A healthy person who fails to distinguish between loss of body fat and loss of water may see this as a desirable effect and start using diuretics for this purpose. Since the only loss induced is water loss, however, the only achievement gained is dehydration.
>
> This theme is taken up again in Chapter 5, where a flag sign of a spurious claim is identified.

So excess water intake cannot by itself cause edema. What can then? One thing is a protein-deficient diet. When protein intake falls below a certain limit, blood proteins become depleted. The water which should be held within the bloodstream then leaks out into the interstitial space. Once there, it is not available to the kidneys to excrete: the kidneys do not "know" there is too much water in the system. Hence the remedy *may* not be less water, but more protein.

In edema, fluid leaks out of the intravascular space making tissue swell, as illustrated at right.

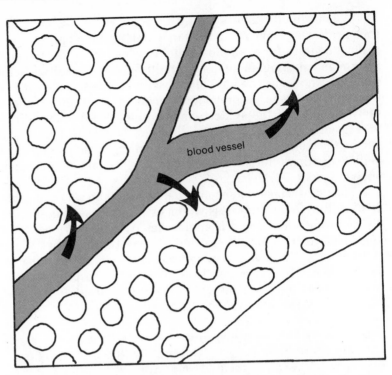

blood vessel

acid-base balance: the balance maintained in the body between too much and too little acid. Blood pH, for example, is regulated normally between 7.38 and 7.42 (pH: see below).

Helper nutrients: minerals (see pages 435-436).

The concentration of H^+ ions is expressed as **pH** (see Appendix B). The lower the pH, the stronger the acid. Thus, pH 2 is a strong acid, pH 6 a weak acid (pH 7 is neutral). A pH above 7 is alkaline or basic (a solution in which OH^- ions predominate).

acidosis: too much acid in the blood and body fluids.

alkalosis: too much base in the blood and body fluids.

lethal: causing death.

sequester (see-KWES-ter): to hide away or take out of circulation.

buffer: a compound which can reversibly combine with H^+ ions to help maintain a constant pH.

Proteins help maintain the acid-base balance. An acid solution is one in which there are hydrogen ions floating around. The more hydrogen ions, the more concentrated the acid. Proteins (and minerals) which have negative charges on their surfaces, attract hydrogen ions, and hydrogen ions in turn attract proteins. As long as the concentration of hydrogen ions—that is to say the strength of the acid—is maintained within certain limits, the proteins will maintain their integrity. If the acid becomes too strong, however, the extra positive charges surrounding the protein molecules deform them and, so to speak, pull them out of shape. When this happens, the proteins can no longer function. Of all the consequences that stem from exceeding the normal limits of acid-base balance in the body, the most direct and serious is that of disturbing the shapes of the proteins that carry out so many of the vital body functions. Acidosis and alkalosis both are lethal if unchecked. The proteins in the plasma help to prevent these conditions from arising. In a sense the proteins protect each by binding or sequestering extra hydrogen ions when there are too many in the surrounding medium and by releasing them when there are too few. This function of regulating the acidity of the medium is known as the buffering action of proteins.

Proteins confer resistance to disease. Other major proteins found in the blood function as anti-disease agents. These proteins are called the antibodies. When a body is invaded by a virus, whether it be a flu virus, the smallpox virus, measles virus, or one that causes a common cold, the virus enters the cells and multiplies there. One virus entering a cell may produce a hundred replicas of itself within an hour or so. These burst out and invade a hundred different cells, soon yielding ten thousand virus particles, which invade ten thousand cells. After several hours there may be a million viruses and then a hundred million, and so on. If they were left free to do their worst they would soon overwhelm the body with the disease they caused.

The antibodies, giant protein molecules circulating in the blood, are a defense against viruses, bacteria, and other "foreign agents." The surface of each antibody molecule has characteristics which enable it to combine with and inactivate a foreign protein like that in a virus coat or bacterial cell membrane. The antibodies work so efficiently that in a normal healthy individual the many disease agents that attempt to attack never have a chance to get started. If a million bacterial cells are injected into the skin of a normal healthy person, fewer than ten are likely to survive at the end of five hours.[1]

Once the body has manufactured antibodies against a disease agent (such as the measles virus, for example), the cells never forget how to produce it. The next time they are infected, they will respond even more quickly than the first time. The immunological response of the antibody-producing cells and the way they achieve their molecular memory of the body's enemies is beyond the scope of this book, but references at the end of this chapter will lead you further, if you like.

Some hormones are proteins. Some hormones are pure protein. Among those made of pure protein are the familiar thyroid hormone and insulin. The roles that these hormones play increase still further the importance of proteins in the body. The thyroid hormone regulates the body's metabolic rate—the rate of the chemical reactions that yield energy. Insulin regulates the concentration of the blood glucose and its transportation into cells, upon which, in turn, the functioning of the brain and the nervous system depend. Hormones have many other profound effects on the body, which will become evident as you read further.

Proteins carry nutrients into and out of cells. There are proteins in the membrane of every cell of the body, each one specific for a certain compound (or group of related compounds). Each of these proteins is confined to the membrane but can rotate or shuttle from one side to the other. Each can pick up a

antibodies

immunology
(im-yoo-NOLL-uh-gee): the study of immunity and the way in which it is achieved by antibodies and other disease-resistance agents.

hormone: see page 157.

Helper nutrients: iodine (part of thyroid hormone), zinc (part of insulin). See page 407.

These membrane-associated proteins are variously called **permeases, vectorial enzymes,** and **transferases.**

[1]Stanier, R. Y., Doudoroff, M. and Adelberg, E. A.: *The Microbial World.* 3rd ed. Prentice-Hall, Inc., Englewood Cliffs, New Jersey, 1970, p. 784.

compound on one side of the membrane and release it on the other, thus enabling the cells to choose what substances to take up and what to release. Examples are the *glucose pump* and *potassium pump*, which transport glucose and potassium into cells faster than they can leak out, and the *sodium pump*, which transports sodium out of cells. Thanks to these pumps, a higher concentration of glucose and potassium is maintained inside than outside the cells, while the reverse is true of sodium. The mineral calcium also enters cells with the help of a protein, the *calcium-binding protein* in the intestinal tract.

It may not be immediately apparent why the cells go to so much trouble to maintain these concentration gradients, but many reasons will become apparent in later chapters. To anticipate one of them very simplistically: the sodium-potassium distribution across the membranes of nerve cells is what makes it possible for nerve impulses to travel, and so for you to think!

Many of these pumps can be switched on or off depending on the body's needs. Often hormones do the switching, with a marvelous precision. Suppose, for example, there is too much glucose in the blood. High blood glucose causes the pancreas to release the hormone insulin; the insulin stimulates the glucose pumps in the membranes of the liver and fat cells (and is destroyed in the process); these cells pick up the excess glucose; then when the blood glucose concentration is normal, the pancreas stops releasing insulin. The absorption of calcium is regulated by hormones (calcitonin and parathormone) in a similar manner. These examples are by no means exhaustive; they simply illustrate how the distribution of nutrients in the various body spaces depends on hundreds of different proteins.

Protein carriers transport nutrients in the circulatory system. Many nutrients travel freely in the vascular system, but others have to be "carried." The lipids are an example. You have already read about the problem these cumbersome molecules pose for the digestive system: they have to be emulsified in order to be made accessible to the enzymes that hydrolyze them. Even after absorption they require special handling. Each major lipid has to be complexed with protein before it can be transported in the blood. These complexes are called lipoproteins. They are giant aggregates, much larger than lipids by themselves, but they travel easily in water because the protein is hydrophilic. (Only the smaller lipids—monoglycerides, glycerol, and fatty acids—can travel freely without carriers.) The fat-soluble vitamins are also carried by special proteins.

The mineral iron is a nutrient whose handling in the body illustrates especially well how precisely proteins operate. On leaving the intestine, iron is picked up by an iron-carrying protein in the bloodstream known as transferrin. Transferrin may, in turn, transfer the iron to a storage protein in the bone mar-

concentration gradient: a difference in concentration of a solute on two sides of a semipermeable membrane. **(solute,** SOLL-yoot: dissolved substance.)

Regulation of calcium absorption, pages 374-375.

emulsification: pages 67-68.

lipoprotein (lip-oh-PRO-tee-in, lip-oh-PRO-teen). See page 187.

hydrophilic (high-dro-FILL-ic): water-loving. See also pages 186-187.

transferrin (trans-FURR-in)

row, known as ferritin. This protein will finally release the iron to make the protein hemoglobin, which is synthesized in new red blood cells as they are formed.

Proteins carry oxygen. The protein hemoglobin is a giant molecule that contains two atoms of iron. The iron can combine with oxygen and then release it. As the red cells flow through the lungs, the hemoglobin iron picks up oxygen. As they together flow through the tissues, the iron releases the oxygen into the body cells, where it can serve the function of oxidizing other nutrients to provide energy. (As a carbon-hydrogen-oxygen compound such as carbohydrate or fat is oxidized, the H combines with O to form water—H_2O—and the C combines with O to form carbon dioxide—CO_2.) The blood then picks up the carbon dioxide released by the cells. As the blood next flows through the lungs, this carbon dioxide is released into the air spaces in the lungs and can be breathed out. The oxygen carrier of muscle, myoglobin, is also a protein.

Proteins are involved in the clotting of blood. Blood is unique and wonderful in its ability to remain a liquid tissue even though it is carrying so many, varied large molecules and cells through the circulatory system, but can also turn solid within seconds when the integrity of that system is disturbed. If it did not clot, a single pinprick could drain your entire body of all its blood, just as a hole in a bucket makes the bucket forever useless for holding water. When you cut yourself, the injured blood cells react immediately by releasing a protein called thrombin. The thrombin encounters another protein already circulating in the fluid part of the blood and converts it to fibrin, a stringy, insoluble mass of fibers that plugs the cut and stops the leak. Later, more slowly, a scar can form to replace the clot and permanently heal the cut.

Proteins help make scar tissue, bones, and teeth. When the construction of a bone or a tooth begins, the shape is first roughed out by laying down a protein matrix known as collagen, which forms a cartilage. Later, crystals of calcium, phosphorus, fluoride, and other minerals are laid down on this matrix, and the hardened bone begins to form. When a bone breaks, again the protein collagen precedes the bony material in the mending process. Collagen is also the mending material in torn tissue, forming scars to hold the separated parts together. It forms the material of ligaments and tendons and is a strengthening constituent between the cells of vein and artery walls, which must be able to withstand the pressure of surging heartbeats.

Proteins are necessary for vision. The light-sensitive pigments in the cells of the retina are molecules of the protein opsin. Opsin responds to light by changing its shape, thus initiating the nerve impulses that convey the sense of sight to the higher centers of the brain.

---

ferritin (FER-it-in)

hemoglobin (HEEM-o-globe-in)

Helper nutrient: iron. See pages 397-399.

myoglobin (MY-o-globe-in)

thrombin: a protein carried by the red blood cells, involved in blood clotting.

thrombo = clot

The protein circulating in the fluid part of the blood ready to react with thrombin is **fibrinogen** (fye-BRIN-o-gen). The reaction between these two and other protein factors produces **fibrin** (FYE-brin), the protein material of the clot.

fibr = fibers
-ogen = gives rise to

Helper nutrients: vitamin K (involved in production of thrombin), calcium (needed for blood to clot). See pages 355, 373.

collagen: see also page 315.

Helper nutrients: vitamin C (needed to form collagen), minerals (to calcify bones and teeth). See pages 315, 404.

opsin: see page 339.

Helper nutrient: vitamin A (see pages 338-340).

Proteins are needed for growth and maintenance. Whenever you take a bath you wash off whole cells from the surface layers of your skin, losing protein. Your hair and fingernails are growing constantly; since you ultimately cut them off (or break or chew them) these processes too result in a net loss of body protein. Inside, similar processes are occurring. When you swallow food, it passes down your intestinal tract and ultimately leaves your body as waste, carrying with it cells that have been shed from the intestinal lining. Both inside and outside you must constantly build new cells to replace those lost from the exposed surfaces. This is what is meant when it is said that a person's skin is totally replaced every seven years.

Given an energy source, either fat or carbohydrate (composed of C, H, and O), the body can construct many of the materials (also composed of C, H, and O) needed to replace these lost cells. But to replace the protein, it must have protein from food, because food protein is its only available source of nitrogen.

If the body is growing, it must manufacture more cells each day than are lost. Children end each day with more blood cells, more muscle cells, more skin cells, than they had at the beginning of the day. So protein is needed both for routine maintenance (replacement) and growth (addition) of body tissue.

The above list of protein functions is by no means exhaustive, but it does give some sense of the immense variety and importance of proteins in the body. With this information as background, you are in a position to appreciate the significance of the world's most serious malnutrition problem: protein deficiency.

Protein Deficiency

protein calorie malnutrition

The most ominous specter haunting the populations of the world's underdeveloped countries is protein calorie malnutrition. Protein and calories (energy) are all-pervasive in human nutrition; they are involved in every body function. When children are deprived of food and suffer a calorie deficit, they will degrade their protein for energy and thus will indirectly suffer a protein deficiency as well as a calorie deficiency.

PCM: protein calorie malnutrition.

Protein- and calorie-deprivation go hand in hand so often that public health officials have adopted an abbreviation for the overlapping deficiency: PCM. Cases are observed at both ends of the spectrum, however, and are given names: the classic calorie deficiency disease is marasmus, and the protein deficiency disease is kwashiorkor.

marasmus: see also page 241.

kwashiorkor (kwash-ee-OR-core, kwash-ee-or-CORE)

Classical marasmus is treated at the end of the chapter on energy balance (Chapter 8), because it can be more easily understood after some facts about energy metabolism have been presented. Kwashiorkor is understandable on the basis of what has been said above about protein, and so is treated here. The two overlapping diseases have a tremendous impact on the world's people and serious implications for the future of humankind. The changing problem on a worldwide scale is so complex that it requires separate emphasis; it is the subject of the Highlight which follows.

The word kwashiorkor originally meant "the evil spirit which infects the first child when the second child is born." It is easy to see how this superstitious belief arose among those Ghanaians who named the disease. When a mother who has been nursing her first child bears a second child, she weans the first and puts the second on the breast. The first child soon begins to sicken and die, just as if an evil spirit had accompanied the new baby into the world and set out to destroy the older child. What actually happens, of course, is that protein deficiency follows soon after weaning, for while breast milk provides these children with sufficient protein, they are generally weaned to a protein-poor gruel.

Kwashiorkor occurs not only in Africa but in Central America, South America, the Near East, the Far East—and in some wealthier countries as well. In all these regions, mother's milk is the only reliable and readily available source of protein for infants. When the infants are weaned they are typically given enough food but this food is in the form of starchy gruel, low in protein. The gruel does not supply enough amino acids to maintain the children's bodies, much less enough to enable them to grow.

Millions of children in the world are affected by kwashiorkor. It typically sets in around the age of two. By the time children with kwashiorkor are four, their growth is stunted; they are no taller than they were at two. Their hair has lost its color; their skin is patchy and scaly, sometimes with ulcers or open sores which fail to heal. Their bellies are swollen with edema; they sicken easily, and are weak, fretful, and apathetic. Figure C4-1 is a picture of such a child.

The body follows a priority system when there is not enough protein supplied to meet all its needs. It abandons its less vital systems first. When it cannot obtain amino acids enough from dietary sources, the body switches to a metabolism of wasting, and begins to digest its own protein tissues in order to supply the amino acids needed to build the most vital internal proteins and keep itself alive. Hair and skin pigments (which are made from amino acids) are dispensable and are not manufactured. The skin needs less integrity in a life-and-death situation than the heart, so its maintenance ceases and skin sores fail to heal. Many of the antibodies are also degraded in order that their

Figure C4.1. Kwashiorkor (left). Without the swelling of edema, the child would appear emaciated. At right, the same child after nutritional therapy.

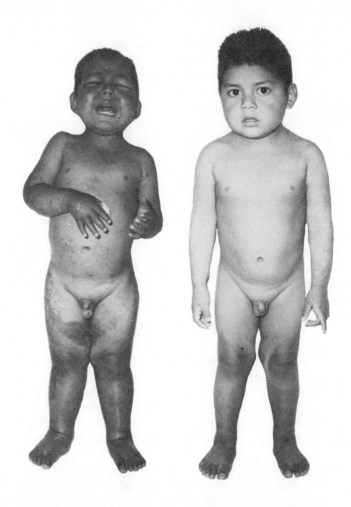

Photograph courtesy of Dr. Robert S. Goodhart, M.D.

dysentery (DIS-en-terry): an infection of the gastrointestinal tract caused by an amoeba or bacterium, giving rise to severe diarrhea.

When two variables interact so that each increases the other, they are said to be acting synergistically.

amino acids may be used as building blocks for heart and lung and brain tissue. Children with a lowered supply of antibodies cannot resist infection and readily contract dysentery, a disease of the digestive tract. Dysentery causes diarrhea, leading to rapid loss of those nutrients—including amino acids—which these children may be receiving in food. Thus dysentery worsens the protein deficiency, and the protein deficiency in turn increases the likelihood of a second or third or tenth attack of dysentery.

The water loss in diarrhea increases losses of the water-soluble B vitamins and vitamin C. The children's inability to manufacture protein carriers for the fat-soluble vitamins makes them deficient in vitamins A and D as well. Their inability to manufacture protein carriers for fat often leaves them with fat accumulated in the liver tissue, from which it would normally be carried away. As the liver clogs with fat, its cells become unable to carry out their other normal functions, and gradually they atrophy and die.

Malnourished children who contract measles cannot fight it off. In our country, where protein deficiency is not a problem, the child with measles may expect to recover within five to seven days; the kwashiorkor child dies within the first two days. Other diseases also take their toll.

The swollen belly of the kwashiorkor child is due to edema; blood protein is so low that fluid leaks out into the body. Since the child is too weak to stand much of the time, the fluid seeks the lowest available space—in this case the belly. The picture of such a child is one of skinny arms and legs and a greatly swollen belly. On first glance you might think the child is fat, but if the fluid could be drawn off, his true condition would be revealed: he is actually a wasted skeleton, just skin and bones.

Kwashiorkor is only one of several diseases associated with protein deficiency. Another, that hits closer to home for most of us, is the nutritional liver disease associated with alcoholism. The alcoholic, like the kwashiorkor child, consumes abundant calories but up to three fourths of his calories may come from alcohol, a nonprotein nutrient. Among the symptoms of protein deficiency in the alcoholic is edema, although in his case it may show up in the abdomen or in the lower extremities—the hands and feet. Also like the kwashiorkor child, the chronic alcoholic develops a fatty liver. If the situation goes unremedied for too long the liver cells ultimately die and are replaced by inert scar tissue. This is the progression to cirrhosis, which is so often caused by alcoholism.

The importance of protein as more than just an energy source must now be abundantly clear. The profound consequences of protein deficiency are suffered by millions of people in the world. They are the subject of the Highlight which follows.

synergism (SIN-er-jism): the effect of two factors operating together in such a way that the sum of their actions is greater than the sum of the actions of the two acting separately.

edema: see pages 118-119.

The "beer belly" of the alcoholic sometimes reflects **ascites** (edema in the abdomen), although it is usually rightly attributed to an excess of calories.

cirrhosis (seer-OH-sis): irreversible liver damage involving death of liver cells and their replacement by scar tissue. See also page 305.

For effects of alcohol on the liver, see Highlight 9.

Summing Up

In addition to acting as enzymes, as described in Chapter 3, proteins perform many other functions in the body. They provide osmotic pressure which regulates the distribution of water in the various body compartments (the water balance). They provide a buffering action in the body fluids which helps to maintain the acid-base balance. Antibodies, which convey immunity, and some hormones, such as thyroid hormone and insulin, are made of protein. In cell membranes, proteins known as permeases, vectorial enzymes, and transferases, confer on the cell the ability to select and take up specific compounds while excluding others, thus establishing concentration gradients. The absorption of many nutrients from the gastrointestinal tract depends on this function. Protein carriers are necessary to transport fats and fat-soluble vitamins in the circulatory system. Proteins are hydrophilic and so can carry these compounds in the watery fluid of the blood. The body's oxygen carriers, the hemoglobin of red blood cells and the myoglobin of muscles, are also proteins. Other important body proteins include collagen—the building material of scar tissue, cartilage, ligaments, bones, and teeth—and the light-sensitive pigments of the retina.

Since all body cells contain protein, routine maintenance and repair of body tissues requires a continual supply of amino acids to synthesize proteins. Growth of new tissue requires additional protein.

Kwashiorkor is the name for the disease in which protein is lacking but calories are adequate. (Calorie deficiency, known as marasmus, is treated at the end of Chapter 8.) It occurs typically in children after weaning, with severest symptoms being observed after the age of two. Symptoms include the stunting of growth, loss of pigment in the hair and skin, ulceration of the skin, edema, weakness, and apathy. The kwashiorkor victim often develops a fatty liver caused by a lack of the protein carriers which transport fat out of the liver. Reduced antibody formation makes the child extremely vulnerable to diseases such as dysentery, measles, and many others. These diseases work synergistically with the malnutrition, leaching nutrients from the body. Similar symptoms are seen in the alcoholic with nutritional liver disease.

Protein deficiency occurs whenever protein itself is lacking in the diet or when calories are inadequate. In the latter case, amino acids are degraded for energy, causing protein deficiency indirectly. The two deficiencies of protein and calories, which often go hand in hand, are together called PCM (protein calorie malnutrition), and are the world's most serious malnutrition problem. PCM afflicts millions of people, especially children. It is the subject of the following Highlight.

To Explore Further—

The chapter on immunology provides a clear and understandable explanation of the way antibodies are constructed and how they work:
Stanier, R. Y., Doudoroff, M. and Adelberg, E. A.: *The Microbial World.* 3rd ed. Prentice-Hall, Inc., Englewood Cliffs, New Jersey, 1970.

A detailed treatment of antibodies written for the layman:
Nossal, G. J. V.: *Antibodies and Immunity.* Basic Books, Inc., Publishers, New York, 1969.

Highlight Four ▬▬▬
World Protein
Calorie Malnutrition

(Man) alone by his own efforts can enlarge the bounds of empire, to the effecting of all things possible, to remolding this sorry scheme of things nearer to the heart's desire. He alone can see himself and his world in width and depth. He alone can choose, out of his vision of the present and the past, his future course.—HOMER SMITH

The story is told of a woman, well educated and beautifully dressed, who parked her car in front of a doctor's office. Late for her appointment, she rushed out of the car and bumped her knee on the door handle. She dabbed at the bleeding knee with a tissue and hurried on into the office. The cut continued to ooze blood; a nurse bandaged it. The doctor, meanwhile, became more interested in the slightly hurt knee than in her original complaint. When an hour had gone by and the knee was still bleeding he admitted her to a hospital for further tests. The diagnosis? Vitamin C deficiency! Prescription? Drink plenty of orange juice. Time to effect recovery? A few days.

While we ordinarily do not expect to find nutritional deficiencies such as this in intelligent, well-to-do persons, we have come to expect that nutritional deficiencies will present easily identifiable symptoms which will be dramatically cured with the addition of the missing nutrient to the diet. The history of nutrition science is filled with such simple and direct stories: the addition of butter to the diet curing infections of the eye, the addition of a lime a day to British sailors' diets preventing scurvy on long voyages, or the addition of the polishings of rice to the diet curing beriberi.

However, the story of protein calorie malnutrition (PCM) does not present a few observable symptoms which would lead to laboratory tests for confirmation. As you have seen in the

129

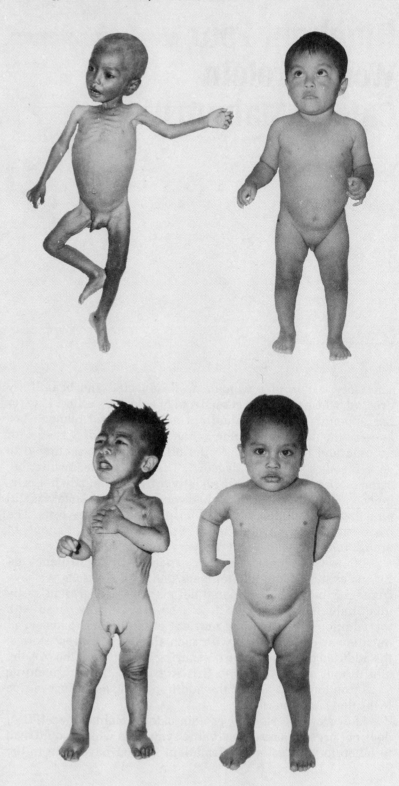

Protein Calorie Malnutrition. The children at left suffer the extreme emaciation of marasmus. At right, the same children after nutritional therapy.

Photos courtesy of Dr. Robert S. Goodhart.

preceding chapter, a lack of protein food reaches into every nook and cranny of the body, causing a vast array of symptoms.

A story about PCM might go like this: a happy little one-year-old girl lives in a shack with several brothers and sisters and her parents in Biafra (or Java or the United States). A new baby has just arrived and is now nestled close to the mother, being fed from the breast where once the little girl was held and fed. She has been banished. She must somehow learn to use a hard utensil to spoon a thin, tasteless cereal into her mouth. She pouts and cries with hunger, but no one listens. Finally, she quits trying to acquire the new skill of eating from a bowl or

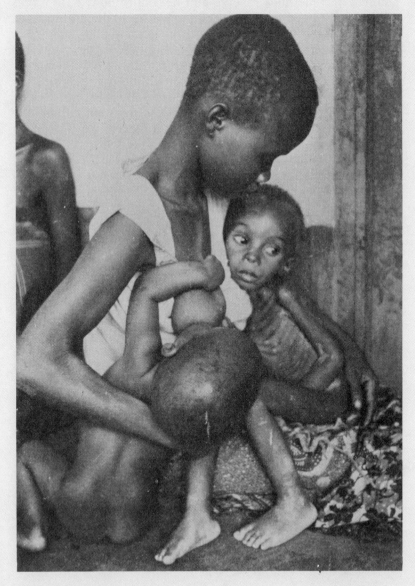

Courtesy of Wide World Photos.

spoon. She doesn't follow her brothers and sisters outside to play but wanders off into a corner and plays alone. The mother is disgusted with her churlishness and doesn't try anymore to entice her to eat. "She will eat when she is hungry," thinks the mother. Sometimes the mother forgets about her altogether, the little girl is so quiet.

This story describes a possible beginning of protein calorie malnutrition. The little girl's body is defending itself from destruction by adapting to the lower energy input with a lower energy output: she keeps still. She ingests few amino acids with which to build body tissue (hormones, enzymes, new cells). The amino acids she does receive and the entire body's resources are being directed toward supplying energy to the brain, heart, and lungs. There is no energy left for the muscular activity of running and playing with her brothers and sisters, or for smiling at her mother, or even for crying for food. Apathy is the body's way of conserving energy. Its danger, in the case of an infant who depends on the mother to give it food, is that apathy can damage the mother-child relationship to the point where the mother rejects the child. The downward spiral which is PCM has thus begun.

Apathy is just one symptom of PCM. Other symptoms result from the disturbance of the water balance (edema), reduced synthesis of key hormones (lowered body temperature), lack of proteins to transport nutrients into and out of the circulatory system (anemia), lack of protein to carry oxygen to the cells (muscular weakness) or to carry away carbon dioxide (sleepiness), and lack of protein to build collagen for scar formation (poor healing of cuts) and for growth of bones and teeth (stunted growth).

Protein calorie malnutrition particularly affects vulnerable groups in the community, such as pregnant and lactating women, nursing infants, just-weaned children, and children in periods of rapid growth. These groups have a greater need for protein than the rest of the population because of the new tissues being formed in their bodies and they need ample calories to protect that protein from degradation, yet in many cultures they are the very ones who are denied protein.

One of the most insidious and far-reaching effects of PCM lies in the possibility of its causing intellectual dysfunction. If the period of insult occurs at a critical period of brain growth, children may never attain their intellectual potential—even if they are well nourished later. It is difficult to determine when observed mental deficiencies in children are due to PCM and when they are due to other disadvantages, since social deprivation often goes hand in hand with malnutrition.[1]

[1]Tizard, J.: Early malnutrition, growth and mental development in man. *British Medical Bulletin* 30(2):169-174, 1974.

In order to study the effects of PCM on brain growth, Winick et al[2] analyzed the brain tissue of young children who died of severe marasmus as well as brain tissue from otherwise healthy, accident victims (children of comparable ages). They found that the number of brain cells of the marasmic children was significantly lower than the number in the well-fed children (Figure H4.1). Since the number of brain cells does not increase after about one year of age, this finding has serious implications for the intellectual development of the child who is deprived of protein and/or calories during gestation and the first year of life.

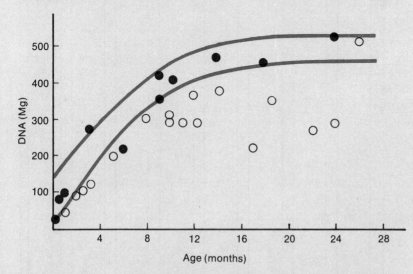

Figure H4.1 DNA content of cerebellum in brain from normal (●) and marasmic (○) children.

M. Winick, P. Rosso, and J. Waterlow. 1970. Cellular Growth of Cerebrum, Cerebellum, and Brain Stem in Normal and Marasmic children. *Experimental Neurology* 26:393-400.

The problems of protein and calorie deficiency did not surface until after World War II. At that time, increasing numbers of health teams sponsored by the United Nations and religious groups carried a message of better sanitation and improved medical care around the world. The post-war development of pesticides and antibiotics also helped raise the standards of health in many countries. Infant mortality was lowered, and recovery from infectious diseases became common. These lowered mortality rates, combined with the already high birth rates, posed a new threat: severe food shortages. There probably had always been a shortage of food, especially protein, but the problem had been masked by the more obvious one of infectious diseases. Figure H4.2 shows the prevalence of PCM in 59 countries in the decade 1963-1973.[3]

[2]Winick, M., Rosso, P. and Waterlow, J.: Cellular growth of cerebrum, cerebellum, and brain stem in normal and marasmic children. *Experimental Neurology* 26:393-400, 1970.

[3]Bengoa, J. M. and Donoso, G.: Prevalence of protein-calorie malnutrition, 1963-1973. *PAG Bulletin* 4(1):24-35, 1974. Nutrition Unit. WHO, Geneva, Switzerland.

Figure H4.2. Prevalence of severe and moderate protein/calorie malnutrition. Compilation of results from 101 surveys in 59 countries. 1963–1973.

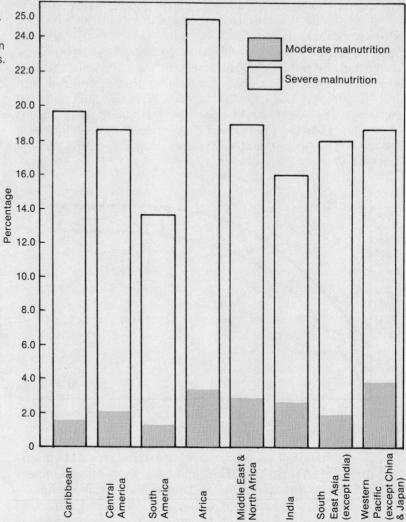

From Bengoa, J. M. and Donoso, G.: Prevalence of protein/calorie malnutrition, 1963–1973. *PAG Bulletin* 4(1): 24–29, 1974. WHO, Geneva

The factors that contribute to the development of PCM are as varied and complex as the physical symptoms observed in persons suffering from it. No one factor can be singled out as the only cause. Geography, education, traditions, economics, and birth rates are involved, all of which are interdependent.

Geography plays a part. The land may be rocky or barren and may require enormous effort to produce the minimum amount of food needed to support human life. Many of the developing countries are in the subtropical or tropical regions. With their high temperatures and rainfall, they may produce an abundant harvest. However, crop pests and bacteria also thrive in a warm, humid climate and act to reduce the harvest. If the region is near the sea, fish may be plentiful but, again, in a warm climate spoilage will take its toll.

Education may seem to be a logical answer to many of the problems. Certainly the *lack of education* is part of the evil cycle. Poorly-nourished people are too sick to use the educational opportunities open to them and so become more poorly nourished. Either they lack knowledge of birth control methods, or they fail to understand that delaying the birth of the next child until the mother has replenished her body's supply of nutrients will be an advantage to the health of subsequent children. In any case, such people continue to produce children destined to die or to live out their lives in a semi-alive condition. The people in the regions of the world where PCM is rampant have no knowledge of efficient ways to plant, fertilize, and harvest crops, and no capital with which to buy technology. Once the crops are harvested, the people do not know how to store them where insects and rodents will not destroy them or how to preserve them by drying or canning. For these people there are alternating periods of plenty and starvation, because one year's bountiful harvest cannot be made to stretch until the next harvest. With no knowledge of nutrition, they greatly reduce, by improper handling, the nutrient levels of the food they do have.

Probably the saddest causal factor of PCM is the *traditions* of the community. In many communities, meat is for males; females are not allowed meat during their reproductive years, which is the very time when they and their future offspring most need the complete spectrum of amino acids offered by meat. Traditions within a group produce food prejudices or beliefs which limit the use of valuable food. For example, some

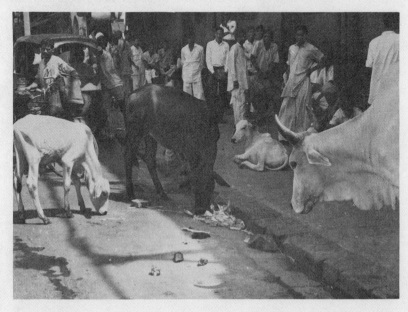

Food prejudices limit the use of a valuable food.

Credit: Courtesy of Wide World Photos.

peoples of Southeast Asia view milk as belonging to the animal's offspring and thus as not rightfully theirs to take. If urged to drink it, they will admit they think of it as an unclean body secretion.[4] Other groups have such a reverence for all life that they refuse to use pesticides, thus a farmer's crop may support the lives of the crop insects while his own children die for lack of food.

The *economic system* may work against an area's having enough food of the best kind for its own people. Countries need to have a marketable export item, even if the item is a food badly needed by their own people, in order to produce a balance of payments with which to import other needed items. Some of these import-export exchanges are difficult to understand. For instance, Africa imports high carbohydrate foods which its own land could produce, and exports pulses (peas or lentils), meat, and groundnuts which its own people need. It has been estimated that a handful of groundnuts per person per day would solve India's protein problem,[5] yet India exports its groundnuts.

An effort by the government of Java to increase its food supply produced a situation in which a large part of its already malnourished population became *less* well fed. Prior to this, about 75 percent of Java's soybeans were grown in East Java during the dry season. Rice was a second crop, grown during the rainy season.

A high yield variety (HYV) of rice seed was developed and hailed as an answer to the need for more food in Java. The government provided tremendous incentives, offering farmers fertilizer, seeds, and technical advisers in order to persuade them to irrigate their lands so that the HYV rice could be grown during the dry season. Once the land was irrigated, however, they could no longer grow soybeans in the dry season; soybean production decreased. Not only that, the farm workers then had no dry land on which to live and on which to raise cassava and other vegetables for their families, as they had done previously. After the introduction of the high yield rice, the entire country had less protein food (soybeans), and the farm workers were forced to live in the cities, paying cash for food they had formerly produced themselves.[5] Thus government intervention in the economy through inducement to use the high yield seed—a move which was thought would be beneficial—produced more PCM, not less.

As mortality from infectious diseases has decreased, more

[4]Simoons, F.: The geographic approach to food prejudices. *Food Technology* 44: 276, 1966.
[5]Palmer, I.: *Food and the New Agricultural Technology.* UNRISD Studies on the "Green Revolution," No. 5 Report No. 72.9. United Nations Research Institute for Social Development, Geneva, 1972.

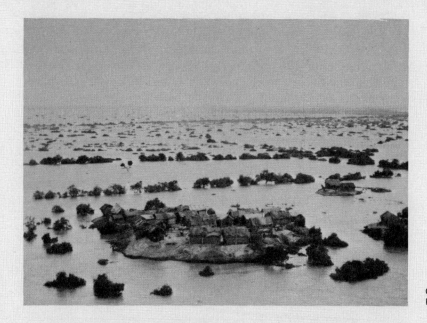

Credit: Courtesy of Wide World Photos.

people have lived more years but have had to be fed from the same amount of land. Thus we can see that a country's *birth rate* contributes to the development of PCM. The late Dr. Grace Goldsmith,[6] Dean of the School of Public Health and Tropical Medicine of Tulane University, and numerous other specialists have stated, "Population growth must be slowed, or all efforts to augment agricultural production will merely postpone mass starvation."

When it became evident in the early 1950s that there was going to be a population explosion, many people were not concerned. "Science will find a solution," we thought, just as it had found the solution to so many other plagues. It was thought that through better fertilizers and higher yield seeds, the "Green Revolution"[5] would produce enough food to take care of the population increase. However, today, in the late 1970s, the picture is even more gloomy than it was in the 50s. The world's grain stores are depleted[6] and since 1971 only three countries—the United States, Canada, and Australia—have had net exports of grain.[7] It is estimated that half the world's people live in perpetual hunger.[6] In spite of the introduction in the 1950s of improved contraceptive methods, which have received worldwide dissemination through the efforts of such organizations as the Planned Parenthood Association, populations have continued to increase faster than food production. The population of

[6]Quimby, F. H. and Chapman, C. B.: National Nutrition Policy: Nutrition and the International Situation. Select Committee on Nutrition and Human Needs. U.S. Government Printing Office, Washington, 1974.
[7]Sanderson, F. H.: The great food fumble. *Science* 188:503-509, 1975.

the United States is still increasing also. The prediction has been made[6] that our population, which in 1973 was 209 million, will be 321 million by the year 2000. This prediction is based on an average of 3 children per family, all other variables remaining the same. If, however, the birth rate declines to 2 children per family, our population size will be 266 million in the year 2000. Figure H4.3 shows how different the size of the U.S. population will be in 2070 if there is a birth rate of 3 children per family or if there is a birth rate of 2 children per family.[6]

Figure H4.3. Comparison of U.S. Population in 2070 between a rate of increase of 3 children/family and 2 children/family.

From F. H. Quimby and C. B. Chapman, 1974. National Nutrition Policy: Nutrition and the International Situation. Select Committee on Nutrition and Human Needs. Washington: U.S. Gov. Printing Office.

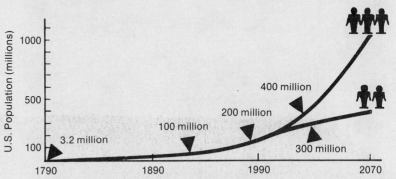

Many have been lulled into thinking that we have stopped population growth in the United States. They have misunderstood headlines that state: "America's Birth Rate Declines." *Birth rate* refers to a *rate of increase*. There continues to be an increase in the number of people to be fed, but the increase *per unit of time* has declined. This difference between an absolute increase and a rate of increase can be illustrated by the changing velocities of automobiles. Two cars are traveling side by side at 30 miles per hour. When the drivers come to the end of the reduced speed zone, they both increase their speeds. One driver increases his speed at the rate of 5 miles per hour per minute; the other driver increases his speed at the rate of 10 miles per hour per minute.

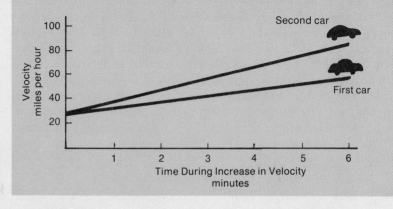

Figure H4.4. Comparison of final velocities of two cars. The first car has a rate of increase of 5 miles/hour/minute. The second car has a rate of increase of 10 miles/hour/minute.

The second driver's *rate of increase* is twice that of the first driver, but the important point for our understanding is that *both have increased their speed.* See Figure H4.4. So it is with birth rates. The United States' population is still growing—more slowly, to be sure, but it is still growing.

The increase in the United States' population from a birth rate of 2 children per family can be likened to placing the population of 7 more New York Cities into the United States between 1973 and 1998. Visualize the land requirement, food distribution, garbage disposal, and other problems connected with feeding 7 new cities that size! If the higher birth rate of 3 children per family prevails, it will be like adding 12 cities the size of New York into the United States of 1973. If you can imagine the problems presented by these increases for a rich country, you can begin to comprehend the impact of increased population on the low income countries.

Figure H4.5 shows that India will need 108 percent more calories in 1985 than it had in 1965 if its birth rate remains the same, or will need 88 percent more calories if its birth rate declines by 30 percent from its 1965 level.[6] Translating numbers of people into numbers of calories needed to feed those people illustrates the contribution which birth rates make to the prevalence of PCM. India's concern over its burgeoning population is presently being expressed in news releases from that country. The government may limit to two the number of children a family may have.

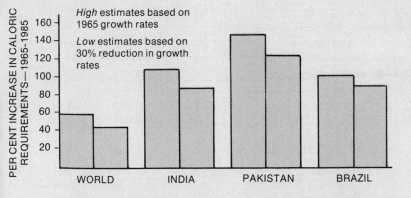

Figure H4.5. Projection of caloric requirements for the world, India, Pakistan and Brazil.

From Bengoa, J. M. and Donoso, G.: Prevalence of protein / calorie malnutrition, 1963-1973. *PAG Bulletin* 4(1): 25-35, 1974. WHO, Geneva.

We have discussed the major factors contributing to world PCM. Two others which are related to them are: *distribution*—food must go from where it is plentiful to where it is in short supply; and *advertising of food products*—mothers in low income groups around the world are beginning to quit breast feeding and are instead buying expensive prepared formulas because the ads have told them "it is better." And there are still other factors.

In this Highlight, we have examined the complexity of the condition known as protein calorie malnutrition and have had a glimpse of the many interlocking factors that produce it. The problem's complexity may give rise to feelings of despair as one wonders how the situation can ever be improved for the millions affected. However, there is hope. The problem is being attacked on a broad front by organizations within the United Nations as well as by individual governments. With the advent of effective contraceptive methods, there is a chance that the population explosion can be brought under control before the food supply runs out.

There are changing attitudes among the affluent countries too, as they realize that the problem is not one they can solve by "do-gooder" methods, the rich giving to the poor; rather, the problem is a mutual, planet-wide one whose solution will determine the survival of all, rich and poor alike. There is a fresh wind blowing, of respect for local food habits and traditions, so that research now is centering on finding food supplements which honor a country's attitudes toward foods. There is a new awareness of the need for research and education in ways of preserving the harvest.[8] Too often in the past agriculture and fishery experts have been sent to low-income countries for the purpose of improving their food economy, without being accompanied by the home economists and allied personnel who could research ways of canning and drying foods and then educate the homemakers in the use of these food products. It is now beginning to be understood that food production and distribution are of such primary importance that they must be disentangled from economic and political systems.

Nutritionists are the professionals who best understand the potential impact of protein calorie malnutrition on the people of the world. It is their responsibility to promote understanding of the problem among medical, agricultural, and other experts —and perhaps most of all among people at the grass roots level where the problem of world hunger must ultimately be solved.

To Explore Further—

Dr. Williams is the person who identified kwashiorkor. She was a pediatrician working in Africa and tells in this article how "eyeballing" techniques must be combined with modern medical practice if we are to help those in this country who are suffering from malnutrition:

Williams, C. D.: Grassroots nutrition or consumer participation. *Journal of the American Dietetic Association* 63:125-129, 1973.

[8]Aylward, F. and Tul, M.: *Protein and Nutrition Policy in Low Income Countries.* John Wiley and Sons, New York, 1975.

These books on the world food problems offer a wide spectrum of viewpoints and expertise:

Aylward, F. and Tul, M.: *Protein and Nutrition Policy in Low Income Countries.* John Wiley and Sons, New York, 1975.

Borgstrom, G.: *World Food Resources.* Intext Educational Publishers, New York, 1973.

Lowenberg, M. E., Todhunter, E. N., Wilson, E. D., Savage, J. R., and Lubawski, J. L.: *Food and Man.* John Wiley and Sons, New York, 1974.

Palmer, I.: *Food and the New Agricultural Technology.* UNRISD Studies on the "Green Revolution," No. 5 Report No. 72.9. United Nations Research Institute for Social Development, Geneva, 1972.

Recheighl, M., editor: *Man, Food, and Nutrition.* CRC Press, Cleveland, Ohio, 1973.

Robson, J.R.K., Larkin, F. A., Sandretto, A. M., and Tadayyon, S.: *Malnutrition, Its Causation and Control with Special Reference to Protein Calorie Malnutrition.* Gordon and Broach, New York, 1972.

Jansen and Howe's article deals with the problem of amino acid supplementation in parts of the world where most food is grown locally; it emphasizes the need for birth control. McPherson discusses the synthetic foods and how they can supplement the diet. Simoons' article and book contribute to an understanding of the problems of imposing one's own foods on another culture:

Jansen, G. R. and Howe, E. E.: World problems in protein nutrition. *American Journal of Clinical Nutrition* 15:262-273, 1964.

McPherson, A. T.: Synthetic foods: their present and potential contributions to the world food supply. *Indian Journal of Nutrition and Dietetics* 9(5):285-308, 1972.

Simoons, F.: The geographic approach to food prejudices. *Food Technology* 44:276, 1966.

Simoons, F.: *Eat Not This Flesh.* University of Wisconsin Press, Madison, Wisconsin, 1960.

In addition to the above, the entire issue of *Science*, May 9, 1975, was devoted to the world food problem, as well as the entire issue of *Scientific American*, September, 1976.

This article shows how the integration of findings from the behavioral sciences and nutritional sciences aids in our understanding of the effect of early malnutrition:

Tizard, J.: Early malnutrition, growth and mental development in man. *British Medical Bulletin* 30(2):169-174, 1974.

Manocha has discussed all aspects of malnutrition from its effects on the brain, to clinical signs and symptoms of kwashiorkor and marasmus, to maternal malnutrition, plus some ways of fighting malnutrition:

Manocha, S. L.: *Malnutrition and Retarded Human Development.* Charles Thomas Publisher, Springfield, Illinois, 1972.

Film, *Hungry Angels* can be ordered from:
        Association Films
        561 Hillgrove Avenue
        LaGrange, Illinois 60525

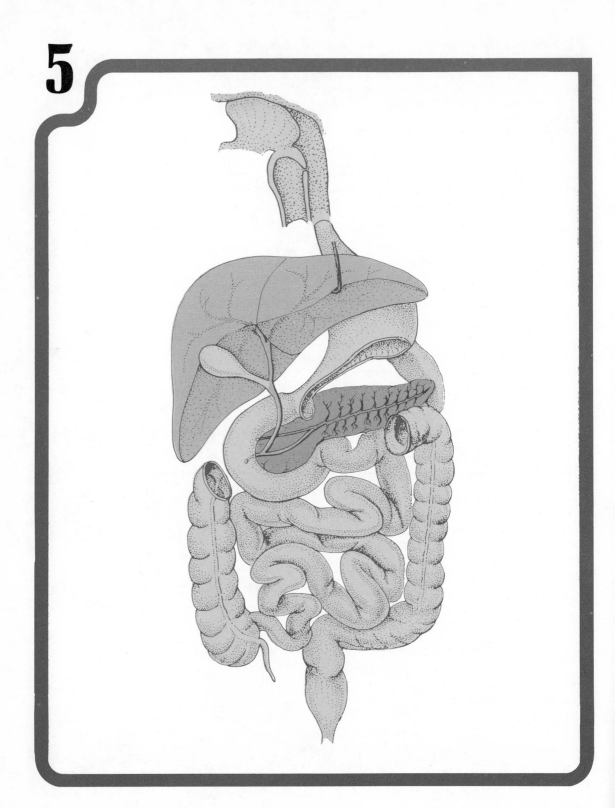

5

Digestion

Food does not become nutrition until it passes the lips.
—RONALD M. DEUTSCH

The Voyage of the Blue Glass Beads

Lynn, age one, is playing with her mother's necklace. As one-year-olds do, she puts it in her mouth and chews on it. The necklace breaks and Lynn begins to put the beads into her mouth one by one and swallows them. An hour later her mother finds her with only a few of the hundred beads left on the table. In a panic, her mother calls the doctor. "Doctor," she says, "my daughter has just swallowed a necklace!" "Don't panic," says the doctor. "What was the necklace made of?" "Glass beads," says the mother. "And how big were the beads?" "About the size of a pea," says the mother. "That's all right then," says the doctor. "You'll get them back. Just watch her diapers for a day or so."

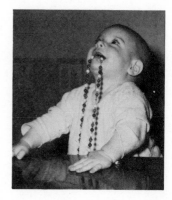

One of the beauties of the digestive tract is that it is selective. Those materials which are nutritive for the body are broken down into particles which can be assimilated into the bloodstream. Those which are not are left undigested and pass out the other end of the digestive tract. In a sense, the human body is doughnut-shaped: the digestive tract is the hole through the doughnut. You can drop beads through the hole indefinitely and none of them will ever enter the material of the doughnut body proper. Two days after Lynn has swallowed them, her mother has recovered and restrung all the beads—and is again wearing the necklace!

The problems associated with those nonnutritive dietary contaminants that can be absorbed are treated in Highlight 13.

143

The Problems of Digestion

As you see, should you ever accidentally swallow a necklace, you would be protected from any serious consequences by the design of your digestive tract. There are many other problems the system solves for you without your having to make any conscious effort. In fact, the digestive tract is the body's ingenious way of solving the problem of getting the nutrients ready for absorption. Let us consider the problems involved first, in order to appreciate the elegance of the solutions.

(1) Human beings breathe as well as eat and drink through their mouths. Air taken in through the mouth must go to the lungs, food and liquid to the stomach. Provision must be made in the throat to ensure that food or liquid do not travel to the lungs.

diaphragm (see page 170).

(2) Below the lungs lies the diaphragm, a dome of muscle which separates the upper half from the lower half of the major body cavity. Food must be conducted through this wall to reach the abdomen.

(3) To pass smoothly through the system, the food must be ground to a paste, and must be lubricated with water. Too much water would cause it to flow too rapidly; too little would make it become too compact, which could cause it to stop moving. The amount of water present should be regulated to keep the intestinal contents at the right consistency.

(4) When digestive enzymes are working on food, it should be very finely divided and suspended in a watery solution so that every particle will be accessible. Once digestion is complete, and all the needed nutrients have been absorbed out of the tract into the body, only a residue remains, which is excreted. It would be both wasteful and messy to excrete large quantities of water with this residue, so some water should be withdrawn, leaving a paste just solid enough to be smooth and easy to pass.

(5) The materials within the tract should be kept moving, slowly but steadily, at a pace that permits all reactions to reach completion. They should not be allowed to back up, except when a poison or like substance has been swallowed. At such a time, reverse flow should be put into effect, to get rid of the poison by the shortest possible route (upwards). If infection sets in further down the tract, the flow should be accelerated, to speed its passage out of the body (downwards).

(6) The enzymes of the digestive tract are designed to digest carbohydrate, fat, and protein. The walls of the tract, being composed of living cells, are made of the same materials. Provision must be made to protect these cells from the action of the powerful juices they themselves secrete.

(7) Once waste matter has reached the end of the tract, it must be excreted, but it would be inconvenient and embarras-

sing if this function occurred continuously. Provision must be made for periodic evacuation.

The following sections show how the body solves these problems.

Anatomy of the Digestive Tract

The GI tract is a flexible muscular tube measuring about 26 feet in length from the mouth to the anus. The voyage of the blue glass beads traces the path followed by food from one end to the other (see Figure C5.1).

When Lynn swallowed the beads, they first slid across her epiglottis, bypassing the entrance to her lungs. This is the body's solution to problem 1: whenever you swallow, the epiglottis closes off your air passages so you do not choke. (You may wonder, however, what happens when a person does choke: that question is answered in the Highlight at the end of this chapter.)

Next, the beads slid down the esophagus, which conducted them through the diaphragm (problem 2) to the stomach. There they were retained for a while. Then one by one they popped through the pylorus into the small intestine. At the top of the small intestine, they bypassed an opening (entrance only, no exit) from a duct which was dripping fluids (problem 3) into the small intestine from two organs outside the GI tract: the gall bladder and the pancreas. They traveled on down the small intestine through its three segments—the duodenum, the jejunum, and the ileum—a total of 20 feet of tubing lying coiled within the abdomen.

Having traveled through these segments of the small intestine, the beads arrived at another sphincter—the ileocecal valve—at the beginning of the large intestine (colon) in the lower right-hand side of the abdomen. As the beads entered the colon they passed another opening. Had they slipped into this opening they would have found themselves in the appendix, a blind sac about the size of your little finger. They bypassed this opening, however, and traveled along the large intestine up the right-hand side of the abdomen, across the front to the left-hand side, down to the lower left-hand side, and finally below the other folds of the intestines to the back side of the body, above the rectum. During passage through the colon, water was withdrawn, leaving semisolid waste (problem 4). There they were held back by the strong muscles of the rectum. When the child chose to defecate, this muscle relaxed (problem 7) and the last sphincter in the system, the anus, opened to allow their passage.

To sum it up, the path followed by the beads was:

GI tract: the gastrointestinal tract or alimentary canal. Principal organs: the stomach and intestines.

gastro = stomach
aliment = food

epiglottis

esophagus

pylorus
common bile duct

gall bladder,
pancreas
duodenum
jejunum
ileum

ileocecal valve

colon
appendix

rectum

anus

see **Figure C5.1.**

To sum it up, the path followed by the beads was:

> mouth (epiglottis) → esophagus → stomach (pylorus) → small intestine (duodenum, with entrance from gall bladder and pancreas → jejunum → ileum) → large intestine (appendix) → rectum (anus).

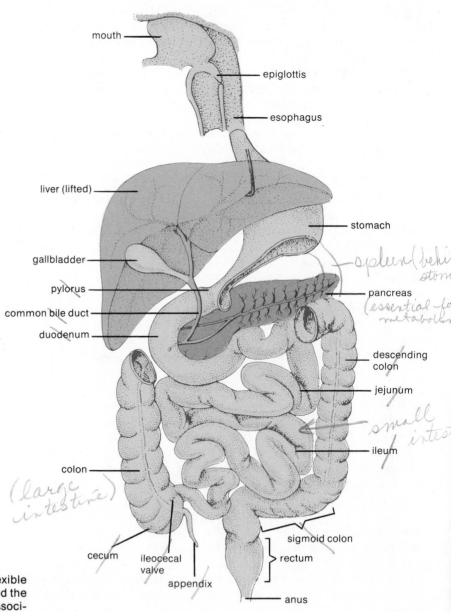

Figure C5.1. The flexible muscular tube called the alimentary canal with associated structures.

epiglottis (epp-ee-GLOT-is): the cartilage in the throat which guards the entrance to the trachea and prevents fluid or food from entering it when a person swallows.

    epi = upon (over)
    glottis = back of tongue (anatomically, the space between the vocal
          folds)

trachea (TRAKE-ee-uh): the windpipe.

esophagus (e-SOFF-uh-gus): the food pipe.

pylorus (pie-LORE-us): a sphincter muscle separating the stomach from the small intestine.

    pylorus = gatekeeper

sphincter (SFINK-ter): a circular muscle surrounding and able to close a body opening.

    sphincter = band (a binder)

gall bladder, pancreas: see pages 154, 153.

duodenum (doo-oh-DEEN-um, doo-ODD-num): the top portion of the small intestine (about "12 fingers' breadth" long).

    duodecim = twelve

jejunum (je-JOON-um): the first two fifths of the small intestine beyond the duodenum.

ileum (ILL-ee-um): the last segment of the small intestine.

ileocecal (ill-ee-oh-SEEK-ul) **valve**: sphincter muscle separating the small and large intestines.

colon (COAL-un): the large intestine. Its segments are called the ascending colon, the transverse colon, the descending colon, and the sigmoid colon.

    sigmoid = shaped like the letter S (sigma)

appendix: a narrow blind sac extending from the beginning of the colon; a vestigial organ with no function.

rectum: the terminal part of the intestine, from the sigmoid colon to the anus.

anus (AY-nus): the terminal sphincter muscle of the GI tract.

Not a very complex route, considering all that happens on the way. If you understand the anatomy of the system, and the way the parts are connected to each other, a number of common experiences can be understood: what happens when you choke on food (and what to do about it), when you vomit, when you get constipated, or when you have an ulcer. These experiences are explained in the Highlight which follows this chapter.

The Involuntary Muscles and the Glands

gland: a cell or group of cells that secretes materials for special uses in the body. The salivary glands are **exocrine** (EX-o-crin) glands, secreting saliva "out" (not into the blood) into the mouth.

exo = outside

endocrine: secreting into the blood.

endo = within

bolus (BOH-lus)

peristalsis (peri-STALL-sis): successive waves of involuntary contraction passing along the walls of the intestine.

peri = around
stellein = to wrap

Individuals are unaware of all the activity that goes on between the time they swallow and the time they defecate. Like so much else that goes on in the body, the muscles and glands of the digestive tract meet internal needs without one's having to exert any conscious effort to get the work done.

Chewing and swallowing are under conscious control, but even in the mouth there are some automatic processes over which we have no control. The salivary glands squirt just enough saliva into each mouthful of food so that it can pass easily down your esophagus (problem 3). (Occasionally, as you have noticed, they will squirt when you definitely do not want them to—when your mouth is open!) After a mouthful of food has been swallowed, it is called a bolus.

At the top of the esophagus, peristalsis begins. The entire GI tract is ringed with muscles that can squeeze it tightly. Within these rings of muscle lie longitudinal muscles. When the rings tighten and the long muscles relax, the tube is constricted. When the rings relax and the long muscles tighten, the tube bulges. These actions follow each other so that the intestinal contents are continuously pushed along (problem 5). (If you have ever watched a lump of food pass along the body of a snake, you have a good picture of how these muscles work.) The waves of contraction follow each other all the time at the rate of about three a minute, whether or not you have just eaten a meal. This prevents anything from backing up.

Diagram of Peristalsis.

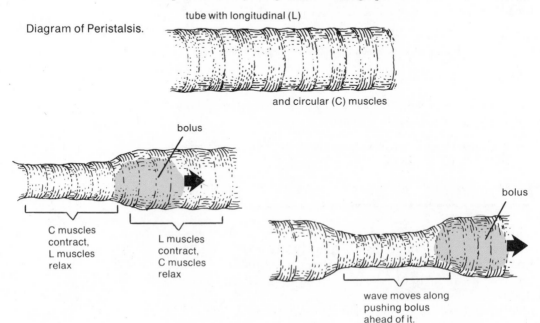

tube with longitudinal (L)

and circular (C) muscles

bolus

C muscles contract, L muscles relax

L muscles contract, C muscles relax

bolus

wave moves along pushing bolus ahead of it.

The pyloric sphincter, which stays closed most of the time, also prevents backup of the intestinal contents into the stomach, and holds the bolus in the stomach long enough so that it can be thoroughly mixed with gastric juice and liquefied. At the end of the small intestine, the ileocecal valve performs a similar function. The tightness of the rectal muscle is a kind of safety device which, together with the anus, prevents elimination until you choose to perform it voluntarily (problem 7).

Smaller and Smaller

Besides forcing the bolus along, the muscles of the GI tract help to liquefy it so that the digestive enzymes will have access to all the nutrients. The first step in this process takes place in the mouth where chewing, the addition of saliva, and the action of the tongue reduce the food to a coarse mash suitable for swallowing. A further grinding action then takes place in the stomach.

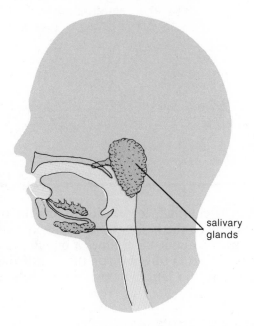

salivary
glands

Of all parts of the GI tract, the stomach has the thickest walls and strongest muscles; in addition to the circular and longitudinal muscles, it has a third layer of transverse muscles which also alternately contract and relax. While these three sets of muscles are all at work forcing the bolus downwards, the pyloric sphincter remains tightly closed most of the time, preventing the bolus from passing into the duodenum. Meanwhile, the gastric glands are releasing juices which mix with the bolus.

gastric glands: exocrine glands in the stomach wall which secrete gastric juice into the stomach.

gastro = stomach

Diagram of stomach muscles.

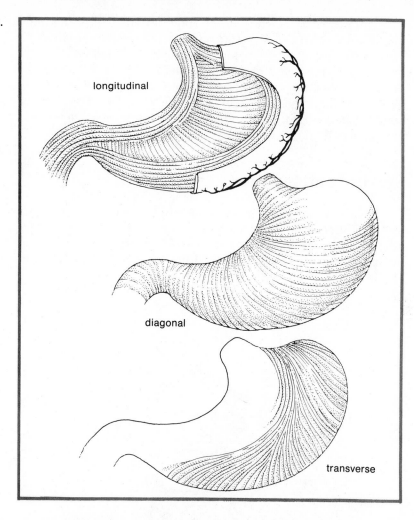

longitudinal

diagonal

transverse

As a result, it is churned, forced down, hits the pylorus, and bounces back. When the bolus is thoroughly liquefied, the pylorus opens briefly, about three times a minute, to allow small portions through. From this point on the intestinal contents are called chyme. They no longer resemble food in the least.

chyme (KIME): the semi-liquid mass of partly digested food expelled by the stomach into the duodenum.

chymos = juice

How Food Becomes You

One person may be a vegetarian, eating only fruit, vegetables, and nuts, while another may be be a meat-and-potatoes eater, avoiding vegetables and fruits entirely. Whatever the diet, people's body composition remains very much the same. It is impossible to tell, from looking at people, whether they have just eaten a bowl of spaghetti and meatballs or a mixed green salad; in either case they have converted the materials in their food into the flesh, skin, and bones they are made of. How do they do it? It all comes down to the fact, of course, that the body renders food—whatever it was to start with—into the basic units of which carbohydrate, fat, and protein are composed. It absorbs these units and builds its tissues from them. The final problem of the GI tract is to digest the food.

For this purpose, there are five body components that contribute digestive juices: the salivary glands, the gastric glands, the intestinal glands, the liver, and the pancreas.

In addition to water and salts, saliva contains amylase, an enzyme which hydrolyzes starch to maltose. The digestion of starch thus begins in your mouth, where, in fact, you can taste the change, if you choose. Starch has very little taste, but maltose has a subtly sweet flavor that you may associate with malted milk. If you hold a piece of starchy food like white bread in your mouth without swallowing it, you can taste it getting sweeter.

saliva: the secretion of the salivary glands. Principal enzyme: salivary amylase.

amylase (AM-uh-lase): an enzyme which hydrolyzes amylose (a form of starch). An older name for salivary amylase is ptyalin (TY-uh-lin).

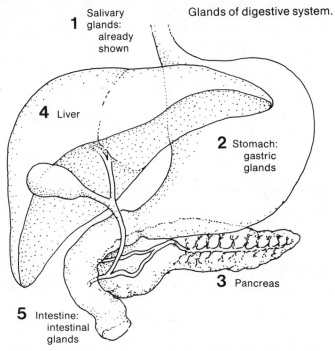

1 Salivary glands: already shown

Glands of digestive system.

4 Liver

2 Stomach: gastric glands

3 Pancreas

5 Intestine: intestinal glands

Mouth:	
Carbohydrate	starch $\xrightarrow{\text{amylase}}$ maltose
Fat	no chemical action
Protein	no chemical action
Vitamins	no chemical action
Minerals	no chemical action
Water	added
Fiber	remains

gastric juice: the secretion of the gastric glands. Principal enzymes: rennin (curdles milk protein, casein, and prepares it for pepsin action); pepsin (acts on proteins); lipase (acts on emulsified fats).

pH: see page 120.

mucus (MYOO-cuss): a mucopolysaccharide secreted by cells of the stomach wall. The cellular lining of the stomach with its coat of mucus is known as the mucous membrane.

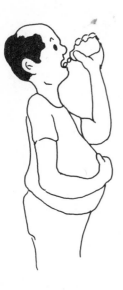

Gastric juice is composed of water, enzymes, and hydrochloric acid. The acid is so strong (pH 2) that if it were spilled on the skin, it would burn. To protect themselves from gastric juice, the cells of the stomach wall secrete mucus, a thick, slimy, white polysaccharide which coats the cells, protecting them from the acid and enzymes which would otherwise digest them (problem 6).

It should be noted here that the strong acidity of the stomach is a desirable condition—television commercials for antacids to the contrary notwithstanding. People who overeat or who bolt their food are likely to suffer from indigestion; the muscular reaction of the stomach to unchewed lumps or to being overfilled may be so violent as to cause regurgitation (reverse peristalsis: another solution to problem 5). When this happens, overeaters or bolters may taste the stomach acid in their mouths and think they are suffering from "acid indigestion." Responding to TV commercials, they may take antacids to neutralize the stomach acid. The consequence of this action is that a demand is placed on the stomach to secrete more acid to counteract the neutralizer, thus enabling the digestive enzymes to do their work.

Antacids are not designed to relieve the digestive discomfort of the hasty eater. Their proper use is to correct an abnormal condition, such as that of the ulcer patient whose stomach or duodenal lining has been attacked by acid (see Highlight 5). Antacid misuse is similar to the misuse of diuretics already described.

A flag sign of a spurious claim is the implication that:

medication designed to correct an abnormal condition is needed for the normal, healthy person.

What our misguided consumers need to do is to chew their food more thoroughly, eat it more slowly, and possibly eat less at a sitting.

All proteins are responsive to acidity; the stomach enzymes work best at pH 2. On the other hand, salivary amylase—which is, of course, swallowed with the food—does not work in this strong acid, so digestion of starch gradually ceases as the acid penetrates the bolus. In fact, the salivary amylase becomes just another protein to be digested; its amino acids end up being recycled into other body proteins.

The major digestive event in the stomach is the hydrolysis of proteins. Both the enzyme pepsin and the stomach acid itself act as catalysts for this reaction. Other events are the hydrolysis of a triglyceride by a gastric lipase and of sucrose by the stomach acid, and the attachment of a protein carrier to vitamin B_{12}.

pepsin: a gastric protease. It circulates as a precursor, pepsinogen, and is converted to pepsin by the action of the acidity of the stomach.

vitamin B_{12} and intrinsic factor: see Chapter 9.

Stomach:

Carbohydrate	(minor action)
Fat	(minor action)
Protein	protein $\xrightarrow[\text{HCl}]{\text{pepsin}}$ smaller polypeptides
Vitamins	(minor action)
Minerals	no chemical action
Water	added
Fiber	remains

By the time food has left the stomach, digestion of all three energy nutrients has begun. But the action really begins in the small intestine, where three more digestive juices are contributed. The intestine itself has glands situated in its wall that secrete a watery juice containing enzymes of all three kinds: carbohydrases, lipases, and proteases, and others as well. In addition, both the pancreas and the liver make contributions by way of ducts leading into the duodenum. The pancreatic juice also contains enzymes of all three kinds, plus others.

Evidently, food needs to be digested completely. The presence of two sets of enzymes for this purpose at this point underscores the body's determination to get the job done. If the pancreas fails, the intestine can, largely, carry on; if the intestine fails, the pancreas will do the job. Such duplication of effort is never seen in nature unless the job is absolutely vital, as in this case it is.

In addition to enzymes, the pancreas secretes sodium bicarbonate, which neutralizes the acid chyme leaving the stomach. From this point on, the contents of the digestive tract are at a neutral or slightly alkaline pH. The enzymes of both the intestine and the pancreas work best at this pH.

Bile, a secretion from the liver, also flows into the duodenum. The liver secretes this material continually, but it is needed only when fat is present in the intestine. At other times, the bile is stored nearby, in the gall bladder, which squirts it into the duodenum on request. As described in Chapter 2, bile is not an enzyme, but an emulsifier; it brings fats into suspension in water where the enzymes can work on them.

Thanks to all these secretions, everything is worked on in the small intestine.

intestinal juice: the secretion of the intestinal glands. Principal enzymes: erepsin (3 peptidases: amino-, carboxy-, and di-); enterokinase (trypsinogen → trypsin); sucrase, maltase, lactase, steapsin (small amount of fats → fatty acids and glycerol).

pancreatic (pank-ree-AT-ic) **juice:** the exocrine secretion of the pancreas (the pancreas also has an endocrine function: the secretion of insulin and other hormones; see page 15). Juice flows from the pancreas into the small intestine through the pancreatic duct. Principal enzymes: trypsin, chymotrypsin, steapsin (lipase), amylopsin (amylase), carboxypeptidase.

When the pancreas fails, fat digestion is seriously impaired, since the intestine has no major lipase.

bicarbonate: an alkaline secretion of the pancreas, part of the pancreatic juice.

bile: an exocrine secretion of the liver (the liver also has many endocrine functions). Bile flows from the liver into the gall bladder, where it is stored.

gall bladder: an organ which stores and concentrates bile. The gall bladder has no secretory function. Bile flows from the gall bladder into the small intestine through the bile duct.

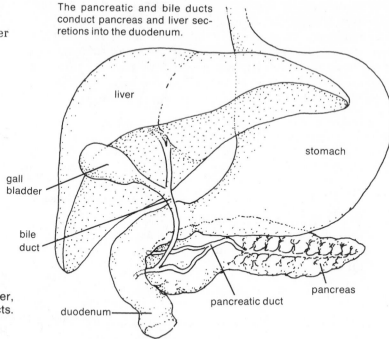

The pancreatic and bile ducts conduct pancreas and liver secretions into the duodenum.

Details of pancreas, liver, gall bladder and ducts.

Small Intestine:

All carbohydrates ⟶ monosaccharides

All fats ⟶ (bile) emulsified fats

Emulsified fats ⟶ monoglycerides or glycerol and fatty acids

All proteins ⟶ amino acids

Vitamins   no chemical action
Minerals   no chemical action
Water   added
Fiber   remains

Most proteins are broken down to amino acids before they are absorbed. With this in mind, you will be in a position to refute certain untrue claims made about foods. For instance:

"Don't eat store-bought beef. They injected a tenderizer into the blood of the steer before they killed it. When it gets into your blood, this enzyme will digest and destroy your tissues."

Just before slaughtering, pancreatic enzymes are sometimes injected into the steer's circulatory system;

they do digest tough connective tissue in the vessel walls and make the meat easier to chew. But when you eat the cooked meat, these enzymes have been denatured and cannot function as enzymes. They are but a few among thousands of different proteins in your digestive tract; they are broken down to amino acids identical to those of the other proteins you eat. Just as your body cannot tell the source of vitamin C, so it cannot tell the source of a particular amino acid.

denaturation: see page 86.

"Eat brains, the materials they are made of will nourish your brain."

Like any other nutrients, the proteins, fats, and carbohydrates in brain tissue will be digested and absorbed and will nourish the body. But they are no better than hamburger, in the sense that both are digested to basic units before absorption. Each body builds its own brain tissue from basic units which can be obtained as well from hamburger as from brains.

This discussion stresses a point that is important for the informed consumer to remember. The arguments that a *food* (tenderized beef) is harmful or that a *food* (brains) is beneficial can be identified as spurious by the flag sign mentioned before (page 65). In addition, although these arguments are logical, they are not based on *evidence*. They sound convincing, as logical statements do, but if you know the facts of nutrition you can see through them. Caution:

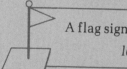

A flag sign of a spurious claim is the use of:

logic, rather than *evidence*.

Such mistaken notions are as old as mankind. Will eating beets build good red blood? Will eating polished rice rather than brown rice give you a clear white complexion? Will you get pregnant from drinking cow's milk? You know these statements are preposterous, but all of them are still believed by thousands of people less well informed than yourself. The level of misleading statements now being circulated to our better-educated public has been raised.

On the other hand, logical statements, once tested, often prove true. In a susceptible system, especially in that of a young infant, whole proteins from an uncooked food such as milk may be absorbed. They may even be beneficial, as in the case where antibodies from mother's milk confer immunity on the infant. They may cause allergy; in fact, the commonest cause of food allergy is milk protein "leaking" into the system. In each case,

milk allergy: see page 380.

when a question such as this is raised, experimental research must be done to ascertain what really happens.

This digression is not intended to review the evidence on protein absorption, but to remind you that questions regarding whether or not a constituent of food is harmful can only be answered by *experimentation*.

The story of food being broken down into nutrients which can be absorbed is now nearly complete. It remains to recall what is left in the GI tract. The three energy nutrients—carbohydrate, fat, and protein—are the only ones which must be disassembled to basic building blocks before they are absorbed. The other nutrients—vitamins, minerals, and water—are mostly absorbable as is. The function of the indigestible residues, such as fiber, is not to be absorbed but is rather to remain in the digestive tract—mainly to provide a semisolid residue which can stimulate the muscles of the tract so that they will stay in tone and perform peristalsis. Fiber also retains water, keeping the stools soft. Furthermore, it carries bile acids, sterols, and fat with it out of the body.[1]

For oxidative changes and the binding of iron, see next chapter; for the B_{12} carrier, or intrinsic factor, see page 293.

Small Intestine:

All carbohydrates	absorbed (as basic units)
All fats	absorbed (as basic units)
All proteins	absorbed (as basic units)
All vitamins	absorbed
Most minerals	absorbed
Water	remains
Fiber	remains

The process of *absorbing* the nutrients presents its own problems, which will be taken up in Chapter 6. For the moment, let us assume that the digested nutrients simply disappear from the GI tract as soon as they are ready. All are gone by the time the GI tract contents reach the end of the small intestine. Little remains but water, a few dissolved salts and body secretions, indigestible materials such as fiber, and an occasional blue glass bead. These remains enter the large intestine, where intestinal bacteria degrade some of the fiber to simpler compounds. The large intestine retrieves from its contents those materials that the conservative body is designed to recycle: much of the water and the dissolved salts (problem 4).

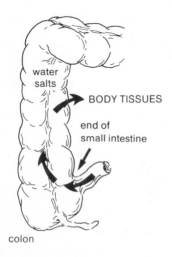

water salts

BODY TISSUES

end of small intestine

colon

Large Intestine:

Minerals	reabsorbed
Water	some reabsorbed
Fiber	some digested by bacteria; remains

[1]Scala, J.: Fiber, the forgotten nutrient. *Food Technology* 28:34-36, 1974.

At the end of the colon what is left is a semi-solid waste of a consistency suitable for excretion.

The Regulation of GI Function

This is the first chapter of the book which takes you inside the body. While you are there, watching the motions of the muscles and the secretion of the digestive juices responding to the presence of food, it is only fair to give you a glimpse of the puppeteers who pull the strings and move these actors. The story of digestion told above, although complete in outline and fair in emphasis, fails to give credit to the two marvelous systems that coordinate all the digestive processes and ensure that nothing goes wrong: the hormonal (or endocrine) system and the nervous system. This is not the place for a detailed description of advanced physiology; accordingly, the five examples given below are only intended as vignettes to illustrate the principles of the body's regulation of its internal environment.

(1) *The stomach normally remains at pH 1.5-1.7. How does it stay that way?* One of the regulators of the stomach pH is a hormone, gastrin, produced by cells in the stomach wall. The entrance of food into the stomach stimulates these glands to release the hormone. The hormone in turn stimulates other stomach glands to secrete hydrochloric acid. When pH 1.5 is reached, the gastrin-producing cells cannot release the hormone, so they stop. (The acid itself turns them off.) The acid-producing glands, lacking the hormonal stimulus, then stop secreting hydrochloric acid. Another regulator consists of nerve receptors in the stomach wall. It responds to the presence of food and stimulates activity by both the gastric glands and muscles. As the stomach empties, the receptors are no longer stimulated, the flow of juices slows, and the stomach quiets down.

hormone: a chemical messenger. Hormones are secreted by a variety of endocrine glands in the body. Each affects a specific target tissue or organ and elicits a specific response.

gastrin: a hormone produced by cells in the stomach wall. Target organ: the stomach itself. Response: secretion of gastric juice.

Gastrin regulation of stomach pH:

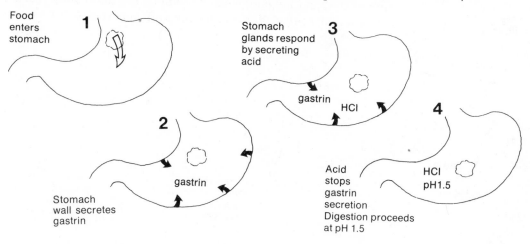

Food enters stomach

1

Stomach glands respond by secreting acid

3

gastrin   HCl

4

2

gastrin

Stomach wall secretes gastrin

Acid stops gastrin secretion

Digestion proceeds at pH 1.5

HCl   pH1.5

(2) *The pylorus opens to let out a little chyme. How does it know when to close?* When the pylorus relaxes, acid chyme slips through. The acid itself causes the pylorus to close tightly. Only after the chyme has been neutralized by pancreatic bicarbonate and the medium surrounding the pylorus is alkaline, can the muscle relax again. This process ensures that the chyme will be released slowly enough to be neutralized as it flows through the small intestine, which is important because the small intestine has less of a mucous coating than the stomach and so is not as well protected from acid.

Acid regulation of pylorus opening:

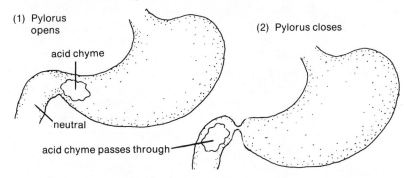

(3) *As the chyme enters the intestine, the pancreas adds bicarbonate to it, so that the intestinal contents always remain at a slightly alkaline pH. How does the pancreas know how much to add?* The duodenal contents stimulate cells of the duodenum wall to release a hormone, secretin, into the blood. This hormone, as it passes through the pancreas, in turn stimulates the pancreas to release its juices. Thus whenever there is an acid in the duodenum, the pancreas responds by sending bicarbonate to neutralize it. When the need has been met, the secretin cells of the duodenal wall are no longer stimulated to release the hormone, the hormone no longer flows through the blood, the pancreas no longer receives the message, and it stops sending pancreatic juice. Nerves also regulate pancreatic secretions.

secretin (see-CREET-in): a hormone produced by cells in the duodenum wall. Target organ: the pancreas. Response: secretion of pancreatic juice.

Secretin regulation of pancreatic secretion:

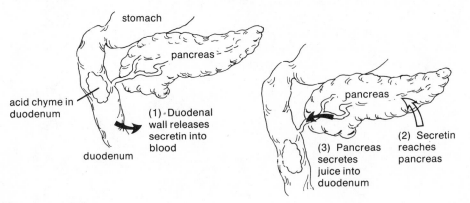

(4) *When fat is present in the intestine, the gall bladder contracts to squirt bile into the intestine, to emulsify the fat. How does the gall bladder get the message that bile is needed?* Fat in the intestine stimulates cells of the intestinal wall to release another hormone, cholecystokinin. This hormone, reaching the gall bladder by way of the blood, stimulates it to contract, releasing bile into the small intestine. Once the fat in the intestine is emulsified, and enzymes have begun to work on it, it no longer provokes release of the hormone, and the message to contract is cancelled.

cholecystokinin (coal-ee-sis-toe-KINE-in): a hormone produced by cells of the intestinal wall. Target organ: the gall bladder. Response: release of bile.

Cholecystokinin regulation of bile secretion:

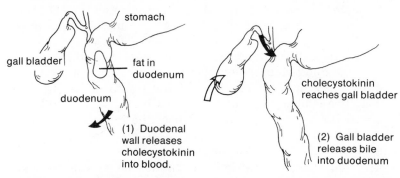

stomach

gall bladder

fat in duodenum

duodenum

cholecystokinin reaches gall bladder

(1) Duodenal wall releases cholecystokinin into blood.

(2) Gall bladder releases bile into duodenum

(3) Fat is emulsified. Cholecystokinin flow stops.

(5) *The digestion of fat takes longer than that of carbohydrate. When fat is present, intestinal motility slows, to allow time for its digestion. How does the intestine know when to slow down?* Fat stimulates the release of a hormone, enterogastrone, which suppresses the nerves that stimulate gastrointestinal motility, thus keeping food in the stomach longer. You may recall that a mixed breakfast of carbohydrate, fat, and protein was recommended in Chapter 1, partly because fat slows the digestion of carbohydrate, helping to keep the blood glucose level steady. Hormonal and nervous mechanisms like these account for much of the body's ability to adapt to changing conditions.

enterogastrone (enter-oh-GAS-trone)

Once you have begun asking questions like those above, you may not want to stop until you have become a full-fledged physiologist. For now, however, these few will be enough to make the point. Throughout the digestive system, and all other body systems, all processes are kept the way they should be, precisely and automatically, without your conscious efforts. This leaves you free to compose a symphony or gaze at the stars, rather than tying up your energy worrying about how much acid to secrete, or when to close your pylorus. This remarkable arrangement once prompted the physiologist Claude Bernard to remark, "Stability of the internal environment is the condition of free life." Walter Cannon, another physiologist, wrote a whole book about these processes, aptly called *The Wisdom of the Body.*

Summing Up

To sum up, let us follow some food through the digestive tract to the point where all needed nutrients have been absorbed. Whether it be a hamburger or a piece of chocolate cake, the same processes occur. The food is lubricated by saliva and broken up into particles by chewing in the mouth; starch digestion proceeds as far as maltose there.

The food is swallowed and carried down the esophagus by peristalsis, a muscular squeezing action which continues throughout the length of the tract. In the stomach further liquefication occurs, and the digestion of proteins begins through the action of pepsin and hydrochloric acid. The pylorus releases small portions of the liquefied contents into the duodenum.

In the duodenum the emulsification of fats occurs—thanks to bile, a secretion of the liver which is stored in the gall bladder until needed. Fat, protein, and carbohydrate digestion all proceed further through the action of the intestinal and pancreatic enzymes, while pancreatic bicarbonate neutralizes the intestinal contents to allow these enzymes to work.

As the liquefied mixture of nutrients passes along the small intestine, the three energy nutrients continue being digested until, by the time the mixture reaches the ileocecal valve, these nutrients have been almost 100 percent rendered into the simpler compounds—the carbohydrates to monosaccharides; the lipids to monoglycerides, glycerol, and fatty acids; and the proteins to amino acids—and have been absorbed. The vitamins and minerals have also largely been absorbed by this time. For the most part, only water, fiber, and some dissolved salts remain.

In the large intestine, water and salts are reabsorbed, leaving a semisolid waste which is excreted from the rectum when the anus opens.

To Explore Further—

A brief exposition of physiology for the beginner. The three pages on the digestive system are unusually clear and concise:

Schmidt-Neilson, K.: *Animal Physiology.* 2nd ed. Prentice-Hall. Inc., Englewood Cliffs, New Jersey, 1964. Paperback.

The early classic in physiology in which Cannon reveals and marvels at the ways in which the body maintains homeostasis:

Cannon, W. B.: *The Wisdom of the Body.* Norton, New York, 1932.

Teaching Aid, *GI Function and Dysfunction* includes four different slide presentations, each with an annotated syllabus. These can be purchased from:

Director, Education Services
Nutrition Today
101 Ridgely Avenue
Annapolis, Maryland 21404

Suggested Activity

Put the story together.

Follow the digestion of a glass of milk through the digestive tract until you have the products monosaccharides, amino acids, fatty acids, and glycerol. Show the steps in the breakdown, where these steps occur, and what enzymes are utilized in making each step possible. Use the chemical equation format:

organ of body: substance to be broken down—(enzyme)→product

Highlight Five ▬▬▬
Common GI Tract Problems

Crazy Quilt Questions and Patchwork Answers

The study of digestion may stimulate questions which have nothing to do directly with nutrition, but are nonetheless interesting. Assembled here are a few of the questions most commonly asked.

Students Ask About Ulcers

What is an ulcer? An ulcer can occur in many places both outside and inside the body but when a person speaks of an ulcer, the term usually means an ulcer in the stomach (a gastric ulcer), or in the duodenum (a duodenal ulcer). The term peptic ulcer includes both of these. An ulcer is an erosion of the top layer of cells from an area, such as the wall of the stomach or duodenum, leaving the second and succeeding underlying layers of cells exposed, without protection; these exposed cells exude fluid, and anything that touches the eroded area elicits pain. The erosion can proceed until the capillaries which feed the area are exposed and bleeding or until there is a perforation, a hole, in the wall.

What foods are allowed on an ulcer diet? Students often phrase this question by saying that someone they know, who has always been very careful about what food he eats because he has an ulcer, has now been told to eat almost anything he wants! Laymen are quite naturally bewildered by this change in philosophy and wonder if they are doing the right thing to once

peptic ulcer: an eroded mucosal lesion in the stomache or duodenum.

mucosal (myoo-COH-sul): of the mucous membrane.

lesion: an abnormal change in structure.

162

again eat all those formerly forbidden foods. Traditionally, the dietary measures that have been used for ulcers in this century have centered around the Sippy Diet or a modification of it, such as the bland diet. Milk, or milk and cream, given every one or two hours in small amounts, formed the basis of the Sippy Diet. Milk was used for its protein, which was thought to have an acid-buffering effect. Cream was included because fat inhibits the secretion of the acid gastric juices that increase the pain and because the fat was thought to coat the walls of the stomach. As the healing took place, low fiber foods were added gradually, but certain foods and condiments which were thought to be stimulating to the secretion of gastric juices, or thought to be mechanically irritating, were totally excluded. Recent research has shown that this rigid, restrictive approach to diet for ulcer patients is based more on tradition and folklore than it is on scientific fact.[1]

Sippy diet

bland diet: the diet traditionally prescribed for peptic ulcer. **Bland** foods are literally dull and insipid, without strong flavor or odor.

buffer: see page 120.

The mucosal layer which has been eroded away in the ulcerous region.

Underlying tissue which has also eroded.

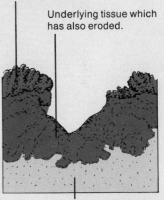

Muscle fibers seen in cross section, are also affected.

A fresh gastric ulcer has formed, eroding several layers of tissue in the stomach wall. This stained section is shown 14 times actual size.

Courtesy of Yearbook Medical Publishers.

Some interesting observations by two doctors, named Wolf and Wolff, set in motion a line of inquiry which was to result in today's controversy over what a peptic ulcer patient should eat. Wolf and Wolff were doctors at a hospital which one day in 1939 admitted a most unusual patient. This patient, remembered in scientific circles only as "Tom," had had since childhood an opening from the outside of his body through the abdominal wall into his stomach. Through this opening, called a fistula, he had learned to feed himself and, keeping his condition a secret, had grown to manhood and had lived a near-normal life. At the age of 53 while performing hard manual labor, he tore the edge of the opening of the fistula and was taken to the hospital where Wolf and Wolff were on the staff. The two doctors managed to gain Tom's confidence. He cooperated with them by allowing them to make observations of his stomach lining through the fistula. As a result, they learned that emotions called forth unique responses from the stomach. Aggressive emotions such as anger and hostility made the capillaries in the stomach lining flush with blood and caused the gastric juices to pour forth as if food had been introduced. On the other hand, when Tom was sad and depressed, there was no secretion of gastric juices, and the capillaries were pale pink instead of red. These emotional states and the stomach's responses to them were entirely independent of Tom's feelings of hunger. This discovery was exceedingly important and was duly reported in the journals. Probably the most important

[1]The American Dietetic Association position paper on bland diet in the treatment of chronic duodenal ulcer disease. *Journal of the American Dietetic Association* 58, 1971. Reprint.

result of these observations was the stimulus to experiment they gave to other doctors who had patients with fistulas. Thus, researchers began to learn exactly which foods were irritating to the lining of the stomach and which foods neutralized the acidity, instead of relying on tradition and logical thinking for this knowledge. For instance, they found that the majority of the foods that had been classified as irritating to the stomach actually had more effect when applied to the skin of the arm! This story should remind you that caution must be applied when decisions are made on the basis of logic (page 155).

CAUTION WHEN YOU READ!
A logical conclusion cannot be accepted as true until it is supported by experimentation.

In 1971 the American Dietetic Association published a paper[1] stating its position on the bland diet in the treatment of duodenal ulcer. The paper contrasted, in clear, concise language, the traditional beliefs with the newer scientific evidence. Following are quotations of some of the points of this paper:

(a) Spices, condiments, and highly seasoned foods are usually omitted on the basis that they irritate the gastric mucosa. However, experiments have indicated that no significant irritation occurs, even when most condiments are applied directly on the gastric mucosa. Exceptions are those items which do cause gastric irritation, including black pepper, chili powder, caffeine, coffee, tea, cocoa, alcohol, and drugs.

(b) Milk has been the basis of diets for duodenal ulcer for many years. One of the primary aims in dietary management of duodenal ulcer disease is to reduce acid secretion and neutralize the acid present. While milk does relieve . . . pain, the acid neutralizing effect is slight. Its buffering action could be outweighed by its ability to stimulate acid production.

(c) Roughage, or coarse food, has been excluded from the diet on the basis that it aggravates the inflamed mucosal area. There is no evidence that such foods as fruit skins, lettuce, nuts, and celery, when they are well masticated and mixed with saliva, will scrape or irritate the duodenal ulcer.

masticate: chew.

(d) The effect of a bland diet on the healing of duodenal

ulcer has been studied extensively . . . . The results indicate that a bland diet [makes] no significant difference in healing the ulcer.

(e) Individualization of the dietary plan [is encouraged] since patients differ as to specific food intolerances, living patterns, life styles, work hours, and education.

(f) [There should be] utilization of small volume, frequent feedings.

(g) It must also be recognized that rest, preferably in bed, rapidly reduces duodenal ulcer symptoms.

(h) [It is suggested that] dietetic practitioners be cognizant of the possible harmful effect of a milk-rich bland diet in patients who have a tendency towards hypercalcemia and/or atherosclerosis.[1]

hypercalcemia (high-per-cal-SEEM-ee-uh): too high a calcium concentration in the blood. See also page 375.

Except for the items listed in the quote above, all irritating items have been found to be the result of individual responses. Meanwhile, evidence[2] shows that a patient's confidence in his doctor may be more important than diet in promoting healing of an ulcer.

The effect of faith in a cure is often therapeutic in and of itself. Called the **placebo effect,** this is discussed in Highlight 10, Vitamin C and the Common Cold.

Students Ask About Vomiting

How is it that food can go in the wrong direction, as in vomiting? Vomiting is a symptom often associated with conditions that are secondary to the principal disease; or it may come from any situation that upsets the body's equilibrium, such as air or sea travel. For whatever the reason, the waves of peristalsis reverse direction, and the contents of the stomach are propelled up through the esophagus to the mouth and expelled. If it continues long enough, or is severe enough, the reverse peristalsis will carry the contents of the duodenum with its green bile salts into the stomach and then up the esophagus. Simple vomiting, while it is certainly unpleasant and wearying for the nauseated person, is no cause for alarm when it starts. It is one of the body's adaptive mechanisms to rid itself of something irritating.

Is vomiting ever serious? Yes. A doctor's care may be needed in some cases. When large quantities of fluid are lost from the gastrointestinal tract, fluid leaves the interstitial spaces to replace it. This interstitial water, in turn, must be replaced from somewhere. The nearest supply is in the capillaries of the circulatory system; it, in turn, is used to replace the interstitial fluid. To resupply the circulatory system, fluid is drawn from the cells. Therefore the crucial point about loss of fluid by vomiting is that eventually fluid is taken from every cell of the body.

interstitial space: see page 118.

[2]Williams, S. R.: *Nutrition and Diet Therapy.* The C. V. Mosby Company, St. Louis, 1973, p. 509.

electrolyte: see page 433.

intravenous (in-tra-VEEN-us): into a vein.

saline (SAY-leen): a salt solution.

Leaving the cells with the fluid are electrolytes, particularly sodium, potassium, chloride, and bicarbonate, which are absolutely essential to the life of the cells. These electrolytes and fluid must be replaced, which is difficult while the vomiting continues. Intravenous feedings of saline and glucose with electrolytes added are frequently necessary while the cause of the vomiting is being diagnosed and corrective therapy is being instituted by the doctor. In an infant, vomiting is especially serious; a doctor should be contacted soon after onset. Babies have a higher proportion of fluid in the interstitial space so that it is much easier to deplete their body water and upset their electrolyte balance than it is with adults.

There is another kind of vomiting that is not the simple type associated with nausea: projectile vomiting. In this type, contents of the stomach are expelled with such force that they leave the mouth in a wide arc, arching far out from the body, similar to the arc followed by a bullet leaving a gun. There are a number of causes for this type of vomiting, and all of them require medical care immediately.

Students Ask About Diarrhea

What is diarrhea? Is it serious? Diarrhea is the name given to the condition characterized by frequent, loose, watery stools. This sort of stool indicates that the intestinal contents have moved too quickly through the intestines for fluid absorption to have taken place or that water has been drawn from the cells lining the intestinal tract and added to the food residue. Diarrhea will be discussed in more detail in Chapter 14, but, briefly, here is an answer to the second part of the student's question: yes, it can become serious if it continues. Diarrhea causes a depletion of the fluid and electrolyte content of the body cells in the same way that vomiting does, and this condition is always serious.

Students Ask About Constipation

How often should I move my bowels? We may joke about or be irritated by the laxative commercials on television that frequently seem to appear on the screen at the dinner hour, but most persons believe the message the advertisements are sending—that is, that our neighbor Mrs. X must have a daily bowel movement or else she will be headachy and irritable and lose all her marvelous personality. The screen then shows Mrs. X the next day feeling her old jovial self because her pharmacist has persuaded her to take a laxative.

Each person's gastrointestinal tract responds to the food he consumes in its own way, with its own rhythm, the fecal matter arriving at the rectal area in a fairly constant number of hours.

Each GI tract then has its own cycle, which is dependent on its "owner's" physical makeup and such environmental considerations as the type of food eaten, when it was eaten, and when a person's schedule allows time to defecate. If several days pass between movements and these movements are experienced without discomfort then the person involved is *not* constipated, nor did he/she absorb any "toxins" which would cause irritable behavior. Nor does anyone need to worry about an inability to have daily movements—TV commercials to the contrary.

What then is constipation? When a person receives the signal that says to defecate and ignores it, the signal may not return for quite a few hours. In the meantime, water will continue being absorbed from the fecal matter so that when the person does decide to defecate, the movement will be drier and harder. If the bowel movement is hard and is passed with difficulty, discomfort, or pain, then it can be said that the person is constipated. Note that in this definition of constipation no mention has been made of the amount of time that has elapsed since the previous bowel movement; that is irrelevant.

What can I do about constipation? If there is discomfort associated with passing the fecal matter, a doctor's help should be sought in order to rule out the presence of organic disease. Once this has been done, dietary or other measures for correction can be considered.

Careful review of daily habits may reveal the causes of the constipation. Being too busy to respond to the defecation signal is a common complaint. One's daily regime may need to be re-examined with the idea of instituting regular eating and sleeping times that will allow time in the day's schedule, at the dictate of the person's body, to have a bowel movement. This may mean going to bed earlier in order to rise earlier so that ample time is allowed for a leisurely breakfast and a bowel movement.

There is a scarcity of laboratory research into the laxative quality of foods. It has been determined, however, that prunes contain a substance shown to be laxative, dihydroxyphenyl isatin. If a morning defecation is desired, prune juice should be drunk at bed time, or the prune juice could be taken at breakfast for an evening bowel movement.

Another cause of constipation that requires some rearrangement of the lifestyle is lack of physical activity. In modern society many people drive cars or ride buses to work, stand at assembly lines or sit behind desks, then sit in front of a television in the evening. Persons who do not have the time or money to work out in a spa are finding that they can park their cars a distance from the office and walk the extra blocks, or they can walk up several flights of stairs rather than take an elevator. With such planning, much exercise can be incorporated into the day. The muscles which are responsible for peristalsis are im-

constipation

defecate (DEF-uh-cate): to move the bowels, eliminate waste.

defaecare = to remove dregs

proved by any activity which increases muscle tone of the entire body.

Recent research[3] has shown that there has been a change in diet as populations have moved from the country to the city and that this has paralleled the increase in constipation. The greatest change has been in the consumption of more sugar, meat, and fat and fewer vegetables and grains which contain fiber.

Fiber from cereals has a much greater laxative effect than that from fruits and vegetables. The fiber in whole grain cereals absorbs water, enlarging its bulk and keeping the fecal matter moist and soft.[4] It is proposed that an increase in fruit, vegetables, and whole grain cereals in the diet would overcome most constipation problems. In addition, there is evidence that the low fiber content of modern diets, especially the fiber of cereals, may be a contributing cause of the increase in incidence of two modern diseases, diverticulitis and cancer of the colon. Some African villagers, who consume an unrefined diet, pass soft stools over four times the volume of those of Westerners,[3] the dietary fiber content of their diets is six times that of Westerners, and they never have diverticular disease.[4]

diverticulitis: see page 106.

Some constipation may be relieved by the addition of fat to the diet. It previously was thought that the success of this regimen was due to its lubricating effect, but it now appears to be due instead to its stimulation of cholecystokinin, which causes bile to be secreted into the duodenum. The bile acts in the same way that a saline laxative does; that is, its high salt content elicits from the intestinal wall an abundance of water which stimulates peristalsis and softens the fecal matter.

cholecystokinin: see page 159.

saline: see page 166.

Another common recommendation for helping to overcome constipation is to increase the fluid intake. Since the fluid is reabsorbed in the lower colon, it has been difficult to understand how a greater intake of fluid would soften the fecal matter. However, it has now been suggested that the beneficial effect comes from the physical stimulation of the increased bulk on the gastrointestinal tract.

These suggested changes in diet or life style should correct chronic constipation without the use of laxatives. One of the fallacies often perpetrated by television commercials is that one person's successful use of a laxative product is a good recommendation for another person to use that product. As a matter of fact, even diet changes that are successful in relieving constipation for one person may increase the constipation of another. For instance, if a person has a spastic type of constipation in which the peristalsis is promoting strong contractions that act to close off a segment of the colon, preventing passage, then

[3]Tunaley, A.: Constipation—the secret national problem. *Nutrition* 28(2): 91-96, 1974.
[4]Scala, J.: Fiber, the forgotten nutrient. *Food Technology* 28: 34-36, 1974.

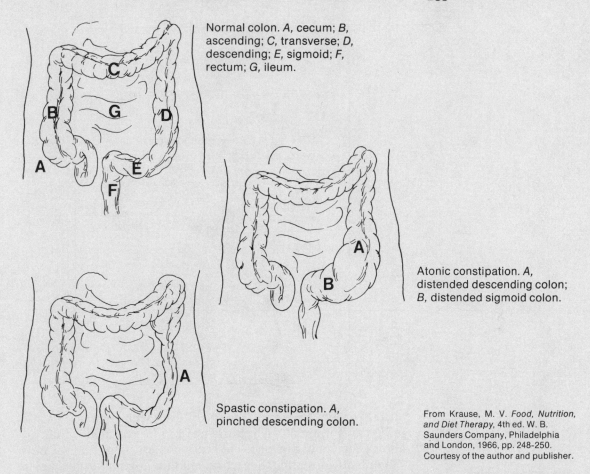

Normal colon. *A*, cecum; *B*, ascending; *C*, transverse; *D*, descending; *E*, sigmoid; *F*, rectum; *G*, ileum.

Atonic constipation. *A*, distended descending colon; *B*, distended sigmoid colon.

Spastic constipation. *A*, pinched descending colon.

From Krause, M. V. *Food, Nutrition, and Diet Therapy*, 4th ed. W. B. Saunders Company, Philadelphia and London, 1966, pp. 248-250. Courtesy of the author and publisher.

increasing the bulk in the diet would be contraindicated. A good rule is that if laxatives seem to be indicated, a doctor's advice should be sought.

Students Ask About Choking on Food

How is it that sometimes people choke on food? At the rear of the mouth there is an area called the pharynx where passageways for air and food cross each other. *Air* enters the nasal passages, goes through the pharynx, crosses to the front of the throat to enter the trachea, passes over the sound box (larynx), and continues into the deeper parts of the lungs. *Food*, readied for swallowing, is guided by the tongue toward the pharynx. When swallowing begins, respiration is stopped by a reflex mechanism which causes the soft palate to push up and close the entrance to the nasal passages and the epiglottis to push forward and close the trachea. The epiglottis' action keeps particles of food out of the trachea, and thus out of the lungs. This mechanism is marvelously effective but occasionally breaks down when a person breathes in, or talks, or laughs while bits

pharynx

soft palate (PAL-ut): the soft part of the roof of the mouth, near the throat.

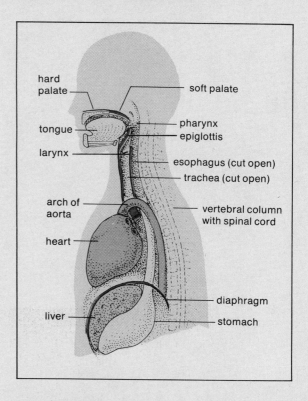

of food are in the mouth. Small children who have not learned to be careful about such things need to be watched if they are allowed to chew gum or to eat hard-to-chew items, such as nuts. When food goes into the trachea, another automatic mechanism attempts to expel it. The trachea and its branches in the upper respiratory tract are lined with cilia which, when touched by foreign particles (such as mucus or food), set up a coughing re-

cilia (singular, **cilium**) (SILL-e-uh, SILL-ee-um): hairlike projections from cells.

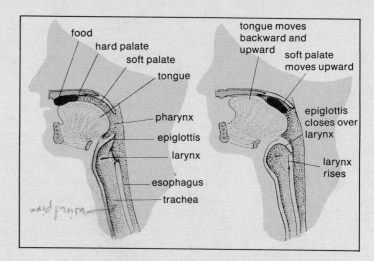

Swallowing action.

action that pushes the offending substance up the trachea to the mouth where it can be expelled.

What should be done for the person who is choking? Don't hit him on the back! If you do, the particle may become lodged more firmly in his air passage. If the choking person is a child, pick him/her up by the ankles so that gravity can aid the coughing mechanism in getting rid of the particle. Also, don't be afraid to probe in the throat for the cause of the choking. If you should scratch the throat tissues with your finger, healing will soon occur. If the choking person is an adult, lay him on his stomach across a table or bed with his head and neck off the support and almost vertical to the floor. Again, gravity will help. Now—and not before—you can slap him sharply between the shoulder blades to help dislodge the particle.

I know someone who got food lodged in his throat who didn't make a sound. He didn't even cough! Yes, food can lodge so securely in the trachea that all air is cut off; no sound can be made, since the larynx is in the trachea and depends on having air pushed across it to make sounds. This has happened often enough so that the event has been given a name: a cafe coronary. The scenario reads like this: a person is dining in a restaurant with friends. A chunk of food, usually meat, becomes lodged in the trachea so firmly that he/she cannot make a sound. Often, the person suffers alone rather than "make a scene in public," or if the victim tries to communicate distress to friends, he/she must depend on pantomime. The friends are bewildered by these antics and when, after a few minutes without air, the victim "faints" they are terribly worried. They call a doctor or an ambulance. However, by the time of arrival at the hospital the victim is dead—from suffocation. In the past, many of these cases were diagnosed as "death by coronary thrombosis"—thus the name, cafe coronary.

larynx: the voice box.

What can I do to help? First, and most importantly, ask this critical question, "Can you make any sound at all?" If the victim makes a sound, relax; you have time to continue with your questioning to see what you can do to help; you are not going to have to make a quick decision. But if the victim should be unable to make a sound, reach into the throat to see if you can pull out the offending food. If this fails, walk behind the victim, put your arms around the lower part of his/her rib cage. Make a fist with one hand and place the fist over the spot shown on the diagram (next page). Grasp the wrist of your balled up hand with your other hand and give a sudden, strong hug. What you are hoping to accomplish with this quick bear hug is to push the diaphragm upward. The diaphragm is a broad band of muscle that separates the chest region from the abdominal region; the brain controls its rise and fall. When it arches, air is pushed out of the lungs, when it flattens, air is caused to flow into the lungs.

The Heimlich Maneuver

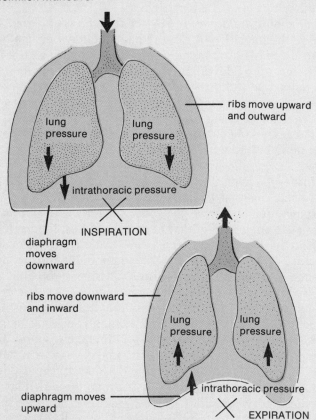

ribs move upward
and outward

lung
pressure

lung
pressure

intrathoracic pressure

INSPIRATION

diaphragm
moves
downward

ribs move downward
and inward

lung
pressure

lung
pressure

diaphragm moves
upward

intrathoracic pressure

EXPIRATION

X marks the spot at the base of
the sternum (breast bone) where
fist should be positioned. This
maneuver credited to Dr. Henry
Heimlich, M.D., Cincinnati, O.

The Heimlich Maneuver
(named for Dr. Henry Heimlich of Cincinnati, Ohio).

When using the Heimlich Maneuver described above, you will
be pushing the diaphragm upward in a sharper-than-normal arc,
giving the residual air in the lungs a push outward. The hope is
that this air will be effective in dislodging the stuck food particle
in the same way that a build-up of gas pressure in a bottle of
wine can push the cork out of the bottle. One word of caution:
be certain that the fist is in position against the person's body
and that you proceed with the hug from that position. There
should be no slamming of the fist against the rib cage; this might
cause the food to be more securely lodged in the trachea. It
would be well to practice this technique at home, for there is
no time to hesitate once you are called upon to perform this
death-defying act.

To Explore Further—

An excellent reference for the way in which various laxatives
work, listing about 90 over-the-counter laxatives by brand name with
classification and site of action:

Corman, M. C., Veidenheimer, M. C., and Coller, J. A. Cathartics.
American Journal of Nursing 75(2): 273-279, 1975.

Film, *The Heimlich Maneuver,* is now being shown by local chapters of the American Red Cross. The film, a 16-minute, 16-millimeter, color film, can be obtained from:

Paramount-Oxford Films
5451 Marathon St.
Hollywood, California 90038

6

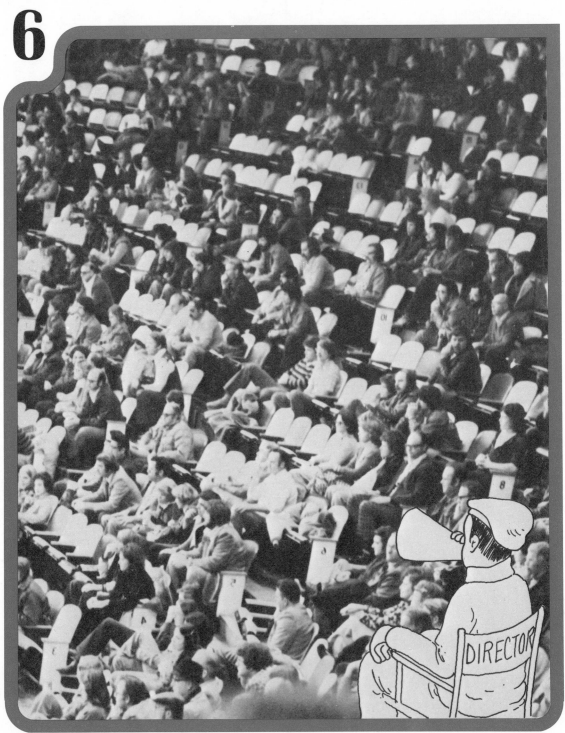

Everyone out of the picture in five minutes!

Absorption

I know there have been
certain philosophers, and
they learned men, who
have held that all bodies
are endowed with sense;
nor do I see, if the nature
of sense be set alongside
reaction solely, how they
can be refuted.
—THOMAS HOBBES

Exit into the Wings

Problem: given an elaborate stage production in which 1,000 actors are on stage at once, provide a means by which all can exit simultaneously! This, simply stated, is the problem of absorption. Within three or four hours after you have eaten a steak dinner with potato, vegetable, salad, and dessert, your body must find a way to absorb some two hundred thousand million, million, million amino acid molecules one by one, to say nothing of the other nutrient molecules! For the stage production, the manager might design multiple wings, into all of which the actors could crowd, twenty at a time. In fantasy, if the manager were a mechanical genius he might somehow design moving wings which would actively engulf the actors as they approached. The absorptive system is no fantasy; in twenty feet of small intestinal wall, this system provides over a quarter acre of surfaces with which the nutrient molecules can come in contact and through which they can be absorbed. To remove them rapidly and provide room for more to be absorbed, a rush of circulation continuously bathes these surfaces, washing away the absorbed nutrients and carrying them to the liver and other parts of the body.

Anatomy of the Absorptive System

Surface features of small intestine:

folds

villi (singular: **villus)** (VILL-ee, VILL-us)

microvilli (singular: **micro-villus)** (MY-cro-VILL-ee, -us)

The inner surface of the small intestine looks smooth to the naked eye, but if looked at through a microscope it is seen to be wrinkled into hundreds of folds. Each of these folds, in turn, is covered with thousands of nipple-like projections, as numerous as the nap hairs on velvet fabric. Each of these small intestine projections is a villus:

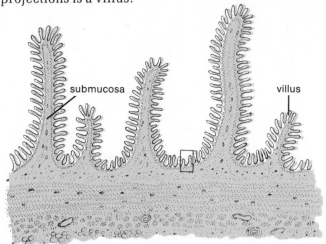

If you could look still closer, you would see that each nipple/villus was in turn covered with minute hairs, the microvilli:

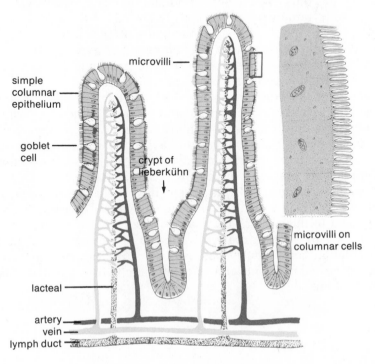

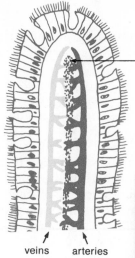

lacteals

veins   arteries

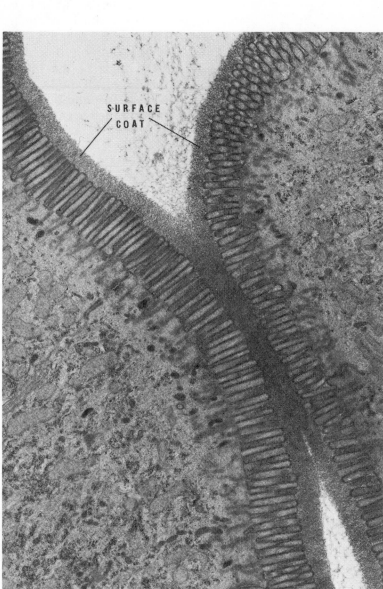

SURFACE
COAT

Microvilli and mucous
coating on two adjacent
intestinal villi. Photographed
through an electron microscope at a magnification of
51,000 x.

Photo courtesy of Dr. Susumu Ito.

A nutrient molecule such as an amino acid, encountering any part of this surface, will be drawn into the cells which compose it.

The villi are in constant motion, waving, squirming and wriggling like the tentacles of a sea anemone. They actively reach for and engulf nutrient molecules, aided by a thin sheet of muscle that lines each of them.

Once a molecule has entered a cell in a villus, the next problem is to transfer it into a circulatory system so that it can be carried away. Surrounding and supporting the stomach and intestines is the strong, flexible mesenteric membrane which enwraps the folds of the intestines. In this membrane are located the vessels of the two circulatory systems of the body: the vascular system and the lymphatic system. Vessels of both systems are supplied to each villus, as shown below:

mesenteric membrane (mesentery) (mez-en-TERR-ic, MEZ-en-terr-ee)

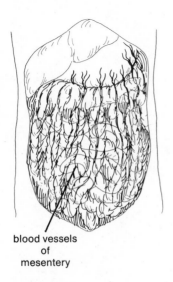

blood vessels
of
mesentery

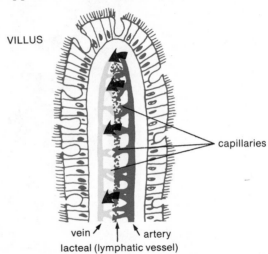

VILLUS

capillaries

vein   artery
lacteal (lymphatic vessel)

When a nutrient molecule has crossed a cell of the villus, it may enter either the lymph or the blood. In either case, the nutrients all end up in the blood, as you will see. In general, at first, water-soluble nutrients are taken directly into the blood stream.

lymph (LIMF): the body's interstitial fluid, between the cells and outside the vascular system. Lymph consists of all those constituents of blood which can escape from the vascular system; it circulates in a loosely organized system of vessels and ducts known as the lymphatic system.

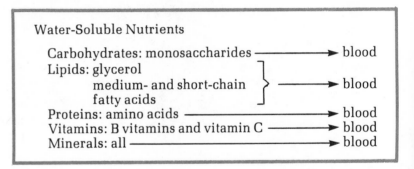

Water-Soluble Nutrients

Carbohydrates: monosaccharides ⟶ blood
Lipids: glycerol
       medium- and short-chain } ⟶ blood
       fatty acids
Proteins: amino acids ⟶ blood
Vitamins: B vitamins and vitamin C ⟶ blood
Minerals: all ⟶ blood

Fat-soluble nutrients travel by way of the lymph to a place where the two fluids mingle; there they enter the blood.

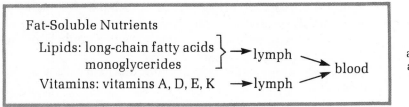

Fat-Soluble Nutrients

Lipids: long-chain fatty acids ⎫ → lymph
        monoglycerides ⎭   → blood
Vitamins: vitamins A, D, E, K → lymph

absorption of lipids: see also pages 186-187.

Where To?

Once a nutrient has entered the blood or lymph circulatory system, it may be transported to any part of the body and thus become available to all the body cells, from the tips of the toes to the roots of the hair. To understand the way in which nutrients arrive at the toes or the hair roots, you must understand the anatomy of the circulatory systems.

The vascular or blood circulatory system is a closed system of vessels through which blood flows continuously in a figure eight, with the heart serving as a pump at the crossover point. The system is diagrammed below. A function of the blood that is familiar to everyone is that of carrying oxygen from the lungs to the tissues and then carrying carbon dioxide back to the

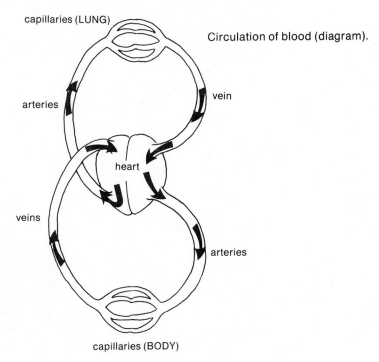

capillaries (LUNG)

Circulation of blood (diagram).

arteries

vein

heart

veins

arteries

capillaries (BODY)

artery: a vessel carrying blood away from the heart.

capillary (CAP-ill-ary): a small vessel at the farthest distance from the heart. Capillaries connect arteries to veins. Exchange of blood and tissue fluids takes place across capillary walls.

vein: a vessel carrying blood back to the heart.

lungs. Blood leaving the right chambers of the heart circulates through the lung capillaries, and then back through the veins to the left chambers of the heart. The left chambers of the heart then pump the blood out through arteries to all parts of the body, where it circulates in the capillaries and then is collected in veins which return the blood again to the right chambers of the heart. Then it starts around again.

In all cases but one, blood leaving the heart travels this simple route:

heart→artery→capillaries→vein→heart.

Only the blood circulating through the mesentery goes through a second capillary bed (in the liver):

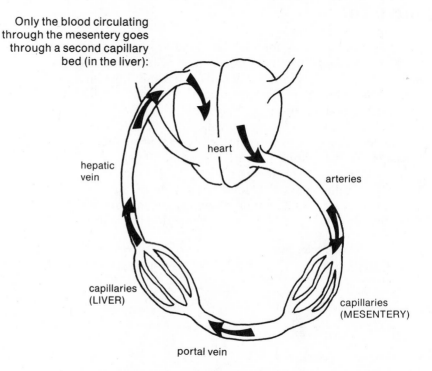

Only in the case of the digestive system does the blood flow twice through a capillary bed:

heart→artery→(mesenteric) capillaries→
(portal) vein→(liver) capillaries→
(hepatic) vein→heart.

portal vein: the vein which collects blood from the mesenteric capillaries and conducts it to capillaries in the liver.

hepatic (he-PAT-ic) **vein:** the vein which collects blood from the liver capillaries and returns it to the heart.

hepat = liver

An anatomist studying this system knows there must be a reason for it. Blood leaving the mesentery must flow through capillaries in the liver before it is returned to the heart. We might guess that the liver is placed in the circulation at this point in order to have the first chance at the materials absorbed from the GI tract. Perhaps the liver stands as a gatekeeper to waylay intruders that might otherwise harm the heart? Perhaps this is

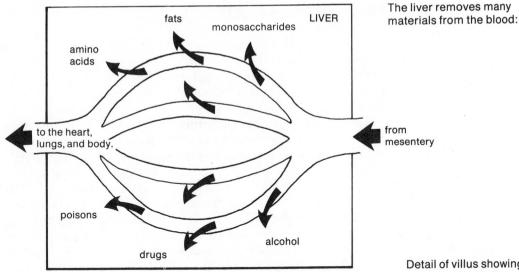

The liver removes many materials from the blood:

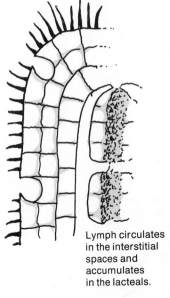

Detail of villus showing lymphatic spaces.

Lymph circulates in the interstitial spaces and accumulates in the lacteals.

why, when we ingest poisons that succeed in passing the first barrier (the GI tract membrane) and enter the blood, it is the liver that suffers the damage—from hepatitis virus, from drugs such as barbiturates, from alcohol, from poisons such as DDT, from toxic metals such as mercury? Perhaps, in fact, we have been undervaluing our livers, not knowing what quiet and heroic tasks they perform for us without seeking thanks or praise? A Highlight following Chapter 9 focuses on the liver, in case you are interested in more information about this organ.

The lymphatic system is an open system that can be pictured simply as being similar to the spaces in a sponge. If you wet a sponge, its spaces fill with water. If you squeeze it, you can force the water from one end of the sponge to the other. Between the cells of the body there are spaces similar to those in the sponge; the fluid circulating in them is the lymph. This fluid is almost identical to the fluid of the blood except that it contains no red blood cells, because they cannot escape through the blood vessel walls. The spaces between the cells are somewhat imprecisely called lymphatic "vessels."

The lymphatic system has no pump; rather, lymph, like the water in a sponge, "squishes" from one portion of the body to another as muscles contract, causing pressure here and there. Ultimately much of the lymph collects in a large duct behind the heart called the thoracic duct. This duct terminates in a vein which conducts the lymph into the heart itself. Thus materials from the GI tract which enter lymphatic vessels in the villi ultimately enter the blood circulatory system and then circulate through arteries, capillaries, and veins like the other nutrients. In other words, nutrients which are absorbed at first into lymph later get into the blood.

thoracic (thor-ASS-ic) **duct:** a duct of the lymphatic system which collects lymph that has circulated to the upper portion of the body. The **subclavian vein** connects this duct with the right auricle of the heart, providing a passageway by which lymph can be returned to the vascular system.

The Problems of Absorption

As the digestive system is the body's way of solving the problems of preparing the nutrients for absorption, so the absorptive system represents the body's solutions to some still more complex problems. It must not only *select* the nutrients that are needed, but must also, as far as possible, *regulate the amounts* of each that are permitted to enter. After all, once they have passed the barriers of the intestinal walls, the compounds are a lot closer to you than they were before. To obtain the right mix, your absorptive system, like a very discriminating hostess, bars the door to some, permits others to enter freely, and provides positive and forceful encouragement for still others to enter.

If the system worked perfectly, the compounds entering your body in a day would be a mixture containing exactly the amount of each that you needed that day. It does work this way for some nutrients, which are absorbed in greater amounts when you need more, and in lesser amounts when you need less. But for others, the absorption system has no defense against excesses. It absorbs water, for example, depending on how much you drink, and salt and fat-soluble vitamins depending on how much you eat. The burden falls on another system to select out those compounds which you have absorbed in too great amounts relative to your needs. This is the excretory system.

The principal excretory system is the renal system, composed of the kidneys, bladder, and associated plumbing. All compounds that circulate in the blood are filtered through the kidneys, which thus have the opportunity to monitor the amounts present and subtract excess amounts from the blood. In the case

Kidneys and excretory system:

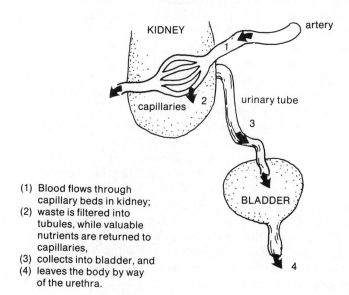

(1) Blood flows through capillary beds in kidney;
(2) waste is filtered into tubules, while valuable nutrients are returned to capillaries,
(3) collects into bladder, and
(4) leaves the body by way of the urethra.

of water and salt, the kidneys thus protect you from excesses by varying the amounts they excrete. Other routes of excretion are the sweat glands, through which (to a limited extent) water, salt, and other minerals can be excreted and the lungs, through which gasses (including carbon dioxide, water vapor, and some alcohol) can exit.

Thus, you absorb the right amount of some nutrients; you absorb more than you need of others but excrete the excess so that you *net* the right amount. This leaves a small but important group of compounds which the absorptive system does not exclude (so that excesses can be taken in), and the excretory system does not excrete efficiently (so that excesses can accumulate in the body). What often happens in this last case is that the compound accumulates in a specific tissue or organ in the body.

The principal organ in which compounds of this last type accumulate is the liver. This organ is strategically located; it is the first station through which blood passes after leaving the intestines where it has picked up absorbed compounds. Other important storage tissues are bone and fat.

Thus there are, broadly speaking, three possible ways for your body to maintain optimal tissue concentrations of the compounds it has access to: (1) by regulating absorption, (2) by absorbing freely but regulating excretion, and (3) by absorbing freely and sequestering or storing the excess. With these three possibilities in mind, we can survey the nutrient classes and see how each, in general, is handled.

Water flows freely into the body fluids from the intestinal tract, and its excretion is closely regulated by the kidneys so that the output exactly equals the input in a given period of time. If you measure the amount of fluid you drink and the volume of the urine you excrete over a twenty-four-hour period you may be amazed to see how accurately this is handled. Only ten percent of the water you drink in a day is lost in the feces.

The energy nutrients. Monosaccharides (from carbohydrate), monoglycerides, glycerol, and fatty acids (from lipids), and amino acids (from proteins) are absorbed actively, so that less than ten percent of each is lost. Energy is precious. Even if not needed today, it may be in short supply tomorrow, so it is stored against a possible future need. From carbohydrate, some of the excess absorbed glucose (that remains after energy needs are met) is stored in the liver and muscles as glycogen; the remainder is converted to fat and stored in adipose cells. From lipid, the excess (that remains after energy needs are met) is stored as fat in adipose cells. From protein, the excess amino acids (that remain after energy needs are met and the needed proteins have been synthesized) undergo removal of their nitrogen (which cannot be deposited in fat) and then are converted

The kidneys depend in turn, however, on the integrity of the vascular system to carry these compounds to them. If the vascular system goes out of order and water and salt leak out into the tissues, then the kidneys cannot "see" the excess accumulation and do not excrete enough to bring the concentrations down to optimum. See edema, page 119.

adipose (AD-i-poce) **cells:** fat cells.

either to glucose or to fat and similarly stored. The nitrogen remaining is excreted by the kidneys.

Vitamins. The vitamins, too, are invited in freely. Excess water-soluble vitamins are then excreted by the kidneys, while the excess fat-soluble vitamins are stored, mostly in liver, bone, and adipose tissue—a fact which has important implications for the overdoser (see pages 272-273).

Minerals. The minerals vary in the extent to which they are taken up by the absorption system. Some, like sodium, potassium, and chlorine, are freely absorbed, placing the burden on the kidneys to excrete the excesses. Others, like calcium and iron, are regulated; that is, the body absorbs more when its stores are less, but never with very great efficiency. Absorption of calcium ranges from 10 to 30 percent of that ingested, while absorption of iron is about 10 percent of the amount available. A consequence of this, of course, is that you must eat three to ten times as much calcium, and ten times as much iron, as your body needs to take in. These absorption factors are taken into consideration by those who calculate the RDA.

The Selective Cell Membranes

The above summaries outline *what* the body does, but not *how* it does it. A closer look at the actual cells of the intestinal walls will show how they bar some compounds, allow others to enter freely, and actively import still others that would not otherwise enter by themselves.

To get into your body after being swallowed, a compound must first get into an intestinal wall cell from the intestinal contents, then leave the cell on the body side, and then either travel through lymph or cross a capillary wall to travel in the blood.

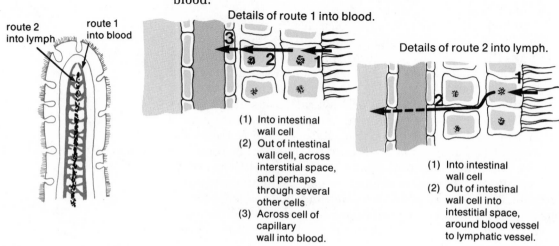

route 2 into lymph   route 1 into blood

Details of route 1 into blood.

Details of route 2 into lymph.

(1) Into intestinal wall cell
(2) Out of intestinal wall cell, across interstitial space, and perhaps through several other cells
(3) Across cell of capillary wall into blood.

(1) Into intestinal wall cell
(2) Out of intestinal wall cell into intestitial space, around blood vessel to lymphatic vessel.

The membranes of the cells in the intestinal walls are the major selective agents for the contents of your GI tract. It is in these membranes that *selection* of the compounds to be absorbed and *regulation of the amount* absorbed occurs.

Several means of absorption are employed by the membranes of these cells. In order of increasing complexity, they are as follows:

(1) *Passive diffusion*. Water crosses the cell membranes freely, without hindrance. The concentration of water tends to equalize on the two sides of the membrane—as long as there is more outside the cell it flows in; if there is more inside the cell it flows out. The cell cannot regulate the entrance and exit of water directly but can control it indirectly by concentrating some other substance to which water is attracted, such as protein or sodium. Thus the cell can pump in sodium, and water will follow passively. This is the way the cells of the large intestinal wall act to retrieve water for the body. Since nearly all the sodium is taken into these cells before waste is excreted, nearly all the water is absorbed too.

(2) *Facilitated diffusion*. Other compounds cannot cross the membranes of the intestinal wall cells unless there is a specific carrier or facilitator in the membrane. The carrier may shuttle back and forth from one side of the membrane to the other, carrying its passengers either way, or it may affect the permeability of the membrane in such a way that the compound is admitted. Insulin probably works the latter way to facilitate the entrance of glucose into liver and other cells. The end result is the same as for passive diffusion: equal concentrations are reached on both sides. By providing carriers only for the desired compounds, the cell effectively bars all others (except those to which it is freely permeable).

(3) *Active transport*. For compounds that must be absorbed actively, the two types of diffusion systems mentioned above will not suffice. The best a cell can do, using diffusion alone, is to take up a compound until the concentration inside the cell is equal to that outside. An effective means of *concentrating* a substance inside the cell is to pump it in by using the permeases, as described on page 121. The monosaccharides, amino acids, and other nutrients are absorbed by intestinal wall cells in this manner.

The three means described above account for the majority of absorptive events in the GI tract. A fourth means of taking up substances that is sometimes employed by cells is pinocytosis. In this process, a large area of the cell membrane is involved, actively engulfing whole

passive diffusion

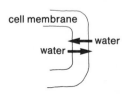

cell membrane

water

water ← water

facilitated diffusion, also called **carrier mediated diffusion** or **passive transport**.

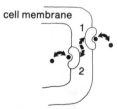

cell membrane

(1) Carrier loads particle on outside of cell,
(2) releases particle on inside of cell, *or the reverse.*

active transport: see also page 227.

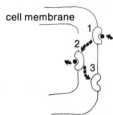

cell membrane

(1) Carrier loads particle on outside of cell,
(2) releases particle on inside of cell,
(3) returns to outside to pick up another. Powered by energy carrier, ATP (see page 227).

pinocytosis (pie-no-sigh-TOE-sis, pin-o-sit-TOE-sis)

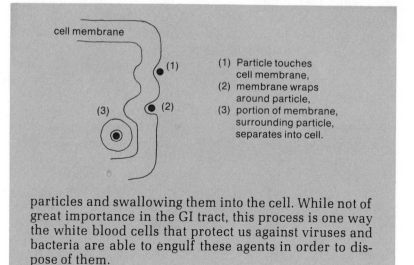

cell membrane

(1) Particle touches cell membrane,
(2) membrane wraps around particle,
(3) portion of membrane, surrounding particle, separates into cell.

particles and swallowing them into the cell. While not of great importance in the GI tract, this process is one way the white blood cells that protect us against viruses and bacteria are able to engulf these agents in order to dispose of them.

The above three mechanisms account for the absorption of the water-soluble nutrients. These mechanisms can now be summed up as follows:

Water-soluble Nutrients

Carbohydrate: monosaccharides actively transported into cells, released by diffusion into blood.

Protein: amino acids, actively transported into cells, released by diffusion into blood.

Water-soluble vitamins and minerals: some diffuse into cells with or without carriers; others are actively transported; all are released into blood.

Water: passive diffusion into cells, often by following sodium which is actively transported, or by attraction to protein which may be concentrated within the cells. Released passively.

The lipids and fat-soluble vitamins represent a special problem for the absorptive system. They can diffuse freely into the intestinal wall cells complexed with bile, since the cell membranes are composed largely of similar materials. Once inside, however, they are trapped. Because they are hydrophobic they cannot be released to travel freely in the watery fluids of the body. To various extents these compounds must therefore undergo chemical rearrangement and attachment to hydrophilic proteins before they can be carried away in the circulation.

hydrophobic: water hating.

hydrophilic: water loving.

To handle monoglycerides and long-chain fatty acids, the intestinal cell combines them into triglycerides, then wraps the triglycerides in protein to form a lipoprotein, known as a chylomicron, which can be released into the lymphatic fluid. The other major lipids (phospholipids and cholesterol) are also packaged in these same chylomicrons. The fat-soluble vitamins have their own protein carriers.

triglyceride: see page 60.

lipoprotein (lip-oh-PRO-tee-in): a complex of lipids with proteins. The lipids apparently orient with their hydrophobic ends in; the proteins associate with the outside of the cluster, rendering the entire complex water soluble. The molecules of a lipoprotein do not bond covalently but associate by hydrogen bonding.[1]

chylomicron (kye-lo-MY-cron): the lipoprotein formed in intestinal wall cells following digestion and absorption of fat. Released from these cells, chylomicrons serve as a means of transporting ingested fats to liver cells. The liver cells dismantle the chylomicrons and construct other lipoproteins for further transport.

Fat-soluble Nutrients

Lipids: *monoglycerides* enter intestinal wall cells; fatty acids are added to make triglycerides; protein is attached to make chylomicrons; released into lymph; *phospholipids, cholesterol,* enter cells, join chylomicrons, released into lymph.

Fat-soluble vitamins: enter cells, are attached to protein carriers, are released into lymph.

hydrophobic lipid
+
hydrophilic protein
= chylomicron:

The provision of protein carriers to remove the lipids from the intestinal wall cells solves one problem but leaves the cells with another: the bile which carried these lipids into the cells. The cells return some of this bile directly to the GI tract and release the rest into the bloodstream. It travels by way of the portal vein to the liver. There the bile is picked up by liver cells and either degraded or returned to the gall bladder for another recycling to the intestine.

Not all the bile is recycled, however. Some travels down the tract along with the waste materials and is excreted with them. Fiber has an affinity for bile, and when the diet is high in fiber, more bile is excreted. Since bile is synthesized from cholesterol, larger amounts of bile excretion effectively reduce body cholesterol. This is one reason for recent interest in the high fiber diet as a means of lowering serum cholesterol and possibly for retarding the development of atherosclerosis.[2]

The circulation of bile from the liver to the gall bladder to the intestine and back to the liver is known as the **enterohepatic circulation** of bile.

enteron = intestines
hepat = liver

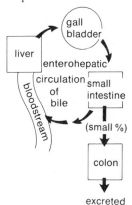

[1]Lehninger, A. L.: *Biochemistry.* Worth Publishers, Inc., New York, 1970, p. 209.
[2]Kritchevsky, D. and Story, J. A.: Binding of biosalts in vitro by nonnutritive fiber. *Journal of Nutrition* 104:458-462, 1974.

As you see, the cells of the intestinal tract wall are beautifully designed to perform their functions. A still further refinement of the system is that the cells of successive portions of the tract are specialized for different absorptive functions, so that the nutrients which are ready for absorption early are absorbed near the top of the tract, while those which take longer to be digested are absorbed further down. Thus the top portion of the duodenum is specialized for the absorption of calcium and several B vitamins such as thiamin and riboflavin; the jejunum accomplishes most of the absorption of triglycerides; and at the end of the ileum, vitamin B_{12}, which has required extensive preparation, is absorbed. The rate of travel of these nutrients is finely adjusted to maximize their availability to the appropriate absorptive segment of the tract when they are ready. The lowly "gut" turns out to be one of the most elegantly designed organ systems in your body.

duodenum, jejunum, ileum: see page 146.

Help, Hindrance, and Regulation

The anatomy of the digestive tract has been described at several levels: the sequence of digestive organs, the structures of the villi and of the cells which compose them, and the selective machinery of the cell membranes. The intricate architecture of the GI tract makes it sensitive and responsive to conditions in its environment. Knowing what the optimal conditions are will help you promote the best functioning of your system. But first a warning: the story you are about to be told is complex. The reader who has not heard it before should perhaps refrain from attempting to learn the details and be encouraged instead to simply appreciate them. The two paragraphs at the end of this chapter explain the relevance of these details to our everyday food choices and life style.

Agents which affect absorption include (1) nonspecific compounds which should be present at certain concentrations in the intestinal contents if the digestive and absorptive machinery is to work at its best and (2) specific hormones and hormone-like agents which affect specific parts of the machinery. A section is devoted to each below.

(1) *Nonspecific agents affecting function of the GI tract.* One of the conditions in the tract which can favor or hinder the absorption of nutrients is its *acidity.* As you recall, many of the nutrients are dependent on proteins for their digestion and absorption, and proteins are responsive to acidity. In addition, the mineral iron is more readily absorbed in the reduced (ferrous ion) than in the oxidized (ferric ion) state, and acid conditions favor reduction of iron. The absorption of calcium is also favored by acid.

acid: see page 60 and Appendix B.

reduced and oxidized iron: see Appendix B.

Fat is a second nonspecific agent affecting GI tract functioning. Fat stimulates the release of bile from the gall bladder, and bile is needed to emulsify and help absorb not only the fats but also to protect vitamin A and other compounds from oxidation. Fat also slows down intestinal motility, permitting time for some of the slower nutrients to be absorbed. Too much fat, however, can form insoluble "soaps" with calcium, and so rob the body of this mineral.

A third nonspecific agent is *fiber*. Fiber stimulates intestinal motility. Too little fiber, and the intestines are likely to be sluggish; they may then fail to mix their contents or to bring materials into contact with the sites on the walls where they can be absorbed. Too much fiber, on the other hand, causes the contents of the intestines to move so fast through the tract that they are not in contact with the walls long enough to be absorbed.

Binders are a fourth nonspecific agent involved in GI tract functioning. Certain compounds, binders, combine chemically with certain nutrients so that they (the nutrients) cannot be absorbed. For example, phytic acid and oxalic acid combine with iron and calcium to prevent their absorption.

(2) *Specific regulators.* For some important nutrients the body regulates not only the kind but also the amount absorbed. Two of the best-understood systems which achieve this kind of adjustment are those for the absorption of iron and calcium. These two systems differ from each other; by describing them both we hope to give you a sense of the variety of ingenious means by which the body achieves its ends.

Iron, to be absorbed, must be carried away from the cells of the intestinal wall by the protein carrier transferrin. Only empty, or unbound transferrin molecules can pick up newly absorbed iron and carry it away. If you lack iron, you will have many unbound transferrin molecules; thus the more iron you need, the more you will absorb.

Phytic (FYE-tic) acid is found in oatmeal and other whole-grain cereals, and oxalic (ox-AL-ic) acid in rhubarb and spinach, rendering some of the calcium and iron in these foods "unavailable."

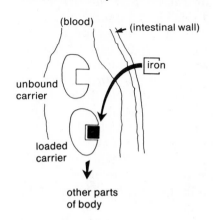

(blood) — (intestinal wall)

iron

unbound
carrier

loaded
carrier

other parts
of body

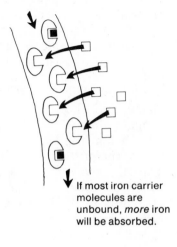

If most iron carrier
molecules are
unbound, *more* iron
will be absorbed.

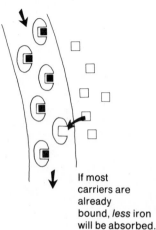

If most
carriers are
already
bound, *less* iron
will be absorbed.

As for calcium, its absorption depends on a calcium-binding protein in the membranes of the intestinal cells, and the synthesis of this protein depends in turn on vitamin D. The synthesis of vitamin D in its own turn is enhanced by a hormone—whose synthesis occurs in response to low blood calcium! Thus the less calcium you have available, the more vitamin D you synthesize, the more calcium-binding protein you synthesize, and the more calcium you absorb.

If you attempt to draw any conclusions from the above myriad details, there is perhaps one general idea that will emerge. It appears that everything depends on everything else. For optimum absorption of any nutrient, several others are needed, many of them at certain optimum concentrations. The nutrients needed for good absorption can be summed up (oversimply) in one long paragraph. You need PROTEIN to attract *water* into cells; to provide pumps and diffusion-mediators for *amino acids, monosaccharides, minerals* and the *water-soluble vitamins*; to provide carriers for *iron*, the *lipids*, and the *fat-soluble vitamins*; and to provide hormone regulators for many of these. You need LIPID to stimulate the release of bile to emulsify *lipids* and *fat-soluble vitamins* and to slow down intestinal motility to allow time for absorption of certain *minerals*. You need CARBOHYDRATE as *glucose* to provide energy for the active transport of many nutrients into cells; as *lactose* to help calcium absorption—after being converted to an acid by bacteria in the intestines; and as *cellulose (fiber)* to stimulate the mixing and moving-along of *all* the nutrients. You need VITAMINS: D, for *calcium* absorption; C, to help provide the acid environment needed for absorption of *iron* and *calcium*, and B_6, to help the transport systems for *amino acids*. You need MINERALS such as *chlorine*, to make the hydrochloric acid which provides the stomach acidity that facilitates the digestion of *protein* and the absorption of *iron* and *calcium*; *sodium*, to provide the sodium bicarbonate secreted by the pancreas to neutralize stomach acid when it reaches the duodenum, to help with the withdrawal of *water* into cells, and to assist the transport system for *glucose*; and *phosphorus*, to assist *vitamin B_6*—which in turn assists the transport systems for *amino acids*. And you need WATER to suspend *all* of the above nutrients in a finely divided state so that they are accessible to the absorptive machinery. The point of all of this must be abundantly clear: to maintain the health and promote the functions of the GI tract, balance and variety should be features of every meal.

one long paragraph

A second general conclusion you might draw from an acquaintance with the facts of digestive physiology may not be so obvious from the information in this chapter. The regulation of events in the GI tract depends largely on hormones and nerves, and your mental state affects their activities. While the interaction between mind and body is not traditionally within the province of an introductory text, we feel that nutrition cannot be properly understood or appreciated without an awareness of the whole-person effects, which can sometimes be very profound. The Highlight which follows this chapter is devoted to some aspects of this interaction.

Summing Up

The last chapter ended at the point where a hamburger or a piece of chocolate cake had been completely digested and the nutrients were ready for absorption. The boxes in the present chapter sum up the next part of the story. From carbohydrates, the monosaccharides—glucose, fructose, and galactose—are absorbed mostly from the small intestinal villi into the capillaries of the mesenteric membrane; the capillaries converge into veins which in turn converge into the single large portal vein. The next stop is the liver.

From lipids, the medium- and short-chain fatty acids and glycerol follow the same route. The long-chain fatty acids and monoglycerides are taken into intestinal cells. There they are put together to form triglycerides, are attached to protein carriers, and are released into the lymph; the lymph later conducts them into the subclavian vein where they join the general circulation.

From proteins, the amino acids follow the same route as the monosaccharides, traveling through the mesenteric capillaries and veins and finally through the portal vein—to the liver.

The water-soluble B vitamins and vitamin C accompany the monosaccharides and amino acids, while the fat-soluble vitamins (A, D, E, K) are attached to carriers and follow the path of the larger fats.

As you will recall (to make the story complete), the water which remains is absorbed into the large intestine, while fiber remains in the GI tract until it is excreted from the body.

The process of absorption is one in which many compounds are interdependent. The absorption of many nutrients depends on protein, of many others on minerals and vitamins. The whole picture is one of complex interrelationships, suggesting that for optimal functioning, a mixture of nutrients should be taken together at each meal.

To Explore Further—

A clear and thorough text for the student who wishes to probe further into physiology:

Macey, R. I.: *Human Physiology.* Prentice-Hall, Inc., Englewood Cliffs, New Jersey. Paperback.

A brief and accurate introduction to endocrinology, which stresses the role of hormones in maintaining homeostasis:

Clegg, P. C. and Clegg, A. C. *Hormones, Cells, and Organisms: The Role of Hormones in Mammals.* Stanford University Press, Stanford, California, 1969.

A superb treatment of the complex relationships which exist between endocrinology, pathology, and vitamins. This is a highly technical book, not for the beginning science student:

Jennings, I. W.: *Vitamins in Endocrine Metabolism.* Charles C. Thomas, Springfield, Illinois, 1970.

An admiring description of the anatomy, physiology, and evolution of the kidney by a man who devoted his life to its study:

Smith, H. W.: *From Fish to Philosopher.* Doubleday & Company, Inc., Garden City, New York, 1959. Paperback.

Highlight Six
Mind and Body

It is natural for students of nutrition to believe that when they have memorized the names of all the digestive enzymes, know whether they break down protein, fat, or carbohydrate, know the pH at which each is active, know where along the GI tract each does its job, know where and how the products of digestion are absorbed, and know how the residue is excreted—that they have an understanding of the digestive and absorptive process. Not so! As Sue R. Williams, with keen insight, states in her textbook, *Nutrition and Diet Therapy*, "Surrounding every stomach there is a person."[1]

It is the person surrounding the digestive tract who has been omitted from the above list of facts. What effect do the pleasures and pains caused by the action of this tract have on the *person*, and what effect does what the *person* thinks or experiences have on the digestion of food? There ought to be at least a "tip of the hat" to this vast area of knowledge.

It is convenient to think of the GI tract as an assembly line (or more correctly, a disassembly line) and to visualize food entering at the mouth and being carried along that assembly line by the force of peristalsis. It makes learning the chemical and physical reactions easier if they are learned in the order in which they occur. However, this GI tract is not a piece of machinery. It has a person around it—a thinking, feeling, re-

[1]Williams, S. R.: *Nutrition and Diet Therapy.* The C. V. Mosby Company, St. Louis, Missouri, 1974. p. 507.

193

acting person. What this person thinks or feels has an effect on the workings of the assembly line, and this assembly line can send out messages of satiety, hunger, or pain which have an effect on how the person reacts to some other event in his life.

As an example, fear or anxiety can shut off the flow of pancreatic juice to the duodenum and can increase peristalsis so that acid contents of the stomach are dumped into the duodenum at a time when the duodenum is unprepared for the acid. The duodenum does not have a thick mucous coating to protect itself against acid; consequently, it relies on hormones to inform the pancreas that acid contents are on the way and that the pancreas must secrete alkaline fluids into the duodenum to neutralize the acid. If the alkaline ions are not present when the chyme mixed with acid arrives, and if this is a frequent occurrence, eventually an erosion of the duodenum mucosa may result: that is, an ulcer may form. The physician tells the patient that *stress* has caused the ulcer to form; often, the patient interprets this remark as an affront to his ability to deal with life's problems, or as an indication that he is a nervous person, or that his illness is psychosomatic and therefore imaginary. These interpretations of the word *stress* indicate a lack of understanding of stress physiology and of the way a person's body responds to life's events.

psychosomatic (sigh-co-so-MAT-ic): relating to the interaction between mental and bodily phenomena. Popular (and incorrect) meaning: imaginary.

   psyche = mind, soul
   soma = body

stress: a physical, chemical, or emotional factor which causes bodily or mental tension and which may be a factor in disease causation.

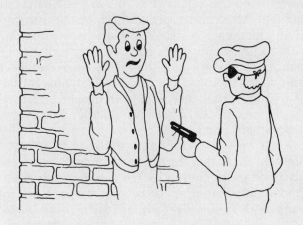

To understand stress there must be an appreciation of the wholeness of the human organism. Sometimes when ulcers form or diarrhea occurs, it seems it would have been desirable during the evolution of the digestive system to have made it into a separate entity, with no communication between it and the person in whom it resides. A person could then have ingested food, digestion would have taken place, nutrients would have been supplied, and never would distress signals have been sent out. (Of course there would have been no pleasure signals either.)

But the systems of the body did not evolve that way. The systems are integrated, meshed into each other, so that they become a whole person. A *whole* person reacts to stress, not just the brain. A woman who is faced with the loss of her husband through death or divorce reacts with her entire body, not just her mind, and illness often follows such a trauma. A little boy who is scolded for not eating his carrots does not merely hear the words and decide mentally that he will not pick up his fork and eat, his entire body feels the effect of the scolding and he *cannot* eat the carrots; if he did, they wouldn't stay in his stomach. All the systems of the body communicate with the other systems and with the environment through neural pathways and by means of the hormones of the endocrine system. This is why the systems of the body react as a unit.

endocrine system: the system of glands which secrete hormones into the blood. See also page 148.

One group of hormones is the catecholamines, epinephrine and norepinephrine, which were first proposed by Cannon early in the twentieth century. They have been dubbed the fight-or-flight hormones because they help people mobilize their defenses to meet danger, either physically or emotionally perceived. Thus the danger presented by a boss who is vindictive or unfair calls forth the same physiological response of the catecholamines as did the danger of an aggressive, large animal in our caveman ancestors.

catecholamines (cat-uh-COAL-uh-meens): epinephrine (ep-in-EFF-rin), norepinephrine (NOR-ep-in-eff-rin). These hormones were formerly called adrenalin and noradrenalin.

When a danger is present, the brain relays a message to the adrenal glands which sit atop the kidneys. The adrenal medulla, the interior of the gland, then secretes epinephrine and norepinephrine into the blood stream where they are carried to target areas all over the body. The result is (1) greater energy through the release of glucose from the liver; (2) greater protection from hemorrhage by a faster clotting time, by a conservation of fluid by the kidneys, and by a retreat of blood from the periphery of the body to the vital organs and the legs; (3) increased ability to see by the widening of the pupils of the eyes; (4) increased ca-

adrenal glands: a pair of endocrine glands situated on the kidneys.

ad = on (to)
renal = kidney

The adrenal cortex produces steroid hormones like the sex hormones; the adrenal medulla produces the catecholamines.

cortex = outer layer
medulla = inner layer

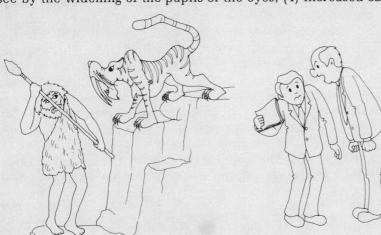

tabolism of body fat for energy during a sustained crisis; (5) faster respiration to bring in more oxygen and get rid of carbon dioxide; and (6) more powerful heart beats to send nutrient- and oxygen-rich blood to the muscles faster. All these events (and there are more) enable the person to escape danger or else to stand and fight the aggressor. At the same time, blood is drawn away from the digestive system, and the flow of digestive juices is halted. In a time of emergency, then, there is interference with the processes of digestion and absorption. This is as it should be for a caveman; these are low priority processes when you are facing a saber-toothed tiger.

In modern urban societies there are not many dangers which require the fight-or-flight set of reactions; rather, modern man, for the most part, faces stresses which demand from him intelligent, rational behavior. Yet he is still encumbered with an overload of glucose, high blood pressure, acid in the duodenum, hyperlipidemia, and all the other reactions brought about by the sense of danger. Armed with this knowledge about ulcers, ulcer patients may be able to institute changes in their lives to relieve stress. Understanding this, they may realize that their illness is not due to a failure to cope and that it is not imaginary.

Study of the actual processes occurring in stress is needed to understand its effects—hence the new area of research on stress. Like a giant jigsaw puzzle that can only be solved by first finding two small pieces that fit together, whole body reactions to stress must be studied by asking questions which concern some small part of the whole. Many of these first questions have now been answered by scientists. In the last decade there has been an explosion of knowledge relating to hormonal action. Since it is difficult to put people in stressful situations in a laboratory, scientists have utilized animal laboratory studies to discover the physiology of particular tissues' responses to threat; they have been limited in their study of human responses largely to observations by doctors of their patients.

It was, therefore, a unique opportunity to study human stress while it was occurring when Kasl and Cobb [2] [3] were privileged to gather data on men who were about to lose their jobs, due to plant closings. The men were visited four times in their homes by public health nurses who conducted interviews, monitored psychological tests, and collected blood and urine for clinical analyses. The four visits occurred about 6 months prior to termination, at the time of the closing of the plant, at 12 months and at 24 months after the closing. The assumption was that with this spacing of the visits the men would be observed

[2]Kasl, S. V.: The experience of losing a job—reported changes in health, symptoms and illness behavior. *Psychosomatic Medicine* 37(2):106-122, 1975.

[3]Cobb, S.: Physiologic changes in men whose jobs were abolished. *Journal of Psychosomatic Research* 18(4):245-258, 1974.

during the stressful times of job-loss anticipation, the actual loss, the period of seeking other employment, and the time of readjustment.

There were a number of psychological and biochemical parameters studied but only two will be discussed here: (1) the psychological test results which showed how the men felt about the support of their families and friends and (2) the biochemical study which revealed the level of stress they were experiencing by measuring amounts of urinary norepinephrine (when more norepinephrine is manufactured, more is excreted). A discussion of these two results should indicate how events in life (outside of the body) affect the body and may establish an appreciation for the type of research undertaken by Kasl and Cobb.

It is not surprising to learn that the rate of norepinephrine excretion was significantly elevated for those whose jobs were abolished. Surely loss of a job should bring forth feelings of distress and anxiety. It is particularly interesting that the elevation lasted from a time 6 months prior to termination until 12 months afterwards. Eighteen months is a long time to suffer stress. By 24 months after termination, the levels had returned to those which the control subjects had maintained throughout the study. (The controls were employees of four plants that were not in danger of closing. The same tests were conducted on them as on the men who lost their jobs. See Figure H6.1.)

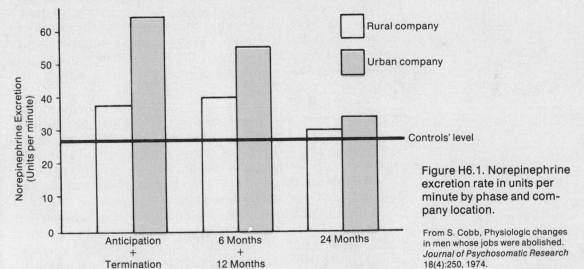

Figure H6.1. Norepinephrine excretion rate in units per minute by phase and company location.

From S. Cobb, Physiologic changes in men whose jobs were abolished. *Journal of Psychosomatic Research* 18(4):250, 1974.

An interesting, unexpected result was the difference in adjustment presumably caused by the locations of the two plants. One plant was in a large city; the other in a small town. The closing resulted in higher norepinephrine production in the city men than in the small town men. At first glance, this finding concerned the experimenters; they wondered if there might be a difference between the two groups of men that would make it impossible to combine the data. However, by the end of 24 months, both groups had returned to the norepinephrine levels of the controls (see Figure H6.1), indicating that the city men were comparable to the others and that their higher elevations were due to a peculiarity in their situation.

A clue to the reason for this difference was found when one of the psychological tests was analyzed. The test was designed to measure support given by family and friends. It showed that the men in the large city plant derived their most important social interaction from fraternization with the other employees at the plant. When terminated, they did not have a social structure on which to rely. In the small town, on the other hand, the men had an active social life centered in the community or in the family; thus their social life continued very much as before. The conclusion was that supportive relationships ease the stress caused by job loss.

At this point, there are a number of questions the reader should ask before accepting these findings as valid (see page 44). How did the researchers know that the elevation of norepinephrine was due to the loss of the job? Maybe some other event in each individual's life caused him to have feelings of crisis, fear, or threat. Maybe he was taking substances—drugs, perhaps—that would cause an elevation. Did the researchers ask the subjects about these things? If you were pondering questions such as these you are to be commended as a critical reader of science articles. If you wish to draw your own conclusions about the validity of this study, the information you need to locate the reports is among the references supplied for this discussion.[2][3]

Research of this kind is bringing our understanding of stress to a deeper level. We have known intuitively that job loss was stressful and that family and community support eased stress. Now we can see that job loss causes a physiological response (increased norepinephrine secretion) and that support reduces the magnitude of this response. Molecular explanations are beginning to lead to an understanding of stress effects.

Kasl and Cobb's study reveals the relationship between the brain's reaction to threatening situations and the body's hormonal responses. If norephinephrine is elevated when a man is about to lose his job, then his digestive system is affected as well as his renal, cardiovascular, and all his other body systems. He has reacted to this threat to his own and his family's survival with his entire body, not with his brain alone. In turn, the reaction of his family and friends towards him and his situation has an effect on the intensity of his reactions to the event, and hence on the physical damage that could result.

The study of nutrition sometimes makes it necessary to take an in-depth look at one small phase or another of the subject; it is equally necessary that the student be reminded that no reaction occurs in isolation. A person is a whole organism and reacts to events in his life with every body system.

To Explore Further—

Frieden and Lippner have written an excellent, readable text intended for college undergraduate chemistry students:

Frieden, E. and Lippner, J.: *Biochemical Endocrinology of the Vertebrates.* Foundations of Modern Biochemistry Series. Prentice-Hall, Inc., Englewood Cliffs, New Jersey, 1971.

This article reports on one vitamin whose metabolism is affected by stress:

Hodges, R. E.: Effect of stress on ascorbic acid metabolism in men. *Nutrition Today* 5:11, 1970.

Teaching Aid, *Stress, on just being sick,* by Selye, H., is a set of 13 slides designed to depict the consequences of stress. The set can be ordered from:

> Director, Education Services
> Nutrition Today
> 101 Ridgely Avenue
> Annapolis, Maryland 21404

Suggested Activities

(1) Put the story together.

Follow the path of absorbed nutrients from a glass of milk into the blood stream, tracing at each step the assistance they receive.

(2) Remember the person.

How could you explain in physiological terms the following statement: "A patient's confidence in his doctor may be more important than diet in promoting healing of an ulcer." (Refer to the definition of placebo effect, page 165.)

7

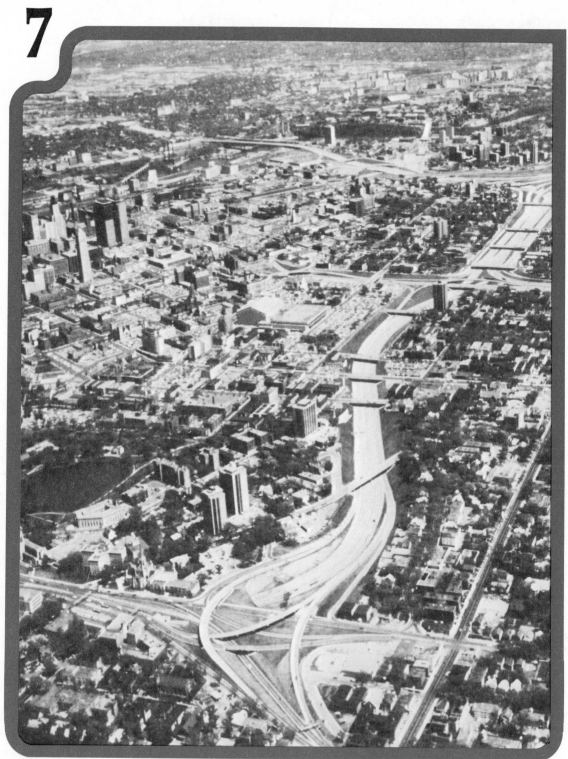

The activities inside the cell are as complex as those of a metropolitan area.　　　Photo by Jerry Miller

Metabolism

... the course of nature ... seems delighted with transmutations ...
—SIR ISAAC NEWTON

The body's cells and the enzymes within them make it their task as far as possible to convert any compound into any other. This is enormously convenient and relieves us of the burden of having to eat exactly the right amount of each type of nutrient at each meal. Given too much glucose in the blood and body stores, the cells convert the extra into fat. Given too few amino acids to make the needed proteins, they convert glucose into amino acids. Given extra amino acids, they convert them into sugar—or fat. And so on. The following pages show some of these extraordinary capabilities.

Starting Points

A brief review may be helpful. The first three chapters introduced the energy nutrients—carbohydrate, fat, and protein—as they are found in foods and in the human body. The next two chapters followed them through digestion to the simpler units of which they are composed and showed these units disappearing into the blood. This chapter follows them into the cells where they lose their identity and become indistinguishable from one another.

The number of chemical reactions that go on in the body is astronomical. The story of metabolism in the largest sense is the story of all these reactions. No attempt will be made here to

201

metabolism: the sum total of all the chemical reactions that go on in living cells.

meta = among
bole = change

tell that story except in the barest outline. At the central core of metabolism the simple units derived from carbohydrate, fat, and protein become interconvertible. For purposes of understanding the principles involved, four of these units will be followed here.

(1) Carbohydrates, as you will recall, come in several varieties in the diet: principally as the polysaccharide starch, the disaccharides, and the monosaccharides. During digestion these units are all broken down to monosaccharides—glucose, fructose, and galactose—and are absorbed into the blood. The latter two are then taken into liver cells and converted to glucose. To continue the story of what happens to carbohydrate thereafter, then, we will simply follow *glucose*.

(2 & 3) Lipids also come in several varieties, but 95 percent of those found in foods are triglycerides. The triglycerides undergo several transformations during digestion and absorption, but many of them end up once again as triglycerides in body cells. There they can be dismantled to *glycerol* and *fatty acids*. Following the further transformations of these two compounds will show the principal fates of dietary fat.

(4) Protein is digested to *amino acids*, absorbed into blood, and carried to the liver where further transformations occur. Thus, to follow protein through metabolism we will trace the steps by which amino acids are further transformed.

At this point we must stop thinking about these compounds as the basic units of the nutrients and remember that they themselves are composed of still more basic units, the atoms. During metabolism, the body goes to work with an electron saw and actually separates the atoms from one another. It will help if you recall the structures of these compounds introduced in the first three chapters. There is no need to remember exactly how they are put together; it is enough to think of them in terms of their "backbones." The structures are repeated here for your convenience.

From carbohydrate, glucose has a 6-carbon backbone with associated —H and —OH groups:

$$-\overset{|}{\underset{|}{C}}-\overset{|}{\underset{|}{C}}-\overset{|}{\underset{|}{C}}-\overset{|}{\underset{|}{C}}-\overset{|}{\underset{|}{C}}-\overset{|}{\underset{|}{C}}-$$

From fat, glycerol has a 3-carbon backbone with associated —H and —OH groups. Fatty acids, on the other hand, are long-chain carbon compounds, many of which contain 18 or more carbon atoms with H's attached:

$$
\begin{array}{c}
| \quad | \quad | \\
-\text{C}-\text{C}-\text{C}- \\
| \quad | \quad |
\end{array}
$$

Glycerol

$$
-\text{C}-\text{C}-\text{C}-\text{C}-\text{C}-\text{C}-\text{C}-\text{C}-\text{C}-\text{C}-\text{C}-\text{C}-\text{C}-\text{C}-\text{C}-\text{C}-\text{C}-\text{C}-
$$

Fatty acid

From protein, an amino acid has a 2-carbon backbone, to which nitrogen is always attached:

$$
\text{N}-\text{C}-\text{C}-
$$

Amino Acid

The story of what happens to these compounds inside of cells can be told most simply by following the fates of the carbon atoms in these backbones: the six in glucose, the three in glycerol, the eighteen in a typical fatty acid, and the two in an amino acid.

Students who have mastered the basic facts of metabolism often look back and report how glad they are that they made the effort to understand. Once the picture is complete, it turns out to be surprisingly simple. The following simple diagram outlines the whole story:

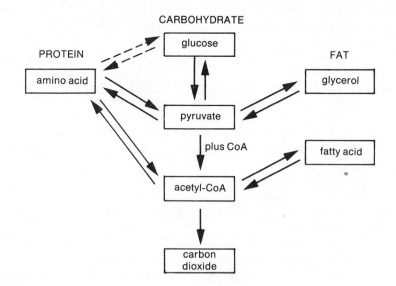

CoA (coh-AY) is the nickname for a compound described further in Chapter 9. As pyruvate loses a carbon and becomes a 2-carbon compound (acetate), a molecule of CoA is attached to it, making acetyl CoA.

Remember, we have four principal actors to follow. Let us follow glucose first. The six carbons of glucose are split into two 3-carbon fragments called pyruvate. Each of these then splits into a 2-carbon fragment called acetate and a 1-carbon compound (carbon dioxide). A molecule called CoA is attached to the acetate, making acetyl CoA. Finally, acetyl CoA loses its CoA again and is broken down to two single carbons (carbon dioxide). Thus one glucose molecule ultimately yields six carbon dioxide molecules.

Once this is understood, the other three principal actors can easily be followed. Glycerol is a 3-carbon compound which can be converted to pyruvate; it follows the same path as glucose from that point on. An amino acid can lose its nitrogen, becoming a carbon compound that can enter this pathway at various levels. For example, glycine is eventually converted to acetyl CoA and follows the same path from that point on. Fatty acids are cleaved into pairs of carbons (acetyl CoA) and then follow the same path from that point on. At the end, every carbon atom in all three nutrients has been combined with oxygen and freed as carbon dioxide.

The remainder of this chapter does little more than repeat this picture and explain it, until each part of it is clear.

These are Catabolic Reactions

catabolism: those reactions in which large molecules are broken down to smaller ones. Catabolic reactions involve oxidation and release energy.

kata = down

When a nutrient molecule is dismantled to smaller, simpler compounds, the process is called catabolic. Generally, catabolic reactions involve oxidation: as each carbon is removed, it is combined with oxygen to form carbon dioxide, which escapes from the body via the lungs. As each hydrogen is removed, it also combines with oxygen to form water, which may recycle or be lost in urine, sweat, or as water vapor from the lungs. The oxygen which formed part of the nutrient may remain with a carbon to help form carbon dioxide or with a hydrogen to help form water. Thus the three principal atoms found in the energy nutrients—C, H, O—can all end up in carbon dioxide or water.

(You may notice an omission here: what happens to the nitrogen in proteins? This question will be answered a few pages later.)

Catabolic reactions also involve the release of energy. When a carbon atom is removed from a molecule, the bonding energy which formerly held it in place becomes available for some other purpose.

Obviously, catabolic reactions are not the only ones, or even the most important ones, which go on in the body. If they were, it would not be long before you would disintegrate and disappear into the atmosphere, leaving nothing but a little puddle of salty water as a reminder that you had existed. Other —anabolic—reactions are simultaneously going on, in which simple compounds are put together to form larger and more complex structures. Anabolic reactions usually involve reduction (addition of hydrogen atoms or removal of oxygen atoms) and require the consumption of energy (which is needed to form the bonds between the atoms in the structures being built).

The way in which the energy in nutrients is captured from them during catabolism and used for anabolic purposes is explained in the next chapter. This chapter is devoted to the fates of the *atoms* during the catabolism of glucose, fats, and protein.

anabolism: those reactions in which small molecules are put together to form larger ones. Anabolic reactions involve reduction and require energy.

ana = up

Six to Three: Glucose to Pyruvate

Glucose molecules are the common energy currency of all cells. Like dollars in the American economy, they are a most convenient unit of exchange. Dollars can be exchanged for ten-dollar or thousand-dollar bills, which may be convenient for temporary storage purposes; they may be broken into small change for purposes of making small purchases.

Glucose molecules are found in all living cells, both plant and animal—from those of lettuce leaves and oak trees to those of the human brain. The process of glucose catabolism, with its attendant release of energy and the production of smaller molecules, is continually going on throughout the living world. As you read this, many billion glucose molecules are being broken down in your brain each second.

The conversion of glucose to pyruvate can be reversed. Thus, two molecules of pyruvate can be recondensed to form a 6-carbon compound, which, in a series of enzymatic rearrangements, can be converted to glucose. The reversibility of the reactions between glucose and pyruvate is shown symbolically as two-way arrows in the diagram:

pyruvate (PIE-roo-vate): a salt of pyruvic acid. Throughout this book the ending -*ate* is used interchangeably with -*ic acid*. Thus acetate = acetic acid.

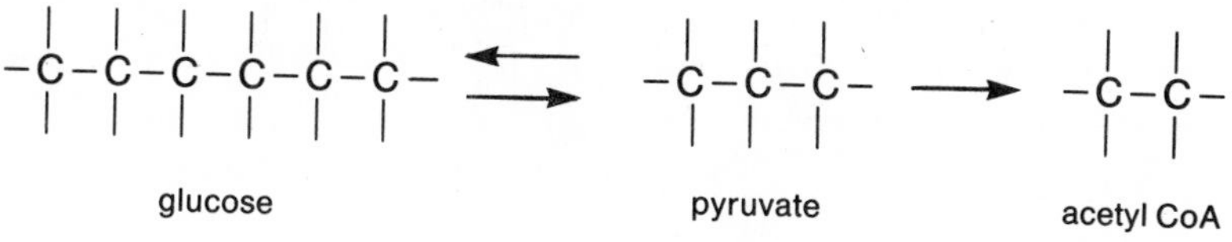

glucose   pyruvate   acetyl CoA

Three to Two: Pyruvate to Acetyl CoA

Pyruvate can be acted on by any of several different enzymes. (Depending upon which enzyme gets hold of it, the pyruvate may have a carbon added to it to make a 4-carbon compound, or may be changed to another 3-carbon compound to be stored temporarily, or may have a carbon removed to reduce its length to two carbons.) In the complete catabolism of glucose, the pyruvate loses a carbon (as carbon dioxide), gains a CoA, and is converted to acetyl CoA.

The enzyme that does this job cannot perform the reverse reaction; the pyruvate cannot be recovered. This fact is shown symbolically by means of a one-way arrow in the diagram. Hence, acetyl CoA molecules cannot be put back together to form glucose.

Fates of Acetyl CoA

As nickels and dimes can be converted into pennies for the purchase of bubble gum, or quarters for cokes, or currency to save or spend on larger items, acetyl CoA is a kind of small change in metabolism that can be converted into many forms for many uses. Among the most important are (1) transformations which lead to synthesis of amino acids, (2) transformations which lead to synthesis of fatty acids, and (3) complete oxidation to carbon dioxide and water, with the release of energy for other uses in the body. The diagram summarizes these metabolic pathways:

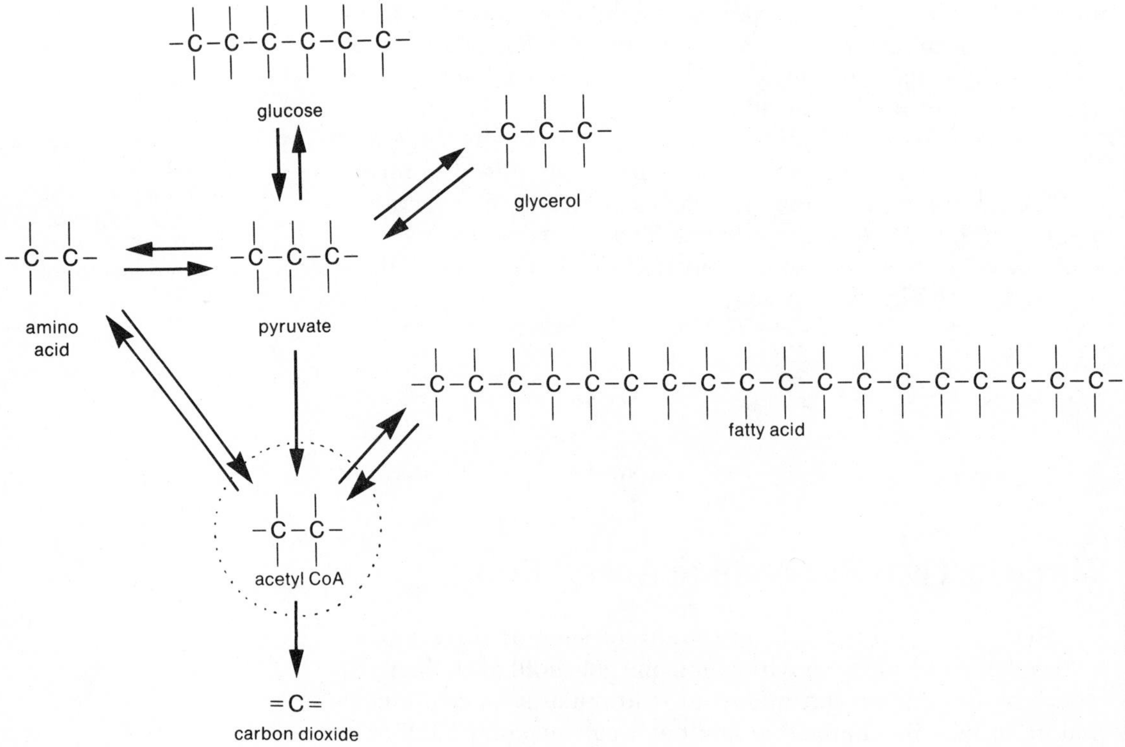

The arrows show that the breakdown of acetyl CoA is irreversible: the enzymes that perform this reaction cannot put carbon dioxide molecules back together to form acetyl CoA. The two-way arrows between acetyl CoA and amino acids, between pyruvate and amino acids, and between acetyl CoA and fatty acids show that these compounds are interconvertible.

So fatty acids and some amino acids enter the central pathway of metabolism at the level of acetyl CoA. As you can see, this puts acetyl CoA at the hub of metabolism; it is a key intermediate. Any compound that can be converted *to* it can ultimately contribute to the formation of any compound that can be made *from* it—as the sale of cokes can yield quarters to be spent on postage stamps, or vice versa.

Glucose to Fat: One Way Only

Glucose and fat live on a one-way street. You can drive from glucose to fat on this street but not from fat to glucose. More technically, you can manufacture body fat from blood glucose (and therefore from carbohydrate in the diet), but you can't manufacture blood glucose from fat, either from the diet or from body stores. Since blood glucose is normally (except after prolonged fasting) the only energy nutrient that can enter nerve and brain cells, those who fast or fad dieters who deprive themselves of carbohydrate are literally starving their brains (see Highlight 8).

carbohydrate → blood glucose — (through acetyl CoA) → body fat

fat ⇸ blood glucose   (IMPOSSIBLE)

There is a minor exception to the statement that you cannot make blood glucose from fat. Whenever a triglyceride is broken down in the intestine, it yields three fatty acids and a molecule of glycerol. As the diagram shows, glycerol enters metabolism at the level of pyruvate, which is reconvertible to glucose. This process is of small significance in the total picture, however, as you will realize if you consider the structure of a triglyceride. Of the 57 carbon atoms in a triglyceride (take one containing three 18-carbon fatty acids as an example),

> only three are in glycerol; the other 54 are in the fatty acids. Hence only about five percent of dietary fat yields a compound that can be converted to glucose.

Amino Acids to Glucose: Both Ways

Another fact is evident from the diagram: you can almost make protein from carbohydrate. More accurately, the *carbons* in a glucose molecule can find their way (through acetyl CoA) into amino acids—although, of course, *nitrogen* is needed to make the amino acids complete. Given an unbalanced protein (one in which there is an abundance of an unneeded amino acid and a shortage of a needed one) this is exactly what the body does: it uses the nitrogen from the amino acid that it can spare plus 2-carbon fragments from the catabolism of glucose to make the amino acid that it needs.

carbohydrate → blood glucose — (through acetyl CoA) (+N) → amino acids

What about the reverse: can the body make glucose from amino acids? Obviously not through acetate. There is another way. Certain amino acids can be converted to pyruvate and thereafter to glucose through a process known as gluconeogenesis. Since glucose is so vital to nerve function, this pathway serves as a backup system in case the two major sources of blood glucose, dietary carbohydrate and liver glycogen, should fail.

gluconeogenesis (gloo-co-nee-o-GEN-uh-sis): synthesis of glucose from noncarbohydrate sources. About 5 percent of fat (the glycerol portion of triglycerides) and about half of the amino acids can be converted to glucose.

gluco = glucose
neo = new
genesis = making

amino acids — (gluconeogenesis) → blood glucose

This is one reason why, as explained in Chapter 1, a high protein breakfast sustains blood sugar levels for much longer than a carbohydrate breakfast; once the carbohydrate is used up, the protein continues supplying glucose by way of gluconeogenesis, which takes longer. Theoretically, body fat should be convertible to glucose too, then, since it can be used to make certain amino acids. In fact, however, the energy required to make glucose from fat is so great that it exceeds the energy the glucose would yield.

```
┌─────────────────────────────────────────────────────────┐
│                                          TOO              │
│   fat — (gluconeogenesis) → blood glucose "EXPENSIVE"     │
│                                                           │
└─────────────────────────────────────────────────────────┘
```

Protein to Fat: Both Ways

Finally, as you can see from the diagram, fat and protein are interconvertible through acetyl CoA. (You can get fat eating protein.)

```
┌─────────────────────────────────────────────────────────┐
│                         (through acetyl CoA)              │
│       amino acids — ───────────────────── → body fat      │
│                              (−N)                         │
└─────────────────────────────────────────────────────────┘
```

```
┌─────────────────────────────────────────────────────────┐
│                    (through acetyl CoA)                   │
│       fat — ──────────────────────── → amino acids        │
│                         (+N)                              │
└─────────────────────────────────────────────────────────┘
```

Perhaps the most important lesson to be learned from this is that you can get fat eating too much of anything: carbohydrate, fat, or protein. It isn't what you eat, it's how much.

As you can see, the magic of body chemistry makes all of the following transformations possible except one:

glucose	→	fat
fat	⇸	glucose
glucose	→	protein
protein	→	glucose
protein	→	fat
fat	→	protein

It almost appears that you could live entirely without one or two of these nutrients. You have to have protein, of course, for the essential amino acids. But why not live on pure protein and fat, dispensing with carbohydrate altogether? You could even—in theory—dispense with fat as well, except for the essential fatty acids.

Don't. The body can perform almost miraculous transformations, but there are limits. The following sections will make some of these limits clear. Carbohydrate, for instance, is "clean" fuel while lipid and protein are not. Activity 2 at the end of Chapter 3 presents a guideline for balancing the carbohydrate, fat, and protein in the diet.

Fat Catabolism and Ketosis

Normally, the catabolism of both lipid and carbohydrate are proceeding simultaneously in the body. Acetyl CoA from the lipids, and a 4-carbon compound derived from carbohydrate (by adding a carbon to pyruvate) are catabolized together completely in a sequence of reactions that yield carbon dioxide and water —"clean" waste, which can be easily excreted:

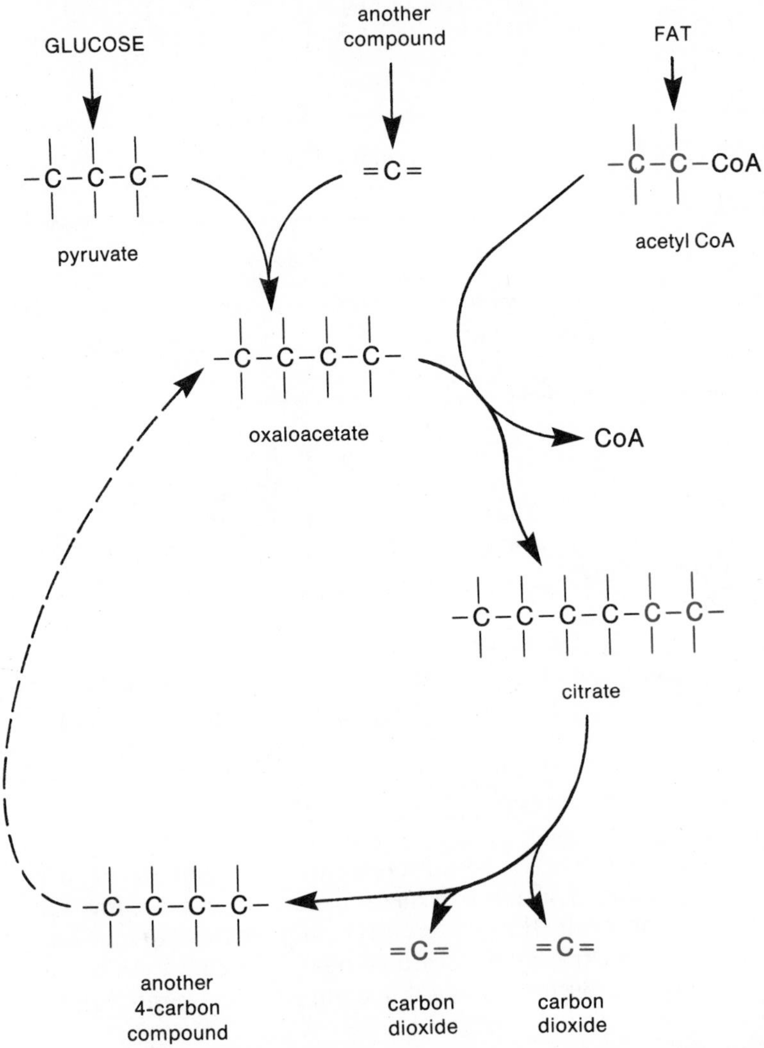

Carbon donated by another compound combines with pyruvate (3 C's) from glucose metabolism to form oxaloacetate (4 C's). Acetyl CoA (2 C's) from fat metabolism joins the oxaloacetate to form citrate (6 C's). This then loses the two carbons from fat as two molecules of carbon dioxide, forming a 4-carbon compound of the Krebs Cycle. These reactions of the Krebs Cycle are shown in more detail in the following Highlight.

However, occasions arise when lipid is being catabolized in the *absence* of carbohydrate as, for example, when a person is on a low-carbohydrate diet, is fasting, or is starving. In these cases, the pyruvate derivative of glucose, essential for complete combustion of acetate, is not available; then the acetate must follow another route. What happens is that an enzyme condenses molecules of acetate together to form ketones such as the one shown at right.

Ketones are always present in the body at a low and tolerable concentration. They are toxic at higher levels but at this low concentration can be handled without harm. One of the functions of the kidneys is to remove ketones from the blood as they pass through and to excrete them into the urine, in which they can leave the body. When the concentration of ketones rises above a certain level, however, they begin to have harmful effects upon cells. The condition in which blood ketone concentration is too high is called ketosis.

Many of the ketones are also acids like the one shown. The accumulation of these keto-acids in the bloodstream throws off the acid-base balance which is vital to the proper functioning of all body systems. The hazards of acidosis have been described in Chapter 4.

The body's principal means of ridding itself of excess ketones is by excreting them in urine; one (acetone) can be thrown off by evaporation in the lungs. Hence ketonuria and acetone breath are both symptoms of ketosis. The need to excrete ketones through the urine explains why it is recommended that you drink plenty of water when fasting or on a low-carbohydrate diet or when ill in any condition where ketosis or acidosis is likely. (We do not mean to imply that we recommend fasting or low-carbohydrate diets any more than we recommend getting ill. Highlight 8 focuses on the risks of these undertakings.)

ketone (KEE-tone): a compound formed during the incomplete oxidation of fatty acids. Ketones contain a—C=O group between other carbons; when they also contain a —COOH, or acid group, they are called keto-acids.

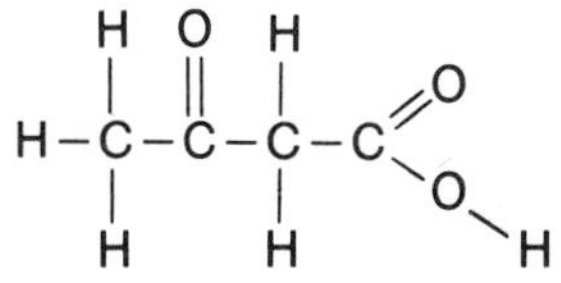

ketosis (kee-TOE-sis): excess ketones in the blood.

acidosis: too much acid in the blood. See page 120.

ketonuria (kee-tone-YOO-ree-uh): the presence of ketones in the urine.

Protein Catabolism, Ammonia, and Urea

As was emphasized in Chapter 3, the amino acids can serve as energy sources, but they are uniquely important as building blocks for body proteins and will ordinarily be used primarily for this purpose. Under certain circumstances, however, amino acids will be used for energy. In other words, IF you have too little carbohydrate and/or fat to meet your body's need for energy, then you will use amino acids for energy, even at the cost of being unable to build important body proteins. (For this reason, it is important to eat ample carbohydrate and fat: to spare protein.) IF you have enough carbohydrate and/or fat to meet your energy needs, then you will use amino acids mostly to build body proteins. IF you then have excess amino acids left over, they will be converted to an energy-storage form.

Excess amino acids cannot be stored in the body. Those not used for building body protein must be converted to compounds that can be metabolized like carbohydrate and fat. The first step in this process is one in which the enzymes convert the amino acid to an intermediate similar to those of carbohydrate and fat: a 2-carbon or 3-carbon chain which can then be converted to acetyl CoA or pyruvate. Since amino acids differ from the sugars and fatty acids in that they contain nitrogen, the first step in this process is removal of the nitrogen-containing amino group, in a reaction called deamination:

deamination: removal of the amino ($-NH_2$) group from a compound such as an amino acid.

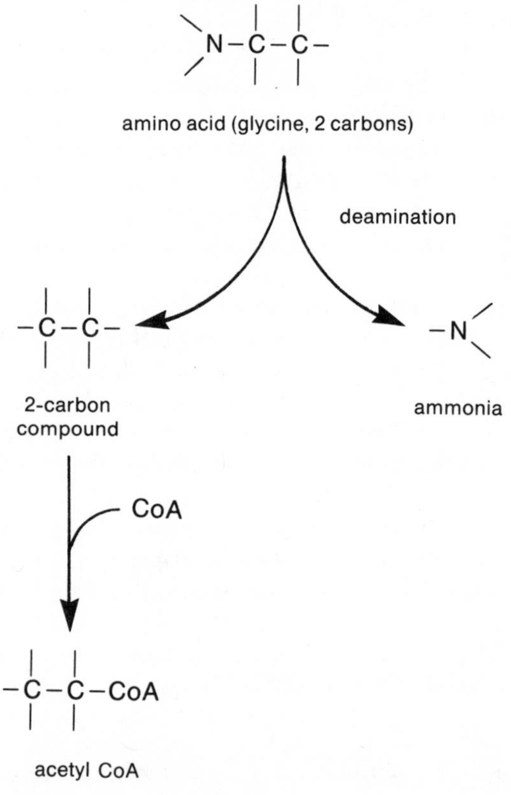

amino acid (glycine, 2 carbons)

deamination

2-carbon compound

ammonia

CoA

acetyl CoA

urea (yoo-REE-uh): the principal nitrogen-excretion product of metabolism. Two ammonia fragments are combined with a carbon-oxygen group to form urea. The diagram greatly oversimplifies the reactions.

The ammonia produced when a liver cell enzyme deaminates an amino acid is identical chemically to the ammonia in the bottled cleaning solutions used in hospitals and in industry; it is a strong-smelling and extremely potent poison. There is always a small amount of ammonia being produced by liver deamination reactions. Some of this ammonia is captured by liver enzymes and used to synthesize other amino acids. The remainder is combined with a carbon-oxygen fragment to make the inert compound urea:

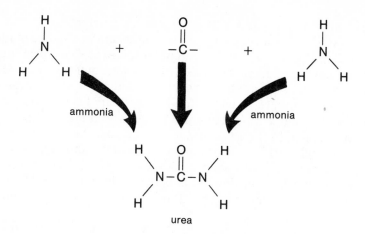

urea

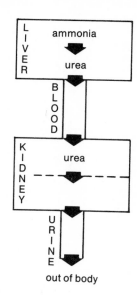

out of body

Urea is released from the liver cells into the blood, where it circulates until it passes through the kidneys. One of the functions of the kidneys is to remove urea from the blood for excretion in the urine. Urea is the body's principal vehicle for excreting unused nitrogen; water is required to keep it in solution and excrete it. This explains why people who consume a high protein diet must drink more water than usual.

After excretion, urea may be converted spontaneously or by bacterial action back to ammonia. This accounts for the ammonia odor of the diaper pail.

Two to One: Acetyl CoA to Carbon Dioxide

If acetyl CoA is not used to manufacture fat, amino acids, or other compounds, it may be completely oxidized. There are several reactions by which this can be accomplished, the details of which are not needed to understand the fates of the nutrients. The end result is that acetyl CoA is broken down. The chemical energy which bound it together is captured and used for the synthesis of other compounds in the body. The carbons are combined with oxygen to make carbon dioxide (CO_2), and the hydrogens that were attached to them are also combined with oxygen to make water (H_2O). Both are ultimately lost from the body through the urine, sweat, or exhaled air.

One Two Three Infinity: Anabolism

The story of metabolism of the nutrients would not be complete without a reminder that the many breakdown processes described above are less than half the total picture. All the intermediates named above—pyruvate, acetyl CoA, glucose, gly-

The discovery of urea by Wohler in 1828 was a momentous event in the history of science, technology, and agriculture. It laid a cornerstone for the science of organic chemistry and made possible the beginnings of the fertilizer industry. See Appendix A.

The reactions by which the complete oxidation of acetyl CoA is accomplished are those of the **Krebs cycle** (named for the biochemist who elucidated them) and **oxidative phosphorylation.** Details are given in the Highlight which follows.

cerol, amino acids, and fatty acids—also participate in anabolic processes in which very large and complex molecules are made, such as those of hair, the pigment of the eyes, the hormones, DNA (the material of the genes), RNA, and many others. Obvious examples of anabolic reactions that have already been described are those in which the four principal compounds derived from food are put together: glucose with more glucose to make glycogen in the liver and muscle; glycerol and fatty acids to make triglycerides (fat) in the adipose cells; and amino acids to make protein. And then of course these elaborate structures may be broken down again when the need arises, providing materials from which still others may be made—or once again providing energy.

The following diagram sums up what has been said about metabolism:

Summing Up

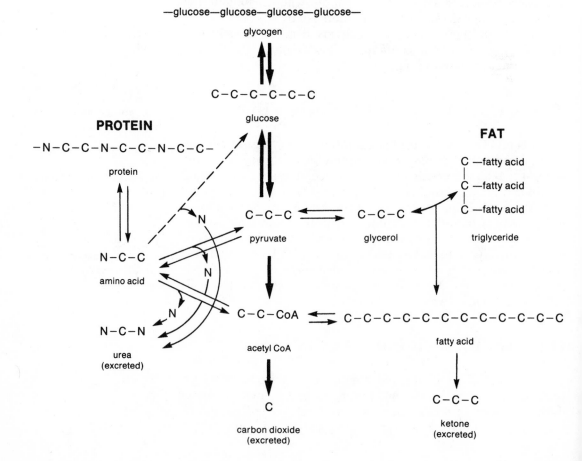

CARBOHYDRATE

—glucose—glucose—glucose—glucose—

glycogen

C–C–C–C–C–C

glucose

PROTEIN

–N–C–C–N–C–C–N–C–C–

protein

N–C–C

amino acid

N–C–N

urea
(excreted)

C–C–C

pyruvate

C–C–CoA

acetyl CoA

C

carbon dioxide
(excreted)

FAT

C —fatty acid
C —fatty acid
C —fatty acid

triglyceride

C–C–C

glycerol

C–C–C–C–C–C–C–C–C–C–C–C

fatty acid

C–C–C

ketone
(excreted)

The principal compounds derived from carbohydrate, fat, and protein in the diet are glucose, glycerol and fatty acids, and amino acids. Glucose may be anabolized to glycogen or catabolized to pyruvate, which in turn yields acetyl CoA. Glycerol and fatty acids may be anabolized to triglycerides or catabolized (glycerol to pyruvate, fatty acids to acetyl CoA). Amino acids may be anabolized to protein or catabolized (after deamination) to pyruvate or acetyl CoA.

Pyruvate is reconvertible to glucose, but the reaction yielding acetyl CoA from pyruvate is irreversible, hence fatty acids cannot ordinarily serve as a source of glucose in the body.

All three nutrients are convertible to acetyl CoA, however, and hence can be used to manufacture body fat.

If fatty acids are catabolized without simultaneous glucose catabolism, a principal product is ketones, which must be excreted. If amino acids are deaminated, the nitrogen removed is combined with carbon in urea and excreted.

The complete oxidation of acetyl CoA yields carbon dioxide, water, and energy.

To Explore Further—

A brief and clear explanation of the ways in which energy flows though living things. Paperback:

Lehninger, A. L.: *Bioenergetics: The Molecular Basis of Biological Energy Transformation.* W. A. Benjamin, Inc., New York, 1965.

An Optional Chapter Extracting Energy from Carbohydrate, Fat, Protein

It is through this structure, in the process of metabolism, that matter and energy flow. Entering in various forms and quantities, they are temporarily shaped exactly to the form and condition of the organism; they conform to the characteristics of the kingdom, class, order, family, genus, species, and variety to which it· belongs, and they assume even the characteristics of the individual itself. Then they depart through the various channels of excretion.
—LAWRENCE J. HENDERSON

The life sciences have come a long way since the oxidation of nutrients was first likened to the burning of fuel, and our knowledge of the processes involved has reached an amazing degree of sophistication. This Highlight provides the option of taking a closer look at that knowledge—of what energy is, and how it is harnessed to do the body's work. The concept that energy can be captured from foodstuffs to do the body's work or to be stored in body compounds is understandable at many levels. The last chapter introduced this concept: the next one describes the uses and measurement of energy in the body. This Highlight is offered as a glimpse at a deeper level of understanding of energy transfer. It is provided for those who wish to probe deeper; the following chapters can be understood without it.

Energy

One of the strangest notions that those human beings who study the nature of things have ever come up with is that there is such a thing as energy. It is a stuff with no concrete existence. It weighs nothing and yet it can move mountains. It makes itself felt over great distances. It is apparent to us sometimes as light, at other times as heat; and one can be turned into the other. It has no mass and yet it possesses a characteristic that physicists call charge—and so it can do the work of electricity. The physicists have measured it and have satisfied themselves that energy is never created or destroyed, that instead, as it is con-

energy: the capacity to do work.

forms of energy: heat, light, electrical, mechanical, chemical.

work: the moving of a mass through a distance.

216

verted from one form to another, it is all conserved. Wherever there is motion there is energy at work, and yet energy may sometimes seem to stand still. Wherever there is the power to move things there is also energy. If you like to ponder the mysteries of the universe, one of the most wonderful (wonder-full) is that energy is real. It exists; it has been measured; it works.

The energy in food, or more properly in the nutrients of which food is composed, is found in what we have somewhat imprecisely called the bonds that hold the atoms of those nutrients together. The glucose molecule, with which you are by now thoroughly familiar, possesses 24 atoms held together by 23 such bonds, each composed of a pair of electrons. As glucose is taken apart during catabolism, some of the electron energy which constitutes those bonds becomes available to form bonds between other atoms. As a glucose molecule is broken down from a 6-carbon compound to two 3-carbon compounds your system can capture the energy which held the two 3-carbon chains together and can use that energy to combine two other molecules (let's call them B and C) to make a new, larger compound (B—C). Later, by breaking this compound, you can use the energy to put together, for example, two amino acids and begin forming a protein: thus is hair made. The proteins of hair are formed by the addition of amino acids to a chain in a process fueled by energy originally released by the breaking of bonds in glucose or other energy nutrients.

Your body and the bodies of other living things, both animals and plants, are specially designed to capture, for their own internal use, much of the chemical bond energy that becomes available as nutrient molecules are disassembled. This characteristic is true only of living things. Breakdown of molecules also occurs in dead, organic systems, but when such a breakdown occurs, as for example when firewood burns, the energy released is not captured in a usable form but is converted to heat and light energy, which radiate away from the burning object. The process by which the body breaks down glucose is ultimately similar to that by which the glucose (cellulose) in firewood is broken down when it burns: the oxygen consumed and energy released are the same amount. But unlike burning firewood, the body doesn't go up in flames. Instead it releases a little energy as heat but retains much of it as chemical bond energy in other body structures.

In some ways, the metabolism of the nutrients is analogous to the transformations which can be performed with tinker toys. The wheels are atoms, the sticks electrons. A toy jungle gym built with these pieces, like a nutrient molecule, can be taken apart, and the same wheels and sticks can be used to build a toy crane (a body structure like hair). There are two important differences, though: a dismantled tinker toy can lie around for

First Law of Thermodynamics: energy is neither created nor destroyed during chemical or physical processes. It may be transformed from one form to another.

days before the pieces are used to build another one, while in organic reactions, the sticks—electrons—never stay still. They either escape—fly off—or they must immediately be associated with atoms, holding them together. So in the body, electron energy removed from glucose and other nutrients is immediately used to form bonds in other compounds.

The other difference is that the sticks may be used over and over again without losing their binding ability, while in chemical reactions a little energy is lost (as heat) in each transfer. The loss of energy from your metabolic system literally heats you up: your body is maintained at 98.6 degrees Fahrenheit by the rate of the metabolic reactions it performs. This continual loss of heat energy from the body surface makes it necessary for people to refuel periodically, that is, to obtain a new energy supply from food to continue their metabolic work.

Second Law of Thermodynamics: the natural tendency of any physical system consisting of a large number of individual units is to go from a state of order to a state of disorder, thus the usable energy decreases.

Where does this heat energy go? The total amount of energy in the *universe* remains constant: in that sense this energy is not lost. But it is lost to you: you can only use energy in forms—such as chemical bonds—that can do your metabolic or mechanical work. Pondering this question has brought physicists to the brink of metaphysics and philosophy, areas outside our province as nutritionists. References at the end of this chapter will carry you further in these directions, should you choose to follow them.

As you read this and try to put together your own mental picture of what happens to energy during metabolism, you may be anticipating that as nutrients are broken down, there must be available somewhere nearby a compound B and a compound C which can be put together whenever energy becomes available to accomplish the task. This is indeed the way the system works. Compounds B and C are floating around in all your body cells; wherever energy is made available to put them together the compound B-C is formed. The energy is captured between them. The combining of B and C is accomplished on the surface of the very same enzyme that takes apart some other molecule, releasing energy.

The enzymes which can perform this energy transfer are those which catalyze coupled reactions. An example will illustrate. Picture an enzyme (a giant molecule whose surface is bristling with positive and negative charges, attractive to other molecules) which has on its surface a place for splitting glucose and elsewhere on its surface a place where B and C can be put together. A molecule of glucose approaches this enzyme and begins to split in half. For the coupled reaction to occur, B and C

coupled reaction: a chemical event in which an enzyme catalyzes two reactions simultaneously, often the breakdown of one compound to two, and the synthesis of another from two.

must also be present at another site on the enzyme surface. As the glucose splits, the electron energy which bonded it together is transferred to bind B and C (losing only a little energy as heat). At no time can the energy which bonded the glucose be freed or lost altogether as heat or light.

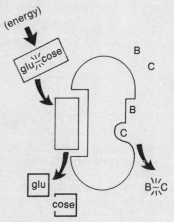

Loading Energy into Carriers

If you have understood the preceding description, you will appreciate the strange paradox that even though energy weighs nothing, it still must be carried. Molecule B and molecule C join together to carry this energy when it is released from an energy nutrient in a coupled reaction. Such a reaction is shown in the figure below. Molecule B is adenosine diphosphate (ADP); molecule C is a phosphate group (P):

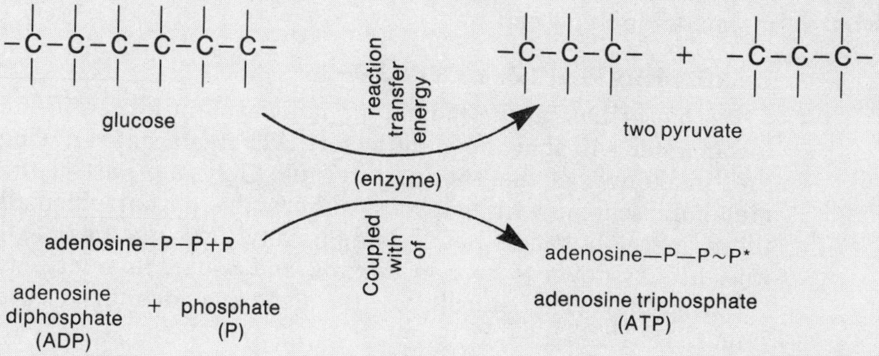

glucose → two pyruvate

reaction transfer energy

(enzyme)

Coupled with of

adenosine–P–P+P

adenosine diphosphate (ADP) + phosphate (P)

adenosine–P—P~P*

adenosine triphosphate (ATP)

*~ denotes a high-energy bond

(It is not important to learn the structures of these compounds. ADP is merely another molecule like others with which you are familiar, composed of C, H, O, and N, and containing two phosphorus—P—atoms derived from the mineral phosphorus in the diet. Free phosphate, also derived from dietary phosphorus, abounds in cells too.)

As energy is released from glucose in this coupled reaction, the phosphate group is attached to ADP to make adenosine triphosphate, ATP. The energy has then been captured between the second and third phosphorus atoms in the ATP molecule.

Not all the bonds in glucose possess enough energy to bind phosphate to ADP. There are high energy bonds and low energy bonds. Hence not every reaction in which a large molecule is broken down yields energy which can be captured in this way; many yield heat only. Then, too, some high energy bonds cannot be used in the body because we do not possess the necessary enzymes to make the transfer. This is why protein, fat, and carbohydrate (and alcohol) are the only molecules which serve

ATP: adenosine triphosphate (ad-DEN-o-sin try-FOS-fate): the commonest energy carrier in cells. (Structure in Appendix C.)

The metabolism of alcohol is described in Highlight 9.

us as energy nutrients: during their breakdown our body cells can extract the energy from them in a usable form, as ATP.

There are billions and billions of molecules of ATP in the body. When you use or spend this energy, what actually happens at the molecular level is that the above reaction is reversed. ATP breaks down to ADP and P once again in a coupled reaction, releasing energy as heat or giving it to some other molecule that is simultaneously being put together.

The reversible reaction between ADP + P and ATP provides an energy-carrying system that is universally used in animal organisms. Any other two molecules could be used in theory, and some are, to a limited extent; the only requirement is that a high energy bond be formed when they are put together. As it happens, animals have evolved to use the ATP system as a most convenient way of carrying and exchanging energy between molecules in living cells.

Generating ATP: A Closer Look

A closer look at the metabolic pathways introduced in the last chapter will show how and where ATP is generated during the breakdown of the energy nutrients. Only one part of the metabolic scheme will be discussed here, that part at which all three energy nutrients have yielded acetyl CoA. As the acetyl CoA breaks down to carbon dioxide and water, its energy is captured into ATP. Let us follow the steps by which this occurs (Figure H7.1).

(1) Acetyl CoA combines with a 4-carbon compound, oxalo-acetate. The CoA comes off, and the product formed is a 6-carbon compound, citrate.

(2) The atoms of citrate are rearranged to form isocitrate.

(3) Now a molecule called NAD^+ reacts with isocitrate. Two H's and two electrons are removed from the isocitrate. One H becomes attached to the NAD^+ with the two electrons; the other H is released as a free proton. Thus NAD^+ becomes NADH + H^+.

> Remember this NADH + H^+. Let us follow the other product first.

A carbon is removed and combined with oxygen, forming carbon dioxide (which diffuses away in the blood and is exhaled). What is left is the 5-carbon compound alpha-ketoglutarate.

(4) Now *two* compounds interact with alpha-ketoglutarate: a molecule of CoA and a molecule of NAD^+. In this complex reaction, a carbon is removed and combined with oxygen (forming carbon dioxide); two H's are removed and one is attached

---

Other energy carriers in animal systems: guanosine (GWON-o-sine) diphosphate (GDP) + phosphate (P) → guanosine triphosphate (GTP) (used in protein synthesis); creatine (CREE-uh-tin) + P ⟷ creatine→P (used in muscle).

The eight reactions described here are those of the **Krebs cycle,** named for the biochemist who elucidated them. This cycle is also known as the **TCA (tricarboxylic acid) cycle,** or **citric acid cycle.**

NAD^+: an organic ion. For ions, see Appendix B. NAD^+ is further defined as a coenzyme in Chapter 9.

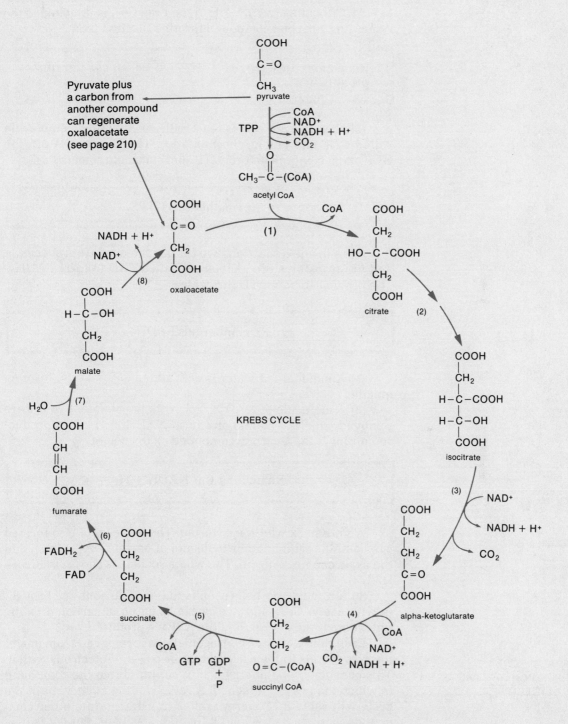

Figure H7.1. The Krebs Cycle.

to NAD⁺ (forming NADH + H⁺), and the CoA is attached to the remaining 4-carbon compound forming succinyl-CoA.

> Remember this NADH + H⁺. Let us follow the other product first.

(5) Now *two* molecules react with succinyl CoA: a molecule called GDP and one of phosphate (P). The CoA comes off, the GDP and P combine to form GTP, and succinate remains.

> Remember this GTP.

(6) In the next reaction, two H's are removed from succinate and are transferred to a molecule called FAD to form FADH₂. The product remaining is fumarate.

> Remember this FADH₂.

(7) A molecule of water is next added to fumarate, forming malate.
(8) A molecule of NAD⁺ reacts with the malate: two H's are removed from the malate and form NADH + H⁺. The product remaining is the 4-carbon compound oxaloacetate.

> Remember this NADH + H⁺.

We are back where we started. The oxaloacetate so formed can combine with another molecule of acetyl CoA (step 1), and the cycle can begin again. The whole scheme is shown in Figure H7.1.

So far, what you have seen is that two carbons are brought in with acetyl CoA, and two carbons end up in carbon dioxide. But where is the energy, and the ATP we promised you?

chemical bond energy: see Appendix B.

Each time a pair of hydrogen atoms is removed from one of the compounds in the cycle, it carries a pair of electrons with it. This chemical bond energy is thus captured into the compound to which the H's are attached. A review of the eight steps of the cycle will show that energy is thus transferred into other compounds in steps 3, 4, 6, and 8. In step 5 as well, energy is harnessed to bind GDP and P together to form GTP. Thus the compounds NADH + H⁺ (three molecules), FADH₂, and GTP are built using energy originally found in acetyl CoA, while the acetyl CoA has been dismantled to two carbon dioxide molecules. To see how this energy ends up in ATP, we must follow the electrons further. Let us take those attached to NAD$^+$ as an example (Figure H7.2).

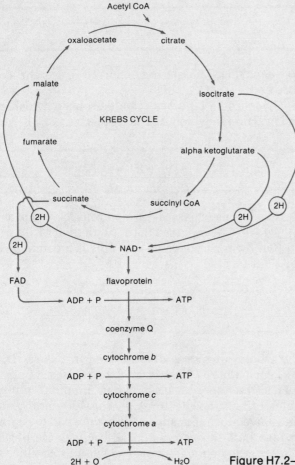

Figure H7.2—The electron transport chain.

An important concept to remember at this point is that an electron is not a fixed amount of energy. The electrons bonding the H to NAD$^+$ in NADH have a relatively large amount of energy. In the series of reactions that follow, they lose this energy in small amounts until at the end they are attached (with H's) to oxygen (O) to make water (H_2O). In some of the steps, the energy they lose is captured into ATP in coupled reactions.

(1) NADH reacts with a molecule called a flavoprotein, losing its electrons (and their H's). The products are NAD$^+$ and reduced flavoprotein. A little energy is lost as heat in this reaction.

The six reactions described here are those of the **electron transport chain.** Since oxygen is required for these reactions and ADP and P are combined to form ATP in several of them (ADP is phosphorylated), they are also called **oxidative phosphorylation.**

(2) The flavoprotein passes on the electrons to a molecule called coenzyme Q. Again they lose some energy as heat, but ADP and P participate in this reaction and gain much of the energy to bond together and form ATP. This is a coupled reaction.

$$ADP + P \;\rightarrow\; ATP$$

(3) Coenzyme Q passes the electrons to cytochrome *b*. Again they lose energy.

(4) Cytochrome *b* passes the electrons to cytochrome *c* in a coupled reaction in which ATP is formed.

$$ADP + P \;\rightarrow\; ATP$$

(5) Cytochrome *c* passes the electrons to cytochrome *a*.

(6) Cytochrome *a* passes them (with their H's) to an atom of oxygen (O), forming water (H_2O). This is a coupled reaction in which ATP is formed.

$$ADP + P \;\rightarrow\; ATP$$

oxidation: see Appendix B.

The whole process is diagrammed in Figure H7.2. As you can see, each time NADH is oxidized (loses its electrons) by this means, the energy it loses is parcelled out into three ATP molecules. When the electrons are passed on to water, at the end, they have much less energy than they had to begin with.

So far, then, the compound with which we began—acetyl CoA—has yielded enough energy to synthesize nine ATP molecules: three for each NADH that was generated by the Krebs cycle (steps 3, 4, 8). In addition, a molecule of GTP was formed (step 5). The GTP can pass on its phosphate group in a coupled reaction:

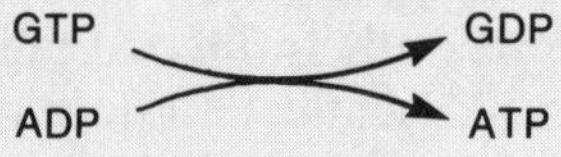

GTP   GDP

ADP   ATP

This reaction forms another ATP. Finally (in step 6), electrons from acetyl CoA were passed to $FADH_2$, which can yield two more ATP (see Figure H7.2). Thus twelve ATP molecules are formed for each molecule of acetyl CoA that is oxidized through the Krebs cycle.

The Krebs cycle and the electron transport chain are the body's major means of taking the energy from nutrients and capturing it in ATP molecules. There are other means (three ATP's are generated in the conversion of pyruvate to acetate, for example) that are similar, and there is much more that biochemists understand about these processes than has been presented here. The suggested readings at the end of this Highlight were selected for the clarity with which they present further details. Some considerations relating to the release of energy from ATP will complete this overview of the way in which energy from food does the body's work.

Unloading Energy from Carriers

Okay—so now you are full of energy. You have just eaten a meal and catabolized the carbohydrate, fat, and protein in it, making billions of molecules of ATP. What do you choose to do with it? Fortunately, you don't have to make all of these decisions consciously. About two-thirds of your energy is spent automatically for you, maintaining your vital functions, and using a priority system that guarantees that you get the most important work done first. The other one-third you are free to spend as you wish, contemplating the mysteries of nature, playing tennis, or doing whatever else you choose to do.

The distinction made above is the distinction between the two major classes of activities that consume human energy each day. The first are the basal metabolic processes, which go on all the time, even during sleep. These are vital processes: the maintenance of the heartbeat, respiration, nerve function, glandular activity, generation of heat and the like, without which you could not be said to be alive. The second are the voluntary activities, over which you have conscious control: sitting, standing, running, eating, playing the piano, and the like. The amount of energy spent on each of these types of activity can be measured, and a total can be found which represents the total amount of energy you must consume each day by eating food in order to stay in balance. These measurements, and the concepts of energy balance, are the subjects of the next chapter. It seems worthwhile here to give a few examples of the way in which the energy taken from nutrients and transferred into ATP is used to power these activities.

ATP provides energy for catabolism. A most vital need is to ensure that you have a continuous influx of energy to replace that which you spend. At certain points during the catabolism of carbohydrate, fat, and protein, energy is needed to power a reaction that otherwise would not occur. At each of these points, a molecule of ATP is split into ADP + P to push the reaction.

One molecule of acetyl CoA oxidized through the Krebs Cycle yields:

$3NADH + H^+$	→	9ATP
1 FADH$_2$	→	2ATP
1 GTP	→	1ATP
Total		12ATP

Basal metabolism is defined and discussed further in Chapter 8.

voluntary activities: see Chapter 8.

ATP energy used for catabolism:

glucose + ATP

glucose—P   ADP

For example, during the breakdown of glucose, an atom of phosphorus must be attached to the glucose molecule to prepare it for the coupled reaction in which it is split by an enzyme into two 3-carbon compounds. The first step in glucose catabolism is one in which ATP donates this phosphorus with its associated energy to glucose. ADP and glucose-phosphate are left.

You can see that catabolism is not a cost-free process. Energy (ATP) must be spent at certain points to keep catabolism going. However, the amount of ATP generated during catabolism is greater than the amount consumed, so that in the end there is a net gain. The catabolism of one molecule of acetyl CoA to carbon dioxide and water generates twelve molecules of ATP. This catabolic action is the most efficient energy-yielding process in the body.

ATP provides energy for anabolism. As already mentioned, anabolic processes require ATP. To make a protein chain, one ATP is split for each amino acid added to the chain. To make glycogen, one ATP provides the energy to add each glucose. To make fatty acids from acetyl CoA, ATP is needed at the rate of one for each acetate added, and so on. Obviously to keep the body's metabolic work going on, energy must be continously supplied.

ATP provides energy for muscle movements. A muscle cell is packed with an orderly array of long, thin, protein molecules lined up side by side. To contract a muscle, what must be done (what you would have to do if you had to think about it) is to let molecule A and molecule B combine chemically, sliding into one

ATP energy used for anabolism:

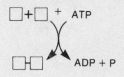

The contractile proteins of muscle are actin and myosin.

creatine phosphate energy used for muscle contraction:

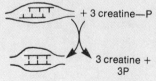

Lipid in muscle. The lipid droplets are stored close to the muscle fiber (bottom), and the mitochondria which generate energy from fatty acids crowd around these droplets. Photographed under an electron microscope at a magnification of 47,000 x.

J. W. Fawcett, *An Atlas of Fine Structure.* Philadelphia and London: W. B. Saunders Company, 1966, Figure 60. Courtesy of the author and publisher.

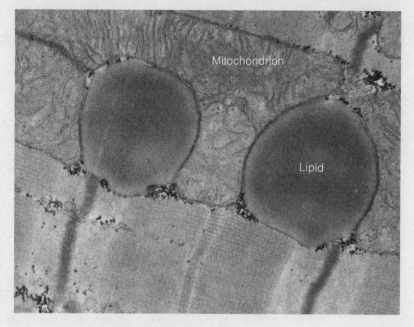

another as they do so. They must then execute another chemical reaction, which slides them still closer together. The reactions which make muscles move are powered by energy carriers similar to ATP. For peristalsis, for the beating of the heart muscle, for the inhalation of air into the lungs, and for many other automatic muscular actions these reactions do the necessary work.

ATP provides energy for the transmission of nerve impulses. Even during sleep, the brain and nerves are active. At the molecular level, what is going on is that the membranes of the nerve cells, which contain protein pumps, are maintaining an electrical charge by pumping sodium ions out and potassium ions in. When a nerve impulse travels along these cells they depolarize: sodium rushes in, and potassium out. To regain the readiness to fire, the membrane pumps go to work to repolarize the cell, sorting out the potassium and sodium ions again. Each protein pump splits one molecule of ATP each time it transfers an ion across the membrane.

The above few examples show the uses of ATP-carried energy for basal metabolic activities. If in addition to simply remaining alive, you wish to use additional energy to compose a poem, knit a sweater, or jog a mile, additional ATP must be available for the extra nervous and muscular activities involved.

Completing the Picture

This Highlight concludes one of nutrition's major stories: the way in which the four principal types of atoms found in food, and the energy which bonds them, flow into the body in food, undergo rearrangements there, and ultimately flow out again. It may be satisfying to you to realize that you can now follow any of these atoms, or the energy connecting them, through the complete cycle around which they flow. Just for fun, let us imagine taking a carbon atom, painting it red, and watching it travel through its cycle. Let us begin at the point where the carbon atom forms part of a molecule of carbon dioxide in the air.

This particular molecule of carbon dioxide enters a potato leaf. There, sparked by a photon from the sun, it is combined with water to become part of a molecule of glucose. This glucose then travels to the root, where it is attached to other glucose molecules to make starch. The starch is stored in the potato until you eat it. After you have swallowed it, the red carbon atom finds itself in your intestine, where the starch is hydrolyzed to glucose again; the glucose enters your bloodstream and is carried to a cell. Inside the cell, the glucose is broken down into two 3-carbon compounds, in one of which our red carbon atom finds itself. This 3-carbon compound loses a carbon to become part of acetyl CoA. Let us suppose that our red carbon atom still finds itself in the acetyl CoA.

ATP energy used to repolarize nerve cell membranes.

The carbon cycle

photon (FOE-ton): a unit of light energy.

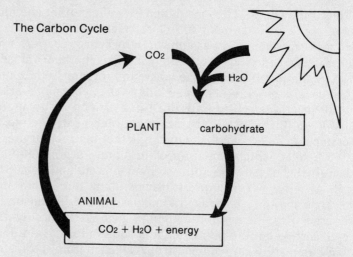

The Carbon Cycle

Now the acetyl CoA may be used to synthesize body fat, in which case our red carbon atom is trapped in a fat cell for a while, or it may be used to synthesize an amino acid and become part of a protein such as hemoglobin, and as such travel in a red blood cell through the circulatory system. Let us suppose in this example that the body's primary need is for energy, and that the acetyl CoA is further broken down to two molecules of carbon dioxide and water. Released in one of these carbon dioxide molecules, our red carbon finds its way back into the blood and ultimately is freed into air spaces in the lungs and breathed back into the atmosphere.

Around again it goes, possibly cycling back through another potato plant and into you again, but far more likely going elsewhere next time—into an acorn on an oak tree, perhaps, and later into a chipmunk's cheek. And around again.

It may prove satisfying to you to follow the path of a hydrogen atom or an oxygen atom in the same way. There is also a nitrogen cycle, although the complete outlines are not apparent from the discussions of nitrogen that have been presented here. But let us take only one more example of the ways in which particles dance: this time an electron.

The electron is born as a photon, released from the sun. It becomes an electron when it enters a potato leaf and is captured into glucose. As one of the bonds in glucose, it enters your body. When the glucose is broken apart, this energy is freed and may be used to put together a molecule of ADP with phosphate to make ATP. It therefore stays behind in your body, while the carbon to which it was connected ends up being breathed out once again. The energy in the ATP is later either spent or stored. Let us consider each of these fates in turn.

If the energy is spent immediately, what happens is that the ATP is broken apart, releasing its energy to help move a

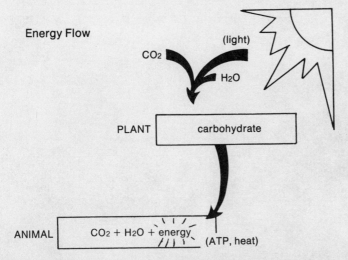

Energy Flow

muscle, or transmit a nerve impulse. The energy ends up as work accomplished and heat radiated away. No longer in the form in which you can use it, it is lost to the body.

If the energy is stored, what happens is that the ATP is split in a coupled reaction during which (let's say) two acetyl CoA molecules are put together to help form a fatty acid. The fatty acid is later connected to a molecule of glycerol together with two others to form a triglyceride, which is stored in a fat cell. For a while, then, our electron is trapped in your body, although at any time when you need it, its energy may become available again as fat breaks down to fuel body processes.

The electron changes forms, unlike the red carbon atom, which can cycle again and again through the atmosphere, to plants, and back to the atmosphere, always remaining recognizable. Beginning as a photon, the electron exists for a while as part of a chemical bond, and later becomes a bit of heat. This heat energy, although still the same in amount as it was when it came from the sun, cannot be used again by plants or animals to fuel their work. Thus, life can go on, on earth, only for as long as the sun continues to burn and flood our plants with light.

The downhill flow of energy is not a cycle.

This discussion has taken us far from the problems of nutrition, although you may agree that the concept of energy must be understood if the very real nutritional problems of underweight and obesity are to be dealt with. Ironically, although energy weighs almost nothing, when you store energy, you weigh more. The reason this is so is clear from the tinker toy analogy, in which energy is represented by the sticks. The sticks weigh nothing, yet in order to keep them in place you must attach them to wheels which weigh something. To capture energy and store it in your body you must trap it in molecules of fat, and thus the more energy you store, the heavier you become. Fat also takes up space, and so the more energy you store, the

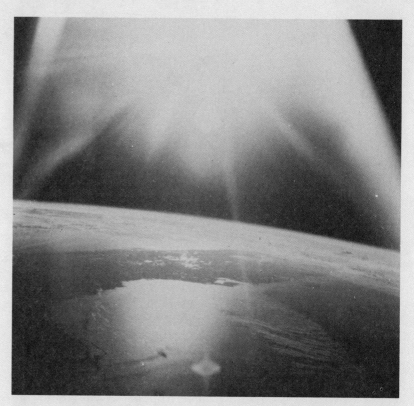

Sunlight provides the energy for life on earth. The photo above, taken from an Apollo spacecraft, shows the Florida peninsula, with the Gulf of Mexico in the foreground.
Photo courtesy of NASA.

bulkier you become. The problems of energy excess, which causes overweight and obesity, and energy deficit, which causes underweight and calorie malnutrition, result from this arrangement. The practical considerations relating to these problems are taken up in the next chapter.

Summing Up

The energy in food resides in the chemical bonds which hold nutrient molecules together. In the body, when these bonds are broken, some of this energy is released as heat, and much is captured through coupled reactions into energy carrier molecules such as ATP. When ATP in turn is broken down to ADP and phosphate, the energy is again released as heat and used to anabolize body compounds. ATP powers all of the energy-requiring processes in the body: metabolic reactions, the transmission of nerve impulses, the contraction of muscles, etc. Ultimately all food energy is expended as work and as heat which is lost from the body. To replace this expenditure, more food must be eaten.

The cell's principal means of generating ATP is the sequence of reactions known as the Krebs cycle and the electron transport chain. In the Krebs cycle, acetyl CoA (from carbohydrate, fat, or protein) is attached to oxaloacetate to form citrate, and citrate is processed in a series of reactions which convert it back to oxaloacetate. During these reactions two carbon dioxide molecules are released, and energy is transferred into other carrier compounds. The major carrier is NAD^+. Each NAD^+ molecule receives two high energy electrons to become NADH $+ H^+$ and then transfers them to a series of other carriers: the electron transport chain. At each step they lose energy, and at several of these steps the energy is transferred, in a coupled reaction, into ATP. The electrons are finally donated to oxygen, yielding water.

The ATP so generated carries a large amount of energy in its terminal phosphate group and participates in other coupled reactions to do the body's work. Among its contributions are energy to power the first step in the catabolism of glucose, energy to synthesize glycogen, fatty acids, and proteins, energy for muscle movements, and for polarization of nerve cells between the transmission of nerve impulses. When the energy originally found in food has been transferred into ATP and used for these purposes, it ultimately leaves the body as heat or work accomplished and is no longer usable.

Thus, while carbon and the other atoms present in nutrients cycle repeatedly through living things, energy flows downhill, being gradually dissipated as heat. Although no net energy is lost in this process, heat energy is not reconvertible to chemical bonds; hence a new supply of usable energy must flow constantly from the sun, through plants, into animals and human beings. This explains the need for food to sustain life.

Energy storage involves the capture of energy which chemically binds organic molecules together, and therefore entails storage of matter which occupies space and has weight. The problem of storing more energy than is needed therefore becomes a problem of storing more weight: obesity, which is taken up in the next chapter.

To Explore Further—

A brief and clear explanation of the ways in which energy flows through living things. Paperback:

Lehninger, A. L.: *Bioenergetics: The Molecular Basis of Biolgical Energy Transformation.* W. A. Benjamin, Inc., New York, 1965.

A more technical, but clear and highly accurate, treatment of biochemical pathways, including the Krebs cycle and the electron transport chain:

Lehninger, A. L.: *Biochemistry.* World Publishers, Inc., New York, 1970.

This entire issue was devoted to energy flow from the sun through living systems, and its relevance to current human problems of pollution and the food supply:

The Biosphere, *Scientific American,* September, 1970.

8

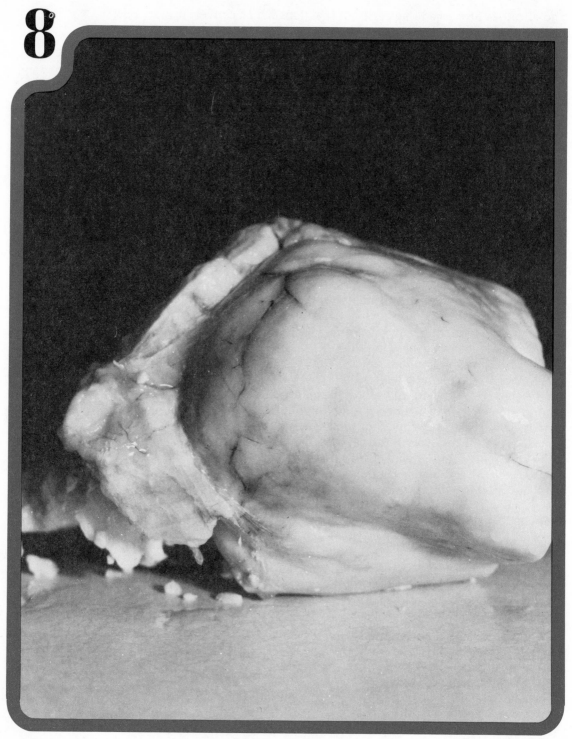

5 pounds of fat.

Energy Balance and Weight Control

The fact that we can become fatter is not, as many people tend to see it, a curse upon the race, or a highly visible punishment for gluttony; it is instead an essential mechanism for human survival.
—RONALD M. DEUTSCH

A promise was made at the start that the information presented in the chapters of this book would be solid information, while the recent or controversial findings would be presented in the Highlights between chapters. Much of the recent important work in the area of obesity (due to positive energy balance) has not yet yielded clear-cut, textbook information, but is so interesting as to demand mention in this chapter. Notes in the margins point the way to suggested readings which cover these areas in depth.

Another mission of this book is to explode myths and fallacies used to beguile the public into adopting costly or unhealthful nutritional nostrums. No area within the science of nutrition is more sorely beset with false and misleading claims than that of weight loss plans. Our decision has been to devote the entire Highlight following this chapter to this problem area.

Chapter 8 itself is devoted to the practical problems of measuring energy intake and output and regulating the balance between them in order to maintain weight. This topic deserves the heaviest emphasis because *prevention* of obesity has important implications for health. Overweight people die younger, contract diabetes, cardiovascular disease, gall bladder disease and gout more readily, and suffer greater risks in surgery than their thinner counterparts.

Methuselah

Methuselah ate what he found on his plate
And never, as people do now,
Did he note the amount of his calorie count—
He ate it because it was chow.
He wasn't disturbed as at dinner he sat
Devouring a roast or a pie
To think it was lacking in unsaturated fat
Or a couple of vitamins shy.
He cheerfully chewed each species of food
Unmindful of troubles or fears
Lest his health might be hurt
By some fancy dessert.
And he lived over nine hundred years!

Unknown

How Much Energy? Calorimetry

calorimetry (cal-o-RIM-uh-tree): the measurement of energy.

calor = heat
metron = measure

Fascinating as the theoretical and molecular study of energy flow may be (see Chapter 7 and Highlight 7), as nutritionists, we must return to the practical goal of making recommendations for human nutrition. Energy is constantly being spent by humans, and there must be a constant influx of new usable energy to replace it. Energy comes into the body in food, as the chemical bonds in the energy nutrients which can be transferred into other compounds during metabolism. It leaves the body, ultimately, as heat. To know how much food energy people need, we must have a way of measuring the energy they spend (lose)—and of measuring the energy they can capture from food. This is what calories are all about.

The infamous calorie: what it is. It is curious to contemplate the fact that we can measure something we cannot see or feel. An object's size is easy to measure. A yardstick tells us that our kitchen table is three feet wide and four feet long. The weight of the table is also easy to measure. We put it on a scale, it stretches a spring, and the spring turns a dial to read twenty kilograms (44 pounds). Energy, which has no dimensions and weighs nothing, can also be measured in ingenious ways. Consider the energy in the table. If we could convert it to light we could measure its brightness. If we could use it to push something, we might measure the distance that that thing was pushed. If we could use it to heat something, we might measure the number of degrees the temperature of the thing being heated is raised. All of these ways of measuring energy are in fact used by physicists. The one which is most convenient to nutritionists is the last described: measuring heat. Nutritionists would be inclined to burn the table in a fireplace under a kettle of water and measure how much the water was heated in the process.

The food energy the nutritionist is interested in is that available to human beings and animals from the chemical bonds in a food's energy nutrients—carbohydrate, fat, and protein. These are the bonds that are broken and ultimately converted to heat when the food is oxidized in the body during metabolism. To determine how much energy can be released from a food this way, nutritionists completely oxidize the food outside the body; that is, they burn it. The chemical bond energy is converted to heat, and they measure the heat released.

weight: the amount that a thing weighs (presses down, as on a scale).

gram (g): the weight of a cubic centimeter (cc) of water under defined conditions of temperature and pressure.

There is nothing absolute about units of measurement; they have no physical existence outside of the human realm. We use them to agree on how much of something we have. In order to agree, we have to adopt a standard. A dollar (a unit of monetary exchange) is an amount of money exchangeable for a certain amount of gold on the international money market. A gram (a unit of weight) is the amount of a substance which weighs as

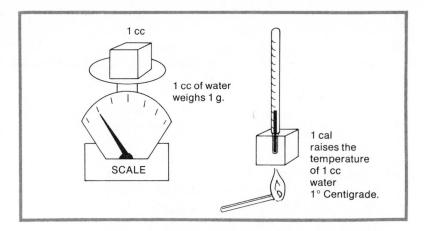

much as a cubic centimeter of water at 4 degrees Centigrade. A calorie (a unit of heat) is the amount of heat energy that will raise the temperature of a gram of water one degree Centigrade. A Centigrade degree (a unit of temperature) is one-hundredth of the difference in temperature between melting ice and boiling water. These definitions are all agreed on among human beings for purposes of communicating about amounts of things.

Energy in food. Equipped with these definitions, we can determine how much energy there is in a food: a potato, for example. All we have to do is to burn the potato in a closed system so that all of the heat released is used to heat a gram of water, put a Centigrade thermometer in the water, and measure the change in temperature. The rise in the temperature tells us the number of calories in the potato.

There is a serious drawback to this method, however: a gram of water is a mere droplet: only a fifth of a teaspoon! Such a tiny amount of water would evaporate before the potato had even begun to burn. Nutritionists find it convenient to use a thousand of these droplets (a kilogram or liter) of water—which

heat: energy that causes substances to rise in temperature.

calorie (cal)

temperature: degree of hotness or coldness measured on a definite scale, as on a thermometer.

degree (°)

kilogram (KILL-o-gram) **(kg):** 1,000 grams. See Appendix D.

liter (LEE-ter) **(l):** 1,000 cubic centimeters. See Appendix D.

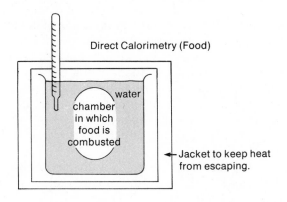

Direct Calorimetry (Food)

Diagram of the Bomb Calorimeter.

kilocalorie (KILL-o-cal-o-ree) **(kcal):** 1,000 calories. A kilocalorie, or **Calorie** (with a capital "C") is the amount of heat energy necessary to raise the temperature of a kilogram (one liter) of water one degree Centigrade. Food energy can also be measured in **kilojoules (kJ)**: a kilojoule is the amount of energy expended when one kilogram is moved one meter by a force of one Newton. One kcal = 4.2 kJ. The kilojoule is now the international unit of energy.

The nutritionists' calorie is a big Calorie.

direct calorimetry

bomb calorimeter

indirect calorimetry

is enough to fill a pot—and measure the heat released in thousands of calories (kilocalories). Putting the potato in a closed system and burning it in oxygen under a liter of water, nutritionists find that the water heats up from zero to 70 degrees Centigrade. They conclude that the potato contained 70,000 calories, or 70 kilocalories.

Thus food energy is measured in kilocalories (Calories). But watch out! While physicists play with their calories, and nutritionists with their Calories, the man on the street fails to make the distinction and envisions "calories" in food when more precisely he should be spelling the word with a capital C. We nutritionists often make the effort to speak about the energy values of foods in kilocalories but we, too, slip. In this book, the kilocalorie is used whenever a quantitative measure of the energy in food is given, while the commoner word calorie is used only to mean energy in general.

The method of measuring food energy described above is known as *direct* calorimetry, since the change in water temperature is a direct measure of the amount of heat energy released from the food. The instrument used is a bomb calorimeter.

There is another convenient way to measure food energy, which is possible because the amount of heat released is always proportional to the amount of oxygen consumed. When a potato is completely oxidized, all of the carbon (C) has combined with oxygen (O) to form carbon dioxide (CO_2), and all of the hydrogen (H) has combined with oxygen (O) to form water (H_2O). In the end, the CO_2 is all released as a gas, and the H_2O as water or water vapor, leaving nothing but mineral ash (and minerals contain no energy usable by humans). Instead of measuring the heat released, it is possible to determine the amount of oxygen consumed while a food is burned, and so obtain an *indirect* measure of the energy in the food.

Energy in people. A goal of this chapter is to make practical recommendations regarding energy consumption by people. The preceding sections have shown that the only energy people can use is that stored in the energy nutrients—carbohydrate, fat, and protein. So the task becomes one of deciding how much carbohydrate-fat-protein energy is needed. It is convenient to make this recommendation as kilocalories, and easy to think in terms of the kilocalories in foods using the Food Exchange System. The only task which remains is to determine how many kilocalories an individual should consume. This of course depends on how many he/she spends. Once again it is necessary to do some measuring: how much energy does a person spend in a day?

It is important to make a distinction here between energy spent and energy stored. Unlike potatoes which when used for food are soon converted to gas and water, people do not disappear; they are still there at the end of the day. At all times they contain some stored energy, as chemical bonds in the carbohydrate, fat, and protein and other large organic molecules in and around their body cells. (Only when they die do they return this energy to the universe from which they borrowed it.) The bonds in these molecules constitute a pool from which the body continuously draws energy and which must be frequently replenished by eating food.

When bond energy enters the body in a nutrient such as glucose and begins to flow through metabolism, it has two possible fates: it may be captured into another bond, or it may be converted to heat energy and dissipated. Each time a bond in glucose is broken, much of the energy is lost as heat. As long as the energy remains in bonds in the body it is unspent; it is stored. Thus the only energy we need to replace is the heat energy we lose. This is the energy we need to measure because this is the energy that must be replaced by eating food.

Energy loss can be measured the same way for a person as for a potato. A person can be put in a closed chamber with water circulating in pipes above. As heat rises from the person's body, the temperature of the water rises: a measure of the change in the water temperature is a *direct* measure of the person's energy expenditure. It is convenient to measure the amount of heat released in an hour, and to multiply by 24 to estimate the number of calories spent per day.

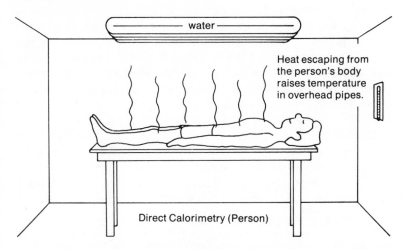

Direct Calorimetry (Person)

Indirectly, the person's oxygen consumption during this hour is a measure of his/her energy expenditure too. This may be obvious, but in case it isn't, the reasoning goes like this: heat-yielding reactions are catabolic, involving the consumption of oxygen. To the same extent as you catabolize compounds and release heat, you are breathing in oxygen and breathing out carbon dioxide.

Energy Balance

As long as your energy intake equals your expenditure, you will neither gain nor lose weight. For many people, this situation prevails. Without any conscious effort, they regulate their calorie intake so that it meets their energy needs exactly. The precision of this regulation is shown by the fact that many people remain at their proper weight throughout their lives without ever counting calories. When asked how they do this, they shrug and reply "I don't know," or explain, "I just eat when I'm hungry and stop when I'm full" — a statement which actually leaves a lot unexplained.

The hunger mechanism must be very precise indeed. A woman of sixty who weighs exactly what she should without ever having to watch her weight has consumed daily the number of calories she needed with virtually no error. If she had dug only a half-inch deeper into the margarine tub each day at breakfast (to the tune of an extra 20 kcalories a day), she would be 120 pounds overweight! Virtually all animals regulate their energy intake with this amazing degree of accuracy. Animals feel hunger when they are experiencing a calorie deficit. They eat in response, and they stop when the hunger signal stops. They only go out of balance when outside circumstances force them to: under experimental laboratory conditions or when food is scarce. It seems that hunger is an inborn biological drive which governs energy intake automatically.

How the hunger mechanism works is still unclear. One hypothesis is that hunger is a response of a part of the brain, the hunger center or hypothalamus, to low blood glucose concentrations; another is that the number of fat cells in the body, determined by the amount of food fed in early life, regulates hunger in some way.

zero energy balance or energy equilibrium: that condition in which calories in = calories out.

A possible explanation for the precision of appetite regulation is the set-point theory of Lepkovsky. See suggested readings.

hunger: the physiological need to eat.

The glucostatic theory of hunger regulation, proposed by Jean Mayer, accounts for many of the observed phenomena. (See suggested readings. For the effect of number of fat cells on hunger, see Chapter 15.)

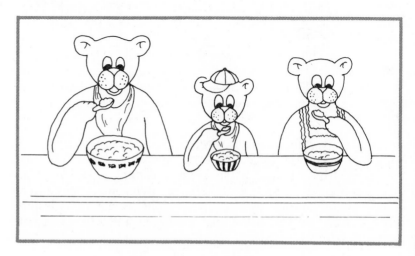

Humans are more complex than other animals. In addition to the innate hunger drive they have a learned response to food: appetite. While hunger is physiological, appetite is psychological, depending partly on people's memories of past experiences with food, partly on their habits. Ideally, appetite and hunger come together. When your body is physiologically hungry you experience appetite — a desire to eat. When your calorie need is met, both turn off together. Your hunger is satisfied and your appetite is quelled. As long as this situation prevails, your body weight is regulated appropriately.

What causes a person to eat habitually too little or too much? The answer to this question, if available, would be worth a million dollars to any person working in the areas of hyperphagia and anorexia. Psychologists and physiologists as well as nutritionists are presently very active in attempting to answer it. Whatever the causes, both of these conditions cause a person's body weight and composition to deviate from the ideal.

Ideal Weight, Underweight and Obesity

Tables of "ideal" weight, available from a variety of sources, are computed from the average weights of persons of each sex of a given height and frame size; one that is commonly used is given in Appendix F. Such tables should more fittingly be entitled weight norms, and the figures in them should not necessarily be taken as ideal for all persons in the categories presented. You should not necessarily weigh the same amount as the average person your age and sex. Nevertheless, the conditions of being under- and overweight are most often defined with reference to these tables: underweight is more than 10 percent below, and overweight is more than 10 percent above the "ideal" weight. A more appropriate criterion for determining actual conditions of undesirably low or high weight would be based on body composition.

Fifty-nine percent of the average man's body weight and 55 percent of a woman's is *water* weight. Excess fluid accumulation (as in edema) or water loss (dehydration) can cause dramatic, but usually temporary, fluctuations in body weight which have nothing to do with body fat. (Many fad diets, which claim to promote losses of "up to five pounds in the first day" actually cause water losses of this magnitude; see the Highlight which follows this chapter.)

Ideally, about 18 percent of a man's body weight and about 22 percent of a woman's should consist of fat. Much of the re-

appetite: the desire to eat, which normally accompanies hunger.

causes of obesity: see suggested readings.

hyperphagia (high-per-FAGE-ee-uh): excessive appetite or eating.

anorexia (an-o-REX-ee-uh): lack of appetite. *Anorexia nervosa* is a severe disturbance of appetite regulation sometimes seen in adolescents.[1]

an = not
orexis = appetite

average: mean.

norm: a standard derived (usually) from the average of a large group.

ideal weight: average weight for a person of a given sex, age, height, and frame size. (For a note on frame size, see Appendix F.)

underweight: more than 10 percent below normal or average ("ideal") weight.

overweight: more than 10 percent above "ideal" weight.

[1]Holt, L. E., Jr. and Snyderman, S. E.: Nutrition in infancy and adolescence. In *Modern Nutrition in Health and Disease.* 4th ed. Wohl, M. G. and Goodhart, R. S., editors. Lea and Febiger, Philadelphia, 1968, p. 1126.

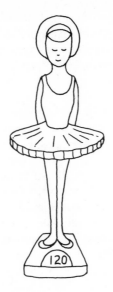
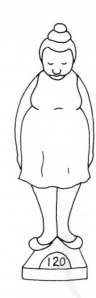

maining body mass is *muscle* and *bone*, which are denser than fat. An athlete or dancer in whom either or both of these tissues are exceptionally well developed may weigh considerably more than the "ideal" weight on the charts, without being overfat. By the same token, a person of "ideal" weight may actually be carrying too much fat. Without regular exercise over the years, the muscles will atrophy to some extent, and fat stores may accumulate. Bones also often become less dense with age. If an eighty-year-old man boasts that he weighs the same as he did on his wedding day, this may not mean that he is at a weight that is ideal for him. He should perhaps be thinner now.

measures of body fatness: densitometry, radioactive potassium distribution, deuterium oxide distribution.

skinfold test:

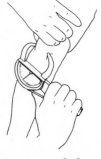

negative energy balance: calories in < calories out.

Weight measures are therefore not the most reliable means of diagnosing excessive body fatness. Since fat is less dense than muscle and bone, a measure based on body density can be used. Since muscle and bone accept water while fat cells take up only fat and fat-soluble substances, measures determining the dilution of water-soluble substances into body tissues provide estimates of body composition. Excess body fat accumulates under the skin so lifting a fold of skin and measuring its thickness is another way of identifying overweight due to overfatness.

With unusual body composition ruled out, most cases of weight deviation from the norm are due to calorie imbalances. This of course means excessive or insufficient intakes of any or all of the three energy nutrients — carbohydrate, fat, and protein.

Calorie deficiency: marasmus. When children are almost totally deprived of food, they cannot obtain the energy necessary to maintain their body systems, much less that necessary for growth. Marasmus, a wasting disease, results. Invariably, protein deficiency occurs with this condition, as available protein is used not to build body protein but to supply energy (which takes priority). As a result, the marasmic child has many, though not all, of the same symptoms as the child with kwashiorkor.

Marasmic children are wizened little old people in appearance, just skin and bones. They are often sick because their resistance to disease is low. Their hearts are weak, and all their muscles are wasted. Their metabolism is slow. They have little or no fat under their skin to insulate against cold. Their body temperatures may be subnormal. The experience of hospital workers with victims of this disease is that their primary need is to be wrapped up and kept warm. They need love, since they have often been deprived of maternal attention as well as food. Unlike the kwashiorkor child, who is fed milk until weaning, the marasmic child may have been neglected from early infancy. The disease occurs most commonly in children from six to eighteen months of age in all the overpopulated city slums of the world. Since the brain normally grows to almost its full adult size within the first two years of life, marasmus impairs brain development and so may have a permanent effect on learning ability.

Marasmus also occurs in adults in countries where calorie deficiency is prevalent. The causes are manifold; in Highlight 4 the attempt was made to sort them out and put them in perspective.

Calorie excess: obesity. When energy nutrient intake exceeds the body's needs, the extra energy is stored in body fat, and results in obesity. Whatever the *indirect* cause (and there are many), the *direct* cause is that obese people eat too much. Their calories in exceed their calories out and have done so for a long time.

Treating obesity requires reversing the balance to achieve and maintain a calorie deficit. One pound of body fat stores 3,500 kcalories. To lose a pound (of body *fat*) you must experience a deficit: the kcalories you take in must be 3,500 less than the kcalories you expend. To lose a pound a week, an average deficit of 500 kcalories a day is therefore needed. Repeat: fat loss always obeys this rule: a person losing weight (fat) is experiencing a deficit of 3,500 kcalories for every pound lost.

Obesity is a prime health problem in this country and is often refractory to treatment, not because the diet plan fails to work when it is applied, but because the subject fails to apply it consistently. This cruel fact is one many

marasmus (ma-RAZ-mus): overt starvation, due to deficiency of calories from any source.

kwashiorkor: see page 124.

For the effect of early malnutrition on brain development, see Highlight 4.

positive energy balance: calories in > calories out.

obesity: excessive body fatness. Often loosely defined as a condition of being overweight by 15 or 20 percent or more.

One pound of body fat (adipose tissue) is actually composed of a mixture of fat, protein, and water, and yields 3,500 kcalories on oxidation. One pound of pure fat (454 grams) would yield (at 9 kcalories per gram) 4,086 kcalories.

refractory: resistant, unresponsive.

of us would like to circumvent. Surely there is an easier way? No, the hard truth is that:

> The only way to lose body fat is to cut calories.

Magical alternatives that have been offered time and again over the centuries—ways to "shrink the stomach," to eat "negative calories," to "eat all you want and lose weight,"—prove to be born of wishful thinking and are effective only when they indirectly affect the calorie balance, as shown in Highlight 8. The success of these plans is not in their achieving their goals, but in their popularity. They sell easily to susceptible people who want something for nothing, who become enthusiastic practitioners (but only briefly), and who pass on the word to the next person. This type of reaction reflects a human characteristic that for all our scientific rationality, we have failed to outgrow: we love magic. Many writers of fallacious books on diets and sellers of fraudulent diet pills and formulas use this characteristic to their advantage.

A flag sign of a spurious claim is the use of:

magical thinking

the promise of something for nothing

The obese person is one with a real problem that happens to be visible. Alcoholics can drink in secret behind closed doors, but foodaholics' problems are obvious: everybody can see that they are too fat. The shame and guilt which sometimes accompany obesity complicate the problem of treatment. To deal successfully with it, all concerned must deal both with the patients' real need to eat, which may be felt very strongly, and with their feelings and emotions. New techniques in the treatment of obesity and the continued use of the timeworn wisdom that a patient must be treated as a whole person are providing hope and solutions for many. (See To Explore Further section.)

One common thread runs through all successful weight control programs, however: negative energy balance. The remainder of this chapter is devoted to the scientific principles and facts needed to understand and achieve this objective. To achieve weight loss or gain it is necessary (1) to know how much energy a person spends in a day (calories out), and (2) to know how much energy the person consumes in a day (calories in),

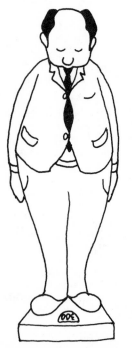

"It must have been the ice cream cone."

and (3) to adjust the balance until the desired weight loss or gain rate is achieved.

Calories Out

Human energy is spent in two major ways—on the basal metabolic processes and on voluntary activities. In order to calculate how much energy a person spends in a day, we must obtain an estimate for the energy spent on each of these types of activity. A third way of spending energy, much smaller but significant, is on digesting, absorbing, and metabolizing food. Let us take these up one by one.

(1) *Basal metabolism*. The ways in which the body spends basal energy include metabolizing nutrients, keeping the heart pumping, transmitting nerve impulses, and the like. The amount of energy spent on these activities can be determined by measuring the heat radiating from the body at rest after fasting for 12 hours. Under normal circumstances, the average adult spends roughly one kcalorie for each kilogram of body weight each hour on metabolism.

(1) **basal metabolism:** the energy output of a body at rest after a twelve-hour fast.

rough *estimate* of basal metabolic energy: one kcalorie/kilogram/hour. For a sample calculation, see Appendix D, example 6.

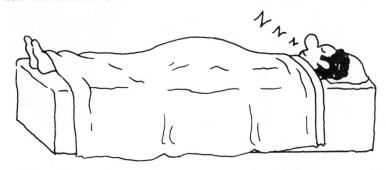

The rate varies, however. The major variables affecting metabolic rate are age and sex. A younger person's metabolic rate is faster; a woman's metabolic rate is slower than that of a man her age and weight. Another factor is the body's shape. Two people of the same weight may radiate different amounts of heat due to differing surface areas. Tall thin people have greater skin surface from which to lose heat than short fat people. To maintain their body temperature at 98.6 degrees F, tall thin people must generate more heat and so will have a faster metabolic rate. A method of calculating basal metabolism based on surface area, age, and sex is given in Appendix D, example 8.

calculation of basal metabolic energy from surface area, taking age and sex into account: see Appendix D, example 7.

(2) *Voluntary activities*. The more active you are, the more energy you need to support your activities. These activities— thinking, writing, running, and the like— involve the nerves and muscles. Nervous activity takes comparatively little energy, while muscular activity requires energy in direct proportion to

(2) energy for activities: the energy expended on activities over and above that needed for basal metabolism.

the amount of muscle being moved. To lie and daydream costs one-tenth of a kcalorie per kilogram per hour; to sit quietly, four-tenths. Fast typing with the back straight and hands and fingers moving rapidly, costs one kcalorie. To sweep the floor you must walk slowly, using your leg muscles a little and your arms more actively; this costs 1.4 kcalories. For a game of tennis or swimming, where all the muscles are active, the cost rises to 4 or more kcalories per kilogram per hour.

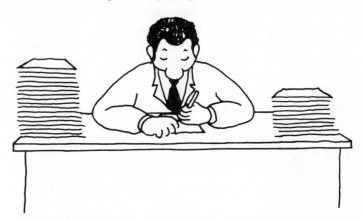

rough *estimate* of activity energy:

for a sedentary person, 20 percent of basal
for light activity, 30 percent of basal
for moderate activity, 40 percent of basal
for heavy activity, 50 percent or more.

calculation of energy for activities by a more accurate method: see Appendix D, example 8.

A rough estimate of the amount of energy needed for voluntary activities can be obtained by adding a percentage to your basal metabolic energy. The percentage varies from 20 percent for a very sedentary person, to 50 percent or more for an active person. A man operating a pneumatic hammer for eight hours a day spends 150-200 percent of his basal energy on this demanding work. A more accurate calculation can be made by adding up the actual activities engaged in for a day, and computing the amount of energy spent on each. This method is demonstrated in Appendix D, example 8.

A question people commonly ask is, "If I want to lose weight, must I exercise?" From the examples above, you can see that an hour of swimming each day, at 5 kcalories/kilogram/hour for a 70 kilogram man would "cost" 350 kcalories, or one-tenth of a pound. To lose a pound this way, he would have to swim an hour each day for ten days without eating any extra food to compensate. From this one example it may be apparent that exercise even in substantial amounts cannot by itself achieve very rapid weight loss—although it helps, and is beneficial in other ways.

There are fringe benefits to exercising, apart from its contribution to weight loss. People who exercise regularly are healthier than those who do not. Their muscles are in better tone, their hearts and lungs are stronger, their circulation is better. Exercise also lowers serum cholesterol and triglyceride levels, reducing the risk of cardiovascular disease.

Another point in favor of regular exercise is that over the long term it makes for a substantial reduction in body weight. One hour of jogging consumes only one-tenth of a pound of body fat, but an hour of jogging every day for a year adds up to more than 35 pounds. Even a very modest amount of exercise, such as walking ten minutes to work from a distant parking space each day will add up to 25 pounds over a ten-year period.

muscle tone: the state of partial contraction characteristic of normal muscle even when it is at rest. More precisely called tonus (TONE-us).

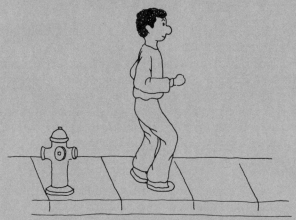

Many a dieter has also found that exercise promotes successful dieting in several ways. It temporarily depresses the appetite, it occupies time that might otherwise be spent eating, and, perhaps most important, it enhances the feeling of well-being and pride that makes weight control worthwhile.

If you have been estimating or calculating your energy needs for a day, you have so far obtained a figure for your basal metabolic energy (say, 1,200 kcalories), and then added a percentage or an amount calculated for your voluntary activities (say, 600 kcalories). It remains now to determine how much energy you spend daily digesting, absorbing, and metabolizing your food.

(3) *The effect of food.* Basal metabolism is conventionally measured for people at rest after a 12-hour fast, when there is no food in their stomachs. Basal metabolism includes the energy needed to maintain the digestive system at rest; that is, to maintain peristalsis and a background secretion of digestive juices. When you eat, your digestive system becomes more active. You secrete additional gastric and intestinal juices, peristalsis

(3) Energy for metabolizing food is called the **specific dynamic energy** (SDE), the specific dynamic effect of food, or the specific dynamic activity (SDA).

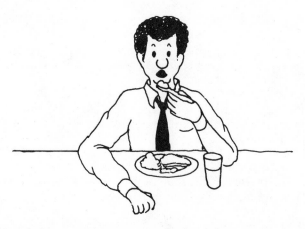

speeds up, the protein pumps which transport nutrients across the intestinal walls into the blood stream go to work. Nutrients must be carried from one place to another in your body, and an additional metabolic burden is placed on every cell, especially those in the liver, to metabolize these freshly assimilated nutrients. The amount of energy spent on these internal activities depends on the amount and type of food you eat.

estimate of specific dynamic energy: 10 percent of the total energy for basal metabolism and activities.

A rough estimate of the amount of energy spent metabolizing food can be obtained by taking 10 percent of the total of basal-metabolic plus voluntary-activity energy.

Total energy expenditure. To conclude, then: to estimate your total energy needs for a day, you first obtain a figure for basal metabolic energy, second obtain an estimate of the energy for voluntary activities, and then subtotal these two. An estimate of the energy for metabolizing food is about 10 percent of this subtotal. Adding this 10 percent and striking a final total gives an approximation of calories out.

sample estimation of energy output of a 60 kilogram person (lightly active):

basal metabolic energy (60 x 24) = 1,440 kcalories
energy for activities (30% of 1,440) = 430

SUBTOTAL = 1,870

energy to metabolize food (10% of 1,870) = 187

TOTAL = 2,057 kcalories

NAS
NRC ⎭ see page 75.
RDA

The method of calculating calories out, given above, is based on assumptions that may not be true for you as an individual. It provides an estimate only. A second way to obtain an estimate of your calorie output is to assume you are average, and to use the averages provided by the NAS-NRC: the calorie RDA. (See boxed section at end of chapter.) Better still, if you are one of those fortunate individuals who maintain weight without conscious effort, you can compute an average day's actual intake, knowing that your intake is automatically regulated to meet your need—but then, you may not need to make the effort!

If you make a serious attempt to lose or gain weight, the problem disappears. After several weeks of consuming a fixed number of calories, you can determine your calorie expenditure from your weight loss or gain rate. If you are losing a pound a week, for example, you must be spending 500 kcalories a day more than you are eating.

Calories In

To calculate the number of kcalories taken in in food, we need not look up every single individual food in a table. While the inexorable fact remains that calories must be controlled, they need not be counted. Exchange systems, like the ADA Food Exchange System presented in Chapters 1, 2, and 3, are the single most useful kind of tool ever devised for diet planning.

Experience with calorimetry has shown food chemists that the amount of energy available from pure carbohydrate is fairly constant, regardless of the food in which it is found. A gram of pure carbohydrate from any source yields about 4 kcalories.

Reminder: to be strictly accurate, we must speak of the energy values of foods in kilocalories. See page 236.

> 1 gram carbohydrate=4 kcalories

Similarly, a gram of pure protein yields about 4, and a gram of pure fat about 9 kcalories.

> 1 gram protein=4 kcalories
> 1 gram fat=9 kcalories

So why bother? If the energy-nutrient composition of a food is known, its calorie content automatically follows. A small apple, for example, which is known to contain 10 grams of carbohydrate, and no protein or fat, must contribute 40 kcalories of energy to the person who eats it.

A weight control program normally includes no alcohol. If alcohol is included, it must be remembered that this compound also can be metabolized to yield energy for the body's use. One gram of pure ethanol yields about 7 kcalories, of which up to 90 percent is available to the body.

ethanol

For the metabolism of ethanol, see Highlight 9.

> 1 gram alcohol=7 kcalories

Since one ounce is about 30 grams, a 12-ounce can of beer containing ½ ounce of alcohol provides 150 kcalories: about 50 from its 14 grams of carbohydrate and about 100 from the alcohol. A cocktail containing one jigger of 100-proof beverage such as gin, rum, vodka, or whiskey supplies 150 kcalories from the alcohol, and additional kcalories if carbohydrate is added. Energy values of other alcoholic beverages are shown in Appendix H (items 553-560).

Other useful numbers:

1 ounce = 28.4 grams (the dietitian often uses 30).

a jigger is a measuring cup for alcoholic drinks, usually measuring 1 ounce or 1½ ounces.

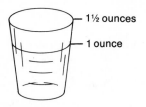

1½ ounces

1 ounce

100 proof means 50% alcohol. Thus a 1½ ounce jigger contains about 43 grams of 50% alcohol, or about 21 grams of pure alcohol. At 7 kcal/gram, this would be about 150 kcal.

It must also be remembered that small differences in the fat content of foods can make large differences in their energy values. To use the Exchange System (pages 33-38) skillfully, one must be familiar with the differences in fat content between skim and other milks (see Milk List), between different kinds of baked goods (see Bread List), and between lean and fat meats (see Meat Lists).

The Food Exchange System with this added information, provides a convenient way to estimate how many kcalories are in a meal or in a day's meals. The table below has been shown before, but this time it emphasizes the energy value of each exchange group.

Exchange Group	Carbohydrate (g)	Protein (g)	Fat (g)	Energy (kcal)
(1) Skim milk	12	8	0	80
(2) Vegetables	5	2	0	25
(3) Fruit	10	0	0	40
(4) Bread	15	2	0	70
(5) Lean meat	0	7	3	55
(6) Fat	0	0	5	45

If you compute the kcalories in each exchange group from the number of grams of each nutrient, you will come up with numbers that differ slightly from the numbers in the energy column. To save effort in adding, the designers of the system have rounded off the number of kcalories in each exchange to the nearest five. The result is a rough but very convenient approximation of the energy values of common foods. Knowing these six numbers in many cases eliminates the necessity of counting calories by looking up individual foods in a table. It also solves the problem often complained of by dieters—that foods lose their appeal when each has a price tag displayed on it. With this system, you can design a pattern of food intake which supplies the number of kcalories you wish to consume. You can then forget the numbers and concentrate on eating food servings that fit the pattern. Having decided to eat three fruit exchanges a day, for example, you can freely select any three of the 37 different fruits listed in the system without doing any calculations. As long as you are careful with serving sizes, you will be consuming 120 kcalories from fruit each day, on the average.

Many highly successful weight control programs are based on this method of diet planning. Most of those handed out in the doctor's office are similar in principle. Any eating plan which consistently restricts calories in to a level below that of calories out will result in loss of body fat.

Weight loss and gain rates. A deficit of 500 kcalories a day

For practice in using these plans, see the Suggested Activities at the end of this chapter.

brings about loss of body fat at the rate of a pound a week; of 1,000, two pounds a week. The absolute limit of the rate of weight loss is set by energy expenditure. For example, a woman who spends 2,000 kcalories a day can lose no more than four pounds of fat a week, and that only if she goes on a total fast. A person who spends more energy can lose more. Extraordinarily active persons, by virtue of their activities, or extremely obese persons, by virtue of the metabolic demands made by the sheer bulk of their body cells, will lose more. For those who are only moderately obese, the maximum recommended rate of weight loss is one to two pounds a week, which for most people means an intake of about 1,000-1,500 kcalories a day. Below 1,200, the diet planner is hard put to achieve adequacy for all the essential nutrients.

The Energy RDA for Adults (kcal)

Age	Males	Females
19-22	3,000	2,100
23-50	2,700	2,000
51+	2,400	1,800

The NAS-NRC has published RDA's for kcalories for a variety of age-sex groups in the United States. The 20-year-old reference woman is 5 feet 5 inches tall, and weighs 128 pounds (58 kilograms). She requires about 2,100 kcalories a day, according to their estimate. The 20-year-old reference man is 5 feet 9 inches tall, weighs 147 pounds (67 kilograms), and requires about 3,000 kcalories a day. Few real persons are identical to the reference woman and reference man used for these purposes, and to the extent that each of us differs from these imaginary figures, we must apply the recommendations to ourselves with a grain of salt.

This is the second time in this book that RDA's have been discussed; the first was in Chapter 3, on protein. You may wish to review the discussion there. In setting the RDA for *protein*, the authorities based their decision on two important facts: first, that protein needs of individuals vary over a wide range; second, that the consequences of a protein deficiency are severe, while those of consuming an excess of protein are not. In deciding what amount of protein to recommend for an individual of a given age-sex group, the NAS-NRC chose to set the RDA rather high, covering 97.5 percent of the population. For an average person, whose protein needs fall near the mean, the RDA recommends half again as much protein in a day as actually needed. For a vital nutrient

reference man, reference woman: a man and woman whose height and weight are the average for U.S. men and women of 20 years of age.

actuarial statistics: statistical calculations of life expectancy.

such as protein, this recommendation makes sense, and it will do no harm to consume more than the actual need.

Calories, on the other hand, are harmful in excess, because they lead to obesity, while a deficit (within reason) is not harmful. The actuarial statistics of insurance companies bear this out, showing that the maximum life expectancy is enjoyed by persons who are about 10 percent under the recommended weight for their height. Obesity is one of the major health problems in this country. It is a contributing cause to our number one killer, heart disease; to our number four killer, diabetes; and is closely related to a host of other ills.

Like protein needs, energy needs of individuals vary, with most people needing some amount of energy near the middle of the range. In setting the RDA for energy, the Food and Nutrition Board elected to draw the line right at the mean. This ensured (if all members of our population were to consume exactly the RDA) that half would be consuming somewhat less than they actually needed as individuals, while half would be consuming somewhat more.

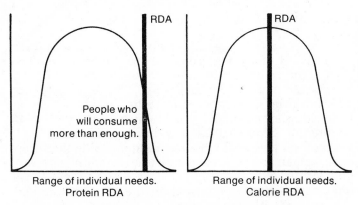

Range of individual needs.
Protein RDA

Range of individual needs.
Calorie RDA

This choice minimizes the risk of encouraging excessive obesity or excessive thinness.

> CAUTION: The energy RDA meets the needs of the average person.

The Food and Nutrition Board has made no recommendation for daily consumption of the energy nutrients (carbohydrate or fat), only for total energy and protein. To understand the reason for this, recall that all three energy nutrients contribute calories, protein being unique among them because it also contributes nitrogen.

You must therefore meet your RDA for protein (to obtain the nitrogen you need). When you have consumed that number of grams of protein, you will have simultaneously consumed a certain number of calories. The remaining calories you need can come from carbohydrate and fat. It is left to you to choose how to balance these two nutrients in meeting your energy allowance.

Suggested guide: not more than 35% of total calories from fat.

Summing Up

The energy in food is contained in the chemical bonds that hold nutrients together. When these bonds are broken in the body, food energy may be released as heat or into other molecules. Ultimately all food energy reappears as heat which is lost from the body. To replace it, more food must be eaten.

A convenient measure of food energy is the kilocalorie: the amount of heat necessary to raise the temperature of one kilogram of water one degree Centigrade. Direct calorimetry measures the heat given off when a food is burned in oxygen in a closed system; the amount of oxygen consumed in this process provides an indirect measure of the food energy. The amount of energy spent by a person over a period of time can be measured in the same two ways: (1) by measuring heat loss or (2) by measuring the oxygen consumed under defined conditions.

As long as energy intake equals expenditure, body weight will remain constant. This situation obtains for many people, whose hunger and appetite regulate their energy intake so that it is in equilibrium with their output. When persons' weights deviate from the norm for their age-sex-height groups by more than 10 percent, they are said to be overweight or underweight. Differences in body composition (water, minerals) account for some of these deviations, but the majority are due to differences in body fatness. Measures of body composition and body fatness in particular include densitometry, radioactive potassium distribution, deuterium oxide distribution, and skinfold thickness.

Calorie deficiency in the extreme reflects overt starvation and causes the wasting disease marasmus common in very young poorly-nourished children, especially in overcrowded city slums throughout the world. Protein deficiency always accompanies this condition because the protein that is available is oxidized for energy rather than used to provide amino acids for body protein synthesis.

Positive energy balance causes accumulation of body fat and obesity. Treatment requires adjustment of calorie input and/or output to achieve a negative calorie balance.

Averages of energy output for various age-sex groups are provided by the RDA. A means of estimating energy output for an individual is to sum three factors: (1) The energy spent in a day on the basal metabolic processes, which require about one kcalorie per kilogram per hour. (These processes generally consume the largest portion of a day's energy output.) (2) The energy spent on voluntary muscular activities. (Frequently this sort of activity requires about half as much energy as metabolism.) (3) The energy needed to digest and metabolize food. (This factor, known as the specific dynamic energy, usually amounts to about one-tenth of the total of the first two factors.)

The energy spent on basal metabolism and on the specific dynamic effect of food is fairly constant, but the energy output for muscular activities can vary widely.

Energy intake depends solely on the amounts of carbohydrate, fat, and protein consumed; that is, on the amounts and types of food eaten. To correct overweight or obesity a negative calorie balance must be achieved and maintained until the desired amount of weight is lost. A deficit of 3,500 kcalories is necessary for the loss of each pound of body fat. The only proven way to lose weight successfully and permanently is to adopt an eating plan that provides balanced nutrition at the appropriate energy level and to stay with such a plan for life.

A means of planning a fixed energy intake without counting calories is provided by the Food Exchange system. It is possible to plan a pattern of exchanges for use each day or each meal and then to select for a day's menus any foods which fit the pattern, thus varying the diet from day to day without changing the average kilocalorie total for the day. To make this system work, it is necessary to be aware of the varying fat contents of foods and (if alcohol is used) to remember that one gram of alcohol yields 7 kcalories for the body's use.

Loss of body fat in excess of two pounds a week can rarely be sustained. A diet supplying fewer than 1,000 kcalories a day can be made adequate only with great difficulty.

To Explore Further—

A brief (57 page) review of the concepts of hunger, appetite, drive, and satiety, and the roles of fat cells and hypothalamus in controlling food intake:

Lepkovski, S.: Regulation of food intake. *Advances in Food Research* 21:1-69, 1975.

A clear explanation, for the layman, of the way in which the hypothalamus is thought to regulate hunger and satiety:

Mayer, J. and Thomas, D. W.: Regulation of food intake and obesity. *Science* 156:328, April, 1967.

Insights of an expert into the causes and remedies of obesity:

Mayer, J.: *Overweight Causes, Cost and Control*. Prentice-Hall, Inc., Englewood Cliffs, New Jersey, 1968.

An example of the better recent work in treating obesity, in this case using the techniques of behavior modification. Paperback:

Stewart, S. and David, B.: *Slim Chance in a Fat World*. Research Press, Champaign, Illinois, 1972.

The ADA Exchange Lists can be ordered from:
    The American Dietetic Association
    420 North Michigan Avenue
    Chicago, Illinois 60611

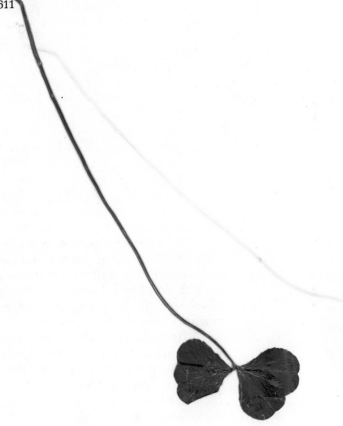

Highlight Eight
Diet Fallacies

fallacy: an argument failing to satisfy the conditions of valid or correct reasoning from evidence. fallacia = deceit

The American public is obsessed with youthfulness and sexiness. It frequently equates these characteristics with a slim and feminine or a powerful and masculine figure. People who seek these physical attributes often begin by searching for an easy way to lose weight—and become willing victims of the diet con artist.

Criminologists tell us that the con game is unique in that its victims are active participants in the crime. The victims want something for nothing so badly they become blind to the possibility that they may lose their life savings. It is often this way for those who long for a slim figure. They do not want to make the effort to change poor eating habits, to give up favorite foods, to count calories, or to study nutrition. Rather, they fall for the advertising of a book or a mail order diet that promises "quick, easy weight loss while you eat all your favorite foods," and do not realize they may lose their good health.

The following are direct quotations from some of this type of advertising in popular magazines (the Suggested Activities following this section list other direct quotations):

CRASH DIET ONLY $1.00—LOSE UP TO 5 POUNDS OVERNIGHT—NO PILLS, NO EXERCISE, ONE DAY RE-

254

DUCING FORMULA. EAT YOUR FILL! GO TO SLEEP, WAKE UP AND YOU HAVE LOST UP TO FIVE POUNDS.

TAKE THAT UGLY FAT OFF THIGHS, NECK, LEGS, WAISTLINE, ALL OVER. WITHOUT PUTTING DOWN YOUR KNIFE AND FORK—EAT THE FOODS YOU LIKE— LIKE VEAL SCALLOPINI, ROAST CHICKEN, STEAK AND LAMB, ROAST BEEF.

NEW FAT BURNING SYSTEM SLIMS YOU DOWN POUNDS IN JUST 10 DAYS.

What scintillating promises to those who want fervently to lose those ugly bulges!

There is nothing magical about weight reduction, despite the promises implied in these ads. From your study of the first eight chapters, you know that the human body has evolved a system whereby calories are given top priority. Calories are never thrown away frivolously just because they are in good supply. Relatively few calories are lost in the excreta, few are used for keeping the body warm or to digest food, more are used to fuel the body's vital organs, and many are used to move the body. If there are some extra calories taken in and not spent on these activities, they are stored in the liver and muscle as glycogen, ready for quick withdrawal when needed. If there exists a larger surplus of calories than can be stored as glycogen, these extra calories are converted to fat and stored in the adipose tissue. The day of the calorie shortage is the day that the stored fat will be withdrawn from the adipose tissue and metabolized for energy. This is the fundamental principle which the willing victims of diet con artists do not understand (or refuse to acknowledge).

One of the oldest and at present the most popular of the reducing diets is the low-carbohydrate diet, currently being advertised as "new" and "revolutionary." However, it is a very old regimen that resurfaces every decade or so under a new name: the Air Force diet, the drinking man's diet, the calories-don't-count diet, for instance. The low-carbohydrate diet consists of cutting down the carbohydrate intake to 60 grams a day or less while allowing dieters to eat all they want of protein or fat foods. "Unlimited food intake while you lose weight!" There are a number of fallacies in this method of losing weight and each will be discussed.

The most striking indictment of the low-carbohydrate diet lies in the fact that *it is dangerous.* It is ketogenic (see page 211). Its high fat content would tend to contribute to atherosclerosis (see Highlight 2). Since this type of diet is currently being promoted by a physician, the public assumes that it will not only result in weight loss but will also be medically safe to follow.

That it is *not* considered medically safe by the majority of the medical profession is evidenced by the statement of the AMA Council on Food and Nutrition[1] which presents experimental proof of its fallacies and dangers. Also, a number of prominent nutritionists have spoken out against it. One of these is Dr. Frederick Stare, Chairman of the Nutrition Department of Harvard University, who testified before a Senate Committee investigating fad diets that "since coronary heart disease is the principal cause of death in the United States, and any diet which tends to be high in saturated fats and cholesterol tends to elevate the chance that the individual will get heart disease, any book that recommends unlimited amounts of meat, butter, and eggs, as this one does, in my opinion is dangerous. The author [a doctor] who makes the suggestion is guilty of malpractice."[2]

As you read this and the following paragraphs exploding the low-carbohydrate diet fallacy, you should be aware that many tools useful for sifting fact from fancy are being used here. In Highlight 2 you were urged, when reading a source of nutrition information, to ask yourself who wrote it, who published it, and why it was published. Clearly in the case of many of these diets, "who wrote it" and "who published it," were people or companies whose major goal was not to further the advancement of science but to earn fame and fortune for themselves. In Highlight 5 it was pointed out that claims based on logic alone must stand the test of experiment. The rationale for many of these diets seems logical enough but proves false on experimental testing, as a scrutiny of the AMA statement[1] will show you. In fact, a perusal of the scientific literature shows that *none* of the claims made by promoters of these diets stands up to testing.

In attempting to sort out fact from fancy, you will find an additional guideline helpful. If the promoters refer to scientific reports in journals such as those referred to in this and other Highlights, you can check them for yourself; if they make no reference to evidence substantiating their claims, you must suspect their word. Also, every creditable institution seems to have a fake counterpart. Watch out for "doctors" without an MD, "universities" with only a post office box address, "nutrition organizations" with no recognized standing, and the like.

[1] A critique of low-carbohydrate ketogenic weight reduction regimens. *Journal of the American Medical Association* 224(10):1415-1419, 1973.
[2] *Nutrition and Diseases—1973*. Hearings before the Select Committee on Nutrition and Human Needs. Part 1, Obesity and Fad Diets, 93rd Congress. U.S. Government Printing Office, Washington, 1973.

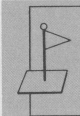

A flag sign of a spurious claim is assertions like:

"Doctors agree"—where the identity of the "doctors" is not revealed.

"Authorities agree"—where no reference to an authoritative publication is provided.

One of the reasons warnings about the danger to health of the low-carbohydrate diet by prominent groups such as the AMA have fallen on deaf ears is that restricting carbohydrates *can* produce a weight loss. However, there is *no experimental evidence* that the weight loss occurs while the dieters are consuming more calories than they are expending, and there is *abundant experimental evidence* that it is damaging to the body. Protein-fat is no magical combination which allows you to eat more energy foods than you need and to oxidize your own body fat at the same time.

The weight loss that occurs appears to come from the toxic effects of the ketones, which produce nausea and thus suppress the appetite, and through a self-restriction of calories. It seems to be nearly impossible to shift from a mixed diet to one totally devoid of carbohydrates and then to eat enough protein and fat to make up the calorie deficit. For example, Yudkin and Corey[3] studied the normal diets of six obese persons, then placed them on a carbohydrate restricted diet in which they could eat all the protein and fat they wanted. When the low-carbohydrate diets which the subjects freely selected were studied, it was found that none of the subjects increased his intake of fat foods and that there had been a reduction of calories ranging from 13 to 55 percent. With reduction in calories came weight loss.

The low-carbohydrate diet also produces weight loss due to excretion of salt, according to the AMA statement.[1] Since water follows salt much of the drop in pounds seen on the bathroom scales may be due to the excretion of salt and water. Not only is it dangerous to upset the water and electrolyte balance (see Highlight 5 and Chapter 14), but also this weight will be regained rapidly when the person resumes carbohydrate ingestion.

In judging any weight reduction program, it is imperative that we speak of the weight loss in terms of a change in body composition, rather than in terms of the change in the reading on the bathroom scales. If on Tuesday you weigh five pounds less than you did on Monday, the next question is, "Was that a loss of fat, which is desirable, or just a loss of water, which is

[3]Yudkin, J. and Corey, M.: The treatment of obesity by the "high-fat" diet. The inevitability of calories. *Lancet* ii:939-941, 1960.

usually undesirable?" Five pounds of fat lost entails a deficit of five times 3,500 kcalories or 17,500 kcalories and will not be regained until you eat 17,500 more kcalories than you expend. Five pounds of water lost, such as an athlete might suffer during a strenuous game or a person with diarrhea may lose, will be regained immediately upon drinking and retaining fluids. A change in body composition, a shift to a lower percentage of body weight in the adipose tissue, is the goal of a valid reducing diet regimen.

There is, however, a water loss that is desirable and represents a change in body composition; that is, oxidation of body fat rather than dehydration of body tissues. As discussed in Chapter 7, when body fat is oxidized for energy, carbon dioxide and water are the end products. Carbon dioxide is absorbed rapidly into the blood stream where it is carried to the lungs for excretion; water, on the other hand, accumulates in the tissues and is more slowly absorbed into the blood stream. When it is finally "seen" by the kidneys as being excess water, it is sent to the bladder to be excreted. Thus, sometimes a person on a calorie deficient diet does not lose weight for several days—may even, in fact, gain a little—then may lose several pounds in one day. Even though this is water loss, it represents a change in body composition, a loss of fat, and is a bona fide weight reduction.

Another claim made by the proponents of the low-carbohydrate diet is that sugar is an "antinutrient" and that starch is the "hidden" source of sugar. Are the writers referring to the sugar, glucose? Glucose is the sugar on which the central nervous system is dependent for energy, therefore it is difficult to see how it could be termed an antinutrient. It is the natural breakdown product of the digestion of carbohydrates (starch) and is so important to the body that if there is no carbohydrate present to supply the blood with glucose, protein will be used for this purpose rather than as a supplier of amino acids. If the writers are referring to the table sugar, sucrose, they should recall that one molecule of sucrose eventually becomes two molecules of glucose after digestion and absorption. Sucrose may be indicted on the grounds that we are using too much of it, but since it yields a vital nutrient, glucose, it cannot be termed an antinutrient—whatever that term means.

In addition to promoting a diet fraught with dangers, the authors of such schemes are acting irresponsibly in the face of today's precarious food situation. By their words, they are intimating to the public that the only way to be slim and healthy is to avoid carbohydrate (plant) foods and to eat meat. (Highlight 4 discusses the world's food crisis.) Plant foods are generally low in cost compared with meat and use much less of the available land. They contribute to the diet many important nutrients in addition to carbohydrates: protein, vitamins, minerals, fiber, and perhaps as-yet-undiscovered substances present in unrefined complex carbohydrate foods. Also, when a layman is told (by a doctor on television or in a book) that to regain his lost figure he must avoid carbohydrates, he interprets this to mean that "carbohydrates are fattening." You know from your study of Chapters 1-3 that carbohydrate calories are no more fattening than any other calories. Gram for gram, carbohydrate produces the same number of calories as protein and less than half as many calories as fat. Additionally, a layman is encouraged to embark on an unwise eating program, often one that includes high cost meat filled with saturated fat and even including other fats, such as cream and butter. During the time the dieter is enthusiastic about losing some "excess baggage," any competent nutritionist would be using that enthusiasm to start an eating program which the dieter could follow for life, without danger.

Following any of the fad diets can be especially dangerous to vulnerable groups, such as persons with a tendency towards diabetes, hyperlipidemia, or heart disease. Of particular interest in this regard is the danger to the developing fetus of ketosis in the pregnant woman on a low-carbohydrate diet. Dr. Karlis Adamsons,[2] Professor of Obstetrics and Gynecology, City University, New York City, testified before the Senate Committee investigating fad diets, and stated that while the fetus is very well protected from harm and will generally get the nutrients it needs from the mother's blood supply, there are two substances critical to its development which the mother's body cannot store: glucose and oxygen. Cellular glucose deprivation occurs in the state of ketosis, which accompanies some diseases (diabetes) and diets lacking carbohydrate foods. The mother may be able to tolerate glucose starvation temporarily, but the fetus may suffer permanent brain damage during such starvation since glucose is the only fuel which the developing central nervous system can use.

It has been pointed out, then, that the low-carbohydrate diet is a ketogenic, high-fat diet and as such is considered dangerous by the AMA and reputable nutritionists. It can, however, produce weight loss through the toxic effects of the ketones and the absence of carbohydrate, which produces an undesirable excretion of salt and water. The resultant weight losses cause many persons to adhere to the diet in spite of the warnings that it is a health hazard.

How are laymen to know that a person or organization is one whose opinion they can trust? What distinguishes the ADA or the AMA from any other organization? And who is a *reputable* nutritionist?

The ADA (American Dietetic Association) and the

AMA (American Medical Association) are two examples of professional organizations. That is, membership in these associations is limited to those persons who have qualified for membership by their education and experience (graduate dietitians or medical doctors, respectively). The journals of these organizations are the vehicles by which scientific information pertinent to their respective fields is disseminated to the membership. These journals constitute the arena in which professional arguments can be resolved. If one of these professional journals speaks out editorially on a controversial topic, laymen can safely assume that the editorial reflects a consensus of member opinions.

There are, also, scientific organizations which any person can join simply by paying the fees. The membership is composed of people who have a common interest or viewpoint. The journals of these organizations do not necessarily publish incorrect scientific information; they just do not have the checks and balances of the journals of the professional organizations. The layman cannot rely on the educational background of the writers, or assume that the articles have been screened by competent professionals before publication, nor can he trust the purpose for which the articles were written (see Highlight 2).

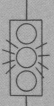

CAUTION WHEN YOU READ!

When an organization's journal speaks out on a controversial topic ask yourself:

Is the organization back of this statement an association of professionals, or can anyone join?

A *reputable* nutritionist is one who is educated in nutrition or a closely allied field. Usually, such nutritionists are associated with a fairly large university or medical center, where they are able to engage in teaching and/or research assignments. Laymen examining the qualifications of a nutritionist should pay no attention to such advertising adjectives as *famous*, or *well known*, or even *reputable*, but should look at the educational background or present affiliations of the person. It is relatively easy to judge the lack of qualifications of movie stars, should they speak on nutrition, but it is much more difficult to make a valid judgment when medical doctors or scientists outside the nutritional field speak on the subject. A careful writer will help the reader make these judgments. For example, on page 256 Dr. Stare is quoted on a nutrition topic. You will note that you were told he is Chairman of the Nutrition Department at Harvard University. On page 259 Dr. Adamsons is quoted on a nutritional topic also. He is a Professor of Obstetrics and Gynecology at City University, New York. Is he then qualified to testify on nutrition? Yes, the topic is concerned with conditions affecting the unborn, the nutrition of the mother.

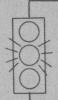

CAUTION WHEN YOU READ!

When an "authority" gives an opinion on a topic, ask yourself:

Does he/she have the educational and experiential background to speak on this topic?

Many diets are variations of the low-carbohydrate diet. For instance, if you are advised to eat a high-protein diet, you are being asked to limit carbohydrates. You have learned that one of the functions of the carbohydrates is to spare the valuable amino acids. Amino acids taken in excess of the need to build or repair tissues are used for energy; amino acids eaten when there is an absolute energy deficit are also used for energy. Since you are extracting energy from the protein, you might as well eat a less expensive source, carbohydrate. Athletes are often urged to eat high-protein diets in the hope that this will stimulate muscle growth, when what they need is calories to support the extra expenditure of energy during games and enough protein for repair and maintenance of tissue.[4]

Other diets are based on equally fallacious reasoning. The "Mayo Diet" which is *not*, and never has been, advocated by the highly reputable Mayo Clinic[5] of Rochester, Minnesota, has many variations—but usually includes nine eggs a day. This diet is a high-cholesterol diet, and therefore may present a danger to vulnerable persons (see Highlight 2). If it results in a weight loss, it is probably because dieters have become bored with the few foods allowed them. Certainly it would not be conducive to learning good eating habits.

The grapefruit diet promises that grapefruit burns up other foods. In this diet, grapefruit is eaten before every meal; the meals themselves are composed of mostly low calorie vegetables and fruit. No one food burns up another food. The diet probably is based on an erroneous understanding of the specific dynamic effect of foods (a few calories are used to fuel the digestive processes; see Chapter 8).

[4]Position paper on food and nutrition misinformation on selected topics. *Journal of the American Dietetic Association* 66:277-279, 1975.
[5]*Mayo Clinic Diet Manual.* Committee on Dietetics, 4th edition. W. B. Saunders Company, Philadelphia, 1971.

One of the oldest ways of reducing which has had a revival in recent years is that of total fasting. With fasting, only non-caloric liquids are allowed. The body has mechanisms by which it can limp along without carbohydrate and fat but it must continually replace amino acids. If the diet does not include amino acids, the body's few amino acid pools will be depleted quickly. The dieter's own protein tissue will then be catabolized to provide the amino acids with which to build vital body proteins. "Metabolic studies of nitrogen balance, performed in obese individuals undergoing total fasting, revealed that 65 percent of their weight loss was due to loss of lean body tissue and only 35 percent was due to loss of adipose tissue," according to Dr. Seymour K. Fineberg, Chief of the Diabetes and Obesity-Diabetes Clinics of the Metropolitan Hospital in New York.[6]

Lean body tissue will be restored at the very first intake of protein. With each pound of protein replaced, three pounds of water must be provided for the intracellular spaces of the protein mass.[6] Dr. Fineberg speaks of *this* weight loss (body protein loss) as an illusionary loss. The only loss that is real is that of adipose tissue.

One of the worst aspects of fasting as a way of reducing is the trauma associated with it—for obese persons to deny themselves totally of food, to then lose a great deal of weight, and then, when they begin to take very low caloric nourishment, to have their weight zoom back up again. They must surely think that no matter how little they eat, they gain weight.

Up to this point we have been discussing fallacies of weight reduction diets. However, there is another type of diet that is receiving a great deal of emphasis today, especially among young people.[7] The Zen Macrobiotic diet is promoted as a means of awakening a spiritual rebirth. This diet actually consists of ten diets, ranging from the lowest which includes cereals, vegetables, animal products, and fruit to the highest which includes only cereals. According to the AMA Council on Foods and Nutrition, "To merely brand as food faddists those individuals whose dietary beliefs are not in accord with what is ordinarily considered sound nutritional practice serves no useful purpose. . . . But, when a diet has been shown to cause irreversible damage to health and ultimately lead to death, it should be roundly condemned as a threat to human health. The Council . . . believes that such is the case with the rigid dietary restrictions placed on the followers of the Zen Macrobiotic philosophy."[8]

In summary, one should always suspect a claim if it is

[6]Fineberg, S. K.: The realities of obesity and fad diets. *Nutrition Today*, July/August:24-26, 1972.
[7]Register, T. D. and Sonnenberg, L. M.: The vegetarian diet. *Journal of the American Dietetic Association* 62:253-261, 1973.
[8]Zen macrobiotic diets. *Journal of the American Medical Association* 218(3): 397, 1971.

couched in terms that sound like magical thinking. In science, one should be wary when a scientist resorts to writing on technical matters in the public arena, unless one can find corroborating testimony in the scientific journals. In nutrition, one should suspect that the claims for any diet are probably unsound if entire classes of food are either eliminated or overemphasized.

To Explore Further—

A help in understanding the problem of obesity and why some diets do not contribute to permanent loss of weight:

Leveille, G. A. and Romsos, D. R.: Meal eating and obesity. *Nutrition Today*, November/December:4-9, 1974.

Fineberg, S. K.: The realities of obesity and fad diets. *Nutrition Today*, July/August:23-26, 1972.

Margolius' book is very well written and very interesting. Deutsch's book has become a classic expose of popular food fads:

Margolius, S.: *Health Foods, Facts and Fakes*. Walker and Company, New York, 1973.

Deutsch, R. M.: *Nuts Among the Berries*. Ballantine Books, New York, 1967.

Pamphlets and reprints, *The Healthy Way to Weigh Less* and *Critique of Low-Carbohydrate Ketogenic Weight Reduction Regimens*, can be ordered from:

> The AMA Council on Foods and Nutrition
> 535 N. Dearborn Street
> Chicago, Illinois 60610

Suggested Activities

(1) Study your own diet.

Review the record you made (Chapter 1, Activity 1) and calculate your average kilocalorie consumption per day. What percentage of your energy comes from carbohydrate? fat? protein? How does your balance compare with the suggested guide on page 113?

(Note: The last Highlight in the book invites you to survey your entire diet for adequacy, balance, and economy. You may wish to save this activity until you have read that Highlight or to read the Highlight now for a sense of perspective.)

(2) Estimate your calories out.

Calculate your energy needs for basal metabolism using the rule of thumb on page 243, and the more accurate surface-area method in Appendix D, example 7. What percentage of your total energy intake is used to support your basal metabolism?

Estimate your energy needs for activities using the rule of thumb on page 244, and the more accurate method demonstrated in Appendix D, example 8. Into what "ball park" do your activities fall? Are you lightly active? moderately active? If the second method gave you a lower figure than the first, ask yourself: did I mistake being busy for being active?

Estimate your energy need for the specific dynamic effect of food. Total the three figures you believe to be most representative of your actual energy expenditure and compare the total with your calories in, obtained from problem 1, above. Account for any discrepancies.

(3) Think about the meaning of energy balance.
Is there any time or situation in people's lives when their energy balance should be positive?

(4) Discover why a fat person can lose weight faster than a thin person.
Estimate the energy needs of a 300 pound (!) woman. If she goes on a 1,000 kcalorie diet, how much weight will she lose per week? Now estimate the energy needs of a 100 pound woman who is the same height and equally active (or inactive). If she goes on a 1,000 kcalorie diet, how much weight will she lose per week? Account for the difference.

(5) Discover the extent to which exercise affects energy out.
Suppose a 70 kilogram man, age 20, plays a game of tennis for an hour. Compared with a similar man who sits around all day, how much extra energy does the first man spend? Now suppose the first man gets a job operating a pneumatic hammer for 8 hours a day (page 244). How much extra energy does this cost him?

(6) Notice another factor that affects basal metabolism.
When people have fevers, their energy needs for basal metabolism increase by 7 percent for each degree (Fahrenheit) of fever. Suppose you had a fever of 103.6° F. How many extra kilocalories does this cost you in a day? (Would there normally be any compensating reduction in activity level so that your overall energy needs might not change?)

(7) Discover the limits of weight loss rates.
Denise, who spends 2,000 kilocalories/day, is getting married six weeks from now, and wants to lose 25 pounds so that she can fit into her wedding dress. Advise her as to the number of kilocalories she may consume per day in order to reach her goal by the deadline (assume no change in activity level).

(8) Devise a weight-loss or weight-gain plan using the Exchange System.
Design an exchange pattern at the appropriate kilocalorie

level for you to lose one pound per week. For example, a 1,200 kcalorie pattern might include: milk exchanges, 2 (160); vegetable, 3 (75); fruit, 4 (160); bread, 5 (350); meat, 5 (275); fat, 4 (180). Make up a sample menu for a day, selecting foods for breakfast, lunch, dinner, and a snack, from the Exchange Lists on pages 33-38. Choose foods you like and combine them into meals you would enjoy. Use seasonings and foods from the Unlimited Foods list freely.

Alternatively, select or design an exchange pattern at a kilocalorie level that would help you to gain a pound a week, and make up a sample menu as above.

(9) Spot the fallacies in crash diet ads.

The following are direct quotes from advertisements in a magazine for teenagers. What can you find in them to criticize, in light of the cautions and warnings offered in this book?

CRASH DIET ONLY $1
LOSE UP TO 5 POUNDS OVERNIGHT!
LEARN THE SECRET OF T.V.'S FANTASTIC NO-PILL, NO-EXERCISE ONE-DAY REDUCING FORMULA! EAT YOUR FILL! GO TO SLEEP! WAKE UP!—AND YOU HAVE LOST UP TO 5 POUNDS. AMAZING? SURE! BUT GUARANTEED TO WORK OR YOUR MONEY BACK! SEND ONLY $1.00. SORRY, NO C.O.D.'S.

WEIGHT LOSS BY THE HOUR! 8 AM . . . 126 POUNDS! 8 PM . . . 124 POUNDS! 8 AM . . . TOMORROW 122 POUNDS! . . . IMAGINE LOSING A FULL POUND IN THE FIRST 6 HOURS! 2 POUNDS BETWEEN MORNING AND NIGHT! UP TO 5 POUNDS IN AS LITTLE AS 24 HOURS! IF THAT SOUNDS UNBELIEVABLE, GET THE ENTIRE PROGRAM NOW AND READ WHAT AN EMINENT DOCTOR SAYS ABOUT IT. READ WHAT PEOPLE WHO HAVE TRIED IT SAY HAPPENED TO THEM! READ THE SCIENTIFIC AND MEDICAL REASONS WHY IT MAY VERY WELL BE THE FASTEST, MOST EFFECTIVE, SAFEST WAY TO LOSE WEIGHT THAT HAS EVER BEEN DISCOVERED.

"THERE'S NO MORE HEALTHFUL WAY TO LOSE SO MUCH WEIGHT SO FAST!"   DR. FRANK R. RICARDO, M.D.

16 TIMES MORE POTENT THAN THE FAMOUS "GRAPEFRUIT DIET." 10 TIMES MORE EFFECTIVE THAN THE POPULAR "HI-PROTEIN" DIET—ABSOLUTELY NO DRUGS OF ANY KIND, NO EXHAUSTIVE EXERCISES, AND NO HUNGER PAINS—EVER. POUNDS AND INCHES BEGIN TO DISAPPEAR WITH YOUR FIRST HEARTY BREAKFAST OF EGGS, HAM, JUICE, TOAST AND COFFEE. WORD OF MOUTH IS SPREADING THE "MEGA-VITAMIN" DIET LIKE UNCONTROLLED WILDFIRE! A NEWLY DEVELOPED SUPER PROTEIN TABLET, CREATED ESPECIALLY FOR THIS DIET, CONTAINS A WHOPPING 570 MILLIGRAMS OF SOLID NATURAL PROTEIN. EACH TINY MILLIGRAM ZEROS IN ON FATTY TISSUES TO BREAK DOWN AND BURN OFF MANY TIMES ITS EQUIVALENT WEIGHT. A DOZEN T-BONE STEAKS COULD NOT PROVIDE AS MUCH UNDILUTED, FAT-FREE, NATURAL PROTEIN AS THIS ONE, TINY, SUPER PROTEIN TABLET. THE QUARTERBACK OF THIS SUPER SUCCESSFUL TEAM, "ULTRA-IRON" CONTAINS THE EXACT AND REQUIRED DOSAGES OF MANGANESE TO ACTIVATE YOUR ENZYMES AND MAINTAIN GOOD GLANDULAR FUNCTIONS, BETAINE TO PREVENT ANY ACCUMULATION OF FAT, ZINC, THE ESSENTIAL INGREDIENT RELATED TO CARBOHYDRATE METABOLISM, AND COPPER, TO PROVIDE CONTINUAL BODY ENERGY, PLUS 25 MICROGRAMS OF THE HIGHLY DESIRABLE B-12 COMPLEX.

PART TWO

VITAMINS,
MINERALS,
WATER

Introduction ━━━━
Supporting Actors

The beginning of Part I introduced the nutrients: carbohydrate, lipid, protein, vitamins, minerals, and water. The next eight chapters were devoted entirely to the first three of these—the principal actors—whose presence in the body accounts for what you are (you are literally made of these three materials and compounds derived from them) and for what you do (because they supply the energy for all your activities).

As you saw, each of those three nutrients is a giant, by molecular standards. A single molecule of carbohydrate may be composed of 300 glucose units, each containing 24 atoms, for a total of some 7,000 atoms. Lipids and proteins are similar in size. Even when they are broken down during digestion, they are absorbed as sizable units—monosaccharides, amino acids, and the like—and these are often reassembled in the cells back into macromolecules. Only if they are oxidized for fuel do they diminish in size to tiny molecules of carbon dioxide and water (three atoms each), and if this occurs, they release tremendous quantities of energy for your use.

Furthermore, you eat (by molecular standards) tremendous quantities of these three nutrients: a hundred or so grams a day of each. If you could purify the carbohydrate, lipid, and protein in your daily diet, you could see that it would fill two or three cups, without any water.

The second three nutrients differ profoundly from the first three in almost every way: in their size and shape, in the roles

carbohydrate, fat, protein: large organic molecules.

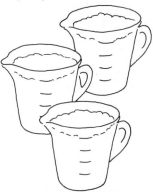

Amount of energy nutrients eaten daily.

carbohydrate, fat, protein: 50-200 grams a day.

269

they play in the body, in the amounts you consume. Perhaps the only characteristics they share with the first three are that they are vital to life and that they are available in food.

The *vitamins* are organic compounds much smaller than the energy nutrients. A molecule of vitamin C, for example, is comparable in size to a single glucose unit. They are never strung together to make body compounds (although each may be attached to a protein), and if they are broken down they yield no usable energy. You consume minute amounts daily—a few micrograms (millionths of a gram) or milligrams (thousandths of a gram), or, at the very most, a few grams. Yet they are vital; in fact, they were named for this characteristic. As you will see, they serve as helpers, making possible the processes by which the first three nutrients are digested, absorbed, and metabolized in the body. There are some fifteen different vitamins, each with its own special roles to play.

The *minerals* are inorganic compounds, smaller than vitamins and found in still more simple forms in foods. Table salt, for example, is the principal source of the minerals sodium and chlorine; it enters the body as a 2-atom pair (NaCl). They may be put together into building blocks for structures such as bones and teeth, but only with the help of the lively enzymes which arrange them in orderly arrays. When they are withdrawn from bone and excreted, they yield no energy. They may also float about in the fluids of the body, by their presence giving the fluids certain characteristics, but they are not metabolized—arranged and rearranged—in the complicated ways or to the same extent as are the energy nutrients. You consume only small amounts of minerals daily, comparable to the amounts of vitamins in your diet. There are some twenty or thirty different minerals important in nutrition.

Then there is *water*, abundant, indispensable, and often ignored because, like air, it is everywhere and we take it for granted. It is inorganic, a single molecule being composed of three atoms (H_2O).[1] The amounts you must consume are enormous, relative to the other nutrients: two to three liters a day, about ten times the amount of the energy nutrients you need.

The next six chapters are devoted to these nutrients: three to the vitamins, two to the minerals, and one to water. A few generalizations presented here will help to put these supporting actors in perspective.

Vitamins are organic. This fact has several consequences. For one, vitamins are destructible. They can be broken down, oxidized, altered in shape. They must be handled with care. The body makes special provisions to absorb them, providing sev-

vitamins: small organic molecules.

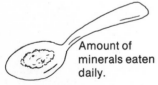

Amount of vitamins eaten daily.

vitamins: yield no energy.

vitamin: an organic compound vital to life, needed in minute amounts. (The first vitamins discovered were amines.)

vita=life
amine=containing nitrogen

minerals: small inorganic molecules.

Na, Cl: symbols for sodium and chlorine. See Appendix B.

minerals: yield no energy.

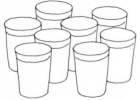

Amount of minerals eaten daily.

water: small inorganic molecule.

water: yields no energy.

Amount of water needed daily.

organic: see page 3.

[1] A more accurate way to describe how water is organized would be to say that while we know that the ratio of hydrogen atoms to oxygen atoms is 2:1 we do not know that water exists as discrete molecules.

eral of them with custom-made protein carriers like those provided for the lipids. A vitamin may be useful in one form here and another there, so special enzymes are also provided which can slightly alter the form of a vitamin to make it active in a given role.

Many vitamins exist in several related forms.

The destructibility of vitamins also has implications for their handling outside the body. The processor of foods, and the cook as well, are well-advised to be aware of the vulnerability of the vitamins in foods, and to treat them with respect.

Vitamins are destructible.

Fat-soluble and water-soluble vitamins. As you may recall, some organic compounds are hydrophilic (water-loving), because positive and negative charges abound on their surfaces and so attract them to the positive (H^+) and negative (OH^-) ions of water. Others are hydrophobic (water-avoiding) and are attracted into the neighborhood of the uncharged, fat-loving compounds. Carbohydrates and proteins are in the first, and lipids in the second, category. The vitamins are divided between these classes: some are water-soluble (the B vitamins and vitamin C), the others are fat-soluble (vitamins A, D, E, and K).

Water-soluble vitamins: B complex and C
Fat-soluble vitamins: A, D, E, K

This fact has several implications for vitamin absorption, transport, and storage.

Absorption of vitamins. The digestive system absorbs these two types of substances differently. Water-soluble substances cross the intestinal and vascular walls directly into the blood, while fat-soluble substances are handled laboriously. Except for the short-chain fatty acids, fat-soluble substances must be emulsified and carried across the membranes of the intestinal cells associated with fat. They cannot cross the blood vessel walls to enter the bloodstream directly but must be transported by way of the lymph to the subclavian vein, through which they enter the bloodstream in the heart.

lymphatic system: see pages 178-179.

> Water-soluble vitamins: absorbed into blood
> Fat-soluble vitamins: absorbed into lymph with bile and
>   fat

Transport of vitamins. The body's principal transportation system is a system of waterways: the bloodstream. Water-soluble vitamins travel freely dissolved in blood; fat-soluble vitamins must be made soluble in water by being attached to carriers.

> Water-soluble vitamins: free in blood
> Fat-soluble vitamins: carried by proteins

Storage and excretion of vitamins. Once the fat-soluble vitamins have been absorbed and transported to cells of the body, they tend to become sequestered there, associated with fat. The water-soluble vitamins, on the other hand, are not held in place. If they are not in use they will circulate freely among all organs of the body, including the kidneys.

The body's principal excretion medium is also water. The kidneys are sensitive to high concentrations of substances in the blood which flow through them. They selectively remove those which are in excess and pass them into the urine. The kidneys will detect and remove excess water-soluble vitamins, but they less readily detect excess fat-soluble vitamins, because these do not accumulate in the blood; they tend to be hidden away in fat-storage places in the body.

> Water-soluble vitamins: excesses excreted
> Fat-soluble vitamins: excesses stored

This difference has two implications. (1) Excess vitamin A eaten today may be stored to meet next month's needs, while blood levels remain normal. But excess vitamin C will lead to a rise in blood levels, the kidneys will respond by excreting the excess, and tomorrow's needs will be met by depleting the vitamin C pool in the blood. (2) Since the water-soluble vitamins are excreted almost as rapidly as they are taken in, toxicity from overdoses occurs transiently if at all. The fat-soluble vitamins, however, can accumulate and reach toxic levels in body stores. This is known to occur with vitamins A and D in particular.

> Water-soluble vitamins: toxicity unlikely
> Fat-soluble vitamins: overdoses dangerous

If you help yourself to a second piece of pecan pie at dinner, you are aware that you are eating more food. The sheer bulk of the energy nutrients and water in the pie makes you feel full. You know, too, that you are eating more calories. But excess vitamin intakes can be indetectable. The amount of vitamin A you need, in pure form, is but a droplet a day. Ten times as much is still only a few drops. This means that it is far easier to take an overdose of vitamins, especially in pure form (pills or drops), than it is of energy nutrients.

Riboflavin is a yellow compound so bright in color that it is easy to see in a water solution. Since excesses of the B vitamins are excreted, a bright yellow color of the urine may signify the presence of this vitamin there. If you are in the habit of taking a multivitamin supplement "to avoid deficiencies," and your diet is otherwise adequate, you may notice this effect.

Some vitamin supplements are inexpensive, but others entail costs far above the value they confer on you in preventing possible deficiencies. The extended activity in Highlight 14 provides you with the opportunity to determine whether your diet, without vitamin supplementation, is adequate by RDA standards. If it is, the following statement may apply to you:

> Overdosing with B vitamins may do nothing for you, and may not hurt you, but it will greatly increase the dollar value of your urine.

9

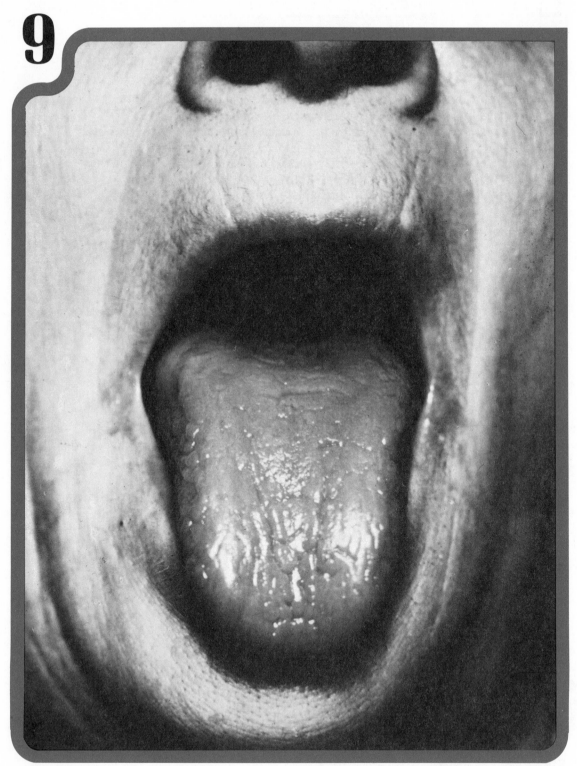

B-vitamin deficiency

The B Vitamins ▬▬▬▬

A television commercial broadcast widely some years ago shows a middle-aged businessman shuffling weakly out of his bedroom with his bathrobe slung loosely around his sagging paunch. He sinks into his chair at the breakfast table and wearily lifts the morning paper to screen his face from the daylight and his bright-eyed, energetic wife. As she places his coffee cup before him, she observes sympathetically, "Sweetie, you look so tired. did you forget to take your vitamin pill today?" (Fadeout, with the voice of the announcer saying "Are you tired in the morning? Do you hate to face the day? What you need is Brand A Vitamins.") Repeat: the same man, transformed, trim and bouncy, waltzes into the breakfast nook, pirouettes gaily around the table, kisses his sweet wife affectionately, takes two hasty sips of coffee, and strides humming out the door. She turns cheerfully to the camera and smiles, "Brand A Vitamins have done wonders for my Harry."

True? No. Poor Harry. If he tries to live on only coffee and vitamins, he will remain a wreck. Like all of the organic nutrients found in foods, the B vitamins are composed of carbon, hydrogen, oxygen, and other atoms linked together by electrons. They do contain energy, but that energy cannot be used to fuel activities or do the body's work. The energy Harry needs comes from carbohydrate, fat, and protein; the vitamins will only help him burn the fuel if he has the fuel to burn.

On the other hand, without B vitamins you would certainly

ATP: the energy-carrier molecule in living cells. See Highlight 7.

feel tired. You would lack energy. Why is this? Some of the B vitamins serve as helpers to the enzymes which release energy from the three energy nutrients—carbohydrate, fat, and protein —to ATP. The B vitamins stand alongside the metabolic pathways and help to keep the disassembly lines moving. In an industrial plant they would be called expeditors. Some of them help to manufacture the red blood cells which carry oxygen to the body's tissues; the oxygen must be present for oxidation and energy release to occur.

As long as B vitamins are present, their presence is not felt. Only when they are missing does their absence manifest itself as a lack of energy. A child, having learned this, defined vitamins on a test as "what if you don't eat you get sick." The definition is one of the most insightful ever given.

Coenzymes

To review the structures and functions of enzymes, see Chapter 3.

coenzyme

prosthetic group

active site: that part of the enzyme surface on which the reaction takes place.

Each of the B vitamins is part of an enzyme helper known as a coenzyme. A coenzyme is a small, nonprotein molecule that associates closely with an enzyme. Some coenzymes form part of the enzyme structure in which case they are known as prosthetic groups; others are associated more loosely with the enzyme. Some participate in the reaction being performed and are chemically altered in the process, but they are always regenerated sooner or later. Some are unaltered but form part of the active site of the enzyme. Thus, while there are differences in details, one thing is true of all: without the coenzymes, the enzymes cannot function.

The consequences of a failure of metabolic enzymes can be catastrophic, as you will realize if you restudy the central pathway of metabolism by which glucose is broken down. The abbreviations for some of the coenzymes needed to keep the processes going are listed beside the reactions they facilitate: NAD^+, TPP, FAD, and CoA:

NAD^+: a coenzyme, nicotinamide (nick-oh-TIN-uh-mide) adenine (ADD-uh-neen) dinucleotide (dye-NOOK-lee-oh-tide). Formerly called DPN (diphosphopyridine (dye-foss-foe-PEER-uh-deen) nucleotide). In many books this coenzyme is abbreviated NAD (without the "+").

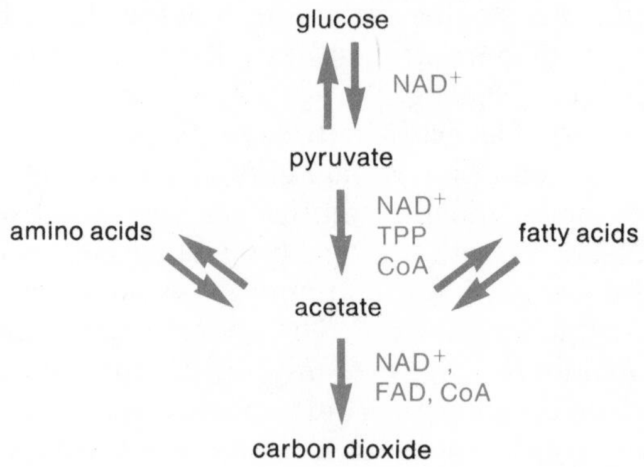

glucose

⇅ NAD^+

pyruvate

NAD^+
TPP
CoA

amino acids   fatty acids

acetate

NAD^+,
FAD, CoA

carbon dioxide

(The examples of coenzyme functions given here are intended to illustrate the way in which these little molecules work to facilitate enzymatic reactions. It is not necessary to memorize the details in order to understand this principle.)

Look at the first step. Some of the enzymes involved in the breakdown of glucose to pyruvate require the coenzyme NAD^+. Part of this molecule is a structure the body cannot make, hence it is an essential nutrient; it must be supplied preformed. This essential part is niacin, a B vitamin.

In other words, to catabolize glucose, the cells must have certain enzymes. For the enzymes to work, they must have the coenzyme, NAD^+. To make NAD^+, the cells must be supplied with niacin (or a closely related compound they can alter to make niacin). The rest of the coenzyme they can make without outside help.

The next step in glucose catabolism is the breakdown of pyruvate to acetate. The enzymes involved in this step require another coenzyme, TPP. The cells can manufacture the TPP they need from thiamin, but thiamin itself is a compound they cannot synthesize, so it must be supplied in the diet. Thiamin is vitamin B_1, the first of the B vitamins to be discovered.

Another coenzyme needed for this step is CoA. As you have probably guessed, the cells can make CoA, except for an essential part of it which must be obtained in the diet. This essential part is pantothenic acid, a B vitamin.

The next step in glucose catabolism is breakdown of acetate to carbon dioxide. The enzymes involved in this process require two of the three coenzymes mentioned above—NAD^+, coenzyme A—and a third in addition: FAD. Again, as before, FAD is synthesized in the body, but a part of its structure must be obtained in the diet: riboflavin. Riboflavin is vitamin B_2.

Now suppose the body's cells lacked any of these B vitamins, niacin, for example. Without niacin, the cells could not make NAD^+. Without NAD^+, the enzymes involved at every step of glucose catabolism would fail to function. Since it is during these steps that energy is transferred into ATP and made available for all of the body's activities, everything would begin to grind to a halt. This is no exaggeration: the symptoms of niacin deficiency are dermatitis (which reflects a failure of the skin to maintain itself), dementia (insanity: a failure of the nervous system), diarrhea (a failure of digestion and absorption), and death! These are only the most obvious, observable symptoms. Every organ in the body, being dependent on glucose catabolism, is profoundly affected by niacin deficiency. As you can see, niacin is a little like the horseshoe nail for want of which a war was lost.

The diagram shows that the complete catabolism of *amino acids* and *fat* as well as glucose depends on the coenzymes

niacin (NIGH-uh-sin): a B vitamin. Part of the structure of NAD^+.

niacin precursor: see page 292.

TPP: a coenzyme, thiamin pyrophosphate (pie-roe-FOSS-fate).

thiamin (THIGH-uh-min): vitamin B_1. Part of the structure of TPP. Alternative spelling: thiamine.

CoA (coh-AY): a coenzyme.

pantothenic (PAN-to-THEN-ic) **acid:** a B vitamin, part of the structure of coenzyme A.

FAD: a coenzyme, flavine (FLAY-vin) adenine dinucleotide.

riboflavin (RIBE-o-flay-vin): vitamin B_2. Part of the structure of FAD.

The 4 D's of niacin deficiency.

*For want of a nail a
   horseshoe was lost.
For want of a horseshoe
   a horse was lost.
For want of a horse, a
   soldier was lost.
For want of a soldier, a
   battle was lost.
For want of a battle, the
   war was lost,
And all for the want of a
   horseshoe nail!*
                —Mother Goose

transamination: the transferring of an amino group from one compound to another, as when nonessential amino acids are manufactured in the body.

pyridoxal-5-phosphate: a coenzyme.

pyridoxine (peer-i-DOX-in): vitamin B_6. Part of the coenzyme pyridoxal-5-phosphate.

Other B vitamins:

folacin (FOLL-uh-sin), also called folic acid

cobalamin (B_{12}) (co-BAL-uh-min)

biotin (BY-o-tin)

NAD^+, FAD, TPP, and CoA. From the point at which they have been converted to acetate, amino acids and fat follow the same path as glucose. This means that the need for the vitamins that go into the making of these coenzymes will be greater if you eat more carbohydrate, fat, or protein. The precise calculation of a person's needs for thiamin, for example, is based on his/her calorie intake. (See boxed section at end of chapter.)

Not only breakdown (catabolism) but also building (anabolism) of compounds in the body requires coenzymes. When nonessential amino acids are made, an amino group is attached to a carbon compound in a process called transamination. Enzymes performing this function require the coenzyme pyridoxal-5-phosphate, which in turn necessitates eating vitamin B_6 (pyridoxine). Other B vitamins needed for the synthesis of coenzymes active in a multitude of body systems are folacin, cobalamin (vitamin B_{12}), and biotin.

Coenzyme Action: A Closer Look

Each coenzyme is specialized for certain kinds of chemical reactions. NAD^+ (containing niacin), for example, can serve as the acceptor of hydrogen atoms removed from other compounds and can lose them to compounds which ultimately pass them to oxygen (see Highlight 7). There are many steps during the catabolism of glucose in which hydrogens are removed and NAD^+ participates in this way. A model of the way NAD^+ works with an enzyme to remove hydrogens is shown below:

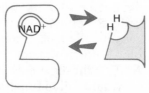

(1) An enzyme with coenzyme NAD^+ encounters a molecule containing two hydrogens.

 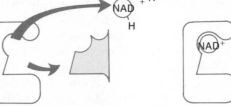

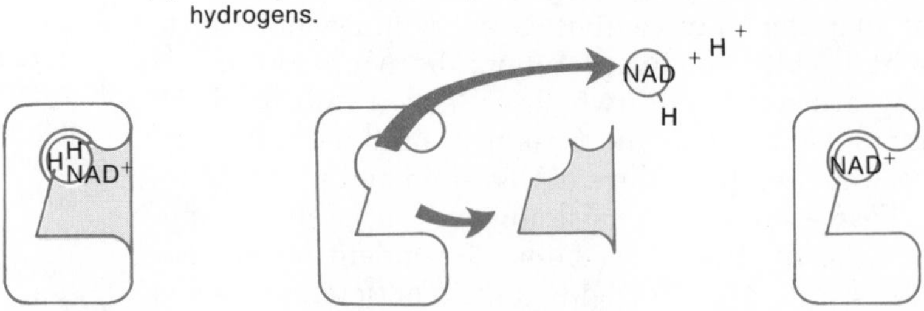

(2) A complex is formed.

(3) The H's are removed from the molecule and attached to NAD^+ forming $NADH + H^+$. The complex releases $NADH + H^+$ and the molecule.

(4) Later the $NADH + H^+$ donates the hydrogens to another compound and returns to its enzyme again.

A very similar compound is the coenzyme NADP, which also contains niacin. NADP accepts hydrogens during similar reactions, and can donate them to the synthesis of fatty acids.

TPP (containing thiamin) is the coenzyme which temporarily accepts keto-acids such as pyruvate, and facilitates the removal of carbon dioxide from them. The reaction in which pyruvate is converted to acetyl CoA is one that requires TPP. Wherever carbon dioxide removal must be performed, TPP is likely to be involved

Coenzyme A (containing pantothenic acid) is a coenzyme which can temporarily accept organic molecules such as acetate and facilitate their transfer to other compounds. This coenzyme is at the hub of metabolism of carbohydrates, fats, and proteins and is needed for the release of energy from them. It also can transfer successive acetates to fatty acids to build longer fatty acid chains and is needed for the synthesis of other major body compounds, such as the steroid hormones.

FAD (containing riboflavin) is a coenzyme which, like NAD^+, can accept hydrogens and pass them on to other compounds. This is important in cellular respiration, as it provides a step in the pathway by which hydrogens removed from the energy nutrients during metabolism are passed to oxygen. A similar coenzyme, FMN (which also contains riboflavin), plays similar roles.

Pyridoxal phosphate (containing pyridoxal) and its relatives are versatile coenzymes which help to catalyze a wide variety of reactions involving amino acids. The step which begins the breakdown of stored glycogen to glucose also depends on these coenzymes.

Biotin is a coenzyme which can accept carbon dioxide molecules removed from one molecule and can add them to another, thus helping to build body structures. An important example of this function is the reaction illustrated on page 210 where a carbon dioxide is added to pyruvate to make oxaloacetate. This is the reaction by which carbohydrate metabolism (yielding pyruvate) makes possible the complete oxidation of acetyl CoA from fat so that ketosis does not occur.

Folacin is a coenzyme which can receive a single-carbon unit from one molecule and transfer it to another. A multitude of such reactions must occur in the body. An example is shown on page 91, where one amino acid is converted to another by removing a $-CH_2OH$ group. Others are needed for the synthesis of DNA and RNA and many other body compounds.

The B_{12} coenzymes (a family of coenzymes containing cobalamin) catalyze reactions that are less well understood but apparently also play key roles in the metabolism of the energy nutrients and the building of body compounds.

Thus each of the B vitamins has specific roles to play in

Structures of NADP and other coenzymes mentioned in this chapter are shown in Appendix C.

keto-acid: see page 211.

These are **decarboxylation** reactions. Another example is that in which alpha-ketoglutarate is converted to succinate (see Highlight 7).

See the diagram of metabolism on page 206.

steroid hormones: see page 70.

See the electron-transport chain, Highlight 7.

FMN: flavine mononucleotide.

Reactions dependent on pyridoxal phosphate include racemization (rearrangement of atoms), transamination, decarboxylation of amino acids, dehydration reactions and others.

The 1-carbon fragment removed by folacin may be a methyl ($-CH_3$) group or a hydroxymethyl ($-CH_2OH$) group.

helping the enzymes do their work of performing thousands of different molecular conversions in the body. These enzymes with their helpers are found in every cell and must be continuously present for the cells to function as they should.

Two other compounds less thoroughly understood are the vitamin-like compounds inositol and choline. These may not be dietary essentials for human beings, but deficiencies can be induced in laboratory animals and their functions can be studied. Like the B vitamins listed above, they serve as coenzymes in metabolism.

inositol (eye-NOSS-i-tal)

choline (KO-leen)

Health food purveyors make much of inositol and choline, insisting that we must supplement our diets with them. This incorrect notion arises from an unjustified application of findings from animal studies to human beings.

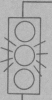

CAUTION WHEN YOU READ!

To weigh the reliability of nutrition information, ask yourself:

Has the finding been proved applicable to human beings?

Highlight 11 enlarges on this theme, which has been a major problem with recent publicity about vitamin E.

B Vitamin Deficiency

Removing a number of "horseshoe nails" can have such disastrous and far-reaching effects that it is difficult to imagine or predict the results. A few generalizations can be made, however, which clarify the principles involved.

First, a B vitamin deficiency seldom shows up in isolation. After all, people do not eat nutrients singly, they eat foods which contain mixtures of nutrients. If a major class of foods is missing from the diet, those nutrients contributed by that class of food will all be lacking to varying extents. In only two cases have dietary deficiencies of single B vitamins been observed on a large scale in human populations, and deficiency diseases named for them. One of these diseases, beriberi, was first observed in the Far East when the custom of polishing rice became widespread. Rice contributed 80 percent of the calories consumed by the people of those areas, and its hulls were their principal source of thiamin. When the hulls were removed, beriberi spread like

beriberi: the thiamin deficiency disease, which led to the discovery of vitamin B_1.

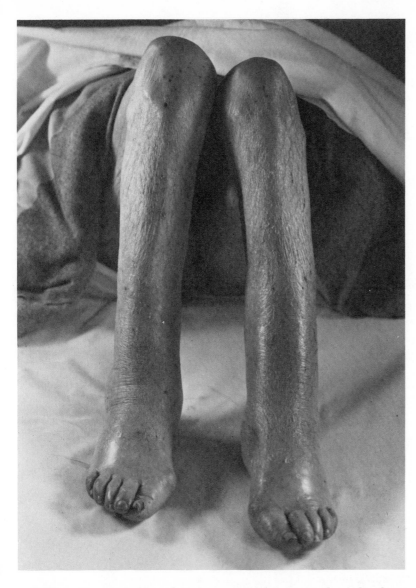

The edema of beriberi.

Photo courtesy of Dr. Samuel
Dreizen, D.D.S., M.D.

wildfire. It was believed to be an epidemic, and medical researchers wasted much time and energy seeking a microbial
cause before they realized that the problem was not what was
present, but what was absent, in the sufferers' intakes.

    The other disease, pellagra, became endemic in the United
States' South in the early part of this century, when the people
were subsisting on a low-protein diet whose staple grain was
corn. They obtained other B vitamins from other foods, but their
diet was uniquely lacking in niacin.

    Even in these cases, the deficiencies were not pure, but
remedying the principal deficiency entailed remedying accom-
panying ones as well.

History of discoveries of
the vitamins: Appendix A.

pellagra (pell-AY-gra): the
niacin deficiency disease.

    pellis=skin
    agra=seizure

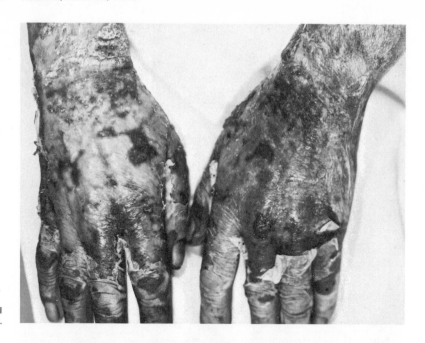

The dermatitis of pellagra.

Photo courtesy of Dr. Samuel
Dreizen, D.D.S., M.D.

mnemonic (ne-MON-ic)
device: a jingle or other
group of words or symbols
which aids in memorizing
information.

mnemos=memory

B vitamin terminology. For historical reasons, some of the B vitamins have both names and numbers, a confusing terminology which prompted one frustrated nutritionist to exclaim, "This riddled paradox causes nightmares for bitty children in pants!" At first glance, his outburst might seem to be a protest against trying to teach vitamin terminology to toddlers who are fresh out of diapers, but on closer examination it turns out that he has invented a mnemonic device that simplifies the task of learning which is which. The first letter(s) of each word stand for a B vitamin. The first four words stand for the numbered vitamins in order: B_1, B_2, B_6, B_{12}. The first six are those for which RDAs have been established.

Mnemonic	Names of Vitamins	Numbers
This	thiamin*	B_1
riddled	riboflavin*	B_2
paradox	pyridoxine*	B_6
causes	cobalamin*	B_{12}
nightmares	niacin*	
for	folacin*	
bitty	biotin	
children	choline	
in	inositol	
pants	pantothenic acid	

*These have RDA's.

Once vitamin research was well under way, and other B vitamins had been discovered, the clarification of their function was often greatly helped by laboratory experiments in which animals or human volunteers were fed diets devoid of one vitamin; the effects of the deficiency of that vitamin could then be studied to determine what functions it normally performed. Other deficiency diseases were discovered in this way and have since been observed to occur outside the laboratory.

Table C9.1 sums up a few of the better established facts about vitamin B deficiency. A look at the table will make another generalization possible. Different body systems depend to different extents on these vitamins. Processes in nerves depend heavily on glucose metabolism and hence on thiamin; thus paralysis sets in when this nutrient is lacking. Synthesis of red blood cells requires folacin and cobalamin; one of the first symptoms of deficiency of either of these nutrients is a type of anemia. But again, each nutrient is important in all systems, and these lists of symptoms are far from complete.

The skin and the tongue appear to be especially sensitive to vitamin B deficiencies. The listing of these items gives them perhaps undue emphasis. Remember that in a medical examination, these are two body parts that the doctor can easily observe. The skin gives an indication of a typical body tissue that may be suffering effects that are also being felt beneath,

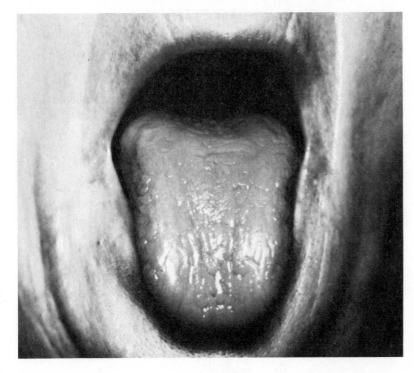

Tongue symptom of B-vitamin deficiency: the tongue is smooth due to atrophy of the tissue (glossitis). This photo is of a person with a folic acid deficiency.

Photo courtesy of Dr. Samuel Dreizen, D.D.S., M.D.

Table C9.1
B Vitamin Deficiency Symptoms in Human Beings

Vitamin	*Deficiency*
Thiamin (B$_1$)	*Beriberi.* Common in the Far East, where polished rice is the staple grain. Main effects on: (1) nervous system: mental confusion, peripheral paralysis (2) muscles: weakness, wasting, painful calf muscles (3) cardiovascular system: edema, enlarged heart, death from cardiac failure
Riboflavin (B$_2$)	*Ariboflavinosis.* Main effects on: (1) facial skin: dermatitis around nose and lips, cracks at the corners of the mouth (2) eyes: hypersensitivity to light, reddening of the cornea
Niacin	*Pellagra.* Observed in the United States' South, where protein was minimal in the diet, and corn was the staple grain. Main effects on: (1) skin: bilateral symmetrical dermatitis, especially on parts of body exposed to sun (2) tongue: smoothness (3) GI tract: diarrhea (4) nervous system: mental confusion, irritability, progressing to psychosis or delirium
Pyridoxine (B$_6$)	*(no name)* Main effects on: (1) skin: dermatitis, cracks at the corners of the mouth, irritation of sweat glands (2) tongue: smoothness (3) nervous system: convulsions, abnormal brain wave pattern
Folacin	*(no name)* Main effects on: (1) tongue: smoothness (2) GI tract: diarrhea (3) blood: anemia (characterized by large cells)
Cobalamin (B$_{12}$)	*Pernicious anemia.* Usually not from dietary lack but from failure to absorb the vitamin (a genetic disease). Main effects on: (1) blood: anemia (characterized by large cells) (2) nervous system: degeneration of peripheral nerves
Pantothenic acid	(deficiency observed only in animals)
Biotin	(has been observed in man under experimental conditions only)

Technical terms for these symptoms are:

cheilosis

photophobia

glossitis

cheilosis

glossitis

glossitis

macrocytic anemia

macrocytic anemia

but less obviously. The mouth and tongue are the foremost parts of the digestive system; if they are abnormal, there may be an abnormality throughout the GI tract. What is really happening, in a vitamin deficiency, is happening inside the cells of the body; what the doctor sees and reports are its outward manifestations.

It is more and more apparent that you cannot observe a symptom and automatically jump to a conclusion regarding its cause. The warning was given earlier (in Chapter 2) about dermatitis: a symptom is not a disease. As you have seen, deficiencies of linoleic acid, riboflavin, niacin, and pyridoxine can all cause dermatitis. As you will see, a deficiency of vitamin A can too. Because skin is on the outside, where you and your doctor can easily look at it, it is a useful indicator of things-going-wrong-in-cells. But by itself, a skin symptom tells you nothing about its possible cause.

The same is true of anemia. We often think of anemia as being caused by an iron deficiency; this is the commonest nutritional cause. But anemia can also be caused by folacin or cobalamin deficiency, by digestive tract failure to absorb any of these nutrients, or by cancer. Bleeding will also cause anemia. A little knowledge is a dangerous thing. Caution:

A flag sign of a spurious claim is:

the implication that a specific nutrient will cure a given symptom

The *nutrient* folacin will clear up the *symptom* tiredness only if the symptom is due to the *disease*, folacin deficiency anemia.

The B Vitamins in Food: First, a Caution

The preceding sections have shown both the great importance of the B vitamins in promoting normal, healthy functioning of all body systems and the severe consequences of deficiency. You may want to know how to be sure you are getting enough of these vital nutrients. This chapter concludes with some practical pointers regarding food intake, but a closer look is possible.

One way to discover whether your intake of a vitamin is sufficient is to calculate the amount you are consuming each day in the foods you eat and to compare your intake with the RDA. (See boxed section at end of chapter.) This is an informative exercise and is recommended repeatedly in Suggested Activities throughout this book. This chapter and those that follow introduce some fifteen nutrients that can be studied this way. However, there are more accurate means of determining whether a deficiency exists, and there are distinct limitations on the reliability of the dietary record method. First, you have to assume that the RDA applies to you. Actually, people's needs for nutrients vary over a wide range; you may not be typical. Of course you may need much less than the RDA, but you may also need more. Second, you have to assume that your body's handling and absorption of the vitamin is normal. This doesn't automatically follow from the fact that you swallowed a food containing it. If your digestive system is disturbed, if you are ill (especially with diarrhea), or if you are emotionally upset, your absorption of certain nutrients may be impaired. Third, when you look up the foods you eat in a table of food composition, you have to assume that the food you ate contained the amount of the nutrient listed in the table. But foods vary too. Not all 200 gram tomatoes contain exactly 1.3 milligrams of niacin. The nutrient contents of foods are averages. Furthermore, the professionals who make up the tables make still a fourth assumption—that the foods are stored and prepared in a normal way, which minimizes losses of vitamins. So there are at least four possible sources of error in assuming that your nutrient intakes calculated this way are meeting your nutrient needs.

The table of food composition most often used is given in Appendix H.

Still, the dietary record is the simplest way to check on a person's nutrient status and is the way most often used by students. Some more precise means of assessing nutritional status (physical examination, anthropometric measures, and biochemical tests) are described at the beginning of Highlight 12.

The B Vitamins in Food

With the above cautions in mind, let us examine the foods for their B vitamin content. A detailed study of the vitamin contents of foods is not necessary to achieve enough understanding to select foods wisely. You only need to be aware of a few general observations in order to avoid the risk of deficiency.

A useful distinction to begin with has to do with the distribution of vitamins in foods. Some are so widely distributed that virtually any food is a good source. Others are found in higher concentrations in certain classes of foods, so that it is important to include these classes in your diet frequently. Of the B vitamins, thiamin and pantothenic acid fall in the first category (widely distributed in foods), while riboflavin, niacin, cobalamin, and folacin fall in the second (found mostly in certain classes of foods).

A second useful fact emerges from surveys done to determine the nutritional status of Americans with respect to these nutrients. It is probably safe to assume that if Americans generally are well-nourished with respect to a certain vitamin, you need not worry about getting enough of it; provided that your diet is not radically different from the average American diet, you no doubt consume this nutrient in adequate amounts. On the other hand, if in the surveys many Americans have been found to be receiving marginal or inadequate amounts of a nutrient, you might want to be aware of the reasons for this, in order to avoid the problem for yourself.

In some cases, the study of nutrient needs and intakes has not progressed to the point where accurate generalizations can be made. This is true of the vitamins pyridoxine (B_6) and biotin.

The following discussion focuses on five of the B vitamins, selected because (1) adequate information about them is available, and because (2) they are found in only certain classes of foods which must, therefore, be included in the diet to ensure adequacy, or (3) Americans are frequently found to be consuming inadequate amounts. As you will see, once a diet has been planned to meet the needs for these vitamins, it meets the general description of "a balanced and varied diet," and is therefore likely to ensure adequacy for other nutrients not considered here.

Thiamin. Surveys of American nutritional status in the 1960s revealed that from ten to twenty percent of those studied had intakes of thiamin below the RDA.[1] Those most affected were girls and women, from the age of nine up. This finding suggests that thiamin is a nutrient to worry about, at least for women, and a look at food sources of thiamin is probably advisable.

It turns out that thiamin has been a problem for as long as dietary studies of this kind have been done in our country. The first national survey, undertaken in 1936, brought this and some other nutritional problems to light and led to governmental action intended to alleviate them.

The enrichment program. The 1936 survey showed our population to be experiencing significantly low intakes of three nutrients in addition to thiamin: two other B vitamins, riboflavin and niacin, and the mineral, iron. The decision was made to take governmental action to improve the nation's nutrition. Nutrition authorities faced with this problem decided to select a food to which these nutrients would be added. Wisely, they chose a food with the following characteristics: it is consumed

enrichment

[1] NAS-NRC: *U.S. Diets of Men, Women, and Children, one day in Spring, 1965.* U.S. Department of Agriculture, Washington, D.C., 1968.

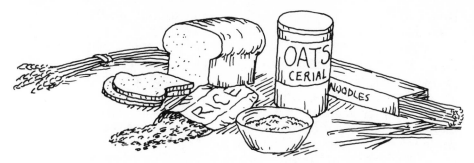

by nearly every American of any racial or cultural background; it is inexpensive; and the amounts consumed are not likely to be excessive. The food group they chose was the bread and cereal group, which includes pasta products such as macaroni, spaghetti, and noodles, and grains such as wheat, corn, and rice.

For years prior to this, nutritionists had been advocating the use of whole-grain products, which contained significant amounts of the B vitamins and iron. The 1936 survey revealed that people truly preferred the refined breads and cereals, from which many of these nutrients were lost during processing. Enrichment standards were therefore set in such a way that the amount of these nutrients added back to the refined products would make them approximately equivalent to the original whole-grain products. Activity 4 at the end of this chapter enables you to compare the two types of foods to see the extent of their similarity.

The enrichment program which developed during the 1940s called for the addition of these four nutrients to foods made from refined grains. As a consequence, the amount of thiamin contributed by these foods to the American diet increased from about 19 percent in the 1930s to over 30 percent in the 1940s. Still, as the more recent surveys have shown, the problem of thiamin deficiency in American girls and women has not been completely solved.

Clearly one important practical suggestion for avoiding a thiamin deficiency is to eat whole-grain or enriched breads and cereals from this food group. An awareness of what other foods contain thiamin is also needed, however. Table C9.2 shows that thiamin is widely distributed in all classes of foods but that very few foods contribute more than 20 percent of the RDA per serving, although many common foods contribute about 10 percent or less. If you study the table while thinking about your own food habits, you will be likely to conclude that many of your favorite foods contain some thiamin. Perhaps a useful guideline is to eat ten or more servings of nutritious foods each day including whole-grain or enriched breads and cereals (assuming that on the average, each food will contribute 10 percent of your thiamin RDA).

enriched: contains thiamin, riboflavin, niacin, and iron in amounts approximately equivalent to those found in whole-grain products.

fortified: see Highlight 13.

thiamin: most nutritious foods contribute about 10 percent RDA per serving.

Table C9.2
Fifty Foods Showing Amounts of Thiamin

The foods listed below are the fifty that rank highest as sources of thiamin from those which are found on the ADA Exchange Lists and which also have been analyzed for nutrient composition. Serving sizes are the sizes listed in the Exchange Lists except for meat, where 3-ounce servings are shown. The numbers 1 through 6 refer to the numbers of the Exchange Lists: 1 = Milk, 2 = Vegetables, 3 = Fruit, 4 = Bread, 5L = Lean Meat, 5M = Medium-Fat Meat, 5H = High-Fat Meat, 6 = Fats and Oils. Numbers in parentheses are the item numbers on the Table of Food Composition (Appendix H).

Exchange Group	Food (Item Number)	Serving Size	Thiamin Milligrams
5L	Ham (113)	3 ounces	.40
5L	Oysters (140)	¾ cup	.25
5M	Liver, beef (112)	3 ounces	.23
4	Green peas (215)	½ cup	.22
5M	Beef heart (104)	3 ounces	.21
4	Lima beans (167)	½ cup	.16
	10% of U.S. RDA of 1.5 milligrams		
2	Collard greens (195)	½ cup	.14
3	Orange (294)	1	.13
4	Dried beans (148)	½ cup	.13
5L	Lamb, leg (108)	3 ounces	.13
2	Dandelion greens (201)	½ cup	.12
4	Rice, enriched (464)	½ cup	.12
2	Asparagus (165)	½ cup	.12
3	Orange juice (298)	½ cup	.11
5L	Veal roast (132)	3 ounces	.11
1	2% fat fortified milk (3)	1 cup	.10
4	Spaghetti, enriched (474)	½ cup	.10
4	Macaroni, enriched (430)	½ cup	.10
4	Cooked cereal (439)	½ cup	.10
4	Corn on cob (196)	1 small	.09
1	Skim milk (2)	1 cup	.09
4	Potato (221)	1 small	.08
4	Mashed potato (226)	½ cup	.08
1	Powdered skim milk (6)	1/3 cup	.08
1	Whole milk (1)	1 cup	.07
1	Yogurt (from whole milk) (72)	1 cup	.07
4	Corn muffin (419)	1	.07
4	Bran flakes (338)	½ cup	.07
4	Puffed rice (468)	1 cup	.07
4	Muffin (435)	1	.07
5M	Hamburger (81)	3 ounces	.07
2	Cooked tomatoes (241)	½ cup	.06
2	Tomato juice (244)	½ cup	.06
2	Brussels sprouts (180)	½ cup	.06
3	Pineapple (314)	½ cup	.06
4	White bread (353)	1 slice	.06
4	Whole wheat bread (372)	1 slice	.06
4	Hamburger bun (471)	½	.06
4	Potato chips (228)	15 chips	.06
4	French fried potato (224)	8	.06

Table C9.2 (continued)

Exchange Group	Food (Item Number)	Serving Size	Thiamin Milligrams
5L	Chipped beef (92)	3 ounces	.06
2	Mustard greens (208)	½ cup	.06
2	Broccoli (179)	½ cup	.06
5M	Egg (73)	1	.05
3	Pink grapefruit (271)	½	.05
2	Summer squash (234)	½ cup	.05
1	Canned evaporated milk (4)	½ cup	.05
2	Green beans (168)	½ cup	.05
5L	Chicken, meat only (95)	3 ounces	.05
5L	Lean beef roast (79)	3 ounces	.05

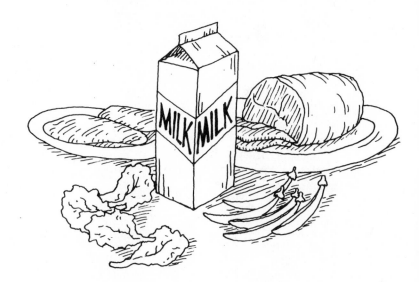

Riboflavin. Another B vitamin found lacking in the American diet in the surveys of the 1960s was riboflavin, and this, too, was a more serious problem for girls and women than for children, boys, or men. Enrichment of breads and cereals with this vitamin makes the choice of these foods advisable, but again in addition one should know what other foods contain this nutrient.

Riboflavin, the light-sensitive vitamin, differs from thiamin in being less evenly distributed among the food groups. About half of the riboflavin in the American diet comes from milk and dairy products, and another 25 percent from the meat group (meat, poultry, and fish). Milk drinkers have little trouble meeting their needs. Table C9.3 shows the amount of riboflavin contributed by servings of foods.

riboflavin: milk contributes about 50 percent, meat about 25 percent, enriched breads and cereals additional.

Table C9.3
Fifty Foods Showing Amounts of Riboflavin

The foods listed below are the fifty that rank highest as sources of riboflavin from those which are found on the ADA Exchange Lists and which also have been analyzed for nutrient composition. Serving sizes are the sizes listed in the Exchange Lists except for meat, where 3-ounce servings are shown. The numbers 1 through 6 refer to the numbers of the Exchange Lists: 1 = Milk, 2 = Vegetables, 3 = Fruit, 4 = Bread, 5L = Lean Meat, 5M = Medium-Fat Meat, 5H = High-Fat Meat, 6 = Fats and Oils. Numbers in parentheses are the item numbers on the Table of Food Composition (Appendix H).

Exchange Group	Food (Item Number)	Serving Size	Riboflavin Milligrams
5M	Beef liver (112)	3 ounces	3.60
5M	Beef heart (104)	3 ounces	1.04
1	2% fat fortified milk (3)	1 cup	.52
1	Skim milk (2)	1 cup	.44
1	Canned evaporated milk (4)	½ cup	.43
1	Whole milk (1)	1 cup	.41
1	Dry skim milk (6)	1/3 cup	.40
1	Yogurt (whole milk) (72)	1 cup	.39
5L	Oysters (140)	¾ cup	.30
5L	Chipped beef (92)	3 ounces	.30
5L	Veal roast (132)	3 ounces	.26
5L	Leg of lamb (108)	3 ounces	.23
5L	Lean roast beef (79)	3 ounces	.19
2	Collard greens (195)	½ cup	.19
5M	Hamburger (81)	3 ounces	.18
	10% of U.S. RDA of 1.7 milligrams		
5L	Sardines (142)	3 ounces	.17
5L	Ham (113)	3 ounces	.16
5L	Chicken, meat only (95)	3 ounces	.16
5L	Canned salmon (141)	3 ounces	.16
2	Dandelion greens (201)	½ cup	.15
5M	Egg (73)	1	.15
5M	Creamed cottage cheese (16)	¼ cup	.15
4	Winter squash (235)	½ cup	.14
2	Asparagus (165)	½ cup	.13
2	Broccoli (179)	½ cup	.12
2	Brussels sprouts (180)	½ cup	.11
2	Spinach (233)	½ cup	.11
5L	Canned tuna (146)	3 ounces	.10
2	Mustard greens (208)	½ cup	.10
4	Lima beans (167)	½ cup	.09
4	Green peas (215)	½ cup	.09
4	Pumpkin (229)	¾ cup	.09
4	Muffin (435)	1	.09
4	Corn muffin (419)	1	.08
3	Strawberries (328)	¾ cup	.08
2	Summer squash (234)	½ cup	.08
4	Corn on cob (196)	1 small	.08
4	Dried beans (148)	½ cup	.07
3	Pear (312)	1	.07

Table C9.3 (continued)

Exchange Groups	Food (Item Number)	Serving Size	Riboflavin Milligrams
4	Spaghetti, enriched (474)	½ cup	.06
4	Macaroni, enriched (430)	½ cup	.06
3	Raspberries (325)	½ cup	.06
4	Pancake (442)	1	.06
2	Green beans (168)	½ cup	.06
4	White bread (353)	1 slice	.05
2	Cauliflower (192)	½ cup	.05
4	Mashed potatoes (226)	½ cup	.05
3	Orange (294)	1	.05
3	Peach (305)	1	.05
4	Hamburger bun (471)	½	.04

A compound which can be converted to a nutrient in the body is known as a **precursor** of that nutrient. Thus, tryptophan is a precursor of niacin.

Niacin. Niacin is unique among the B vitamins in being obtainable from another nutrient source: protein. The amino acid tryptophan can be converted to niacin in the body. If you eat more than enough protein, chances are that you will be meeting your niacin needs as well. Since American diets are high in animal protein, niacin deficiency is not a problem in this country, being seen instead wherever protein deficiency occurs. The widespread pellagra that was seen during the early part of this century in the United States' South was due to the fact that the cornmeal-salt pork-corn syrup based diet of the people of that area was lacking in both niacin and protein and was unusually low in tryptophan. Symptoms of niacin deficiency are no longer often observed in this country except in persons whose protein intake is unacceptably low (alcoholics).

niacin equivalents

No table of niacin contents of foods is given here. The amount of this vitamin available in a food can be expressed in niacin equivalents; that is, the amount of preformed niacin available from the food plus the amount available if the tryptophan in the food is converted to niacin. Sixty milligrams of tryptophan yield one milligram of niacin, hence a food containing one milligram of niacin and 60 milligrams of tryptophan would contain two niacin equivalents.

Until 1973 the niacin RDA was also expressed in niacin equivalents. This terminology was then abandoned in favor of recommending amounts of preformed niacin in milligrams. For any given individual it is impossible to guess how much of the tryptophan consumed is converted to niacin in the body, and hence how much niacin the diet actually supplies. In any case, the point to remember is that a diet supplying abundant meat and milk will be adequate in niacin.

About one-half of the niacin equivalents consumed by Americans comes from milk, eggs, meat, poultry, and fish, and about one-fourth from enriched breads and cereals. Vegetarians who lack some of these important food sources are well advised to emphasize nuts and legumes in their diets, as these are good sources of niacin and protein. A look at the nutrient contents of foods (Appendix H) will reveal other good sources.

Cobalamin (vitamin B_{12}). Vitamin B_{12} is unique among the nutrients in being found only in animal flesh and animal products. Anyone who eats ample amounts of meat and drinks plenty of milk is guaranteed an adequate consumption of this vitamin; the strict vegetarian must take a supplement.

A second special characteristic of B_{12} is that it requires a protein factor for transportation from the intestinal tract into the bloodstream. As with all proteins, the design for this protein is carried in the genes. Certain people have in their genetic makeup a defective gene for this factor and so cannot make the protein. These people may fail to absorb the vitamin, even though they are taking enough in their diets. They risk developing pernicious anemia. In such a case, or when the stomach has been injured and cannot produce enough intrinsic factor, the vitamin must be supplied to the body by injection, bypassing the block in the intestinal tract.

Early research on pernicious anemia revealed that the disease could be aided but not cured by eating large amounts of raw calves' liver. The researchers concluded that liver contained a factor needed to prevent the disease. This was of course B_{12}. The concentration of B_{12} in liver was so great that some was absorbed even without the carrier protein. Later it appeared that something within the body itself was also needed: the protein to help absorb the vitamin. Hence liver was said to contain an extrinsic factor, while the body product was called an intrinsic factor. Intrinsic factor is now known to be synthesized in the stomach, where it attaches to the vitamin; the complex then passes to the small intestine and is gradually absorbed.

The anemia caused by vitamin B_{12} deficiency can be mistaken for that caused by folacin deficiency because both are characterized by large red blood cells that are indistinguishable under the microscope. As a result, the B_{12} deficiency anemia can be misdiagnosed as folacin deficiency anemia, and the wrong vitamin administered to correct the disorder. In fact, folacin does clear up the blood symptoms of B_{12} deficiency, but it fails to correct the neurological damage, which may persist and advance while the obvious symptoms are masked.

The masking of pernicious anemia by administration of folacin underlines a point already made several

niacin: adequate if protein is adequate.

cobalamin (B_{12}): adequate if animal foods are ample.

extrinsic factor

intrinsic factor

neurological: having to do with the nerves or nervous system.

times: it takes a skilled diagnostician to make a correct diagnosis, and the risk laymen take when they diagnose themselves on the basis of a single observed *symptom* is clearly a serious one.

A second point should also be underlined here. Since B_{12} deficiency in the body may be caused *either* by B_{12} lack in the diet *or* by genetically caused inability to absorb the vitamin, a change in diet alone may not suffice to correct it. You might wish to think about this in relation to the cautions offered on pages 64 and 285.

For the effects of oral contraceptives on nutrient needs, see suggested readings at the end of Chapter 15.

folacin: the "foliage" vitamin.

Folacin. Folacin deficiency may result from an inadequate intake of folacin, impaired absorption, or unusual metabolic need for the vitamin. A significant number of cases of anemia develop from these causes, especially among pregnant women and women taking oral contraceptives, whose needs for this vitamin are unusually high.

The best food sources of this vitamin are organ meats (such as liver), green leafy vegetables (the name of the vitamin is related to the word *foliage*), beets, and members of the cabbage family (such as cauliflower, broccoli, and Brussels sprouts). Among the fruits, oranges, orange juice, and cantaloupe melon are the best sources, while among the starchy vegetables corn, lima beans, parsnips, green peas, pumpkin, and sweet potato are good sources. Whole wheat bread, wheat germ, and milk also supply folacin.

Putting it all together. If you wanted to plan a diet that was adequate for the five B vitamins discussed above, you would be well advised to include daily: two or more cups of milk or dairy products (for riboflavin and niacin equivalents), two or more servings of meat, fish, poultry, or eggs, including liver and pork occasionally (for thiamin, riboflavin, and niacin), whole-grain or enriched breads and cereals (for thiamin, riboflavin, and niacin), and green leafy vegetables (for folacin). The animal products would supply cobalamin, and all would supply thiamin. What foods would then be missing? Other vegetables, fruits, and fats—but as you will see in the following chapters, these latter foods are rich in vitamins A, C, D, and E. The conclusion is unavoidable: a balanced and varied diet is the best guarantee of adequacy for the essential nutrients. Such a diet would include selections from all six groups of the Food Exchange System.

Minimizing Losses in Food Handling

The B vitamins are all water-soluble. Whenever a vegetable is soaked or cooked in water and the water is thrown away, significant losses of these vitamins occur. In addition, each of the B vitamins is sensitive to heat to some extent, and riboflavin can be destroyed by light.

Moralizing is tiresome. Let us for fun play the devil's advocate instead, and devise a means of maximizing *losses* of the B vitamins. First, cook meats at high temperatures for long periods of time and throw away the juices which leak out of them. Leave milk in a transparent container on the countertop in the sunlight for several hours to destroy the riboflavin before storing it in the refrigerator. When baking, bake at high temperatures for long periods of time, using unenriched refined flour for your recipes. Buy unenriched bread and cereal products. When buying vegetables, select those that are several days old and that have been sitting at room temperature in the market since they came in. On bringing them home, put them in the sink, cover them with water, and let them soak for half a day before washing them. When cooking them, slice them thinly, cover them completely with water, bring the water slowly to a boil and cook them for a long time. Discard the cooking water. If leftover vegetables are to be reheated, pour off the old water and add fresh water. Losses of up to 50 or 60 percent of the B vitamin content of foods can be achieved in this way.

Bad advice

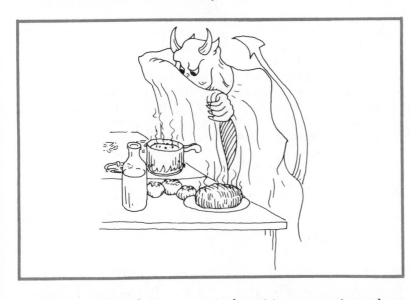

Lest you fear that no practical positive suggestions about storage and cooking of foods will be offered, you may be reassured to learn that these are given at the end of the next chapter. Of all the water-soluble vitamins, vitamin C is the most vulnerable—to losses in cooking water, to heat, and to several other agents as well. Recommendations for the preservation of this most sensitive of the vitamins apply to the B vitamins as well.

The B Vitamin RDA's for Adults

Vitamin	Adult Female	Adult Male
Thiamin (B_1)	1.1 mg*	1.5 mg
Riboflavin (B_2)	1.4 mg	1.8 mg
Pyridoxine (B_6)	2.0 mg	2.0 mg
Cobalamin (B_{12})	3.0 μg†	3.0 μg
Niacin	14 mg	20 mg
Folacin	400 μg	400 μg

*mg = milligrams

†μg = micrograms (see Appendix D).

This is the third time RDA's have been mentioned in this book. You may wish to recall the points made previously (pages 96, 249). Like the RDA's for protein, the B vitamin RDA's are set high, leaving a margin of safety so that nearly all individuals who use them as a guideline will be covered. Like the protein RDA's also, they are intended to apply only to healthy individuals. Some additional clarification may be in order here.

A man's needs for thiamin, riboflavin and niacin are higher than a woman's. The reason for this is readily apparent: men consume more calories. Since these vitamins are needed to help extract energy from the energy nutrients, recommended intakes depend on the number of calories consumed.

The recommendations above are for average women and men, age 19-22, who consume 2,100 and 3,000 calories a day, respectively. As they grow older and their intake of calories decreases (we hope), they will need smaller amounts of the B vitamins. The complete RDA table (Appendix I) lists twelve different adult age-sex groups separately with recommendations tailored to each.

Summing Up

The B vitamins serve as coenzymes assisting many enzymes in the body. Thiamin (B_1), riboflavin (B_2), niacin and pantothenic acid are especially important in the glucose → energy pathway, being active as the coenzymes TPP, FAD, NAD+, and CoA respectively. Pyridoxine (B_6) facilitates amino acid transformations and thus protein metabolism, while folacin and cobalamin (B_{12}) are involved in pathways leading to red blood cell synthesis. Other B vitamins less well understood are biotin, choline, and inositol.

Since men's needs for energy are higher than women's, their RDA's for thiamin, riboflavin, and niacin are set higher. The RDA's for the other B vitamins are equal for all adults.

B vitamin deficiencies seldom occur in isolation; all have multiple symptomatology affecting each body organ and tissue in proportion to the roles they play there. Deficiency diseases are named for three of them and are well known. A lack of thiamin causes beriberi; a lack of niacin causes pellagra; and a lack of vitamin B_{12} causes pernicious anemia.

The detection of deficiencies from an individual's food intake alone rests on several assumptions: (1) that the individual is average (that the RDA's are applicable), (2) that body absorption is normal, (3) that the foods consumed are typical (that nutrient values found in tables of food composition are accurate), and (4) that food preparation has been done with reasonable care. Biochemical assessments of nutritional status, described in Highlight 12, are more accurate means of pinpointing nutritional problems. The above cautions are offered to provide a context within which to consider food sources and intakes of the nutrients.

Thiamin is widely distributed in foods, but no food contributes a very great amount of it; a balanced and varied diet of nutritious food will best assure an adequate amount of this nutrient. Riboflavin is primarily concentrated in milk and secondarily in meats, which makes inclusion of members of these two food groups advisable. Niacin is found wherever protein is found, and in addition can be made from the amino acid tryptophan. It is therefore supplied in proportion to the amounts of protein in all common foods, except corn (which lacks tryptophan). These three vitamins are added to all enriched breads and cereals, together with iron, making the thiamin, niacin, riboflavin content of these foods equivalent to that of whole-grain products. Vitamin B_{12} is found only in animal products, while folacin is supplied best by green leafy vegetables. Any diet plan which recommends moderate amounts of all these foods assures probable adequacy for these nutrients.

alcohol dehydrogenase: an enzyme found in liver which converts ethanol to acetaldehyde (ass-et-AL-duh-hide).

Highlight Nine
Alcohol and the Liver

The Disruptive Molecule, Ethanol

The drama of alcohol abuse and malnutrition takes place in the cells of the liver where the director, an enzyme called alcohol dehydrogenase, makes the decisions as to what action shall take place and with what speed. Alcohol must be converted to acetaldehyde before the body can use it for energy,[1] and alcohol dehydrogenase must be present for this conversion to take place.

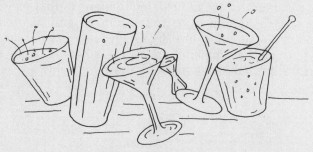

The only tissue in the body that can metabolize alcohol is the liver. No other cells can use the potential calories of alcohol. There is a limited number of molecules of the enzyme alcohol dehydrogenase. If they are at work metabolizing alcohol when

[1]Iber, F.: In alcoholism, the liver sets the pace. *Nutrition Today*, January/February:2-9, 1971.

298

more alcohol molecules come by in the bloodstream those later-arriving alcohol molecules will have to keep on traveling around and around the body until some enzyme molecules are free to process them. Truly, alcohol dehydrogenase is the director, the rate-limiting factor, in the metabolism of alcohol.

To the chemist, "alcohol" refers to a group of compounds, such as glycerol (at right), which contain a reactive hydroxyl (−OH) group. To the person interested in alcoholic beverages, "alcohol" refers to ethanol, C_2H_5OH (at right). This molecule is the intoxicating molecule present in beer, wine, or whiskey. To the liver cell, ethanol is a disruptive, demanding, egocentric molecule. Ethanol demands that it be used as fuel instead of the fatty acids which the liver cells usually prefer.[2] The rest of the body may be screaming for some glucose for energy, but ethanol uses up the available supply of the vitamins (niacin and thiamin) to convert itself to acetaldehyde (Figure H9.1) and then to energy in liver cells. Meanwhile, the glucose remains glucose; the other cells of the body may have ample glucose but no coenzymes with which to convert it to energy for their use.

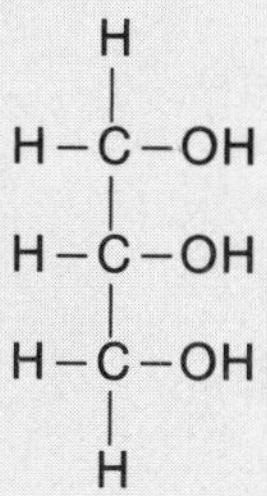

Glycerol is an alcohol.

Ethanol is the alcohol in beer, wine, or whisky.

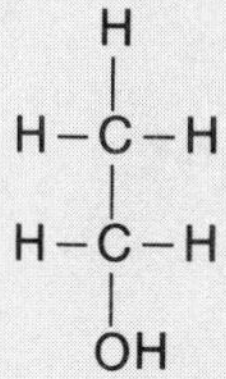

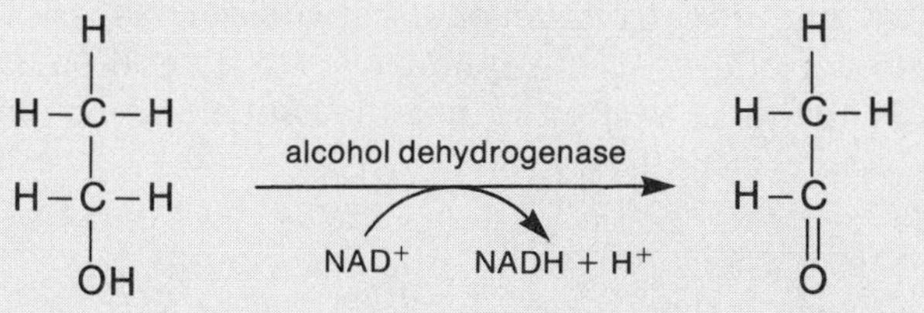

ethanol   acetaldehyde

Figure H9.1. Ethanol must be converted to acetaldehyde by the enzyme alcohol dehydrogenase and the coenzyme NAD⁺ before it can enter the glucose → energy pathway.

The pathway shown in Figure H9.2 is a simplified version of the steps from glucose to energy and includes some of the substances that must be present to make these reactions go in the direction indicated. Of particular importance to the understanding of the way alcohol is metabolized are the coenzymes, NAD^+ and TPP.

NAD^+ is the active form of niacin, one of the B vitamins which, because it is water soluble, is not stored in the body and must be constantly resupplied by the diet. NAD^+ acts as a hydrogen carrier, picking up hydrogen from a substance and forming $NADH + H^+$. The curved arrows show NAD^+ being used and $NADH + H^+$ resulting, in the steps where NAD^+ is

[2]Lieber, C. S.: Liver adaptation and injury in alcoholism. *The New England Journal of Medicine* 288(7):356, 1973.

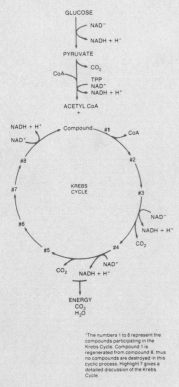

The numbers 1 to 8 represent the compounds participating in the Krebs Cycle. Compound 1 is regenerated from compound 8, thus no compounds are destroyed in this cyclic process. Highlight 7 gives a detailed discussion of the Krebs Cycle.

**Figure H9.2. Glucose →
energy pathway.**

involved. NADH is then available to donate a hydrogen to another substance; when this happens, NAD^+ will be reformed. However, in the direct path from glucose → energy, this reformation does not occur.

Thiamin in the form of thiamin pyrophosphate (TPP) acts as a coenzyme in the metabolism of pyruvic acid to acetyl CoA. Thiamin, like niacin, must be constantly replenished by the diet, for reactions requiring TPP to take place.

Upon examination of the pathway, it can be seen that glucose on its way to becoming energy uses up niacin and thiamin. When these vitamins are depleted, no more glucose can be used for energy, no matter how ample the supply in the blood and in the cells.

When ethanol enters the cells of the liver, alcohol dehydrogenase is required to convert it to acetaldehyde (Figure H9.1). NAD^+ must also be present to pick up two hydrogens. The acetaldehyde formed will enter the glucose → energy pathway at the site of the complex set of reactions between pyruvic acid and acetyl CoA and will use up TPP and NAD^+, leaving behind $NADH + H^+$ (Figure H9.3). Strangely, most other reactions going on in the cell will be slowed to make way for this conversion.[1] The manufacture of alcohol dehydrogenase will take precedence over other protein syntheses; NAD^+ will be used preferentially for this reaction rather than for the reactions in the glucose → energy pathway.

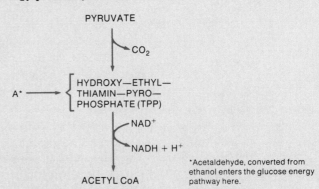

*Acetaldehyde, converted from ethanol enters the glucose energy pathway here.

**Figure H9.3. The complex
reactions between pyruvate
and acetyl CoA.**

If the two sets of reactions (Figures H9.2 and H9.3) are shown together, it becomes apparent that NADH is going to accumulate in the cells. Examine the pathways in Figure H9.4 and note the numerous times it shows, with the curved arrow, that NAD^+ is being converted to $NADH + H^+$. As you can see, in only one reaction is NAD^+ recycled from NADH — when pyruvic acid cannot get into the Krebs cycle but must go to lactic acid. This is a mixed blessing, however, as other problems are created by the higher levels of these two acids, as will be shown later.

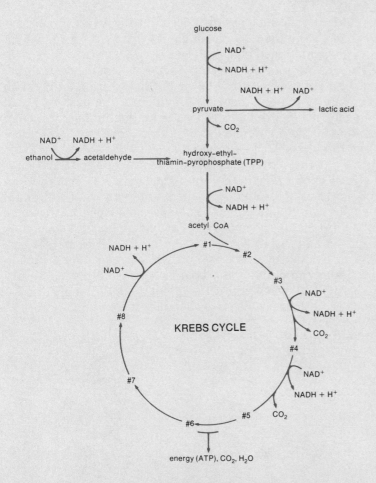

Figure H9.4. A simplified version of the glucose → energy pathway showing the entry of ethanol into the pathway. The coenzymes which are the active forms of thiamin and niacin are the only ones included. For a more detailed diagram see Figure H7.1.

With even a small amount of knowledge of what happens inside liver cells when ethanol enters, some of the physical difficulties (malnutrition included) which the alcoholic encounters can be understood.

If the pathways are blocked by depletion of niacin and thiamin, pyruvic acid and lactic acid will accumulate. This will tend to lower the pH, perhaps to a dangerous level. Acidosis will develop.

Lactic acid interferes with the excretion of uric acid in the urine. About eight percent of all alcoholics have a diagnosis of gout because of the high serum levels of uric acid. This is not true gout, will clear up with abstinence, and explains the common observation that gout symptoms are aggravated by the drinking of alcohol.[1]

Alcoholics frequently have hypoglycemia. If the alcoholic has fasted for as little as eight hours the shortage of NAD^+ can be severe enough for him to go into a coma and die because of the lack of glucose to the brain. Sudden death due to massive

pH: see page 120.

acidosis: see page 120.

gout (GOWT): a disease in which uric acid and salts are deposited around joints. It causes swelling and severe pain, especially in the big toe.

hypoglycemia: see page 14.

intakes of ethanol, such as might occur during drinking contests, have been explained by the high NADH:NAD$^+$ ratio which blocks the oxidation of glucose.[2]

Persons who attend cocktail parties but don't want to become inebriated have learned to space their drinks, to sip them, and to enjoy the high fat snacks provided by the host. As noted previously, alcohol dehydrogenase is limited in amount; when all of it is in use the molecules of ethanol continue to circulate around the body. As they travel they are a part of all the body fluids; when they enter cells they excite the cells and have varying effects upon them. In the brain, the molecules first anesthetize the cells of the frontal lobe, the reasoning part. If additional molecules continue to enter the bloodstream from the digestive tract before the liver has had time to oxidize the first ones, then the speech and vision centers of the brain will be narcotized, and the area that governs reasoning will become more incapacitated. Later the cells of the brain controlling the voluntary muscles will be affected; at this point, people "under the influence" will stagger or weave when they try to walk.

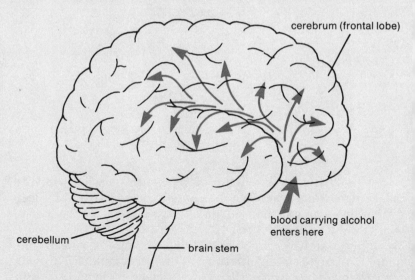

cerebrum (frontal lobe)

blood carrying alcohol enters here

cerebellum

brain stem

The sipping of drinks, then, is a technique for staying relatively sober, since it allows the ethanol to drip into the bloodstream at a rate the liver is more likely to be able to handle. A common practice, according to novels and movies, is to walk drunks to sober them. This technique is ineffective for two reasons. The muscle cells have no alcohol dehydrogenase with which to oxidize the ethanol so walking is not going to speed up oxidation; also, the liver oxidizes alcohol at a steady rate, therefore time, proportional to the amount consumed, is the absolute necessity for becoming sober.

Time between onslaughts of ethanol molecules is needed so

that the liver can oxidize the alcohol and release the enzyme supply. It has been estimated that for most persons the liver can completely metabolize about 10 milliliters (about 1/3 ounce) of alcohol per hour. This would mean that it would take five or six hours to oxidize the ethanol in three 12-ounce bottles of beer or in 4 ounces of whiskey.[1] Responsible pilots understand the necessity of allowing time for the body to metabolize alcohol. They refuse to fly if they have had cocktails in the previous 24 hours; they know that they need time to recover their judgment and that the body's ability to keep the brain supplied with glucose is impaired until all alcohol has been metabolized.[3]

Another technique for reducing the amount of unoxidized alcohol circulating in the blood is to eat while drinking. Ethanol receives preferred treatment in the stomach and duodenum; it is the only substance that can be absorbed through the walls of the stomach into the bloodstream. This explains the speed with which a euphoric state can be reached after imbibing a drink. The more food there is in the stomach, the less chance there is that the molecules of ethanol will touch the stomach walls and diffuse through them to the capillaries beyond.

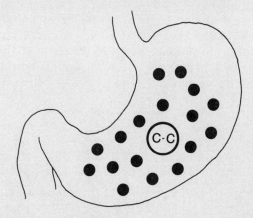

The alcohol C-C in a stomach filled with food has a low probability of touching the walls and diffusing through.

No matter how much food is with the alcohol when it arrives in the duodenum, however, the alcohol is absorbed quickly and completely,[1] as if, again, it is receiving preferential treatment. Therefore, any method which keeps the alcohol in the stomach longer will serve to keep the flood of alcohol molecules from reaching the brain and anesthetizing it. High fat snacks slow down gastric motility and thus are helpful in regulating the amount of unoxidized alcohol circulating in the blood.

It is interesting that sociological studies have shown that in those countries where the drinking of alcoholic beverages is customarily a part of meals in the home, there is a relatively

[3]Private communication from Captain Francis J. Black, Senior Eastern Airlines Pilot, retired after 35 years service, now residing in Tallahassee, Florida.

Keep the food in the stomach as long as possible for when it enters the duodenum it will be quickly absorbed. The longer alcohol is in the stomach, the greater the delay in narcotizing the brain.

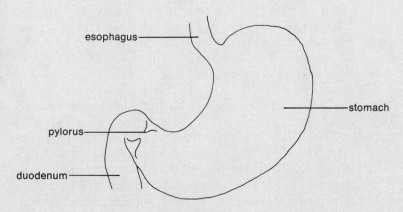

low rate of drunkenness in the population. The converse also seems to be true: that where alcohol characteristically is drunk in public places such as a pub and not usually with meals, the incidence of drunkenness is extremely high.

The high level of NADH caused by the liver cells oxidizing ethanol to acetaldehyde and then into the glucose → energy pathway to produce ATP has the effect of increasing fatty acid synthesis.[2] The 2-carbon fragments are left stranded when all the NAD^+ has been converted to NADH and the Krebs cycle has slowed to a stop until some more NAD^+ is available. Nature always works to conserve valuable resources; therefore the 2-carbon fragments become building blocks for fatty acids.

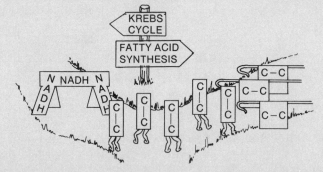

Two-carbon fragments are blocked from getting into the Krebs Cycle by the high level of NADH. Instead of being used for energy they become building blocks for fatty acids.

Simultaneously, protein synthesis is depressed, except for the synthesis of alcohol dehydrogenase, which means that the protein carriers which would normally transport the fatty acids away from the liver are not being manufactured. Also, you will recall from an earlier statement that liver cells seem to want to burn alcohol for fuel when it is present but normally prefer fatty acids. Thus the stage is set for the condition common to alcoholics known as *fatty liver*. This condition prevails when: (1) fatty acid synthesis is stepped up, (2) protein carrier synthesis is depressed, and (3) the fatty acids are not being burned for fuel.

fatty liver

In this condition, fats accumulate in the liver tissue and interfere with the flow of blood from the capillaries to the cells. As the fat infiltration becomes more extensive, liver cells die for lack of nutrients and oxygen. This condition is called *necrosis*. Wherever dead cells occur, fibrous scars invade the area. In the liver, this fibrous tissue and the preceding condition of fatty liver can be corrected with good nutrition and abstinence from alcohol consumption.[1] However, if allowed to continue developing, this condition results in *cirrhosis* of the liver, which is not reversible. Cirrhosis can only be controlled with proper food and abstinence.

necrosis (neck-RO-sis): death of tissue.

The invasion of scar tissue into the necrotic area is called **fibrosis**.

Liver cells are not the only cells that die with excessive exposure to alcohol; brain cells are particularly sensitive. When liver cells have died, others may later multiply to replace them, but there is no regeneration of nerve cells. Hence the permanent brain damage observed in some alcoholics.

cirrhosis (seer-OH-sis): irreversible hardening of liver tissue. The cirrhotic liver is nodular and orange in color. See also page 127.

cirrhos = orange

About 90 percent of ethanol ingested is metabolized in the liver and, as stated previously, only about 10 milliters per hour can be handled. In many cases, if there is an abundance of a nutrient, the oxidation of that nutrient is speeded up, but this is not true for ethanol. The rate for oxidizing it to acetaldehyde is a constant, no matter what amount is entering the bloodstream from the digestive tract at any one time.

The remaining 10 percent of alcohol not metabolized in the liver is excreted through the lungs and kidneys. The concentration of alcohol in the breath and in the urine is proportional to the concentration of unmetabolized alcohol circulating in the blood. Breathalyzers used by police departments to determine legal drunkenness operate on this principle.

It is the *average* person's liver which takes about five or six hours to handle three bottles of beer, not the alcoholic's liver. Alcoholics do better than that! Steady and prolonged consumption of alcohol increases the cells' ability to synthesize alcohol dehydrogenase and to clear the blood of ethanol, even to doubling the amount they can clear in an hour.[1] This fact provides a partial explanation for the fact that steady drinkers must take increasingly larger amounts of alcohol to produce the euphoria they desire. It may even be one of the factors leading to alcohol addiction.

In the United States it has been estimated that there are more than nine million persons who abuse the use of alcohol to the point that their personal relationships, their jobs, or their health are impaired. One of the health hazards is malnutrition. Ethanol depresses the appetite through the euphoria it produces as well as by its attack on the mucosa of the stomach[1] so that heavy drinkers usually eat poorly, if at all. With a large portion of their calories coming from the empty calories of alcohol, it is difficult for them to obtain the essential nutrients in the remaining calories. Thus some of the alcoholic's malnutrition is due to lack of food. If alcoholics eat well during the times they are not drinking, they may survive for many years without clinical evidence of deficiencies.

The other cause of malnutrition, however, is produced by the alcohol itself: the B vitamin depletion which has been the principal topic of this Highlight.

As a way of summarizing, let us examine the deficiencies which are seen in long time drinkers or in alcoholics.

Obviously, niacin will be lacking. It is used in the metabolism of alcohol and glucose and must be replenished through the diet.

Thiamin, also, will be in short supply since it is needed in one vital step by which the acetaldehyde gets into the Krebs cycle. In fact, clinical signs of thiamin deficiency are the symptoms most often seen in the long time drinker.[1]

Protein deficiency would be expected to develop, partly from the poor diet, but also from the depression of protein synthesis in the cells which would ordinarily use the amino acids that do happen to be eaten by the alcoholic. Instead, the alcoholic's liver deaminates the amino acids and channels their carbon backbones into fat or into the Krebs cycle to be used for energy. Alcohol's interference with glucose metabolism tends to increase the body's use of amino acids for energy.

Two additional deficiencies which research has shown are present even in well-nourished alcoholics are iron deficiency[4] and folic acid deficiency.[5] Abstaining from alcohol cures both deficiencies very quickly; at the most it takes only two or three days in the hospital eating ordinary hospital diets. But with continued use of alcohol, even with extra supplementation, the deficiencies continue.[4]

There has been no attempt in this Highlight to enumerate all the effects of the presence of alcohol on systems of the body. Rather, the emphasis has been on the interference of alcohol with glucose metabolism. The details were selected with the intention of showing the student how understanding nutrition at the molecular level clarifies related physiological and even sociological problems. There is, however, one additional effect of alcohol that is nutrition related. Its importance demands that it be mentioned.

Alcohol depresses the antidiuretic hormone (ADH). All people who drink have observed the increase in urination that accompanies drinking, but they may not realize that they are eliminating more than just water and some alcohol. With water

antidiuretic hormone
(ADH): a hormone produced by the pituitary gland in response to dehydration (or high sodium concentration in the blood) which stimulates the kidneys to reabsorb more water and so excrete less. This ADH should not be confused with the enzyme, alcohol dehydrogenase, which is sometimes also abbreviated ADH. (See diuretic, page 119.)

[4]Eichner, E. R.: The hematological disorders of alcoholism. *American Journal of Medicine* 54(5):621-630, 1973.
[5]Southmayd, E. B.: The role of the dietitian in team therapy for chronic alcoholics. *Journal of the American Dietetic Association* 64:184-186, 1974.

loss there is a loss of important minerals, such as magnesium, potassium, and zinc[1] (see Chapter 14). These minerals are vital to the maintenance of fluid balance and to many chemical reactions in the cells, including muscle contraction. Repletion therapy is often instituted in the recovering alcoholic to bring magnesium and potassium levels back to normal as quickly as possible.

In summary, ethanol, the 2-carbon alcohol present in beer, wine, and distilled alcoholic beverages, interferes with many chemical and hormonal reactions in the body. In particular, this disruptive molecule depresses protein synthesis, increases fatty acid synthesis, increases mineral loss through increased urinary excretion, and interferes with the metabolism of glucose to energy by grabbing all the niacin and thiamin for its own metabolism. Its calories are available only to the liver cells, and since it uses up the niacin and thiamin needed for the metabolism of glucose to energy in the other cells of the body, it effectively blocks the utilization of glucose by the rest of the body. Protein, the B vitamins, and minerals (especially magnesium and potassium), are the principal nutritional deficiencies found in heavy drinkers.

To Explore Further—

In both these articles, the metabolism of alcohol in the body is clearly enunciated. Iber's article is especially well suited for laymen:

Lieber, C. S.: The metabolism of alcohol. *Scientific American* 234(3):25-33, 1976.

Iber, F.: In alcoholism, the liver sets the pace. *Nutrition Today*, January/February:2-9, 1971.

One of the possible explanations for the reason some persons do not become alcoholic while others with seemingly similar backgrounds do, is studied in this report:

Wolff, P. H.: Ethnic differences in alcohol sensitivity. *Science* 175:449, 1972.

Teaching Aid, *Alcoholic Malnutrition* by Iber, F., is a set of 16 slides illustrating the way in which the liver sets the pace in the nutritional troubles that beset the alcoholic. This aid can be ordered from:

> Director, Education Services
> Nutrition Today
> 101 Ridgely Avenue
> Annapolis, Maryland 21404

Suggested Activities

(1) Study your own diet.

Review the record you made in Activity 1 of Chapter 1 and record from Appendix H your thiamin and riboflavin intakes.

Which foods made the greatest contribution of thiamin to your diet? Which contributed the most riboflavin?

Compare your intakes of these vitamins with the RDA for a person your age and sex. What *percent* of the RDA did you consume of each? Was this enough? (See page 98.)

If your intake was less than 2/3 of the RDA for either of these nutrients, find foods or beverages in the Table of Food Composition you would be willing to eat or drink daily that would correct this deficiency.

(Note: The last Highlight in the book invites you to survey your entire diet for adequacy, balance, and economy. You may wish to save this activity until you have read that Highlight, or you may wish to read the Highlight now for a sense of perspective.)

(2) Find alternative B vitamin sources for the nonmilk drinker.

Many non-Caucasians avoid drinking milk because of lactose intolerance. How can such persons meet their riboflavin needs without drinking milk? Plan a day's menus around the favorite foods of the United States' South (pork, fish, chicken, greens, corn bread, hominy grits, and sweet potatoes) that provides adequacy for thiamin and riboflavin. Is it necessary to eat *enriched* corn bread and grits in order to get enough of these nutrients?

(3) Consider the problem of alcoholism.

From your reading of Highlight 9, would you say that the nutritional deficiencies caused by alcoholism and the alcoholic's habit of heavy drinking work synergistically (see page 127) to promote ill health? Explain.

(4) Is whole-grain bread superior to enriched white bread?

The following table compares a loaf of whole-grain bread (whole wheat) with two loaves of refined white bread, one enriched and one unenriched:

Nutrient Content of a 1-Pound Loaf of Bread:	*Appendix H Item Number*		
	(368) Whole wheat	*(345)* Italian (white) enriched	*(346)* Italian (white) unenriched
Food energy (kcal)	1095	1250	1250
Protein (g)	41	41	41
Fat (g)	12	4	4
Carbohydrate (g)	224	256	256
Calcium (mg)	381	77	77
Iron (mg)	13.6	10	3.2

Nutrient Content of a 1-Pound Loaf of Bread:	Appendix H Item Number		
	(368) Whole wheat	*(345)* Italian *(white)* enriched	*(346)* Italian *(white)* unenriched
Vitamin A value (IU)	trace	0	0
Thiamin (mg)	1.36	1.32	.41
Riboflavin (mg)	.45	.91	.27
Niacin (mg)	12.7	11.8	3.6
Ascorbic acid (mg)	trace	0	0

Consider each of the following questions: Does the refining process cause the loss of nutrients? Does enrichment replace those that are lost? (Important: remember that not all nutrients are listed in tables of food composition.) Given that one chooses to eat refined bread, is the contribution it makes of the enrichment nutrients (thiamin, riboflavin, iron, and niacin) significantly different from the contribution of these nutrients made by whole-grain bread? Another component of whole-grain bread not listed in the table is fiber, which is largely lost in the refining process. Should this influence your choice of which type of bread to use regularly? (What other fiber sources are staples in your diet?)

10

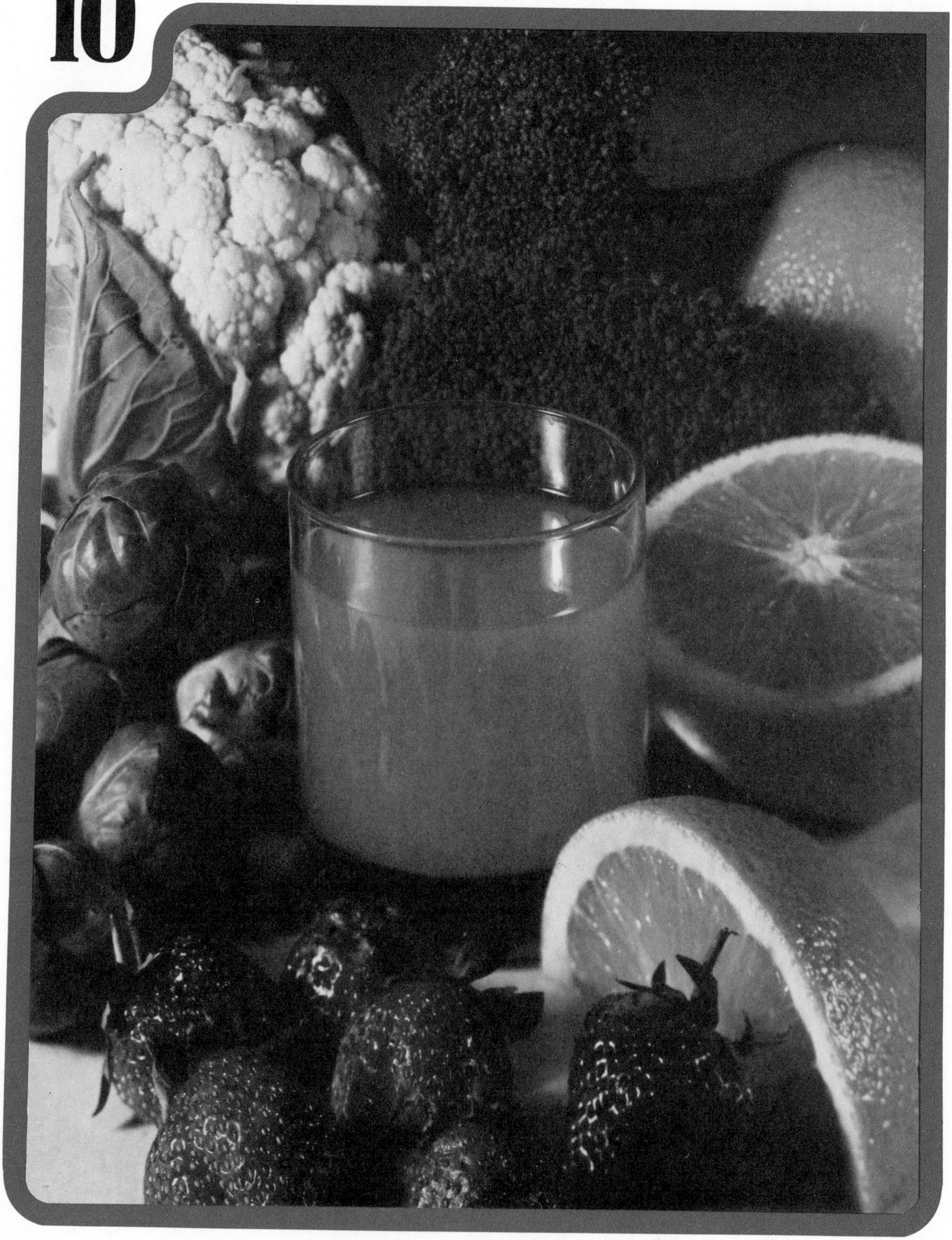

Vitamin C: Ascorbic Acid

It is often felt that only the discovery of a micro-theory affords real scientific understanding of any type of phenomenon, because only it gives us insight into the inner mechanism of the phenomenon, so to speak.
—*C. G. HEMPEL and P. OPPENHEIM*

The recent furor over the role of vitamin C in preventing the common cold cast this vitamin into the limelight during the 1960s. Its advocates said it was needed by human beings in far larger quantities than its RDA; its opponents argued that these claims were unfounded and cited evidence refuting them. The controversy has largely died down in the popular press, although the issue is still under discussion, as shown in the Highlight following this chapter.

Meanwhile, studies of vitamin C are continuing to reveal and account for the roles this little vitamin plays in the body and to explain the symptoms that result from vitamin C deficiency.

A hundred years ago, all that was known about vitamin C was that there was something present in certain foods which prevented scurvy, a disease that afflicted sailors whose provisions on long voyages at sea included no fresh fruits or vegetables. This "something" was dubbed the antiscorbutic factor. Fifty years ago, the factor was isolated from orange juice and found to be a 6-carbon compound similar to glucose. Shortly thereafter it was synthesized.

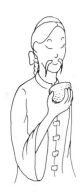

History of discoveries of the vitamins: Appendix A.

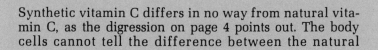

Synthetic vitamin C differs in no way from natural vitamin C, as the digression on page 4 points out. The body cells cannot tell the difference between the natural ascorbic acid purified from an orange and the synthetic ascorbic acid from a chemists's laboratory. The only benefits conferred by "natural" vitamin C pills are the dollar benefits reaped by those who sell these preparations.

One way to distinguish between true and suspect nutrition information is to ask who gains from it. If the people spreading the word about a product stand to gain financially from its sale, their claim warrants skepticism. You cannot believe what they say until you have seen (more than one) confirmation from an unbiased scientific source.

 A flag sign of a spurious claim is:

financial investment of the person making the claim.

Then came the molecular biology revolution. Thousands of observations meticulously collected by scientists over the preceding centuries yielded to explanations of life processes at the molecular level. The structure of DNA explained the genes and heredity; protein structure revealed how enzymes work and accounted for metabolism. Among recent advances has been the elucidation of the roles of vitamins.

The reward of persistent curiosity is the satisfaction that comes with a "real" explanation. In nutrition, as in the other life sciences, a type of explanation that feels especially real is one that is based on atoms and molecules. Many of the characteristics and functions of carbohydrate, fat, and protein were explained in this way in Part One. In the preceding chapter you saw that the functions of the B vitamins are largely accounted for by their roles as coenzymes. With vitamin C, as it is currently understood, some explanations of this kind are also possible, while others are yet to come. Looking at the molecule itself and reasoning from its characteristics, it is possible to see why it behaves as it does and what implications this has for you: why, for example, you need it to prevent anemia and heal wounds; why you can tolerate large doses often without ill effect. Other whys are still unexplained: why you need more if you are a smoker or if you are under stress. This chapter shows wherever possible how vitamin C's structure accounts for its functions.

To put this nutrient in perspective as a member of the vitamin family, it will be helpful to note how it resembles the other vitamins, what properties it shares with the B vitamins, in particular, and finally what characteristics make it unique.

Properties of Vitamin C

Like all the vitamins, vitamin C is a small, organic compound needed by human beings in minute amounts daily. Being organic, it is convertible to several different forms, two of which are active. To use it properly, the body must be functioning normally, providing the enzymes and the fluid environment needed to keep it in its active forms.

Like the B vitamins, vitamin C is water soluble, a fact which has implications for its handling both inside and outside your body. Inside, you absorb it readily and directly into your blood along with other water-soluble nutrients. With an adequate intake, you maintain a fixed pool and excrete any excess rapidly in your urine. With an inadequate intake, the pool becomes depleted (at the rate of about 3 percent a day). Overt deficiency symptoms begin to appear when the pool has been reduced to about a fifth of its optimal size.

Outside the body, the water solubility of vitamin C has implications for the handling of foods containing it. Other properties of the vitamin are also relevant to its handling. A consideration of these properties is saved for the end of this chapter.

It is not clear whether vitamin C is also like the B vitamins in that it forms part of a coenzyme. If it does, the coenzyme is so unstable that it has, to date, eluded efforts to isolate it. If not, it apparently functions as a catalyst all by itself. What *is* clear is that vitamin C is essential for several metabolic processes in the body.

Vitamin C as an Acid and Antioxidant

Unlike the B vitamins, vitamin C also has nonspecific roles in the body as both an acid and an antioxidant. A look at its chemical structure will show how it works:

Ascorbic Acid
(vitamin C)

An acid is a compound which in a water solution can release hydrogen (H^+) ions into the water. As the concentration of H^+ ions increases, the strength of the acid increases. Ascorbic acid has this property.

acid, pH: these terms are defined on page 120 and explained in Appendix B.

Vitamin C is stable in strong acids (pH 4); as long as there are plenty of H^+ ions floating around, it tends to hold on to its own hydrogens. But if H^+ ions are not abundant in the medium, the vitamin will lose two of its H's, becoming dehydroascorbic acid:

Dehydroascorbic Acid

This is a reversible reaction. Replaced in a strong acid, vitamin C will recapture its H's and become ascorbic acid again.

If the acid solution is still weaker (fewer H^+), the dehydroascorbic acid ring is broken, and a derivative is produced which no longer has vitamin C activity. Thus vitamin C is destroyed. Patients (for example, ulcer patients) taking acid-neutralizing medications may tend to become deficient in vitamin C because irreversible destruction of the vitamin occurs when the normal acidity of the stomach is neutralized.

antioxidant: a compound that protects others from oxidation by being oxidized itself.

When there is another compound nearby that can accept H's, vitamin C can serve as a hydrogen donor; this is its role as an antioxidant. Oxygen itself can accept H's, becoming water (H_2O). Many compounds in the body are sensitive to and can be destroyed by oxygen; if ascorbic acid is present in sufficient amounts it will protect these compounds by being oxidized itself. By the same token, these other compounds can protect vitamin C in the same way. Three vitamins—C, A, and E— share this property; each can protect the others. Of course if oxidation is going to occur, it will affect some of each of them, but there is safety in numbers. Thus, it is advisable to have adequate intakes of all three.

Because of its antioxidant property, vitamin C is sometimes added to food products, not only to improve their nutritional value, but also to protect important constituents from oxidation.

ion: see Appendix B. Iron is an atom which can exist in two ionic states, ferric (Fe^{+++}, lacking 3 electrons) or ferrous (Fe^{++}, lacking 2).

The acidic and antioxidant properties of vitamin C also enable it to assist in the absorption of the mineral, iron. Iron can exist in two forms: an oxidized (ferric ion) form, which is not readily absorbed in the GI tract, and a reduced (ferrous) form, which is more readily absorbed. Vitamin C and other acids, including most importantly the stomach acid (hydrochloric acid) itself, help to keep iron in the more absorbable state. A vitamin C deficiency therefore often indirectly causes or contributes to iron-deficiency anemia.

Another mineral, calcium, tends to form insoluble complexes which cannot be absorbed. The possibility is minimized when calcium is kept in an acid solution. Because it is an acid, vitamin C eaten at the same time as calcium facilitates calcium absorption.

You can see from these examples how the nutrients co-operate. The mineral chlorine, by forming part of hydrochloric acid, helps provide an environment in which vitamin C is stable. Vitamin C and hydrochloric acid both help promote the absorption of iron and calcium. Vitamins C, A, and E protect each other from oxidation and, as you will see later, by virtue of its association with polyunsaturated fatty acids, vitamin E also protects the essential fatty acid, linoleic acid, from destruction.

oxidation of linoleic acid: see page 66.

In the body proper, vitamin C plays roles similar to those it plays in the GI tract. At least one enzyme in amino acid metabolism can be destroyed by oxidation and is protected by vitamin C. Iron, which is stored attached to a protein in many body organs, is released into the blood in the presence of vitamin C, thus becoming available for use where it is needed. Additional examples of this vitamin's roles as an acid and antioxidant are accumulating as research into its mode of action continues.

Metabolic Roles of Vitamin C

Vitamin C wears several hats. As an acid and antioxidant its roles are nonspecific, and are shared with other compounds. The following metabolic roles are unique to vitamin C.

Collagen formation. The best understood metabolic role of vitamin C is its function in helping to form the protein, collagen. Brief mention was made of this protein in Chapter 4; it is the single most important connective tissue protein in the body. It serves as the matrix on which bone is formed. It is the material of scars. When you have been wounded, the protein collagen forms and glues the separated tissue faces together, forming a scar. The cement which holds cells together is largely made of collagen (and calcium); this function is especially important in the artery walls, which must expand and contract with each beat of the heart, and in the walls of the capillaries which are thin and fragile and must withstand a pulse of blood every second or so without giving way.

collagen (COLL-uh-gen): a water-insoluble protein. For roles, see Chapter 4.

kolla = glue
gennan = to produce

Collagen, like all proteins, is formed by stringing together a chain of amino acids. One amino acid which is found in unusual abundance in collagen is proline. After the proline has been added to the chain, it is altered by an enzyme which adds an —OH group to it, making hydroxyproline. This step, which completes the manufacture of collagen, requires ascorbic acid and oxygen, although it is not known whether the vitamin functions as a coenzyme or in some other way.

proline: see Appendix C.

Epinephrine and norepi-
nephrine were formerly
called adrenalin and
noradrenalin.

thyroxine (thigh-ROX-in)

atherosclerotic plaques
(PLAKS): patchy, nodular
thickenings of the artery
walls. See page 72.

Adrenal hormone production. A person under stress needs more vitamin C. Stress causes the release of large quantities of the hormones epinephrine and norepinephrine from the adrenal gland, where a large amount of the vitamin is also stored. The gland makes more of these hormones to replace those it has secreted; their production is accelerated by vitamin C.

Thyroid hormone production. Vitamin C is also needed for the synthesis of thyroid hormone, thyroxine, which regulates the metabolic rate. Your metabolic rate speeds up when you are under stress and also when you need to produce more heat: when you have a fever, or when you are out in the cold. Thus infections and exposure to cold increase your needs for vitamin C.

Deposition of calcium. Bones and teeth were long believed to be inert, like stones, but they are actually very active. Calcium is continually being withdrawn and redeposited in these structures, another process for which vitamin C is essential.

Other roles. Information on other roles of the vitamin is coming out monthly, but no final statements can be made about its mode of action. Heavy cigarette smoking lowers blood levels of vitamin C for reasons as yet unknown. Formation of atherosclerotic plaques seems to occur more readily when vitamin C levels are low; perhaps the loss of intercellular cement from the artery walls favors plaque formation.

Vitamin C Deficiency

scurvy: the vitamin C
deficiency disease.

The National Nutrition Survey (see Highlight 12) showed evidence of unacceptable serum levels of the vitamin in about 15 percent of all age groups studied, with symptoms of outright scurvy showing up in 4 percent. Especially in infants, teenagers, and people over 60 years of age, intakes of the vitamin were much lower than the RDA (less than 50 percent). Perhaps it is wise for all Americans to be alerted to the symptoms that can result and to make efforts to obtain enough of this vitamin.

Knowing from the above two sections how vitamin C functions in the body, you can largely anticipate what the symptoms will be when inadequate amounts are obtained from the diet. As serum levels fall, latent scurvy appears. Two of the earliest signs have to do with the role of the vitamin in maintaining capillary integrity: the gums bleed easily and spontaneous breakage of capillaries under the skin produces pinpoint hemorrhages. If the vitamin levels continue to fall, the full set of symptoms of overt scurvy appears. Failure to promote normal ﹐collagen synthesis causes further hemorrhaging to occur. Muscles, including the heart muscle, may degenerate. The skin becomes rough, brown, scaly, and dry. Wounds fail to heal be-

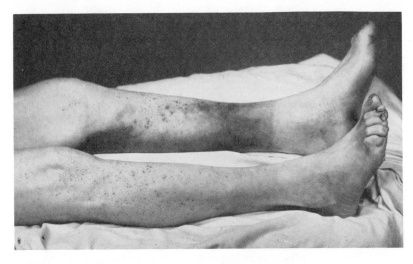

Skin symptoms of scurvy.

Photo courtesy of Dr. Samuel
Dreizen, D.D.S., M.D.

cause scar tissue will not form. Bone rebuilding is not maintained; the ends of the long bones become softened, malformed,
and painful, and fractures appear. The teeth, receiving less
than the needed amounts of calcium, lose their integrity, soften,
and may become loose in the jawbone. Iron deficiency may
occur, causing anemia.

If you are tired all the time, this may mean that you have
iron-deficiency anemia, as any television viewer is
aware. As you can see from the above, however, it
doesn't necessarily follow that you need to take iron
supplements; a vitamin C deficiency can indirectly
cause the same symptoms. Still more indirect causes are
lack of stomach acid (due to failure to secrete enough)
and too frequent use of acid neutralizers which can rob
you of vitamin C and in turn reduce iron absorption,
causing anemia.

You may notice too that the skin seems to be involved whenever there is a nutrient deficiency. It was
mentioned first in connection with linoleic acid (Chapter 2), then with protein (Chapter 3), then with the B
vitamins (Chapter 9), and now with vitamin C. It comes
up again when deficiencies of fat-soluble vitamins
(Chapter 11) are encountered. Evidently a skin symptom
by itself points to no particular cause.

On the other hand, with so many nutrients—and
other factors—involved in maintaining the health of the
skin, it is not surprising that many people's complexions
are less than perfect. A prescription for a beautiful complexion might be "eat a balanced and varied diet, take
regular exercise, get plenty of sleep, and enjoy life."
Even then, certain skin disorders would persist.

clinical tests: see discussion
on pages 386-387.

Although no cause of bleeding gums other than vitamin C deficiency has been described in this book, would it be safe to conclude that this symptom necessarily points to a vitamin C deficiency? This point has been made before (page 294).

How can you really tell if you have a vitamin C deficiency? As you will see in Highlight 12 a clinical test would provide the most reliable evidence.

The present RDA for vitamin C is 45 milligrams a day for adults, both male and female. As noted above, however, vitamin C needs may be increased by stress, heavy cigarette smoking, fevers, infections, and other conditions. (See boxed section at end of chapter.)

Vitamin C is found in high concentrations in a limited group of foods. Rather than risking deficiency, it makes sense to be aware of what these foods are and to include them in your diet daily.

Vitamin C in Fruits and Vegetables

citrus fruit: so-called
because these fruits contain
an organic acid, citric acid.

The citrus fruits are rightly famous for their high content of vitamin C, as Table C10.1 shows. Less well known is the fact that certain vegetables, such as broccoli and Brussels sprouts, and other fruits, such as cantaloupe melon and strawberries, are excellent sources. A single serving a day of any of these provides over 100 percent of the RDA.

Table C10.1
Fifty Foods Showing Amounts of Ascorbic Acid

The foods listed below are the fifty that rank highest as food sources of ascorbic acid from those which are found on the ADA Exchange Lists and which also have been analyzed for nutrient composition. Serving sizes are the sizes listed in the Exchange Lists except for meat, where 3-ounce servings are shown. The numbers 1 through 6 refer to the numbers of the Exchange Lists: 1 = Milk, 2 = Vegetables, 3 = Fruit, 4 = Bread, 5L = Lean Meat, 5M = Medium-Fat Meat, 5H = High-Fat Meat, 6 = Fats and Oils. Numbers in parentheses are the item numbers on the Table of Food Composition (Appendix H).

Exchange Group	Food (Item Number)	Serving Size	Ascorbic Acid Milligrams
2	Brussels sprouts (180)	½ cup	68
3	Strawberries (328)	¾ cup	66
3	Orange (294)	1	66
3	Orange juice (298)	½ cup	60

Table C10.1 (continued)

Exchange Group	Food (Item Number)	Serving Size	Ascorbic Acid Milligrams
2	Broccoli (179)	½ cup	52
3	Grapefruit juice (277)	½ cup	48
3	White grapefruit (270)	½	44
3	Pink grapefruit (271)	½	44
2	Collard greens (195)	½ cup	44
2	Mustard greens (208)	½ cup	34
2	Cauliflower (192)	½ cup	33
3	Cantaloupe (263)	¼	32
	50% of U.S. RDA of 60 milligrams		
3	Tangerine (330)	1	27
2	Cabbage (183)	½ cup	24
5M	Beef liver (112)	3 ounces	23
2	Cooked tomatoes (241)	½ cup	21
2	Tomato juice (244)	½ cup	20
2	Asparagus (165)	½ cup	19
4	Green peas (215)	½ cup	17
2	Turnips (246)	½ cup	17
2	Dandelion greens (201)	½ cup	16
3	Raspberries (325)	½ cup	16
4	Potato (221)	1 small	15
3	Blackberries (261)	½ cup	15
4	Lima beans (167)	½ cup	15
4	Winter squash (235)	½ cup	14
3	Pineapple (314)	½ cup	12
2	Spinach (233)	½ cup	12
2	Summer squash (234)	½ cup	11
4	French fried potatoes (224)	8	10
2	Radishes (230)	4	10
4	Mashed potatoes (226)	½ cup	10
3	Blueberries (262)	½ cup	10
4	Pumpkin (229)	¾ cup	9
2	Green beans (168)	½ cup	8
4	Sweet potatoes (239)	¼ cup	8
4	Corn on cob (196)	1 small	7
3	Pear (312)	1	7
3	Peach (305)	1	7
2	Onions (211)	½ cup	7
3	Pineapple juice (317)	1/3 cup	7
3	Bananas (259)	½ medium	6
4	Potato chips (228)	15	5
2	Beets (174)	½ cup	5
2	Carrots (190)	½ cup	5
4	Corn (197)	1/3 cup	4
1	2% fat fortified milk (3)	1 cup	2
1	Skim milk (2)	1 cup	2
1	Whole milk (1)	1 cup	2
1	Yogurt (72)	1 cup	2

The humble potato is an important source of the vitamin, not because a potato by itself supplies the daily need, but because potatoes are a staple so popular in this country and eaten

staple: a food kept on hand at all times and used daily or almost daily in meal preparation.

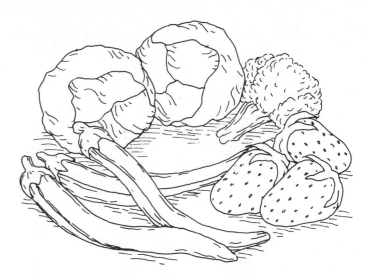

so frequently that overall they provide about 20 percent of all the vitamin C Americans consume.

Vitamin C contents of individual foods vary widely, as a look at various types of oranges (Appendix H) will show. One factor influencing the amount of vitamin C found in a fruit or vegetable is the amount of sun to which it is exposed. The reason for this may be clear to you if you recall that the vitamin, being a hexose, is a member of the carbohydrate family and that carbohydrates are produced by photosynthesis. No vitamin C is found in seeds, only in growing plants. Thus grains (breads and cereals) contain negligible amounts of the vitamin. Milk is also a notoriously poor source.

hexose: see page 20.

No animal foods other than the organ meats contain vitamin C. For this reason, if for no other, fruits and vegetables must be included in any diet to make it nutritionally adequate.

Protecting Vitamin C

Vitamin C is an organic compound synthesized and broken down by enzymes found in the fruits and vegetables that contain it. Like all enzymes, these have a temperature optimum: they work best at temperatures at which the plants grow, normally about 70° F, which is also the room temperature in most homes. When a fruit has been picked, synthesizing activity which has depended on a continued influx of energy from sunlight largely stops, while degradative activity which releases energy, continues. Chilling the fruit will slow down these processes. To maximize and protect vitamin C content, fruits and vegetables should be sun ripened, chilled immediately after picking, and kept cold until they are used.

An example is ascorbic acid oxidase.

Because it is an acid and antioxidant, vitamin C is most stable in an acid solution, away from air. Citrus fruits, tomatoes, and many fruit beverages containing the vitamin are acid enough to favor its stability. As long as the skin is uncut or the can is unopened, the vitamin is protected from air. If you store a cut vegetable or fruit or an opened container of juice, you should cover it tightly with a wrapper that excludes air, and store it in the refrigerator.

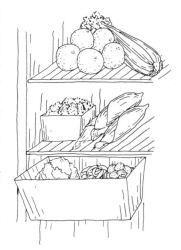

Being water soluble, vitamin C readily dissolves into water in which vegetables are washed or boiled. If the water is later discarded, the vitamin is poured down the drain with it. Cooking methods which minimize this kind of loss are steaming vegetables over water rather than in it, or boiling them in a volume of water small enough to be reabsorbed into the vegetables by the time they are cooked. Of course if the water is kept with the food, as in the making of preserves or fruit pies, a larger volume of water can be used.

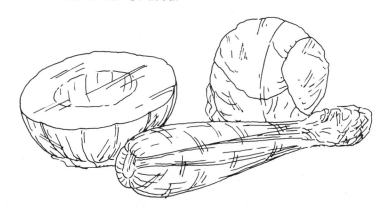

Unlike many of the B vitamins, vitamin C is relatively stable to heat, but very high temperatures and long cooking times should be avoided. Iron, like oxygen, destroys vitamin C by oxidizing it, but perhaps the benefits of cooking with iron utensils outweigh this disadvantage. Another agent which destroys C is copper.

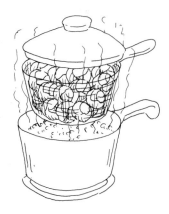

Let's be reasonable. All of the factors mentioned above represent legitimate concerns to which industrial food processors rightly pay attention. Awareness of them has brought about changes in many commercial products; for instance, fortification of instant mashed potatoes with vitamin C to replace that lost during processing, quick freezing of vegetables to minimize losses, display of fresh produce in crushed ice cases in the grocery stores, and many others. Saving a small percentage of the vitamin C activity in foods can mean saving several hundred pounds of the vitamin a day; when some of it goes to people whose intakes are otherwise marginal, this can make a crucial difference.

Meanwhile, in your own kitchen, a law of diminishing returns operates. You have other things to do besides hovering over your precious ascorbic acid, shielding it from all harm. If you turn the devil loose in your kitchen, as suggested in the last chapter, you can indeed suffer undesirably high losses of this nutrient, but you can tolerate some losses if you make sure to start with foods containing ample amounts of vitamin C. To be on the side of the angels, perhaps all you need is a little common sense.

Ascorbic Acid RDA for Adults: 45 mg

Two cautions must be kept in mind when RDA's are applied to individuals; they both apply to the vitamin C RDA.

(1) They provide a margin of safety, being set high (except for the calorie RDA) so they cover nearly all normal individuals. In the case of vitamin C, the RDA of 45 mg is more than four times the amount (10 mg/day) necessary to prevent scurvy.

(2) They are derived from studying the needs of normal, healthy individuals whose overall nutrition is good. In cases of illness or malnutrition, the indicated dose of a nutrient may be much higher than its RDA. The recommended dose of vitamin C for treatment of scurvy is about 300 mg/day. After a major operation (such as removal of a breast) or extensive burns, when a tremendous amount of scar tissue must form during healing, the amount needed may be as high as 1,000 milligrams (one gram) a day or even more.

Summing Up

Vitamin C (ascorbic acid) acts like other acids and antioxidants in the body: as an acid it promotes the absorption of calcium and the reduction of iron to its absorbable ferrous form; as an antioxidant it protects vitamins A and E from oxidation. The vitamin also plays specific roles: it promotes the formation of the protein collagen which is needed for scar tissue, intercellular cement, connective tissues (especially those of capillaries and other blood vessels), and the matrix of bones and teeth; it is involved in the production of the hormones from the adrenal cortex, and in thyroxine production.

Deficiency of vitamin C causes scurvy, characterized by bleeding from capillaries in the gums and under the skin, degeneration of muscles, failure of wounds to heal, and malformations of bones and teeth; a secondary iron deficiency may also result.

The RDA for vitamin C (45 milligrams a day for adults) is set at four times the level necessary to prevent scurvy, although higher doses are needed to recover from scurvy, major operations, burns, or fractures.

Best food sources of vitamin C are the citrus fruits, strawberries and cantaloupe, broccoli and other members of the cabbage family, and greens. Important fair sources include tomatoes, green peas, and (because they are eaten frequently by many people) potatoes. Preparation of foods to protect their vitamin C contents is best done away from air and alkaline solutions, and without the use of large volumes of water.

Highlight Ten
Vitamin C and the Common Cold: The Importance of Controlled Research

When Linus Pauling published his book *Vitamin C and the Common Cold*[1] in 1970, he started a storm of controversy that has been raging ever since. Newspaper headlines screamed VITAMIN C CURES COLDS, others yelled back VITAMIN C NO EFFECT. One "famous scientist" said this, another that. Meanwhile, behind the scenes, teams of researchers in laboratories and hospitals across the world went to work designing and executing experiments to determine whether in fact ascorbic acid had any therapeutic or preventive effect against the viruses which cause the myriad disorders collectively called the cold.

Since then some hundreds of articles have been published in the research journals, numbering several thousands of pages. Hundreds of people have been tested in a variety of experimental designs and still the answer is not completely clear.

The purpose of this Highlight is twofold: first, to make you aware of the difficulties inherent in attempting to discover whether a nutrient (or any therapeutic approach) remediates symptoms or cures a disease, and secondly, to bring you up to date on the story of vitamin C.

In most studies on the efficacy of vitamin C, the research design was as follows: two groups of people were selected. Only one group was given vitamin C; both were followed to determine whether the vitamin C group had fewer or less severe

[1]Pauling, L. C.: *Vitamin C and the Common Cold.* W. H. Freeman and Company, San Francisco, 1970.

324

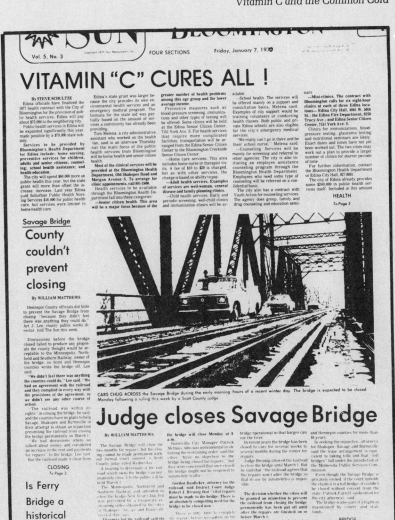

colds than the control group. A number of pitfalls are inherent in an experiment of this kind; they must be avoided if the results are to be believed.

Controls. First, the two groups must be similar in all respects except for vitamin C dosages. Most importantly, both must be equally susceptible to colds to rule out the possibility that an observed difference might have occurred anyway. (If group A gets twice as many colds as group B anyway, then the fact that group B received the vitamin proves nothing.) Also, in experiments involving a nutrient, it is imperative that the diets of both groups be similar, especially with respect to that

control: in any experiment in which a variable is being tested, one group of subjects must be studied for the effect of that variable while a second group must be followed that is similar in all respects to the first except for that variable. This rules out the possibility that any variable other than the one under study is causing the effect. Then if a difference is observed between the experimental and the control group, it is a significant result. (Without a control group, a change may be observed in the experimental group alone, but this cannot definitely be attributed to the variable under study.)

variable: see page 44.

nutrient. (If those in group B were receiving less vitamin C from their diet, this fact might cancel the effects of the supplement.) Similarity of the experimental and control groups is one of the characteristics of a well-controlled experiment.

Sample size. To ensure that chance variation between the two groups does not influence the results, the groups must be large. (If one member of a group of five people catches a bad cold by chance, the whole group will have a spuriously high "cold severity," but if one member of a group of 500 catches a bad cold, it will not unduly affect the group average.) In reviewing the results of experiments of this kind, a question to ask, always, is: was the number of people tested large enough to rule out chance variation? Statistical methods are useful for determining the significance of differences between groups of various sizes.

Placebos. There is a mind-body effect that must also be ruled out. If one group of people receives vitamin C, they may believe that they will be protected from colds, and their faith in the vitamin may actually affect their experience of their illness. (Recall from Highlight 5 that a patient's confidence in the doctor has been experimentally shown to have a beneficial effect on the healing of an ulcer, while Highlight 6 showed the effect of mental anguish—mind—on hormone secretion and physical symptoms—body.) Even if there is no absolute difference between the two groups, group members receiving vitamin C may report fewer or less severe colds because their belief influences their experience of the reality. Self-report is a notoriously imprecise source of information anyway, although it is often the only available means of collecting needed data.

To control for this effect, the experimenters must give pills to *all* participants, some containing vitamin C and others of similar appearance and taste but containing an inert ingredient (placebos). All subjects must believe they are receiving the vitamin so that the effects of faith will work equally in both groups.

placebo (See also page 165.)

As the public has become more sophisticated and better acquainted with research designs of this kind, more and more people have learned about the use of placebos and have become suspicious when they are offered pills that purport to contain a certain substance. If it is not possible to convince all subjects that they are receiving vitamin C, then the extent of unbelief must be the same in both groups. An experiment conducted under these conditions is called *blind*.

A **blind** experiment is one in which the subjects do not know whether they are members of the experimental or the control group.

Double blind. With all of these precautions a further pitfall exists in experiments of this kind. It turns out that the expectations of the experimenters can also influence the results. They, too, must not know which subjects are receiving the placebo and which are receiving the vitamin C. Being fallible human beings, and having an emotional investment in a successful outcome, they tend to hear what they want to hear, and so to interpret and record results with a bias in the expected direction. This is not dishonest, but is an unconscious shifting of the experimenters' perception of reality to agree with their expectations. To avoid it, the pills given to the subjects must be coded by a third party, who does not reveal to the experimenters which subjects received which medication until all results have been recorded quantitatively.

A **double blind** experiment is one in which neither the subjects nor those conducting the experiment know which subjects are members of the experimental group and which are serving as control subjects, until after the experiment is over.

In discussing all of these subtleties of experimental design, the intent is not to make a research scientist out of you but to show you what a far cry real scientific validity is from the experience of your neighbor, Mary (sample size, one, no control group), who says she takes vitamin C when she feels a cold coming on and "it works every time." (She knows what she is taking, and she has faith in its efficacy.)

CAUTION WHEN YOU READ!

Before concluding that an experiment has shown that a nutrient cures a disease or alleviates a symptom, ask yourself:

Was there a *control group* similar in all important ways to the experimental group?

Was the *sample size* large enough to rule out chance variation?

Was a *placebo* effectively administered (blind)?

Was the experiment *double blind*?

These are a few, but not all, of the important variables involved in researching a "cure." With them in mind, let us review the literature to see how successfully Pauling's vitamin C theory has stood the test of experiment.

Thomas C. Chalmers, a physician at Mount Sinai Medical Center, New York City, reviewed the data from 14 clinical trials of ascorbic acid in the treatment and prevention of the common cold in the April, 1975, issue of the *American Journal of Medicine*.[2] Of the 14 clinical trials reviewed, five were poorly con-

[2]Chalmers, T. C.: Effects of ascorbic acid on the common cold. *American Journal of Medicine* 58:532-536, 1975.

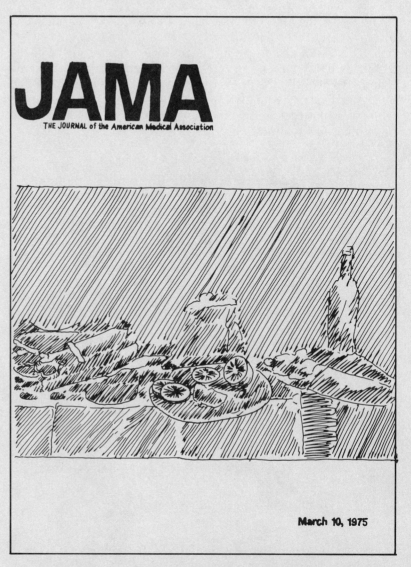

Modified from *The Journal of the American Medical Association.*

trolled, in Chalmers' judgment, and eight were reasonably well controlled in that the subjects given ascorbic acid and those given placebos were randomly chosen. In addition, these eight studies were double blind. When the data from these eight studies were pooled, there was a difference of 1/10 of a cold per year and an average difference in duration of 1/10 of a day per cold in those subjects taking ascorbic acid over those taking the placebo. In two studies, the effects on the symptoms seemed to be more striking in girls than in boys.

In one study, a questionnaire given at the conclusion revealed that a number of the subjects had correctly guessed the contents of their capsules. A reanalysis of the results showed that those who received the placebo *who thought they were receiving ascorbic acid* had fewer colds than the group receiving ascorbic acid *who thought they were receiving placebos!* In this study there were no differences in duration of colds among those who did not know which medication they were taking.

Independently, Michael H. M. Dykes, Senior Scientist with the American Medical Association Department of Drugs, and Paul Meier, Professor in the Department of Statistics and Pharmacological and Physiological Sciences, University of Chicago, authored a review of literature entitled "Ascorbic Acid and the Common Cold" in the March 10, 1975, issue of the *Journal of the American Medical Association.*[3] In evaluating the studies on the efficacy of vitamin C on the incidence and alleviation of symptoms of the common cold, these authors reviewed essentially the same literature as Chalmers, and noted the same strengths and weaknesses in the design of the studies as regards good control. A student of science would find this review valuable for its analysis of experimental design and the discussion of the importance of accurate reporting of all a study's details so that the research can be reproduced in another laboratory. It appears from this review, also, that by the summer of 1976, a definitive experiment had not yet been reported.

In Highlight 2, where the differing viewpoints of scientists on the causes of atherosclerosis were discussed, it was noted that each scientist defends his own point of view and that consequently, a reader cannot discern the total picture from a report of one experiment appearing in a scientific journal. There was an implication, not voiced, that the scientists were being dishonest. Not so. *The purpose of reports in journals is to present the results of one experiment,* not to present a total picture.

In this Highlight, we have been looking at a different kind of article, which is also found in scientific journals: the review of literature. These articles are just what their name implies—candid, objective reviews of all, or nearly all, of the experimental work on a theory that has been reported in the professional journals. *The purpose of a review is to present a balanced picture of the research in an area.* The reviewers are scientists first and writers second. They put their knowledge and skill to work in analyzing the various reports of research. They analyze the reports, then make judgments as to the validity of the data and of the conclusions drawn from the data. Sometimes they gather together several studies that have comparable designs in order to pool the data to

[3]Dykes, M.H.M. and Meier, P.: Ascorbic acid and the common cold. Evaluation of its efficacy and toxicity. *Journal of the American Medical Association* 231(10):1073-1079, 1975.

to form a larger sample. Their work makes a valuable contribution because it compiles the critical points from a number of reports, allowing the busy person to gain an overview of what is being written on a subject. Probably the most appreciated section of a review of literature for students is the list of references. Without having to research the indexes on a topic, they can find a large number of (perhaps as many as fifty or sixty) references listed in one place and in addition may read a critique of each.

The popular writer of science articles rarely reports on these reviews of literature because they are cold, objective, and give many viewpoints, rarely stressing one. They are not, therefore, sensational enough to sell in the marketplace. Who wants to read both sides of a question in the newspaper?

indexes: books in which the articles published in journals are indexed by author, title, or topic.

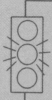

CAUTION WHEN YOU READ!

To weigh the reliability of nutrition information, ask yourself:

Is this one viewpoint? or is it a balanced picture?

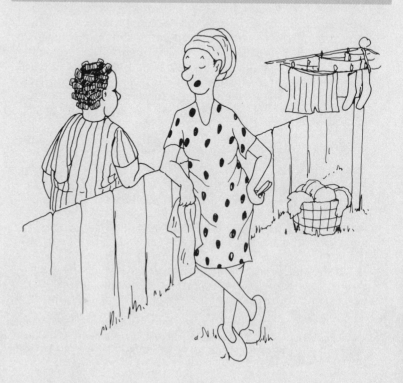

References and Notes

1. V. J. Chapman, Seaweeds and Their Uses (Methuen, London, 1950).
2. M. Schwimmer and D. Schwimmer, The Role of Algae and Plankton in Medicine (Grune Stratton, New York, 1955).
3. Pliny (Caius Plinius Secundus, A.D. 23 to 79), See Pliny's Natural History (Bohn, London, 1855 to 1857), six volumes.
4. R. F. Nigrelli, Ed., Ann. N.Y. Acad. Sci. 90, 615 (1960).
5. Proceedings of the Food-Drugs from the Sea Conference (Marine Technology Society, Washington, D.C., 1967, 1969, 1972, 1974).
6. P. J. Scheuer, Chemistry of Marine Natural Products (Academic Press, New York, 1973); J. T. Baker and V. Murphy, in Handbook of Marine Science, vol. 1, Compounds from Marine Organisms (CRC Press, Cleveland, Ohio, 1976); E. Premuzic, in Fortschr. Chem. Org. Naturst. 29, 417 (1971); D. J. Faulkner and R. J. Andersen, in The Sea, E. D. Goldberg, Ed. (Wiley, New York, 1974), vol. 5, p. 679.
7. B. W. Halstead, Poisonous and Venomous Animals of the World (Government Printing Office, Washington, D.C., 1965), vols. 1–3; F. E. Russell, in International Encyclopedia of Pharmacology and Therapeutics (Pergamon, New York, 1971), vol. 2, sect. 71, p. 3.
8. Cited and translated by G. W. Fraenkel, Science 129, 1466 (1959).
9. M. O. Stallard and D. J. Faulkner, Comp. Biochem. Physiol. 49, 25 (1974); ibid., p. 37.
10. A. R. Kriegstein, V. Castellucci, E. R. Kandel, Proc. Natl. Acad. Sci. U.S.A. 71, 3654 (1974).
11. J. S. Kittredge, in Proceedings of the Food-Drugs from the Sea Conference 1974, H. H. Webber and G. D. Ruggieri, Eds. (Marine Technology Society, Washington, D.C., in press).
12. J. McN. Sieburth, J. Bacteriol. 77, 521 (1959); Limnol. Oceanogr. 4, 419 (1959); Science 132, 676 (1960).
13. A. Hardy, The Open Sea. Its Natural History: The World of Plankton (Collins, London, 1956).
14. R. F. Nigrelli, Trans. N.Y. Acad. Sci. 20, 248 (1958).
15. R. Pratt, H. Mautner, G. M. Gardner, Y. Sha, J. Dufrenoy, J. Am. Pharm. Assoc. 40, 575 (1951).
16. E. Steemann-Nielsen, Deep-Sea Res. 3 (Suppl.), 281 (1955).
17. P. R. Burkholder and L. M. Burkholder, Science 127, 1174 (1958); L. S. Ciereszko, Trans. N.Y. Acad. Sci. 24, 502 (1962).
18. A. M. Welch, J. Bacteriol. 83, 97 (1962); W. Fenical, J. J. Sims, D. Squatrito, R. W. Wing, P. Radlick, J. Org. Chem. 38, 2383 (1973).
19. N. G. M. Nadal, L. V. Rodriguez, C. Casillas, in Antimicrobial Agents and Chemotherapy (Williams & Wilkins, Baltimore, 1964), p. 68.
20. K. C. Hong, R. L. Cruess, S. C. Skoryna, Proc. Int. Seaweed Symp. 7, 566 (1972).
21. Cited in The Merck Index, an Encyclopedia of Chemicals and Drugs (Merck & Company, Rahway, N.J., ed. 8, 1968).
22. S. Murakami, T. Takemoto, Z. Shimizu, Yakugaku Zasshi (J. Pharm. Soc. Jpn.) 73, 1026 (1953).
23. K. K. Takemoto and S. S. Spicer, Ann. N.Y. Acad. Sci. 130, 365 (1965).
24. P. Gerber, J. D. Dutcher, E. V. Adams, J. H. Sherman, Proc. Soc. Exp. Biol. Med. 99, 590 (1958).
25. F. Claudio and B. Stendardo, Proc. Int. Seaweed Symp. 5, 369 (1965).
26. L. C. Houch, J. Bhayana, T. Lee, Gastroen-

38. K. Czapke, Proc. Int. Seaweed Symp. 5, 371 (1965).
39. Y. Tanaka, A. J. Hurlburt, L. Angeloff, S. C. Skoryna, J. F. Stara, ibid. 7, 602 (1972).
40. G. D. Ruggieri, Ann. N.Y. Acad. Sci. 245, 39 (1975).
41. R. F. Nigrelli and G. D. Ruggieri, in Proceedings of the Food-Drugs from the Sea Conference 1974, H. H. Webber and G. D. Ruggieri, Eds. (Marine Technology Society, Washington, D.C., in press).
42. R. J. Andersen and D. J. Faulkner, in Proceedings of the Food-Drugs from the Sea Conference 1972, L. R. Worthen, Ed. (Marine Technology Society, Washington, D.C., 1972), p. 111; Tetrahedron Lett. 14, 1175 (1973); A. K. Bose, J. Kryschuk, R. F. Nigrelli, in Proceedings of the Food-Drugs from the Sea Conference 1972, L. R. Worthen, Ed. (Marine Technology Society, Washington, D.C., 1972), p. 217; P. R. Burkholder and K. Ruetzler, Nature (London) 222, 983 (1969); D. B. Cosulich and F. M. Lovell, J. Chem. Soc. Chem. Commun. 397 (1971); S. Jakowska and R. F. Nigrelli, Ann. N.Y. Acad. Sci. 90, 913 (1960); L. Minale, G. Sodano, W. R. Chen, Chem. Commun. 674 (1972); R. F. Nigrelli, S. Jakowska, I. Calventi, Zoologica 44, 173 (1959); R. F. Nigrelli, M. Baslow, S. Jakowska, Am. Soc. Microbiol. 1st Interscience Conference on Antimicrobial Agents and Chemotherapy (1961), p. 83; B. N. Ravi, T. R. Erdman, P. J. Scheuer, in Proceedings of the Food-Drugs from the Sea Conference 1974, H. H. Webber and G. D. Ruggieri, Eds. (Marine Technology Society, Washington, D.C., in press); I. Rothberg and P. Schubiak, Tetrahedron Lett. 10, 769 (1975); G. M. Sharma and P. R. Burkholder, ibid., 42, 4147 (1967); G. M. Sharma, B. Vig, P. R. Burkholder, in Proceedings of the Food-Drugs from the Sea Conference 1969, H. W. Youngken, Jr., Ed. (Marine Technology Society, Washington, D.C., 1969), p. 307; M. F. Stempien, Jr., G. D. Ruggieri, R. F. Nigrelli, J. T. Cecil, in ibid., p. 295; M. F. Stempien, Jr., J. S. Chib, R. F. Nigrelli, R. A. Mierzwa, in Proceedings of the Food-Drugs from the Sea Conference 1972, L. R. Worthen, Ed. (Marine Technology Society, Washington, D.C., 1972), p. 105; M. F. Stempien, Jr., J. S. Chib, R. A. Mierzwa, in Proceedings of the Food-Drugs from the Sea Conference 1974, H. H. Webber and G. D. Ruggieri, Eds. (Marine Technology Society, Washington, D.C., in press); G. E. Van Lear, G. O. Morton, W. Fulmor, Tetrahedron Lett. 4, 299 (1973).
43. J. T. Cecil, M. F. Stempien, Jr., G. D. Ruggieri, R. F. Nigrelli, in Aspects of Sponge Biology, F. W. Harrison and R. R. Cowden, Eds. (Academic Press, New York, 1976), p. 171; C. H. Tan, C. K. Tan, Y. F. Teh, Experientia 29, 1373 (1973).
44. M. H. Baslow and P. Turlapaty, Proc. West. Pharmacol. Soc. 12, 6 (1969).
45. M. M. Sigel, L. L. Wellham, W. Lichter, L. E. Dudeck, J. L. Gargus, A. H. Lucas, in Proceedings of the Food-Drugs from the Sea Conference 1969, H. W. Youngken, Jr., Ed. (Marine Technology Society, Washington, D.C., 1969), p. 281.
46. W. Bergmann and R. J. Feeney, J. Org. Chem. 16, 981 (1951); W. Bergmann and D. C. Burke, ibid. 20, 1501 (1955).
47. S. S. Cohen, Perspect. Biol. Med. 6, 215 (1963).
48. J. S. Evans, E. A. Musser, G. D. Mengel, K. R. Forsblad, J. H. Hunter, Proc. Soc. Exp. Biol. Med. 106, 350 (1961).

calculi (CAL-kyoo-lee): "stones."

withdrawal reaction: a reaction to withdrawal (usually of a drug) that reveals that the user has become dependent, as for example when an infant born of a mother who took massive doses of ascorbic acid develops scurvy on an intake that would be adequate for the average infant,[2] or when an infant born of an alcoholic mother suffers from the symptoms of withdrawal from alcohol (fetal alcohol syndrome).

A pharmacological dose is higher than the intake needed to prevent deficiency symptoms and may have unexpected effects, as it may be working by a different mechanism than that by which the preventive or physiological dose works. See the discussion on pages 408–409.

leucocytes (LOO-ka-sites): white blood cells which engulf foreign particles by phagocytosis and destroy them.

    leukos=white
    kytos=cell

phagocytosis (fag-o-sigh-TOE-sis): engulfing of large particles by a cell, similar to pinocytosis (see page 186).

    phagein=to eat
    kytos=cell
    osis=intensive

Experts in one area, presenting opinions in another, are outside their field; their word must be interpreted with caution, as suggested in Highlight 8.

The balanced picture emerging from the 1975 reviews of literature seemed to indicate that when all the results of the experiments on vitamin C and the cold were pooled, the effects of the pill on the common cold, if any, were small.

Meanwhile, another question has been raised: does the taking of large doses of vitamin C constitute a risk to the taker? Evidence on this question is scanty. Chalmers' review states that "since there are no data on the longterm toxicity of ascorbic acid when given in doses of 1 gram or more per day, it is concluded that the minor benefits of questionable validity are not worth the potential risk, no matter how small that might be."[2] Dykes and Meier[3] also reviewed the recent literature concerning toxicity of massive doses and reached a similar conclusion. It was formerly accepted, they state, that ascorbic acid is nontoxic, and that even massive doses have no harmful effects because the excess is excreted in the urine. Recently reports of toxic effects have been cropping up, although it is apparently too early to generalize. Possible harmful reactions to massive doses, 2-5 grams,[4] of the vitamin are formation of urinary tract calculi, effect on fertility and the fetus (an animal study), effect on carbohydrate metabolism (an animal study), withdrawal reactions, and drug interactions such as the effect of vitamin C on vitamin B_{12}.[5] Dykes and Meier conclude that we cannot be sure there are no harmful effects of massive doses of vitamin C. They believe that "until such time as pharmacological doses of ascorbic acid have been shown to have obvious important clinical value in the prevention and treatment of the common cold, and to be safe in a large, varied population we cannot advocate its unrestricted use for such purposes."[3]

Meanwhile, the scientist who started it all, Linus Pauling, has repeated in an editorial in the *Proceedings of the National Academy of Sciences*, November, 1974,[6] that the Recommended Daily Allowance for vitamin C of 45 milligrams a day should be called the Minimum Daily Allowance and that the RDA should lie somewhere between 250 and 4,000 milligrams a day. He believes that ascorbic acid has antiviral and antibacterial activity and is required for the phagocytic activity of leucocytes. Pauling is a chemist of world renown, winner of the Nobel Peace Prize in 1954 for his work on elucidating chemical bonding. But this writing is an editorial—a place for presenting opinions—and not a presentation of evidence.

One disturbing feature of Pauling's book, *Vitamin C and the Common Cold*,[1] is his frequent use of the phrase, "I am

[4]Lewin, S.: Evaluation of potential effects of high intakes of ascorbic acid. *Comparative Biochemistry, Physiology* 37(B):681-695, 1973.
[5]Herbert, V. and Jacob, E.: Destruction of B_{12} by ascorbic acid. *Journal of the American Medical Association* 224:1529-1530, 1974.
[6]Pauling, L. C.: Are recommended daily allowances for vitamin C adequate? *Proceedings of the National Academy of Sciences* 71(11):4442-4446, 1974.

sure," in reference to his theory, following which he does not present corroborating evidence. Also, he fails to report conflicting testimony. On the other hand, Coulehan, et al, when reporting on research using 641 children to test the effectiveness of vitamin C in curing colds, phrased the results this way: "The actual clinical meaning of these findings is unclear . . . but there are enough data suggesting a beneficial influence of vitamin C on respiratory infections to warrant further investigation."[7] Laymen may be made uneasy by scientists who think their data are unclear, but the scientific community prefers total honesty to dogmatic statements.

Was Pauling wrong to present his ideas to the world? No one is wrong who presents a theory as a theory only. One of the characteristics of a "good" theory, from the scientific point of view, is that it stimulates research from which new knowledge comes. Even if the theory is proved wrong, it has had value in inspiring experiments that further the progress of science.

Out of the vast research that is taking place in an attempt to discern the effectiveness of vitamin C in curing the common cold will eventually come better understanding, and we will all be indebted to Pauling for his vigorous defense of his ideas. In the meantime, the best evidence seems to be that vitamin C *may* have such an effect, but that in massive doses, such as 2-5 grams, there is a danger of toxic side effects.

To Explore Further—

The National Institutes of Health supplied 311 employees for this study. The conclusion was that vitamin C at best had only a minor influence on duration and severity of colds and the effects demonstrated might be explained equally well by a break in the double blind of the experiment:

Karlowski, T. R., Chalmers, T. C., Frendel, L. D., Kapikian, A. Z., Lewis, T. L. and Lynch, J. M.: Ascorbic acid for the common cold. A prophylactic and therapeutic trial. *Journal of the American Medical Association* 231:1038-1042, 1975.

This is a report of a study which took place in four boarding schools in Dublin during 1967-68. The conclusion was that vitamin C significantly reduced the severity and total intensity of colds in girls but did not benefit cold symptoms in boys:

Wilson, C.W.M. and Loh, H. S.: Common cold and vitamin C. *Lancet* i:638-641, 1973.

The stress effect on vitamin C is explained in this article for the lay reader:

Hodges, R. E.: Effect of stress on ascorbic acid metabolism in man. *Nutrition Today* 5:11, 1970.

[7]Coulehan, J. L., Reisinger, K. S., Rogers, K. D. and Bradley, D. W.: Vitamin C prophylaxis in a boarding school. *The New England Journal of Medicine* 290: 6-10, 1974.

Suggested Activities

(1) Study your own diet.

Review the record you made in Activity 1 of Chapter 1. Look up each food you ate in Appendix H and record its ascorbic acid contribution to your diet. Which foods provided most of this nutrient? Compare your intake of ascorbic acid with the RDA for a person your age and sex. What *percent* of the RDA did you consume? Was this enough? (See page 98.)

If your intake was less than 2/3 of the RDA, find foods or beverages in the Table of Food Composition you would be willing to eat or drink daily that would correct this deficiency.

(Note: The last Highlight in the book invites you to survey your entire diet for adequacy, balance, and economy. You may wish to save this activity until you have read that Highlight, or you may wish to read the Highlight now for a sense of perspective.)

(2) Find a substitute for fruit sources of vitamin C.

If a person dislikes fruits but likes vegetables, how much of a serving of greens would he/she have to consume daily to meet the vitamin C RDA? How many servings of potatoes would meet the RDA?

Cabbage is a favorite vegetable of the Chinese. How much cabbage must a person eat to consume 2/3 RDA for vitamin C? to consume 100 percent RDA?

Mexicans eat citrus fruits infrequently but use chili peppers and tomatoes daily. Can they meet their ascorbic acid needs this way?

(3) Discover a generalization about the vitamin C contents of foods.

What do the foods at the top of the list in Table C10.1 (above 25 milligrams ascorbic acid per serving) have in common? (Hint: consider whether they are from animal or vegetable sources. If vegetable, which part—that above the ground or under the ground?) With this in mind, would you expect the outer leaves of a cabbage to contain more ascorbic acid than the inner leaves?

(4) Caution when you read!

Start a collection of newspaper articles in which a claim is made that a specific nutrient cures a disease or alleviates a symptom. Make a trip to the library and use the indexes or check Nutrition Reviews to find review articles giving a balanced picture of research in one of these areas. Note the differences between the approaches and implications made by the writers of the newspaper articles and those of the authors of a review article. (Suggestion: vitamin A and vitamin E are two recent headline makers of this kind.)

(5) Make up your own mind.

In the light of what is known about the efficacy of massive doses of vitamin C as opposed to the risks of these doses, what is your decision regarding the use of this nutrient as a supplement? Defend your position.

11

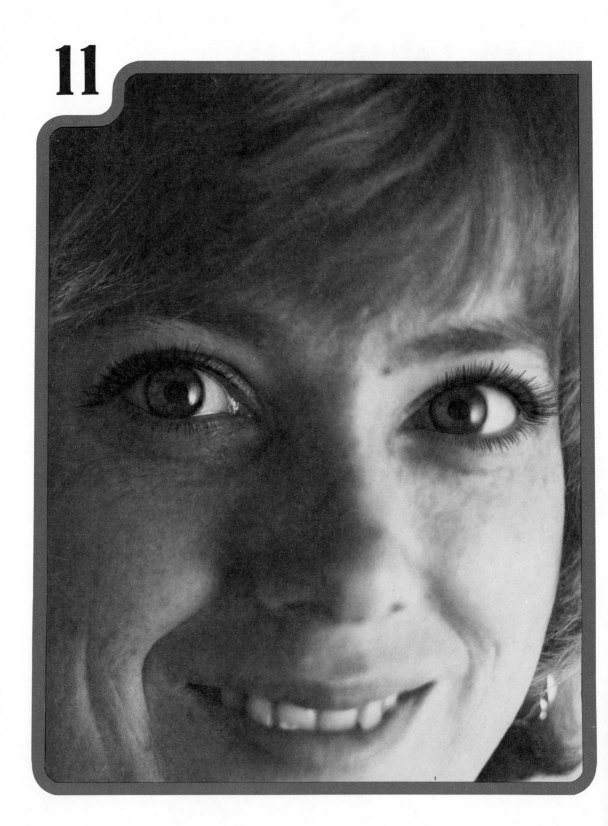

The Fat-Soluble Vitamins: A, D, E, K

I remember well the time when the thought of the eye made me cold all over.
—CHARLES DARWIN

Has it ever occurred to you how remarkable it is that you can see things? As an infant you were enchanted with the power this gave you. You closed your eyes and the world disappeared. You opened them and made everything come back again. Later you forgot the wonder of this phenomenon, but the fact remains: your ability to see does bring everything into being for you, more so than do any of your other senses. Light reaching your eyes puts you in touch with things outside your body, from your friend sitting on the couch near you to stars in other galaxies.

Has it ever occurred to you how extraordinary it is that a child grows? From a mere nothing, a speck so tiny that it is invisible to the naked eye, each person develops into a full-sized human being with arms and legs, teeth and fingernails, a beating heart and tingling nerves. Years go into the making of an adult human being, with each day bringing changes so gradual they seem indetectable. Only if you are absent during a part of this process do you notice it on your return and remark to a child, "My, how you've grown!"

And when did you last think about your breathing? In, out, in, out, day and night, year after year, you take in the oxygen you need, and release it, carrying away used-up carbons whose energy moves you and keeps you alive. The nutrients discussed in this chapter are vital for these and other processes which we often take for granted.

Roles of Vitamin A: (1) Vision

retina (RET-in-uh): the layer of light-sensitive cells lining the back of the inside of the eye, consisting of rods and cones.

At the place where light hits the retina of the eye, profoundly informative communication occurs between the environment and the person. The eye receives the signal—light—and transforms it into informational signals which travel to the interior of the brain:

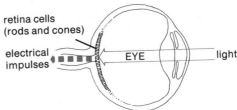

There, a mental picture is formed of what the light conveys. For this to happen, the eye performs a remarkable transformation of light energy into nerve impulses. The transformers are the molecules of pigment (rhodopsin, iodopsin, and others) in the cells of the retina.

pigment: a molecule capable of absorbing certain wavelengths of light.

rhodopsin (ro-DOP-sin): the light-sensitive pigment of the rods in the retina.

iodopsin (eye-o-DOP-sin): another light-sensitive pigment in the retina.

Experts have written whole volumes about the eye, and it is not our intent to convey more than the briefest summary of the way that remarkable organ works. (A beautiful, simple explanation is given in one of the references suggested at the end of this chapter.) From the standpoint of nutrition, what is important is to know that this extraordinary capability of the body, like so many others already discussed, depends first on the perfect structures and functions of protein and other molecules which are synthesized following instructions coded in the genes, and second on obtaining in the diet pieces of those molecules that the body cannot synthesize—the essential nutrients. The description which follows in the next four paragraphs identifies the cells in the retina which respond to light by day and by night, the pigments within those cells which absorb the light, and the way in which they convert light into nerve impulses which are interpreted in the brain as a picture. The punchline is that a portion of each pigment molecule is the compound retinal, a compound which the body cannot synthesize; retinal is destroyed during the process of converting light into nerve impulses and must be replaced by vitamin A from the diet.

retinal (RET-in-al): an active form of vitamin A. For the structure of this and other forms, see Appendix C.

A mechanical genius could not have designed such a system better. Light itself cannot be conducted through the solid material of the brain, so it is changed into signals transmitted by nerves. But light comes in different colors (wavelengths), which reveal a lot about the environment. To keep the colors sorted out, the eye uses different light-sensitive cells (cones) to receive them. Blue light is absorbed by one set of cells, green by another, and yellow-red by a third. By day, combinations of these give

cones: the cells of the retina that respond to light by day.

the full range of color vision. By night, the light entering the eye is of low intensity, and the set of cells (rods) which can receive this light are of one kind only, so that by night a person can normally discern only the presence of light but not its color.

What absorbs the light is the pigment molecules inside the cells. Each pigment molecule is composed of a protein called opsin bonded to a molecule of retinal. When a particle of light (a photon) enters the eye, it is absorbed into the retinal molecule, which responds by changing shape (it actually changes color, too: is bleached). In its altered form it cannot remain bonded to opsin and so is released. This in turn disturbs the shape of the opsin molecule:

rods: the cells of the retina that respond to light by night.

opsin (OP-sin): the protein portion of the visual pigment molecule.

photon (FOE-ton): a particle of light energy. Depending on its wavelength, a photon conveys different colors of light.

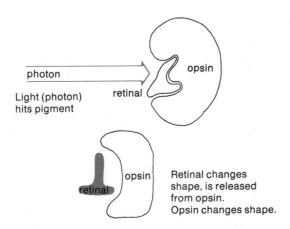

photon → opsin / retinal

Light (photon) hits pigment

opsin / retinal

Retinal changes shape, is released from opsin. Opsin changes shape.

At this point, the light energy has caused disarrangement in the shape of a protein molecule. It remains to use this shape change to send a message saying, in effect, "Green light has entered here." By a mechanism not completely understood, the cell membrane is disturbed by the pigment's change in shape and permits charged ions to enter and leave the cell. The cell *hyperpolarizes* (that is, the electrical charge across its membrane changes), and an electrical impulse is generated which travels along the cell's length. At the other end of the cell, the impulse is transmitted to a nerve cell, which conveys it deeper into the brain. Thus the message is sent.

Meanwhile, back in the retina, a pigment molecule has been destroyed. In absorbing a photon, retinal changed shape and was split off from the protein opsin. Many molecules of retinal are destroyed during this process. There are about 6-7 million cone cells and 100 million rod cells in the retina, and each cell contains about 30 million molecules of visual pigment. Ultimately, vitamin A and its relatives in foods are the source of all the retinal which replaces that destroyed in the eye by light.

Bright light seen at night destroys much more retinal than light seen by day, for three reasons. First, the pupil is wide open at night, to allow as much light as possible to enter the eye. Second, there is an adaptation in the retina itself: a shadowing pigment protects the rods by day (they are not needed in bright light) but withdraws at night, leaving them exposed. Third, there are many more rods than cones. Hence if a bright light suddenly shines through the wide open pupil onto the unprotected rods, much of the pigment in them is bleached and the retinal is destroyed. A moment passes before the pigments regenerate and sight returns. You no doubt recall experiencing this when you were "blinded" by a flashlight shining directly into your eyes. People who must do a lot of night driving, facing headlights from oncoming cars, thus need an increased amount of vitamin A.

The eye is not designed for night driving, or in general, for accommodating itself to bright light at night. The mechanisms of vision evolved over millions of years, before humankind had harnessed electricity and lit up the night with headlights, beacons, and streetlights. In nature, animals in the wilderness have no need to adapt to sudden flashes of bright light at night, because they occur so seldom.

Vitamin A is undeniably an important nutrient, if for no other reason than that it plays a vital role in vision, but only one-thousandth of the vitamin A in the body is in the retina. It does other things as well. A look at one of its humbler functions follows.

mucosa (myoo-COH-suh): the membranes, composed of cells, that line the surfaces of the body tisuses.

urethra (you-REE-thruh): the tube through which urine from the bladder passes out of the body.

The cells are known as **epithelial** (ep-i-THEE-lee-ul) **cells**.

mucus (adjective **mucous**): a substance secreted by the epithelial cells of the mucosa, mucopolysaccharide. See also page 152.

cilia: see page 170.

Roles of Vitamin A: (2) Mucous Membranes

Fortunately for you, your mucosa are all intact. You may not properly appreciate what these membranes do for you, but consider how important it is that each of these surfaces should be smooth: the linings of the mouth, stomach, and intestines, the linings of the lungs and the passages leading to them, the linings of the urinary bladder and urethra, the linings of the uterus and vagina, the linings of the eyelids and sinus passageways. The cells of all these surfaces secrete a smooth and slippery substance (mucus) which coats and protects them from invasive microorganisms and other harmful particles. The mucous lining of the stomach also shields its cells from digestion by the gastric juices. In the upper part of the lungs these cells also possess little whiplike hairs (cilia) which continuously sweep the coating of mucus up and out, so that any foreign particles that chance to get in are carried up and away by the flow. (When you clear your throat and swallow, you are excreting this waste by way of your digestive tract.) In the vagina, similar cells sweep the mucus down and out. During an infection in any of these organs, these surface cells secrete more mucus and become more active, so that a noticeable discharge occurs; when you cough it up, blow your nose, or wash it away, you help to rid your body of the infective agent.

Vitamin A plays a role in maintaining the integrity of all these membranes. When vitamin A is not present, the cells cannot produce the carbohydrate normally found in mucus, and produce a protein instead, called keratin. As you might predict, greater losses of the vitamin occur during infection than under normal conditions.

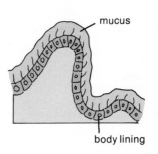

keratin: see below, page 342.

This mucous membrane function accounts for the use of much of the vitamin A in the body. There is over a quarter of an acre of mucous membranes to maintain. And as if this weren't enough, vitamin A is also essential for healthy skin, another one or two square meters of body surface. Thus all surfaces, both inside and out, are maintained with the help of vitamin A.

Besides its roles in vision and in the maintenance of internal and external linings, vitamin A has an important part to play during growth, as the following section shows.

Roles of Vitamin A: (3) Bone Growth

"Growth is when everything gets bigger all together," is the definition given by a five-year-old. Certainly that is how it looks from the outside. A baby's hands, feet, arms, legs, and internal organs are all baby-sized; an adult's are all relatively larger. Actually, however, the organs and body parts all grow at different rates and experience growth spurts at different times. The brain, for instance, reaches 80 percent of its adult size by the time a child is two, while the testes are still baby-sized when a male enters his teens. Also, they do not just "get bigger": bones are a case in point.

To enlarge the interior of a brick fireplace, the first thing you have to do is remove some of the old bricks. Similarly, to make a bone larger requires remodeling, as the picture below shows: to convert small bone (A) into large bone (B) it is necessary to "undo" some parts of the small bone first:

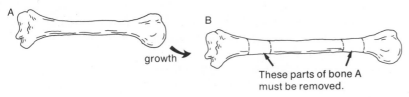

These parts of bone A must be removed.

It is in the undoing that vitamin A is involved. Some of the cells involved in bone formation are packed with sacs of degradative enzymes which can take apart the structures from which bone is made. With the help of vitamin A, in a carefully controlled process, these cells release their enzymes, which gradually eat away at selected sites in the bone, removing the parts of its structure that are not needed as the bone grows longer. (A similar process occurs when a tadpole loses its tail and becomes a frog. As you know, the tail doesn't simply fall off, rather it is resorbed, growing shorter and shorter until it disappears. As a fetus you also had a tail and lost it, a process which depended on vitamin A.)

The functions of vitamin A in promoting good night vision, the health of mucous membranes and skin, and the growth of bone are well known, although still not completely understood. Others, less well understood, include roles it plays in reproduction, in maintaining the stability of cell membranes, in helping the adrenal gland to synthesize a hormone (corticosterone) and the thyroid gland to secrete thyroid hormone, helping to maintain nerve cell sheaths, and many others. Vitamin A research is still in progress and is yielding many new answers to the questions of how this nutrient functions in the body.

These sacs of degradative enzymes are **lysosomes** (LYE-so-zomes).

lyso = to break
soma = body

The cells are osteoclasts. See page 346.

Vitamin A Deficiency

Up to a year's supply of vitamin A may be stored in the body, 90 percent of it in the liver. If you stop eating good food sources of the vitamin, deficiency symptoms will not begin to appear until after your stores are depleted. Then, however, the consequences are profound and severe. Table C11.1 itemizes some of them.

From what has been said above, it is clear why many of these symptoms appear. Some have to do with the role of vitamin A in vision, some with its functions in epithelial tissue, some with its part in growth; others are as yet unexplained.

Vision is impaired. If sufficient retinal is not available (from the blood bathing the cells of the retina) to rapidly regenerate visual pigments bleached by light, then a flash of bright light at night will be followed by a prolonged spell of night blindness. This is one of the first detectable signs of vitamin A deficiency. Because it is easy to test, it is a symptom that aids in diagnosis of the condition.

Smooth surfaces become rough. Instead of staying smooth and well rounded and producing normal mucus, the epithelial cells flatten and harden, losing their protective mucous coating. In the eye this leads to drying and hardening of the cornea, which may progress all the way to blindness. In the mouth, the

night blindness

The epithelial cells fill with keratin, in a process known as **hyperkeratinization**. *The progression of this condition to the extreme in the eye is* **xerophthalmia** (ze-roff-THAL-mee-a) *and causes blindness.*

hyper = too much

keratin (KER-uh-tin): *a water-insoluble protein.*

cornea (KOR-nee-uh): *the transparent membrane covering the outside of the front of the eye.*

Table C11.1
Vitamin A Deficiency

Main effect upon:

Eye, retina: night blindness

Membranes: failure to secrete mucopolysaccharide causes changes in epithelial tissue and hyperkeratinization

Eye—mildest form—opaqueness
more severe—drying
most severe—irreversible drying and degeneration of the cornea—causes blindness

Skin—hair follicles plug with keratin forming white lumps

GI tract—changes in lining; diarrhea

Respiratory tract—changes in lining; infections

Urinogenital tract—changes in lining favor calcium deposition resulting in kidney stones, bladder disorders

Bones: bone growth ceases; shapes of bones change

Teeth: enamel-forming cells malfunction, teeth develop cracks and tend to decay; dentin forming cells atrophy

Nervous system: brain and spinal cord grow too fast for stunted skull and spine. Injury to brain and nerves causes paralysis

hyperkeratinization: see page 342.

Bitot's spots

xerosis (zer-OH-sis)

xerophthalmia: see page 342.

follicular hyperkeratosis: see page 344.

enamel: the hard mineral coating of the outside of the tooth, composed of calcium carbonate and calcium phosphate embedded in a fine network of keratin fibers.

dentin: the softer material underlying the enamel of the tooth, composed of calcium phosphate and carbonate embedded in a network of collagen fibers.

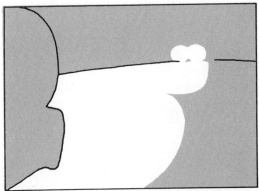

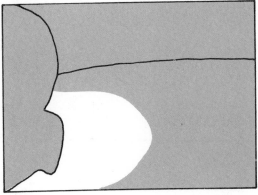

The headlights of an approaching car tend to momentarily blind a driver.

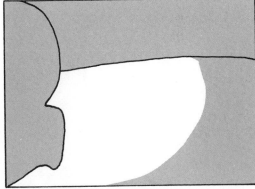

The eyes of a driver not suffering from vitamin A deficiency will be able to adapt to this and will have a good view of the road after the car has passed.

The eyes of a driver suffering night blindness will not adjust to the change and will not be able to see the road for several minutes after the car has passed.

The accumulation of this hard material, keratin, around each hair follicle is **follicular hyperkeratosis.**

follicle (FOLL-i-cul): a group of cells in the skin from which a hair grows.

drying and hardening of the salivary glands makes them susceptible to infection; failure of mucus secretion in the mouth may lead to loss of appetite. Mucus secretion in the stomach and intestines is reduced, hindering normal digestion and absorption of nutrients, causing diarrhea, and so indirectly worsening the deficiency. Infections of the respiratory tract, the urinary tract, and the vagina are made more likely by the same cause. On the outer body surface, the cells also harden and flatten, making the skin dry, rough, scaly, and hard. Around each hair follicle an accumulation of hard material makes a lump.

Growth is abnormal. Because growth and the development of the brain and eyes are most rapid in the unborn and in the very young baby, the effects of vitamin A deficiency are most severe in and around the time of birth. For example, in a child of one or two, abnormal growth of the skull may cause crowding of the brain (which is growing rapidly at that age). Damage to the eyes is also most pronounced in the young, with blindness resulting in thousands of cases of vitamin A deficiency throughout the world. Vitamin A deficiency is second only to protein calorie malnutrition as a nutritional problem afflicting the young of the world.

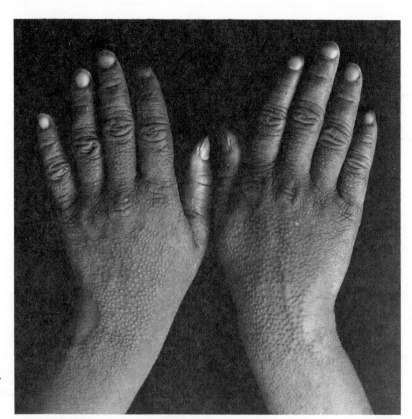

Follicular hyperkeratosis.

Photo courtesy of Dr. Samuel Dreizen, D.D.S., M.D.

Naivete on the part of the well intentioned can cause more harm than good, as is often observed when attempts are made to remedy the problem of malnutrition in the underdeveloped countries. An awareness of the way in which nutrients function in the body, and of their interdependency, must precede efforts to correct malnutrition problems, as the case of vitamin A illustrates. The vitamin depends on proteins for its functions and transport in the body. In protein calorie malnutrition, when vitamin A stores are also low, there is a balance of a kind. When protein is given without supplemental vitamin A, protein carriers may be synthesized and deplete the liver of the last available stores of the vitamin, thus precipitating a deficiency. Administration of protein has been observed to cause an epidemic of blindness, as when skim milk was offered by UNICEF to children in Brazil (1961). Vitamin A capsules were supplied with the milk, but the parents ate the capsules or sold them for money, giving only the milk to the children.[1]

Knowledge of nutrition must accompany the giving of nutritional help.

In the United States as well, the problem of vitamin A deficiency is all too common. The Ten-State Nutrition Survey revealed that one-third of the children under six who were examined had less than the recommended vitamin A intakes.[2] Spanish Americans and Blacks exhibited the most pronounced evidence of deficiency. Since the major sources of this vitamin for children are vegetables and fruits, especially green and yellow vegetables, a probable reason for the high incidence of this disease in children is their refusal to eat these foods. A section of Chapter 15 emphasizes the importance of encouraging children to like vegetables and suggests practical ways to ease their acceptance.

Results of surveys must be interpreted with caution. See Highlight 12.

Vitamin A Toxicity

Too much vitamin A is as bad as too little, having serious effects on many of the same body systems it helps when ingested

[1]Roels, O. A.: Vitamin A physiology. *Journal of the American Medical Association* 214(6):1097-1102, 1970.
[2]*Ten-State Nutrition Survey 1968-1970*. U.S. Department of Health, Education, and Welfare. DHEW Publication No. (HSM) 72-8130. Center for Disease Control, Atlanta, Georgia.

in proper amounts. (See Table C11.2). Again, it is children who are most affected: they need less, they are smaller and more sensitive to overdoses, and it is easy to make the mistake of giving them too much in pill form or in other concentrates. The availability of breakfast cereals, instant meals, fortified milk, and chewable, candy-like vitamins each containing 100 percent of the vitamin A RDA makes it possible for a well-meaning parent to provide several times the daily allowance of this vitamin to a child in a few hours, while the children, liking vitamin pills and believing they are good for them, may eat several, reasoning that if one is good for them, four or five are sure to be even better.

There is a wide range of vitamin A intakes over which neither deficiency nor toxicity symptoms appear. The RDA is set at double the minimum necessary to prevent deficiency. (See boxed section at end of chapter.) Thus intakes below the RDA may be more than adequate for many people. Toxicity symptoms appear, in many cases, only after intakes for several months of ten times the RDA or more. Infants, pregnant women, and children are more sensitive to high vitamin A intakes. One month of daily doses of 25,000 IU has been reported as having toxic effects.[3] Another susceptible group is adolescents being

[3]Yaffe, S. J. and Filer, L. J., Jr.: American Academy of Pediatrics, Joint Committee Statement on Drugs and on Nutrition. The use and abuse of vitamin A. *Pediatrics* 48:655-656, 1971.

Table C11.2
Vitamin A Toxicity

Hypervitaminosis A

Main effect upon:

osteoclasts: the cells which destroy bone during its growth. Those which build bone are **osteoblasts**.

osteo = bone
clast = break
blast = build

Bones: increased activity of osteoclasts causes decalcification, joint pain, fragility, stunted growth, thickening of long bones; pressure increases inside skull

Blood: red blood cells lose hemoglobin and potassium; menstruation ceases

Nervous system: loss of appetite, irritability, fatigue, restlessness, headache, nausea, vomiting

GI tract: nausea, vomiting, abdominal pain, diarrhea, weight loss

Skin: rashes, dry scaling lips, loss of hair, brittle nails

jaundice: yellowing of the skin, a symptom of liver disease, in which bile and related pigments spill over into the bloodstream.

hypercarotenemia: see page 347.

Liver: jaundice, enlargement

Spleen: enlargement

Hypercarotenemia

Main effect upon:

Skin: yellow color

---

treated with massive doses of vitamin A for acne. Evidence is lacking that this treatment is effective against acne, and cases of toxic overdosing have been reported.[1][3]

It is possible to suffer toxicity symptoms only when excess amounts of the preformed vitamin from animal foods or supplements are taken. The precursor, beta-carotene, which is available from plant foods, is not converted to vitamin A rapidly enough in the body to cause toxicity but is instead stored in fat depots as carotene. Being yellow in color, it may accumulate under the skin to such an extent that the overdoser actually turns yellow! It makes sense, therefore, to get one's vitamin A from plant sources; if supplements are taken they should not exceed 6,000 IU per day.[3]

preformed vitamin A: vitamin A in its active form, which needs no conversion in the body.

precursor: a compound which can be converted into active vitamin A. See page 292.

beta-carotene: the vitamin A precursor found in plants. (For structures, see Appendix C.)

hypercarotenemia

Vitamin A in Foods

It is easy to get ample amounts of vitamin A from foods rather than from dietary supplements, as a look at Table C11.3 will show. For example, let us aim at an intake of 3,000 IU a day, which is about ¾ of a woman's RDA, or 3/5 of a man's. Since the body stores the vitamin, a 2-ounce piece of beef liver eaten only once every ten days is sufficient without any other food sources. (A moment's reflection will tell you why liver is the best of all food sources of this vitamin. Livers vary, of course, depending how much of the vitamin the animal had in storage at the time of slaughter, but all are excellent sources. Polar bear liver is notorious for containing too much, as explorers in the Arctic learned the hard way.) Other than liver, according to the Table of Food Composition (Appendix H), one cup of spinach will provide enough beta carotene to meet vitamin A needs for five days, while beta carotene is so concentrated in carrots that one carrot every other day should suffice. However, absorption and digestion of the carotenes are inefficient and the values in the Table are probably spuriously high. No doubt you can find food sources of the vitamin that appeal to you and can easily calculate the minimum amounts you should eat in order to meet your needs.

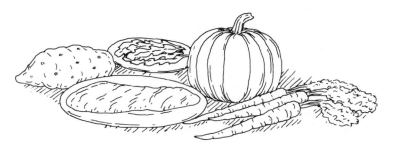

Table C11.3
Fifty Foods Showing Amounts of Vitamin A

The foods listed below are the fifty that rank highest as sources of vitamin A from those which are found on the ADA Exchange Lists and which also have been analyzed for nutrient composition. Serving sizes are the sizes listed in the Exchange Lists except for meat, where 3-ounce servings are shown. The numbers 1 through 6 refer to the numbers of the Exchange Lists: 1 = Milk, 2 = Vegetables, 3 = Fruit, 4 = Bread, 5L = Lean Meat, 5M = Medium-Fat Meat, 5H = High-Fat Meat, 6 = Fats and Oils. Numbers in parentheses are the item numbers on the Table of Food Composition (Appendix H).

Exchange Group	Food (Item Number)	Serving Size	Vitamin A International Units
5M	Beef liver (112)	3 ounces	45,420
4	Pumpkin (229)	¾ cup	10,943*
2	Dandelion greens (201)	½ cup	10,530
2	Carrots (190)	½ cup	7,610
2	Spinach (233)	½ cup	7,200
2	Collard greens (195)	½ cup	5,130
			5,000 = U.S. RDA
4	Winter squash (235)	½ cup	4,305
4	Sweet potatoes (239)	¼ cup	4,250
2	Mustard greens (208)	½ cup	4,060
3	Cantaloupe (263)	¼	3,270
2	Broccoli (179)	½ cup	2,363
3	Dried apricots (254)	4 halves	1,635
3	Peach (305)	1	1,320
2	Cooked tomatoes (241)	½ cup	1,085
2	Tomato juice (244)	½ cup	970
2	Asparagus (165)	½ cup	605
5M	Egg (73)	1	590
5L	Oysters (140)	15, ¾ cup	555
3	Pink grapefruit (271)	½	540
4	Green peas (215)	½ cup	430
2	Summer squash (234)	½ cup	410
2	Brussels sprouts (180)	½ cup	405
1	Canned evaporated milk (4)	½ cup	405
3	Tangerine (330)	1	360
1	Whole milk (1)	1 cup	350
1	Yogurt (made w/whole milk) (72)	1 cup	340
2	Green beans (168)	½ cup	340
4	Corn on cob (196)	1 small	310
3	Orange juice (298)	½ cup	275
3	Orange (294)	1	260
6	Cream, light (37)	2 tbsp	260
4	Lima beans (167)	½ cup	240
6	Cream, heavy (45)	1 tbsp	230
4	Corn (197)	1/3 cup	230
1	2% fat fortified milk (3)	1 cup	200
5L	Sardines (142)	3 ounces	190

*Recall that vitamin A activity reported in plants may be spuriously high.

Table C11.3 (continued)

Exchange Group	Food (Item Number)	Serving Size	Vitamin A International Units
6	Soft margarine (504)	1 tsp	156
3	Blackberries (261)	½ cup	145
3	Banana (259)	½ medium	115
5M	Creamed cottage cheese (16)	¼ cup	105
4	Corn muffin (419)	1	100
3	Raspberries (325)	½ cup	80
5L	Chicken, meat only (95)	3 ounces	80
4	Yellow grits (410)	½ cup	75
4	Pancake (442)	1	70
5L	Canned tuna (146)	3 ounces	70
3	Blueberries (262)	½ cup	70
3	Strawberries (328)	¾ cup	68
5L	Canned salmon (141)	3 ounces	60
3	Pineapple (314)	½ cup	50

Color is a key to the vitamin A and carotene contents of foods. The top fifteen items in Table C11.3 are all brightly colored foods: green, yellow, orange, or red. Any food with significant vitamin A activity must have some color, since the vitamin and its plant precursor carotene are colored compounds themselves (vitamin A is a very pale yellow, carotene is a rich, deep yellow, almost orange). The dark green leafy vegetables contain abundant amounts of the green pigment chlorophyll, which masks the carotene in them. A skilled hostess or restauranteur knows that to make a meal attractive she/he should provide foods of different colors that complement each other, but may not be aware that doing so probably ensures a good supply of vitamin A as well.

On the other hand, food with a yellow or orange color does not invariably reflect the presence of vitamin A or carotene. Many of the compounds which give foods their colors, such as the yellow and red xanthophylls, are unrelated to the vitamin and have no nutritional value.

On the third hand (this chapter has three hands), if a food is white or colorless, it contains little or no vitamin A. Notice that many of the foods at the bottom of Table C11.3 are in this category.

About half of the vitamin A activity in foods consumed in the United States comes from fruits and vegetables, and half of this in turn from the dark leafy greens (not iceberg lettuce or green beans) and the yellow or orange vegetables, such as yellow squash, carrots, and sweet potatoes. The other half comes from milk, cheese, butter and other dairy products, eggs, and meats. Since the vitamin is fat-soluble, it is lost when milk is

chlorophyll: the green pigment of plants, which absorbs photons and transfers their energy to other molecules, initiating photosynthesis.

photosynthesis: the synthesis of carbohydrates by plants from carbon dioxide and water, using the sun's energy.

fortified: see page 422.

skimmed, and skim milk is often fortified with 5,000 IU (the male RDA—see boxed section at end of chapter) of vitamin A per quart to compensate. The butter substitute, margarine, is usually fortified with 15,000 IU per pound.

The Bone Vitamin: D

Vitamin A helps to remodel bones; vitamin D helps to grow them. Vitamin A is versatile and important in many body systems; vitamin D seems to play its part only in connection with the minerals of the bone system. That part is considerable, however, and the vitamin is indispensable to keep the system working during periods of bone growth or remodeling. Vitamin D is a member of a large and cooperative bone-making and maintaining team made up of nutrients and other compounds, including vitamins C and A and the hormones parathormone and calcitonin, the protein collagen, which precedes bone, and the minerals calcium, phosphorus, magnesium, fluoride, and others, of which the bone is finally composed.

parathormone, calcitonin: see page 375.

collagen: see pages 123, 315.

Bones are very active metabolically. It has been estimated that about ¼ of the calcium in the blood is exchanged with bone calcium every minute. The special function of vitamin D is to help make the minerals calcium and phosphorus available in the blood which bathes the bones so that they can be deposited there as the bones grow (harden or mineralize).

One way in which vitamin D raises blood concentrations of these minerals is by stimulating their absorption from the gastrointestinal tract; a second way is by helping to withdraw calcium from bones into the blood. The star of this particular show is calcium itself, while vitamin D is a supporting actor. A description of how calcium moves from food into the blood and into and out of bone is reserved for Chapter 12, where a closer view of the whole system will be given. What is important here is to be aware of the importance of vitamin D, the risks of deficiency and toxicity, and the ways in which it can be obtained from foods.

mineralization (calcification): the process in which calcium, phosphorus, and other minerals crystallize on the collagen matrix of a growing bone, hardening the bone.

precursor: see page 292.

animal precursor:
7-dehydrocholesterol
|
sun
↓
cholecalciferol (D₃)

plant (bacterial) precursor:
ergosterol
|
sun
↓
ergocalciferol
(D₂, calciferol)

(For structures, see Appendix C.)

But is D a vitamin? A note should be made here of one way in which this nutrient is unique: the body can synthesize its own vitamin D in the skin with the help of sunlight. In this sense it is not an essential nutrient. Given enough sun, you need consume no vitamin D at all in the foods you eat. Rather, it is like a hormone: a compound manufactured by one organ of the body, having effects on another.

The liver manufactures a vitamin D precursor which is released into the blood and circulates to the skin. When ultraviolet rays from the sun hit this compound it is converted to vitamin D₃. Similarly, plants and microorganisms manufacture a related vitamin D precursor, and this too is converted to a form of the vitamin, D_2. Both D_2 and D_3 are active in human beings. Theoretically, then, you could obtain enough of this vitamin to meet your needs in any of three ways: by eating good plant sources of D_2, or good animal sources of D_3, or by making your own D_3. Actually, however, only animal foods and self-synthesis provide appreciable amounts of the active vitamin for human beings.

Microorganism sources are used to make vitamin D supplements.

Vitamin D Deficiency and Toxicity

Both inadequate and excessive vitamin D intakes take their toll in the United States, despite the fact that the vitamin has been known for decades to be essential for growth and toxic in excess. The Ten-State Nutrition Survey revealed that nearly 4 percent of the children under six who were examined showed evidence of vitamin D deficiency, with several cases of overt rickets. Worldwide, rickets still afflicts large numbers of children.

Results of surveys must be interpreted with caution. See Highlight 12.

rickets: the vitamin D deficiency disease in children.

A rare type of rickets, not caused by vitamin D deficiency, is known as **vitamin D-refractory rickets.**

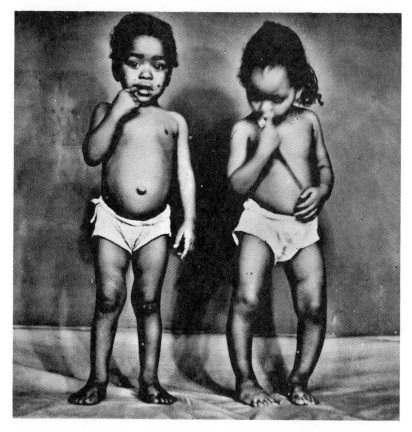

Rickets

Photo courtesy of Parke-Davis & Company.

The symptoms of an inadequate intake of vitamin D are those of calcium deficiency, as shown in Table C11.4. The bones fail to calcify normally and may be so weak that they become bent when they have to support the body's weight: a child with rickets who is old enough to walk characteristically develops bowed legs, often the most obvious sign of the disease.

Adult rickets, or osteomalacia, occurs most often in women who have little exposure to sun and who go through repeated pregnancies and periods of lactation. The bones of the legs may soften to such an extent that a woman who was tall and straight before her first pregnancy becomes bent over, bowlegged, and stooped after her second or third.

While vitamin D deficiency depresses calcium absorption and results in low blood calcium levels and abnormal mineralization of bone, an excess of the vitamin does the opposite, as

osteomalacia (os-tee-o-mal-AY-shuh): the vitamin D deficiency disease in adults.

osteo = bone
mal = bad (soft)

Osteomalacia may also occur in calcium deficiency; see Chapter 12.

**Table C11.4
Vitamin D Deficiency**

Rickets

Main effect upon:

Bones: faulty calcification resulting in misshapen bones (bowing of legs) and retarded growth
  enlargement of ends of long bones (knock knees)
  deformities of ribs (they become bowed, and beads or knobs form on them)
  delayed closing of fontanel results in rapid enlargement of head

Blood: decreased calcium and/or phosphorus

Teeth: slow eruption; teeth not well formed; tendency to decay

Muscles: lax muscles resulting in protrusion of the abdomen

Excretory system: increased calcium in stools, decreased calcium in urine

Glandular system: abnormally high secretion of parathyroid hormone

Osteomalacia

Main effect upon:

Bones: softening effect: deformities of limbs, spine, thorax, and pelvis; demineralization; pain in the pelvis, lower back, and legs; bone fractures

Blood: decreased calcium and/or phosphorus
  increased alkaline phosphatase

Muscles: involuntary twitching, muscle spasms

Bowing of the ribs causes the symptom known as **pigeon breast.** The beads which form on the ribs resemble rosary beads; this symptom is known as **rachitic** (ra-KIT-ik) **rosary** (the rosary of rickets).

fontanel: the open space in the top of a baby's skull before the skull bones have grown together.

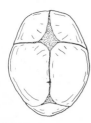

thorax: the part of the body between the neck and the abdomen.

alkaline phosphatase: an enzyme in blood.

shown in Table C11.5: it increases calcium absorption, causing abnormally high concentrations of the mineral in the blood, and promotes return of bone calcium into the blood as well. The excess calcium in the blood tends to precipitate in the soft tissues, forming stones. This is especially likely to happen in the kidneys, which are concentrating calcium in the effort to excrete it. Calcification or hardening of the blood vessels may also occur. This process is especially dangerous in the major arteries of the heart and lungs, where it can cause death.

Table C11.5
Vitamin D Toxicity

Hypervitaminosis D

Main effect upon:

Bones: increased calcium withdrawal

Blood: increased calcium and phosphorus concentration

Nervous system: loss of appetite, headache, excessive thirst, irritability

Excretory system: increased excretion of calcium in urine; kidney stones; irreversible renal damage

Tissues: calcification of soft tissues (blood vessels, kidneys, lungs), death

---

The range of safe intakes of vitamin D appears to be narrower than that for vitamin A. One-half the RDA is too little, while over a few times the RDA may be too much. Intakes of 4,000 IU per day cause high blood calcium levels in infants, but some are sensitive to lower doses than this. Intakes of 10,000 IU cause toxicity in children and, if prolonged, in adults. The amounts of the vitamin found in foods available in the United States are well within these limits, but pills containing the vitamin in concentrated form should definitely be kept out of the reach of children. It used to be possible to obtain over-the-counter preparations of vitamin D such as halibut-liver oil containing 10,000 IU per teaspoon (and concentrates of this oil containing 250 times as much!), but the sale of such concentrated preparations is now strictly limited by law and the risks are correspondingly reduced.

vitamin D RDA = 400 IU.

Vitamin D from Sun and Foods

In rapidly growing children an intake of close to 400 IU of vitamin D a day is needed, the same amount as for adults. Only a few animal foods supply significant amounts of the vitamin, notably eggs, liver, and some fish, and even these vary greatly depending on the animal's exposure to sun and on its consumption of the vitamin in its foods. The fortification of milk with 400 IU per quart is the best guarantee that children (at least those who drink milk each day) will meet their vitamin D needs.

Significant amounts of vitamin D can be made with the help of sunlight. This is why most U.S. adults need not make special efforts to obtain it in food. The vitamin is manufactured on, not in, the skin, and it is afterwards gradually absorbed into the blood. (If you swim or shower too soon after sunbathing, you can wash off a substantial amount of the vitamin!)[4]

Exposure to sun should be reasonable. Excessive exposure to sun predisposes to skin cancer.

The Miracle Vitamin: E

The theater lights darken, a hush falls over the audience. Silence—and suspense. Slowly, the heavy curtains open revealing a giant stage. The drum roll begins, rising in volume, the audience waits with bated breath. Suddenly, with a flare of trumpets, a bright circle of light spots at center stage the One, the Only, the Magnificient . . . Vitamin E! (applause, swelling to thunderous ovation). Here it is, the vitamin that can do everything!

Like Broadway stars, many wonder nutrients have had their moments of glory, but most have returned rapidly to obscurity. Only those with real talent, versatility, and dedication to their art have managed to stay in the limelight for long. Vitamin E looks like a winner, but it is still too early to predict what its greatest roles will be.

As stated at the start, this book is intended to give you a sense of what to believe and what not to believe, presenting well-known and documented research in the chapters, and reserving recent, speculative, and controversial material for the Highlights. Much of what is presently being said about vitamin E is too uncertain to have won the security of a textual presentation and so is addressed in the Highlight at the end of this chapter. There is one role vitamin E plays—as an antioxidant—that is quite well understood; this and the food sources of the vitamin are treated in the following paragraphs.

Antioxidant properties of vitamin E. Like vitamin C, vitamin E is readily oxidized. If there is plenty of vitamin E in a mixture of compounds exposed to an oxidant, chances are this vitamin will take the brunt of the oxidative attack, protecting the others. Because it is soluble in fat, vitamin E is found in

antioxidant: see page 314.

oxidant: a compound (such as oxygen itself) which oxidizes other compounds.

[4]Williams, S. R.: *Nutrition and Diet Therapy.* The C. V. Mosby Company, St. Louis, 1973, p. 81.

fat-rich fluids and tissues of the body in association with the lipids of cell membranes and with the other fat-soluble vitamins. Because of this and its relative abundance in the diet (RDA 15 milligrams as compared with about one-tenth as much vitamin A and about one-thousandth as much vitamin D), it is especially effective in preventing the oxidation of vitamin A and the polyunsaturated fatty acids.

Vitamin E deficiency. Of twelve possible diseases associated with vitamin E deficiency in animals, only one has been demonstrated in human beings. When serum levels of the vitamin fall below about 100 milligrams per 100 milliliters of blood, the red blood cells tend to break open and spill their contents, probably due to oxidation of the polyunsaturated fatty acids (PUFA) in their membranes. (Cell membranes are rich in PUFA, and those of the red blood cells in particular are exposed to high concentrations of oxygen because of their repeated circulation through the lungs.) In animals, this action tends to occur more readily if the diet is high in PUFA, suggesting that it is indeed the vitamin's role in protecting PUFA from oxidation that prevents the deficiency disease. A person's need for vitamin E may therefore depend on the amount of PUFA consumed. Fortunately, the vitamin and the polyunsaturates tend to occur together in the same foods. (See boxed section at end of chapter.)

Vitamin E is the only one of the fat-soluble vitamins for which toxicity symptoms are unknown in human beings, even prolonged intakes of many times the RDA having no observable effects.

Vitamin E in Foods. About 60 percent of the vitamin E in the diet of Americans comes directly or indirectly from vegetable oils in the form of margarine, salad dressings and shortenings; another 10 percent comes from fruits and vegetables, and smaller percentages come from grains and other products. Soybean oil and wheat germ oil have especially high concentrations of E; cottonseed, corn, and safflower oils rank second to these as superior sources, with a tablespoon of any of these supplying more than 15 milligrams (the RDA) of the vitamin. Other oils contain less (for example, peanut oil supplies about ½ the RDA per tablespoon). Animal fats such as butter and milk fat have negligible amounts of vitamin E.

milligrams, milliliters: see Appendix D.

erythrocyte (eh-REETH-ro-cite) **hemolysis** (he-MOLL-uh-sis): the vitamin E deficiency disease in human beings.

erythrocyte: red blood cell.

> erythro = red
> cyte = cell

hemolysis: bursting of red blood cells.

> hemo = blood
> lysis = breaking

The tocopherol form of the vitamin is readily converted to tocopheronic acid and excreted in the urine.

The Blood Clotting Vitamin: K

Role of vitamin K. Like vitamin D, vitamin K seems to be limited in its versatility. Like D also, however, its presence can make the difference between life and death. At least thirteen different proteins as well as the mineral calcium are involved in the making of a blood clot, and vitamin K is essential for the

K stands for the Danish word Koagulazion (coagulation or clotting).

thrombin: see page 123.

hemorrhagic (hem-o-RAJ-ik) **disease:** the vitamin K deficiency disease.

hemophilia: a hereditary disease having no relation to vitamin K but caused by a genetic defect which renders the blood unable to clot because of lack of ability to synthesize certain clotting factors.

The bacterial inhabitants of the digestive tract are known as the **intestinal flora**.

flora = plant inhabitants

sterile: free of micro-organisms, such as bacteria.

The synthetic substitute usually given for vitamin K is **menadione** (men-uh-DYE-own). See Appendix C.

synthesis of at least four of these proteins, among them the protein thrombin.

Deficiency and toxicity of vitamin K. When any of these factors is lacking, blood clotting cannot occur, and hemorrhagic disease results; when this occurs, if an artery or vein is cut or broken, bleeding goes unchecked. (As usual, this is not to say that the cause of hemorrhaging is always vitamin K deficiency. Another cause is hemophilia, which is not curable by K.) Deficiency of vitamin K may occur under abnormal circumstances when absorption of fat is impaired; that is, when bile production is faulty, or in diarrhea. The vitamin is sometimes administered preoperatively to reduce bleeding in surgery, but is only of value at this time if a vitamin K deficiency exists.

Toxicity can result when too much vitamin K is given, especially to an infant or to a pregnant woman.

Sources of vitamin K. Like vitamin D also, vitamin K is made within your body—but not by you! In your intestinal tract there are billions of bacteria, which normally live in perfect harmony with you, doing their thing while you do yours. One of their "things" is synthesizing vitamin K, which you can absorb. You are not dependent on bacterial synthesis for your K, however, since many foods also contain ample amounts of the vitamin, notably green leafy vegetables, members of the cabbage family, and milk. Brand new babies are commonly susceptible to a K deficiency, for two reasons. First, they are born with a sterile digestive tract; they have their first contact with intestinal bacteria as they pass down their mothers' birth canals, and it takes the bacteria a day or so to establish themselves in babies' intestines. Second, babies may not be fed at the very outset (and breast milk is a poorer source of vitamin K than cow's milk). A dose of vitamin K (usually in a synthetic form similar, but not identical, to the natural vitamin) may therefore be given at birth to prevent hemorrhagic disease of the newborn; it must be carefully administered to avoid toxic overdosing.

Persons taking sulfa drugs, which destroy intestinal bacteria, may also become deficient in vitamin K.

Putting It All Together

ADA Food Exchange System, see pages 33-38.

This chapter concludes the treatment of the vitamins. Another look at diet adequacy and balance is in order at this point. For the B vitamins, meat, milk, breads, cereals, and vegetables are good sources; for vitamin C, the fruits are important. With this consideration of the fat-soluble vitamins, the sixth group of foods in the Exchange System, namely the fat group, assumes significance. The diagram below shows how selections of foods from all six exchange groups will ensure that each nutrient so far discussed will be consumed in the recommended amounts.

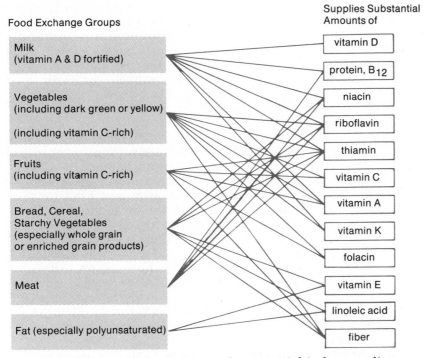

Note: some vitamins known to be essential in human diets have not been studied sufficiently to permit setting a Recommended Daily Allowance. Food sources of these nutrients are less well known than those for the RDA nutrients. However, the variety of selections suggested above is so great that chances are good they will supply most nutrients in amounts sufficient to meet the needs of virtually all members of a healthy population. This diagram will be repeated at the end of the next chapter, where it will be shown that some modifications are necessary to ensure adequacy for certain minerals.

The RDA's for Adults: The Fat-Soluble Vitamins

	Females	*Males*
Vitamin A Activity:	800 RE or 4,000 IU	1,000 RE or 5,000 IU
Vitamin D:	400 IU up to age 22	400 IU up to age 22
Vitamin E Activity:	12 IU	15 IU

The meaning of the RDA has largely been summed up in previous treatments (Chapters 3, 8, 9, 10). A few additional points about measures need to be made here.
RE: retinol equivalents. Vitamin A, like niacin, can

retinol, retinal: see Appendix C.

Beta-carotene yields vitamin A with about 50% efficiency. For structure and conversion, see Appendix C.

assay

all-trans: an alternating arrangement of the H— and —OH groups on the molecule.

d: having a molecular configuration that rotates light clockwise.

be made in the body from precursors (related forms) consumed in foods. Rather than measuring the amount of each different form of the vitamin found in plant and animal foods, the amount of retinol to which each form can be converted is calculated. Thus what is measured is not the actual vitamin A in the food, but the *vitamin A activity* which results when the various related forms are converted to the active form, retinol. The same is true of vitamin E: several related forms are available in the diet, and are converted to the active form, alpha-tocopherol.

IU: international units. Before the chemical structures of these vitamins were known, amounts of them were determined indirectly by seeing how much work they could do. The reasoning of the investigators who needed to make these measurements must have gone like this: "I know I have a certain amount of this vitamin here. If I feed it to test animals who lack only this one vitamin in order to grow, I know that the more I have, the more they'll grow. I'll define as a 'unit' the amount of the vitamin that makes my test animals grow a certain amount." Tests of this kind (assays) were developed for each of the fat-soluble vitamins and the conditions agreed upon among scientists across the world. Thus the originally arbitrary units became standardized and international.

Later, when the vitamins were purified and the structures of their active forms were known, it was possible to find out how much of the purified vitamin actually constituted a unit. It turned out that an IU of vitamin A is equivalent to 0.344 micrograms of crystalline vitamin A acetate, or 0.6 micrograms of (all-trans) beta carotene. An IU of vitamin D is 0.025 micrograms of pure vitamin D_3. An IU of vitamin E is equivalent to one milligram of synthetic *d*-alpha-tocopherol.

U.S.P. units. One other unit sometimes used on labels to describe the amount of vitamin A is the United States Pharmacopeia Unit, which is the same as the IU. Perhaps in the future, both the RDA and the amounts of these vitamins found in foods will be expressed in metric units (micrograms or milligrams), or equivalents, rather than as IU. The transition to this more standardized type of measurement is presently occurring with the vitamin A RDA which was expressed as RE as well as IU for the first time in the 1973 version of the RDA.

Levels chosen for the RDA. The RDA for vitamin A is set at double the minimum necessary to prevent deficiency symptoms; this amount reflects the belief that a liberal intake of this vitamin is to be recommended. For vitamin D the allowance is known to prevent the occurrence of rickets in young children, but how generous this amount may be is hard to say, since people's exposure to sun varies so greatly. The lack of a recommendation for a vitamin D intake from foods after age 22 does not imply that no vitamin D is needed by people above this age, but rather reflects the belief that their needs are largely met by sun-mediated synthesis of the vitamin from its precursors within the body. The vitamin E RDA is still under study, having first been set at 30 IU for adult males in 1968, and then reduced to half that amount in 1973. It is known to vary with the PUFA (polyunsaturated fatty acids) in the diet, but since vitamin E and PUFA occur naturally together in foods, people's intakes of the vitamin will normally keep pace with their PUFA intakes.

polyunsaturated fatty acids (PUFA): see pages 62, 66.

Summing Up

Vitamin A as part of the visual pigment rhodopsin is essential for vision, especially in dim light. Vitamin A is involved in maintaining the integrity of mucous membranes throughout the internal linings of the body and thus in promoting resistance to infection. It helps maintain the health of the skin and is essential for the remodeling of bones during their growth or mending; it plays a part in cell membrane functions, in hormone synthesis, in reproduction, and other functions.

Deficiency of vitamin A causes (1) night blindness due to failure to regenerate rhodopsin, (2) a failure of mucus secretion, which can lead by way of keratinization of the cornea to blindness, (3) disorders of the respiratory, urinogenital, reproductive, and nervous systems, and (4) abnormalities of bones and teeth. Toxicity symptoms are caused by large excesses (10 x RDA) taken over a prolonged period and result only from the preformed vitamin (from supplements or animal products such as liver), not from the precursor carotene, a yellow pigment found in plants.

The Vitamin A RDA (4,000 IU for adult females, 5,000 IU for males), is easily met by periodically consuming the vitamin's richest food sources, such as liver or dark green leafy vegetables, or by consuming daily small amounts of other concentrated sources, such as carrots, cantaloupe, yellow squash, or broccoli. All food sources of vitamin A or carotene have some color.

Vitamin D promotes intestinal absorption of calcium and mobilization of calcium from bone stores (trabeculae), and is therefore essential for the calcification of bones and teeth. Given reasonable exposure to sun, human beings can synthesize this vitamin on the skin from a precursor manufactured by the liver. Deficiency of vitamin D causes the calcium deficiency diseases (rickets in children and osteomalacia in adults); excesses cause abnormally high blood-calcium levels, due to excessive GI absorption and withdrawal from bone, and result in deposition of calcium crystals in soft tissues, such as the kidney and major blood vessels. The U.S. RDA of 400 IU/day is best met by drinking fortified milk; food sources of the vitamin are unreliable. Exposure to sunlight probably ensures vitamin D adequacy for the average adult.

The best substantiated role of vitamin E in human beings is as an antioxidant which protects vitamin A and the polyunsaturated fatty acids (PUFA) from destruction by oxygen. While many E deficiency symptoms have been observed in animals, only one has been confirmed in human beings: hemolysis of red blood cells due to oxidative destruction of the PUFA in their membranes. The RDA of 15 mg/day is more than adequate to prevent this. The human requirement for vitamin E is known to vary with PUFA intake; since the vitamin occurs in proportion to the PUFA in foods it is normally supplied in the needed amounts and deficiencies are seldom observed. Toxicity symptoms are unknown.

Vitamin K, the coagulation vitamin, promotes normal blood clotting; deficiency causes hemorrhagic disease. The vitamin is synthesized by intestinal bacteria and is available from foods such as green vegetables and milk; deficiency is normally seen only in newborns whose intestinal flora have not become established, in people taking sulfa drugs, or in conditions where fat absorption is impaired.

Adequate intakes of all the nutrients so far discussed are ensured by selecting a variety of foods from all six of the Food Exchange Groups, as shown in the diagram on page 357; inclusion of polyunsaturated oils such as those in margarine promotes ample intakes of both linoleic acid and vitamin E.

To Explore Further—

Three interesting articles. The first one takes up the entire issue of the *Journal of Nutrition* and has the up-to-date research on vitamin A:

Rodriquez, M. S. and Irwin, M. I.: A conspectus of research on vitamin A requirements of man. *Journal of Nutrition* 102(17):909-968, 1972.

Kusin, J. A., Reddy, V. and Sivakumar, B.: Vitamin E supplements and the absorption of a massive dose of vitamin A. *American Journal of Clinical Nutrition* 27:774-776, 1974.

Roels, O. A.: Vitamin A physiology. *Journal of the American Medical Association* 214(6):1097-1102, 1970.

This beautifully illustrated biology textbook provides in Chapter 26 a clear, accurate, and detailed explanation of the way the eye works:

Biology Today (a CRM book). Communications Research Machines, Inc., Del Mar, California, 1972.

Highlight Eleven ▬▬▬▬
Vitamin E: A Cure-all?

Is it likely that the RDA Committee is grossly in error about the amounts of vitamin E needed for optimum health? One "common sense" way of approaching such questions (which might be called a "biological" approach) is to consider that mankind evolved on the food it could readily obtain, and that one should not expect to find large natural barriers blocking access to foods needed for health. Let us see what one would have to eat to get 1,500 IU of vitamin E each day . . . (It) would require some eight or nine pounds of oil, something over a gallon a day.
—RONALD M.
    DEUTSCH

You are watching a movie about the early days in the Old West. A wagon is parked in the woods. A man is mixing a batch of something in a washtub and then ladling it into medicine bottles. The scene shifts to the nearby town. The man is now dressed in a high silk hat and swallow-tail coat and is hawking the "medicine" from a makeshift stage on the rear of the wagon. The camera shows the faces in the crowd, mesmerized by the man's tale

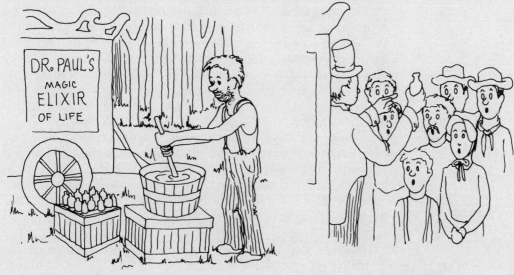

lumbago (lum-BAY-go): rheumatic pain in the joints.

ague (AY-gyoo): a chill, a fit of shivering.

of the wonderful cures this medicine has effected. "Step right up, folks, and buy this time-tested medicine, only a dollar for the giant bottle, and it will cure lumbago, the ague, and rheumatism." The faces in the crowd register concern over some private ailment they wish could be cured by this magical medicine. As you watch the film, you wonder how the people could have been duped by such a show.

Today's magical medicine barkers don't wear high silk hats or mix their potions in washtubs. Those props have gone out of style along with the ailments the old barkers sought to cure. Only the faces in the crowd remain the same. They listen avidly now as the authors of a book on vitamin E hawk their wares on a television talk show. The authors sound knowledgeable, sure of the truth of what they are saying.

There must be some reasonable explanation for so many honest persons believing the many claims of the curative powers of vitamin E, especially as research shows that human beings are rarely deficient in this vitamin. Let us examine what is known about this vitamin that has caught the public's fancy as a cure for everything from impotence in males to the healing of burns.

Male rats, deprived of vitamin E, cease to manufacture sperm. Their testes become atrophied, brownish, and flabby. The rabbit, dog, and monkey show similar damage but the mouse seems remarkably resistant, taking a great deal longer to exhibit these signs.[1]

In pregnant female rats, on a diet lacking vitamin E, the fetus dies during the first week. If vitamin E is restored to the diet during the first week of pregnancy, the fetus can be saved, indicating that the damage from vitamin E deficiency is to the blood supply between the uterus and the placenta.[1]

In animals on a vitamin E deficient diet, the muscles become weak and a kind of muscular paralysis sets in which can be reversed upon restoration of the vitamin to the diet. The extent of the paralysis seems to be related to the amount of polyunsaturated fat in the tissues. The heart muscles of rabbits, sheep, and cattle (plant-eating animals) seem to be especially vulnerable. Fatal heart attacks are not uncommon, taking place before overt signs of the deficiency have developed.[1]

These results of studies of vitamin E deficient animals indicate a possible role for the vitamin in prolonging virility in males, carrying a fetus to full term in females, and keeping muscles healthy, particularly heart muscles. The next logical quest is to see if the vitamin is necessary for maintenance of these functions in human beings.

[1]Horwitt, M. K.: Vitamin E. In *Modern Nutrition in Health and Disease*, 5th ed. Goodhart, R. S. and Shils, M. E., editors. Lea and Febiger, Philadelphia, 1973.

The search to find such a role for vitamin E in human beings has continued for over thirty years and, thus far, has produced negative results. However, the "faces in the crowd" continue to look to vitamin E as the potion which will prolong virility, abolish miscarriages, and cure muscular weakness like that in muscular dystrophy.

Why is it that laboratory findings on vitamin E deficiencies in animals cannot be applied to human beings? To answer this question, we must examine nutrition research on animals in order to understand why we are unable to apply these same methods to research on human beings.

There are two steps necessary in both animal and human research to show that a lack of a nutrient is causing a certain symptom. First, a diet lacking that nutrient, and *only* that nutrient, must be fed. The administration of this diet must result consistently in the appearance of the deficiency symptom. Then when the nutrient is returned to the diet, the deficiency symptom must disappear. In nutrient research using animals, several preparatory steps must be taken before the feeding of the deficient diet can take place.

(1) An animal must be found that does not synthesize the nutrient. For example, vitamin C deficiency research cannot be carried out on rats because rats synthesize vitamin C.

(2) A laboratory feed must be prepared which contains all essential nutrients except the one under study. This is not the simple task of finding a food for the animal; it rather entails the mixing of nutrients in the correct proportion. The result is usually a mixture of synthetic nutrients, since natural foods would very likely contain traces of the nutrient being excluded. Moreover, chemical analysis must show that the mixture is indeed free from the nutrient and that it is not lacking in another essential nutrient.

(3) The animals must have a common heredity and be maintained on similar diets for the same length of time prior to the start of the experiment.

(4) Other variables may need to be controlled for specific nutrients. For example, if it has been shown in other work that a nutrient's absorption is under seasonal hormone control, that fact will need to be considered in the design of the experiment.

When the deficiency symptom has been produced in the laboratory animal and alleviated with the addition of the missing nutrient, researchers can say that *in that species* they have found the lack of a particular nutrient caused a particular symptom. When other laboratories have duplicated these results, they are accepted—*for that species.* Until the laboratory research has shown this relationship to be true for another species

seasonal hormone control: the levels of some hormones vary in a regular cycle. Some of these hormones have an effect on the absorption of nutrients.[2]

[2]Weindling, H. and Henry, J. B.: Laboratory test results altered by the pill. *Journal of the American Medical Association* 229(13):1762-1768, 1974.

of animal, researchers can only theorize that the relationship *may* be true in both.

If one wishes to apply knowledge gained from laboratory animal research to human beings, it is much trickier than to transfer knowledge gained from one species to another in the laboratory. The experimental animal is caged, thus assuring that feed, fluid, temperature, and most of the factors in his environment will be controlled. Also, it is possible to allow the experiment to continue until death intervenes, after which an autopsy can show the effects of the nutritional deficiency on the internal organs.

In human beings, all intake of food and fluid cannot be controlled except in very short-term experiments. In addition, there is no way of knowing that each subject is in a similar nutritional state prior to the beginning of the experiment. This fact necessitates the use of large numbers of human subjects so that the results can be averaged. Finding a large enough population hinders the launching of the experiment and adds to the cost.

Experimentation on human beings must depend on subjects who are free to break the restrictions of the diet or to drop out of the experiment at any time, even if they are being paid to be subjects.

In the case of vitamin E research on human beings, there have been several unique obstacles in addition to these.

(1) Vitamin E is widely distributed in foods. It is, therefore, difficult to compose a diet totally devoid of it.[3]

(2) Vitamin E is one of the fat-soluble vitamins and as such is stored in abundance in the tissues of the body, particularly in adipose tissue. Therefore, it takes a long period of deficiency for the body to be depleted.[3]

Another type of study that can be carried out in human beings is that in which results from many case studies involving a possible vitamin E deficiency are pooled to see if there is a common thread of truth. For the most part these pools have been unproductive. Vitamin E has been shown to be ineffective in the treatment of such diseases as muscular dystrophy, reproductive failure, and heart disease. It seems that these conditions in humans are not the result of vitamin E deficiency states.[4]

In summary, when a symptom has been shown to be caused by a deficiency of a nutrient in several species of laboratory animals, this fact can be used as a pointer toward the existence of the same relationship in human beings. However, until a deficiency symptom can be produced in human subjects by a diet deficient in the nutrient, and then cured by the restoration of

---

[3]The Committee on Nutritional Misinformation of the Food and Nutrition Board, NAS-NRC: Who needs vitamin E? *Journal of the American Dietetic Association* 64:365-366, 1974.
[4]Editorial: Vitamin E in clinical medicine. *Lancet* i:18, 1974.

that nutrient, it cannot be claimed that the symptom is caused by the lack of that nutrient.

The Committee on Nutritional Misinformation of the Food and Nutrition Board of the NAS-NRC prepared a statement[3] which reads in part, "How did these claims (for vitamin E) come about? To some extent, they arose from a misinterpretation of the results of research on experimental animals. . . . The widespread presence of the vitamin in human diets has prevented a deficiency, such as seen in animals under experimental conditions."

The amount of misinformation that has arisen out of the public's failure to understand these distinctions and the profit-making incentive of those who promote misunderstandings of this kind has cost the American public millions of dollars every year.

A flag sign of a spurious claim is the use of: animal research findings misapplied to humans.

There would seem to be another factor operating in the public's ready acceptance of these claims that cannot be substantiated in human beings. The areas where animal research suggests a possible role for vitamin E in the human body are the same which currently are of the greatest concern to people. Emotional appeals for belief in the efficacy of vitamin E fall on willing ears when claims are made that supplements of it will cure, for example, muscular dystrophy. *Muscular dystrophy* is the term given to a hereditary disease afflicting children who usually die at an early age when the respiratory muscles cease to function properly. *Nutritional muscular dystrophy*, on the other hand, is a term that is not in everyday use which denotes the muscular weakness produced in many animals by a deficiency of vitamin E. This deficiency develops an atrophy of the muscles; it can be cured by reintroducing vitamin E into the diet. At no time has there been any evidence in the reliable literature which links this condition to hereditary muscular dystrophy.

It is easy to understand how a layman might be confused by the use of these similar terms for separate conditions, but a nutritionist should be aware of the difference. Some years ago a popular writer[5] on nutrition published in her book an account

muscular dystrophy (DIS-tro-fee)

nutritional muscular dystrophy

[5]Davis, A.: *Let's Eat Right to Keep Fit.* Harcourt, Brace, Jovanovich, Inc., New York, 1970, chapter 20.

of curing a child who had muscular dystrophy with early administration of vitamin E. Throughout the several pages devoted to vitamin E it was apparent that she was not aware of the difference between the two conditions, muscular dystrophy and nutritional muscular dystrophy. The cruelty of such a promise being held out to parents of children with the disease is unconscionable.

Luckily, none of the work that has been done on human beings indicates that toxicity develops at the levels usually taken in supplements.[4] It may be that a person's belief that vitamin E is helping to alleviate a condition, for instance the aging process, may provide a helpful psychological boost which in itself is worth the price of the vitamin. There is one dangerous aspect that should be noted, however: if the taking of the vitamin lulls a user into not seeking the medical help necessary to establish the correct diagnosis and treatment of a serious condition, the vitamin supplement may cost more than anyone can afford to pay.

In the meantime, the modern day hawkers of vitamin E supplements get richer, and as far as is known, no one gets healthier.

To Explore Further—

Teaching Aid, *Vitamin E* by Tappel, A. L., contains 12 slides and explores the cellular function of vitamin E. It can be ordered from:

Director, Education Services
Nutrition Today
101 Ridgely Avenue
Annapolis, Maryland 21404

Suggested Activities

(1) Study your own diet.

Review the record you made in Activity 1 of Chapter 1. Look up each food you ate in Appendix H and record its vitamin A contributions to your diet. (Since vitamin A is highly concentrated in a few foods, you will get a more accurate estimate of your average consumption by averaging three days' intakes.) Which foods make the greatest contribution of this vitamin to your diet?

Compare your intake of vitamin A with the RDA. What percent of the RDA did you consume? Was this enough? If your intake was less than 2/3 of the RDA, find foods or beverages in Appendix H or in Table C11.3 that you would be willing to eat or drink daily to correct this deficiency.

For vitamin D, answer the following questions: did you drink fortified milk (read the label)? eat eggs? liver? Are you in the sun frequently? (Remember, though, excessive exposure to sun can cause skin cancer in susceptible individuals.)

For vitamin E, consider the foods you ate in 24 hours: which of them contained polyunsaturated fatty acids? Vitamin E often accompanies linoleic acid in foods; how much linoleic acid did you consume (Chapter 2, Activity 2)?

(Note: The last Highlight in the book invites you to survey your entire diet for adequacy, balance, and economy. You may wish to save this activity until you have read that Highlight, or you may wish to read the Highlight now for a sense of perspective.)

(2) Be a discriminating listener.

Make a collection of all the statements you read and hear about vitamin E for a week (solicit some from acquaintances, if necessary). What questions would you want to ask the persons making these statements before accepting or rejecting them?

(3) Collect some fallacies of your own.

Go to a health food store and interview the owner or sales person regarding the virtues of the products being sold there. Jot down the claims made and the evidence cited to substantiate them. Which claims would you be inclined to believe on the basis of the evidence? What flag signs of spurious claims can you identify?

12

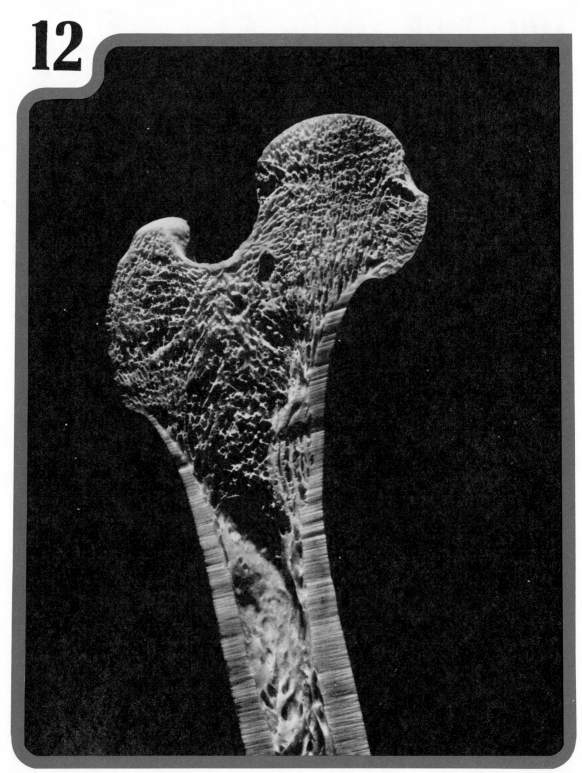

Photo courtesy of Gjon Mili.

The Major Minerals ▬

Professor C. Culmann of
Zurich was . . . designing
a crane, and during a
visit to the laboratory of
his friend and colleague,
Professor Meyer, the
anatomist, he saw the
trabeculae in the head of
a bisected femur. With a
sudden flash of insight he
exclaimed, "That's my
crane!" . . . the cells
which deposit the bone
(are) sensitive to tensions
and compressions . . .
they deposit bone with
respect to these lines of
force.
—JOHN TYLER BONNER

The preceding eleven chapters have been devoted to the first four of the six classes of nutrients: carbohydrate, fat, protein, and the vitamins. Now we move on to the minerals. Before taking up some of the more interesting minerals and presenting the more important details about them, it is possible to make a few generalizations that hold for all of them and by doing so to distinguish them from vitamins.

Minerals are inorganic. The minerals are *elements* like carbon, hydrogen, oxygen, and nitrogen of which the previous four classes of nutrients are composed, and so are simpler than the vitamins, which are *compounds.* Because they contain no carbon, minerals are inorganic; they need never have been part of a living thing. This means that the variety of forms in which they can appear is more limited than for the vitamins; that is, minerals cannot have different chemical structures. Calcium, for example, enters the body as an ion with two positive charges. It may be combined with any of a number of negative ions (phosphate, sulfate, etc.) to form salts in food, and may be more absorbable in these combinations, but in the body these dissociate, and the calcium ion itself is what is used. Iron may enter the body as an ion with either two or three positive charges: this variation (differences in ionic state) is the only variation possible for a mineral element.

element, compound: see Appendix B.

ion: see Appendix B.

salt: a compound composed of two ions other than H^+ and OH^-, such as $CaCl_2$ or $NaCl$ ($Ca^{++}Cl_2^-$ or Na^+Cl^-), held together by an ionic bond (electrostatic attraction). See Chapter 14 and Appendix B.

ionic state: the number of positive or negative charges that an ion may carry. The two states of iron are explained in Appendix B.

369

> Minerals exist as inorganic ions.

Minerals are indestructible. An atom of iron may exist in two different ionic states, and it may be reversibly combined with a variety of other ions in salts, but it never loses its identity —it is always iron. Cooking it, exposing it to air or acid, or mixing it with other substances has no effect on it. In fact, if you burn a food until only the ash is left, and eat the ash, you will be eating all the minerals that were in the food before it was burned! Once they have entered the body proper they are there until excreted; they cannot be changed into anything else.

> Minerals retain their chemical identity.

Because they are indestructible, minerals need no special handling in food to preserve them. You need only make sure that you don't soak them out of the food or throw them away in cooking water. As long as they are kept in the food, they may be handled in any way whatever without any effect on the amount of the mineral present.

By virtue of being ionic, minerals tend to associate with water, and so to form either acid or basic solutions.

> Mineral ions are water soluble.

---

acid-base balance: see page 120. See also Chapter 14.

water balance: see page 118. See also Chapter 14.

Because minerals are water soluble, they influence the acid-base balance of the body, and in associating with other ions in the body fluids they affect the distribution of water into the various body compartments.

Like the water-soluble vitamins, some minerals are readily absorbed into the blood, transported freely there, and readily excreted by the kidneys. There are exceptions, however. Each mineral differs in amounts the body can absorb, and the extent to which they must be specially handled and transported by protein carriers.

> Minerals vary in the amounts absorbed and in the routes and ease of excretion.

Some minerals, like fat-soluble vitamins, must be carried by proteins in the body; others travel freely as ions in the blood and other fluids.

Some are stored like the fat-soluble vitamins, and like them, therefore, are toxic if taken in excess.

Because their presence is not obvious in foods, overdosing with toxic minerals is a real possibility. Other minerals do not accumulate in the body but instead are readily excreted; toxicity with these minerals is not a risk.

The amount of minerals needed in the daily diet varies greatly from a few micrograms for the trace minerals, such as cobalt, to a million times as much, a gram or more, for the major minerals, such as calcium, phosphorus, and sodium. The amounts of each mineral found in the body vary equally widely. Many authorities, therefore, divide them for treatment into two categories: the major minerals and the trace minerals. Both are listed in Table C12.1.

Toxic in excess: iron, copper, mercury, chlorine, magnesium, manganese, iodine, fluorine and others.

> Some minerals require protein carriers.

> Some minerals are toxic in excess.

Table C12.1
The Minerals

Major Minerals	*Trace Minerals*
Calcium	Iron
Phosphorus	Zinc
Potassium	Selenium
Sulfur	Manganese
Sodium	Copper
Chlorine	Iodine
Magnesium	Molybdenum
	Cobalt
	Chromium
	Fluorine

The major minerals are sometimes called the **macronutrient elements**, and are needed in amounts on the order of 1/10 gram or more each day. They comprise 1/10 of 1% of the body weight or more.

The influence of the minerals on the acid-base balance of the body fluids is proportional to the amounts found in the body; thus the major minerals have a much greater effect than the trace minerals on this balance. The special roles of minerals in regulating the pH of body fluids depend on their interaction with water, the last of the nutrients to be discussed in this book.

The trace minerals are the **micronutrient elements**, needed in amounts on the order of 1/100 gram or less each day, and comprising 1/100 of 1% of the body weight or less.

Chapter 14 is reserved for a discussion of these roles, and Table C14.1 in that chapter shows the major minerals divided into the acid- and base-forming classes.

In addition to the mineral elements listed in Table C12.1, most of which have long been familiar to nutritionists, others of which very tiny amounts are needed in the daily diet, have recently come to light. The list of needed mineral elements is lengthening each year as present research continues. Perhaps when all is known the number of minerals proven to be essential in the human diet may number thirty or more. This means that the amount of information available on the minerals, like that on the vitamins, is overwhelmingly great and cannot be treated exhaustively in an introductory text. What is probably most important for the beginning student is to be aware of those minerals which are presently known to be lacking in the diets of significant numbers of people in the United States or in the world. Those most needing emphasis by this criterion are calcium, iron, iodine, and fluorine. Calcium will be discussed here; the next chapter is devoted to the trace minerals.

Calcium, the Wonder Nutrient

A popular book on nutrition[1] which has enjoyed wide sales over the past thirty years makes extravagant claims for calcium. The writer implies that even a very slight decrease in dietary intake will cause these symptoms: air swallowing and indigestion, insomnia and other forms of inability to relax, irritability of the muscles including cramps and spasms, menstrual cramps, hypersensitivity to pain, a tendency to hemorrhage, cataracts, tooth decay, and complications in childbirth. Since there is hardly anyone in the world who is free of all of these symptoms, the naive reader might be led to believe that calcium is a virtual cure-all and that people must make special efforts to procure adequate amounts of this extremely important, even miraculous, nutrient.

The claims made for this wonderful nutrient are based on misunderstanding of the facts about the roles it plays in the body. A deficiency of calcium caused by failure of the *body* to maintain a proper concentration can cause some of these symptoms, but a *dietary* deficiency cannot. The following sections will give you a few details about the known roles of calcium

---

[1]Davis, A.: *Let's Eat Right to Keep Fit.* Harcourt, Brace, Jovanovich, Inc., New York, 1970, chapter 21. This and other unreliable books are on a list of not recommended nutrition books available on request from:
The American Medical Association
530 N. Dearborn Street
Chicago, Illinois 60611.

in the body and will explain why it is that a dietary calcium deficiency has little or no effect on its blood concentration, or on functions mentioned above.

Roles of Calcium

Calcium's most obvious role is as a component of bones and teeth: 99 percent of the calcium in the body is found in these structures. The remaining one percent circulates in the watery fluids of the body, where it performs a number of important functions. Some calcium is found in close association with cell membranes; it appears to be essential for their integrity. The calcium found between and among cells is essential for keeping them in association with each other. In some way it helps to support or maintain the intercellular cement, collagen. In association with cell membranes, calcium helps to regulate the transport of other ions into and out of cells. In association with the membranes of muscle cells, calcium is essential for muscle relaxation. Between nerve and nerve, and between nerve and muscle, calcium must be present for nerve impulse transmission.

collagen: see pages 123, 315.

The mineral must be present if blood clotting is to occur, being one of the fourteen factors directly involved in this process (the other thirteen are proteins; also vitamins, such as vitamin K, are needed for the synthesis of some of these proteins). Calcium is also needed as a cofactor for several enzymes, acting like a coenzyme.

An awareness of all these functions might lead you to believe that *dietary* deficiency of calcium would cause nerve and muscle irritability and possibly nervous tension, hemorrhaging, and the other symptoms mentioned in the first paragraph of this section. Yet in fact none of these things happens with a dietary deficiency of calcium. The reason for this is that the amount of calcium found in the *blood* remains remarkably constant over a wide range of dietary intakes, while deficiency affects the calcium stores in *bones*.

Why the Blood Calcium Level Does Not Change

It is an axiom of nature that if a function is vital to life it will be maintained against tremendous odds. Breathing is such a function; there is no way you can stop breathing voluntarily, as you may remember learning when you were a very small child. Children having tantrums will make furious efforts to hold their breath until they are blue in the face. But even as they begin to lose consciousness, their automatic, instinctive reflexes take over and they begin to breathe again. In the same way, if the beating of the heart is stopped by a heart attack, affecting the node of cells in the heart muscle known as the pacemaker, it turns out that there is a second node of cells nearby, which takes over and keeps the heartbeat going, albeit at a slower pace. As a third example: if the secretion of pancreatic enzymes fails, it turns out that a second set of enzymes similar to the pancreatic ones, produced by the small intestine, continue to work so that some digestion will still proceed.

These examples could be multiplied many hundredfold to show that wherever there is a vital function, backup systems provide for it to be carried out in emergencies. You can tell how important a body function is for survival by observing how many different systems serve the backup function. By this criterion it is obvious that the maintenance of the blood calcium concentration is extremely important for overall health and even life, for calcium is the most closely regulated ion in the body.

The bones hold the body upright, supporting the other tissues of which it is composed, but from the point of view of the blood, this is not their primary role. The bones are a storage place for calcium and other minerals. The minerals can be readily withdrawn from bone in case amounts in the blood begin to fall, and they can be redeposited into bone if blood levels rise too high. The 99 percent of the body's calcium stored in bone constitutes a tremendous reserve.

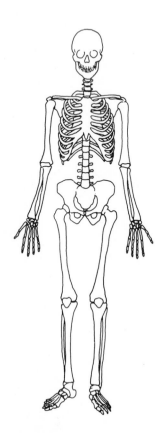

albumins (al-BYOO-mins), **globulins** (GLOB-yoo-lins): two major classes of blood proteins.

The concentration of ionic calcium in the blood is maintained within very narrow limits, around 10 milligrams per 100 milliliters of blood. If it falls or rises ever so slightly, it is immediately corrected. There are four separate systems serving to maintain the blood calcium level. Some calcium in the blood itself is reversibly bound to blood proteins such as the albumins and globulins. The first line of defense against a fall of blood calcium is release of this bound calcium from these proteins. The other three systems are regulated with the help of vitamin D and the hormones.

Other factors influencing calcium absorption are summarized in Chapter 6.

One of these systems is the absorption system. The amount of calcium absorbed from the diet depends on the amount that is needed; that is to say, you will absorb more when you need more. This is most obviously reflected in the increased absorption by a pregnant woman. She may drink the same amount of milk that she did before she was pregnant but will absorb 50 percent of the calcium from it, whereas she formerly absorbed only 30 percent. Thus her body's calcium supply almost doubles, even if her food intake does not change at all. Similarly, growing children will absorb 50 or 60 percent of ingested calcium; when their growth slows or stops (and their bones are no longer demanding a net increase in calcium content each day), their absorption falls to the adult level of about 30 percent.

The second system is a storage system. Calcium is reversibly stored in the trabeculae of the bones. When blood calcium concentration rises, more is put away inside these lacy filaments. When calcium is needed in the blood, the trabeculae break down again. The exquisite photograph at the opening of this chapter shows the architecture of bone.

The third system involves the kidneys. The kidneys are sensitive to blood calcium concentrations and will excrete more when they experience a rise in blood calcium above the acceptable level and less when they experience a fall.

These three systems are regulated by two hormones, one secreted by the parathyroid glands, the other by the thyroid gland. The first, parathormone, is released whenever blood calcium falls below 7 milligrams per 100 milliliters. Parathormone affects all three systems, stimulating (1) increased absorption in the intestines, (2) release of calcium from bone trabeculae, and (3) increased retention by the kidneys. The other, calcitonin, is secreted by the thyroid gland when blood calcium rises above tolerance and inhibits the release of calcium from bone. For these reasons, *blood* calcium concentrations are very little affected by varying dietary intakes.

To say that *dietary* calcium deficiency is never reflected in abnormal blood levels of this mineral is not to say that abnormal blood levels of calcium are never observed. In fact, sometimes blood calcium does rise above normal, causing a condition known as calcium rigor. When this happens, the muscle fibers contract and cannot relax. Similarly, calcium levels may fall below normal in the blood, causing calcium tetany—also a situation in which uncontrolled contraction of muscle tissue occurs, due to a change in the stimulation of nerve cells. These conditions do not reflect dietary lack or excess of calcium, but are due to lack of vitamin D or to glandular malfunctions resulting in abnormal amounts of the hormones which regulate blood calcium concentration.

On the other hand, a chronic dietary deficiency of calcium or a chronic deficiency due to poor absorption can, over the course of years, have a pronounced effect on the structure of the bones. It is on the bones, not on the blood, that calcium deficiency has its impact.

Calcium Deficiency

The disease rickets has already been mentioned in connection with vitamin D deficiency. In rickets, often the amount of calcium available from the diet may be adequate, but it passes

trabeculae (singular, **trabecula**) (tra-BECK-you-lee, tra-BECK-yoo-luh): lacy filaments inside bone which serve as a storage site for calcium and phosphorus. They are readily broken down and built up again in response to the body's changing needs for these minerals.

parathyroid (para-THIGH-royd) **glands:** four small glands situated on the surface of the thyroid gland, two on each side, which produce the hormone parathormone.

thyroid gland: gland in the neck, which produces the hormones thyroxine (see page 316) and calcitonin (see below).

parathormone (para-THOR-mone): hormone secreted by parathyroid glands in response to low blood calcium concentrations, causing increased intestinal absorption, release from bones, and increased renal resorption of calcium.

calcitonin (cal-si-TONE-in): actually there are two calcitonins, one secreted by the thyroid gland in response to high blood calcium concentration, inhibiting release of calcium from bone, and the other secreted by the parathyroid. The former is more properly called **thyrocalcitonin.**

calcium rigor: hardness or stiffness of the muscles.

calcium tetany: intermittent spasms of the extremities due to nervous and muscular excitability.

rickets

through the intestinal tract without being absorbed into the body, thus leaving the bones undersupplied. Vitamin D deficiency is the most common cause of this condition. The symptoms of rickets have been described (Table C11.4); in children, the failure to deposit sufficient calcium in bone causes growth retardation and skeletal abnormalities. In adults, the disease may set in after a normal childhood during which calcium intake and absorption were adequate, and the skeleton has become fully calcified. A prolonged inadequate calcium uptake during adulthood, often due to vitamin D deficiency, may cause the gradual and insidious removal of calcium from the bones, resulting in altered composition or reduced density of the bones in old age, making them fragile.

Altered composition of the bones is reflected in **osteomalacia**, the condition in which the bones become soft. See page 352.

The fragility of the bones is most severe in the pelvic bone, which may become so brittle that it breaks when the person is walking. You may have heard of an old person who fell and broke her hip. What often actually happens is that while she is walking, her hip breaks and then she falls.

Reduced density of the bones results in **osteoporosis** (oss-tee-oh-pore-OH-sis), literally "porous bones."

osteo = bone

While rickets in children and osteomalacia in adults appear to be vitamin D- and calcium-related, the causes of osteoporosis are unclear. A net calcium loss occurs in many adults, especially in women after menopause or hysterectomy, suggesting that hormonal changes are responsible. Many minerals and vitamins are required to form and stabilize the structure of bones, including magnesium, fluoride, vitamin A, and others. Any of these may be essential for preventing osteoporosis. One obvious line of defense, however, is to maintain a lifelong adequate intake of calcium.

Food Sources of Calcium

calcium RDA for adults: 800 mg/day (= 0.8 grams/day).

Calcium is found almost exclusively in a single class of foods—milk and dairy products—as shown in Table C12.2. For this reason, if for no other, members of this group must be included in the diet daily. Since one cup of milk contains almost 300 milligrams of calcium while the RDA for adults is 800 milligrams, an intake of two cups of milk each day provides more than 2/3 RDA, an amount which is adequate for most people. The other dairy food source of calcium which contains comparable amounts is cheese. One slice of cheese (one ounce) contains about two-thirds as much calcium as a cup of milk. For nonmilk drinkers, greens are an important food, a one cup serving providing as much calcium (and riboflavin) as a cup of milk.

The absurdity of attempting to meet the calcium RDA in any way other than by consuming two servings a day of these foods can be demonstrated by listing the amounts of other foods you would have to consume instead: six heads of iceberg lettuce,

ten cups of cooked green beans, twelve oranges or eggs, or
twenty cups of strawberries!

Table C12.2
Fifty Foods Showing Amounts of Calcium

The foods listed below are the fifty that rank highest as sources of
calcium from those which are found on the ADA Exchange Lists and
which also have been analyzed for nutrient composition. Serving sizes
are the sizes listed in the Exchange Lists except for meat, where 3-
ounce servings are shown. The numbers 1 through 6 refer to the numbers of the Exchange Lists: 1 = Milk, 2= Vegetables, 3 = Fruit, 4 =
Bread, 5L = Lean Meat, 5M = Medium-Fat Meat, 5H = High-Fat Meat,
6 = Fats and Oils. Numbers in parentheses are the item numbers on
the Table of Food Composition (Appendix H).

Exchange Group	Food (Item Number)	Serving Size	Calcium Milligrams
5L	Sardines with bones (142)	3 ounces	372
1	2% fat fortified milk (3)	1 cup	352
1	Canned evaporated milk (4)	½ cup	318
1	Skim milk (2)	1 cup	296
1	Dry skim milk (6)	1/3 cup	293
1	Whole milk (1)	1 cup	288
1	Yogurt (72)	1 cup	272
5L	Oysters (140)	¾ cup	170
5L	Canned salmon with bones (141)	3 ounces	167
2	Collard greens (195)	½ cup	145
2	Dandelion greens (201)	½ cup	126
2	Spinach (233)	½ cup	106
		10% of U.S. RDA of 1 gram	
2	Mustard greens (208)	½ cup	97
4	Corn muffin (419)	1	96
5M	Creamed cottage cheese (16)	¼ cup	58
4	Pancake (442)	1	58
3	Orange (294)	1	54
2	Broccoli (179)	½ cup	49
4	Dried beans (148)	½ cup	45
4	Pumpkin (229)	¾ cup	43
4	Muffin (435)	1	42
4	Lima beans (167)	½ cup	40
3	Tangerine (330)	1	34
2	Cabbage (183)	½ cup	32
2	Green beans (168)	½ cup	32
6	Cream, light (37)	2 tbsp	30
4	Winter squash (235)	½ cup	29
2	Turnips (246)	½ cup	27
5M	Egg (73)	1	27
2	Summer squash (234)	½ cup	26
3	Dried fig (268)	1	26
2	Onions (211)	½ cup	25
4	Whole wheat bread (372)	1 slice	25
2	Brussels sprouts (180)	½ cup	25
4	Mashed potato (226)	½ cup	24
2	Carrots (190)	½ cup	24

Table C12.2 (continued)

Exchange Group	Food (Item Number)	Serving Size	Calcium Milligrams
3	Blackberries (261)	½ cup	23
4	White bread (353)	1 slice	21
3	Pink grapefruit (271)	½	20
3	White grapefruit (270)	½	19
4	Rye bread (350)	1 slice	19
4	Green peas (215)	½ cup	19
5M	Peanut butter (160)	2 tbsp	18
3	Strawberries (328)	¾ cup	17
5L	Chipped beef (92)	3 ounces	17
2	Asparagus (165)	½ cup	15
4	Hamburger bun (471)	½	15
3	Raspberries (325)	½ cup	14
3	Cantaloupe (263)	¼	14
4	Sweet potatoes (239)	¼ cup	14

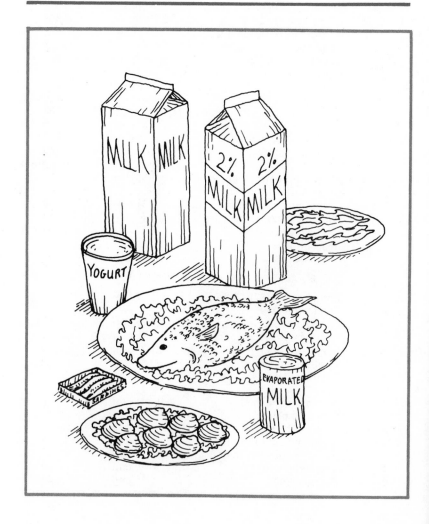

The amount of calcium recommended for the daily diet is so great that it cannot be packaged in a single pill that could be swallowed. To be absorbed, calcium is combined into an organic salt, such as calcium gluconate or calcium lactate, this process makes the pill extremely bulky. Six hundred milligrams of calcium in this salt comprises six pills, each the diameter of a quarter and the thickness of four quarters. You therefore never find significant amounts of calcium in vitamin-mineral supplements of the type that are to be taken once a day.

Many vitamin-mineral supplements do contain some calcium, however. There are two ways to read a label: one is to read what it contains; the other is to read how much. A reading of a list of ingredients in a pill that contains calcium might mislead unaware consumers into believing their calcium needs would be met by the pill. However, a reading of the amount, "10 milligrams," coupled with the knowledge that the calcium RDA is 800 milligrams, would reveal that the pill supplied only one-eightieth of the amount recommended for daily intake. This discussion should remind you of a point made once before (page 107): use a yardstick.

It is important to remember, too, that pills do not supply the relative amounts of nutrients that are in the best balance for your overall health. A typical calcium supplement, for example, is labeled with the instructions to take six a day. Yet six pills a day will supply less than 50 percent of your calcium RDA, and 500 percent of your vitamin D! (Vitamin D is added to the pill to enhance the absorption of calcium.)

On the other hand, two cups of fortified skim milk would supply the following percentages of the U.S. RDA: calcium, 60 percent; vitamin D, 50 percent; protein, 40 percent; vitamin A, 50 percent; thiamin, 12 percent; and riboflavin, 50 percent; plus 24 grams of carbohydrate in the form of lactose. You will recall from Chapter 6 that calcium absorption is favored by some of these other nutrients. Once again, a point made previously (page 4) is relevant: there are fringe benefits to eating a nutrient in a natural food as opposed to a purified nutrient preparation.

U.S. RDA: see page 419.

For most people, the obvious way to meet calcium needs is to include milk and dairy products in the diet daily. This is especially important for pregnant or lactating women and for children in the growing years (their calcium balance must be positive to permit good skeletal growth). Adults concerned with the feeding of children who dislike milk will find it helpful to learn how to conceal milk in foods. Ice cream and ice milk are often

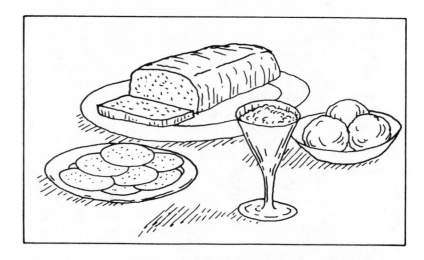

acceptable substitutes for regular milk, while puddings, custards, and baked goods can be prepared in such a way that they also contain appreciable amounts of milk. Powdered skim milk, which is an excellent and inexpensive source of protein and other nutrients including calcium, can be added to many foods (such as cookies and meatloaf) in preparation. For children with a milk allergy, a calcium-rich substitute such as fortified soy milk must be found.

The word *daily* should be stressed with respect to food sources of this mineral. Because of its limited ability to absorb calcium, the body cannot handle massive doses periodically but rather needs frequent opportunities to take in small amounts.

A generalization that has been gaining strength throughout this book is supported by the information given here about calcium: a balanced diet that supplies a variety of foods is one which best guarantees adequacy for all essential nutrients. Calcium is found lacking wherever milk is underemphasized in the diet—whether through ignorance, simple dislike, lactose intolerance, or allergy. By contrast, iron is found lacking whenever milk is overemphasized, as the next chapter will show.

milk allergy: the commonest food allergy in people caused by the protein in raw milk. Sometimes overcome by cooking the milk to denature the protein; sometimes "cured" by abstinence from, and gradual reintroduction to, milk. See also lactose intolerance, page 27.

When iron deficiency is caused by overemphasis on milk, the resulting anemia is called **milk anemia.**

Other Major Minerals

The other major minerals are as interesting and as vital to life as calcium and iron. Recalling the principle with which we began, however, that it is more important to understand how and why certain generalizations are true about nutrition than to learn many isolated details, we are choosing to present the essential facts about the other major minerals in table form (Table C12.3). The prevalence of nutritional deficiencies in America is the subject of the following Highlight.

Table C12.3
Summary of Facts About Major Minerals

Mineral	Adult RDA	Roles in Body	Deficiency	Major Food Sources
Calcium	800 mg	(see page 376)	rickets osteoporosis osteomalacia (see Table C11.4)	milk cheese greens
Phosphorus	800 mg	bones: associates with calcium in structure of bones and teeth; ATP: part of the energy carrier; DNA, RNA: part of the genetic material; enzymes: part of many enzymes; a major intracellular electrolyte (see Chapter 14)	unlikely	protein-rich foods grains
Potassium	(none)	a major intracellular electrolyte (see Chapter 14)	occurs in dehydration (see Chapter 14)	many
Sulfur	(none)	part of many body compounds (certain amino acids, thiamin)	unlikely	protein-rich foods
Sodium	(none)	bones: large amounts found there; a major extracellular electrolyte (see Chapter 14)	occurs in dehydration (see Chapter 14)	salt, salty foods, seafood other animal foods
Chlorine	(none)	a major extracellular electrolyte (see Chapter 14)	occurs in dehydration (see Chapter 14)	see sodium
Magnesium	350 mg (M) 300 mg (F)	bones: large amounts found there; cofactor for many enzyme systems including those involved in protein synthesis, also necessary for photosynthesis in plants where it forms part of the chlorophyll molecule	occurs in PCM, alcoholism, and disorders of calcium metabolism	seeds, grains, nuts, greens

Summing Up

Of the major minerals or macronutrient elements—calcium, phosphorus, potassium, sulfur, sodium, chlorine, and magnesium—calcium was selected for emphasis in this chapter. Ninety-nine percent of the body's calcium is a structural component of the bones and teeth; these structures, in addition to their obvious roles, serve as a reserve to help maintain blood calcium at a constant concentration. The one percent of body calcium found in body fluids helps maintain cell membrane integrity, intercellular cohesion, transport of substances into and out of cells, and transmission of nerve impulses. It is also a factor essential for blood clotting and acts as a cofactor in some enzyme systems.

Ionic calcium concentration in the blood is held constant by equilibrium between free and bound calcium, and by the hormones parathormone and calcitonin with the help of vitamin D. Parathormone is secreted in response to low calcium concentration, and, with the help of vitamin D, enhances calcium absorption from the GI tract, resorption by the kidney, and release from the stores in bone trabeculae. Calcitonin is secreted in response to high calcium concentration and enhances deposit of calcium into bone. Abnormal calcium concentrations in blood reflect abnormal amounts of these hormones or of vitamin D in the system; dietary calcium lack has its impact on bone.

Calcium deficiency in the body may be caused directly by inadequate calcium intakes over a prolonged period of time, or indirectly by vitamin D deficiency, which suppresses calcium absorption. The diseases which result are rickets and osteomalacia, already described in Chapter 11.

The calcium RDA (800 mg a day for adults) is easily met by consuming two or more cups of milk or equivalent dairy products such as cheese; fortified soy milk is an alternative in the case of milk allergy or lactose intolerance. The only other rich food source of calcium is dark green leafy vegetables, one cup of cooked greens being equivalent to a cup of milk in calcium content. Daily consumption of calcium-containing foods is preferable to infrequent large amounts. Overconsumption of milk, if it displaces foods rich in iron, can cause iron-deficiency anemia.

Phosphorus is abundant in foods, and therefore deficiencies are highly unlikely. It participates with calcium in forming the crystals of bone, and therefore composes a large proportion of the minerals found in the body. Unlike calcium, it is not difficult to absorb and tends to follow calcium passively into the bloodstream. *Sulfur*, similarly, while a major mineral constituent of body tissues, is abundant in the diet, and deficiencies are unknown.

Magnesium, whose role in the synthesis of body proteins places it in a key position with respect to all body functions (recall the ubiquity and importance of proteins from Chapter 4), is seldom found lacking in human beings, except in conditions which aggravate dietary protein deficiency, such as kwashiorker or alcoholism. However, persons on low-calorie diets may have trouble meeting the magnesium RDA. The deficiency of magnesium causes severe renal, neuromuscular, and cardio-vascular disorders.

Potassium, sodium, phosphorus, and chlorine are the main participants (with protein) in maintaining the water balance and body fluid pH; they are treated in Chapter 14.

Highlight Twelve
Hunger in America

Hunger is a very personal matter. You cannot feel compassion and concern over a statistic—"X number of children go to school in the United States each day with no breakfast." Until that figure is translated in your mind into a child who must sit in a classroom and perform intellectual tasks on an empty stomach, it is difficult to comprehend the agony of hunger.

Hunger is hidden today. Every day middle class Americans drive on superhighways over and around the very poor and forget that the poor are there, because they reside in the back roads and in the inner city slums. In the depression of the thir-

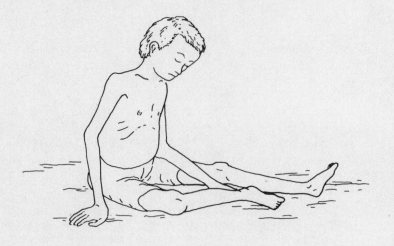

384

ties the hungry were visible. They stood in long lines outside soup kitchens set up in church basements and said by their presence, "Look, I am hungry. I have no money to buy food." Today, newspapers report daily the immense sums spent on food stamps and welfare programs and the American people say to themselves, "Surely, there are no hungry people in the United States today!"

How do we know if there is hunger in America? What can we do to find out? Also, what do we mean by *hunger*? Are we speaking of an empty stomach or of the malnutrition of imbalance? The nutritionist is concerned with both these definitions of hunger: the no-food hunger of the child who goes without breakfast and the hunger caused by the limited variety or amount of food that results in malnutrition. A nutrition survey is the only known way of discovering the hungry in a population. This Highlight is intended to show you first, how the Ten-State Survey was conducted; second, what kinds of hunger were found; and third, to give you some examples of the kinds of people who were hungry.

In 1968-70, the Federal Government mandated a nutritional survey for the United States. Dr. Arnold E. Shaefer, who had conducted many such surveys for the ICNND in other countries, was selected to head the project. Ten states (California, Kentucky, Louisiana, Massachusetts, Michigan, South Carolina, Texas, Washington, New York State, and West Virginia) and New York City were chosen to represent geographic, ethnic, economic, and other features of the whole United States. In all, 62,532 people were surveyed.

Prior to describing the Ten-State Nutrition Survey, let us briefly examine the ways in which the level of a nutrient in the body can be measured. If we look at the route the nutrient follows from ingestion to metabolism, storage, or excretion, we can see that there are places where the nutrient or its metabolite are accessible to the diagnostician. When a nutrient comes into the body, the amount of the intake can be calculated; and after digestion and absorption into the blood stream, the nutrient level in the blood can be measured. Furthermore, if other tissues are in need of the nutrient so that they pick it up from the blood and metabolize it, the metabolites will be put back into the bloodstream, filtered out by the kidney, and excreted in the urine; therefore, presence of both the unused nutrient and the metabolite can be measured in the urine. Also, if the tissues of the body are able to store an excess of the nutrient, this storage form of the nutrient can be measured. The level of the nutrient then can be measured on intake, in the blood, in the urine, and in the storage sites.

One of the methods of determining the nutritional status of a population is to study its food intake. The amount and kinds

undernutrition: across-the-board deficiency of nutrients that accompanies calorie deficiency, or "hunger."

malnutrition: deficiency, excess, or imbalance of nutrients or calories.

ICNND: Interdepartmental Committee on Nutrition for National Defense.

Means of assessing nutritional status:

(1) dietary intake records

of food consumed by a person can be recorded either by keeping a diet record or in reply to an interviewer's questions. The tables of food composition are used to calculate the nutrient content of the diet, which is then compared to the RDA. The assumption is made, when this method is employed, that the RDA applies to the persons studied. There are wide variations between individuals in their need for specific nutrients, so the larger the sample of the population the more validity there is in the use of the RDA as the yardstick. Two other assumptions are also made: that everyone absorbs the same amount of the nutrient and that the foods analyzed in the Food Composition Tables have the same nutrient content as the food consumed by the subject. It must be remembered, also, that the RDA's are based on the nutrient needs of healthy persons, thus a survey team would need to include a medical examination for the presence of such conditions as intestinal parasites before it can properly compare the nutrient intake with the RDA. Inherent in the process of obtaining a diet record is the matter of honesty on the part of those being interviewed and of the interviewer's skill.

(2) clinical tests

In the same way that the RDA's have been established as yardsticks for measuring the level of nutrient intake, standards for normal plasma and serum levels of many nutrients have been established against which the level of the nutrient in the blood can be compared. Some of the blood tests require sophisticated equipment and techniques and so are unsuitable for field surveys; but many, such as the test for protein, are simple to perform and are widely used.

A urine sample can furnish a wealth of information about what is happening in the cells. The urine can be used to tell if the cells had no need of the nutrient or if the cells hungrily used all that they could obtain from the bloodstream. For example, a test load of a vitamin, such as thiamin, can be given and the amount of it that is excreted in the urine can be measured. If a large percentage is excreted, we say the tissues must have been saturated and the dietary intake must have been adequate. On the other hand, if very little is excreted, the tissues must have been in need of it, and, therefore, the diet must have been inadequate. If, in children, less than 10 percent of a test load of thiamin is excreted it is understood that there is a dietary deficiency which has probably extended over many months.[1] Sometimes the end product of the metabolism of the nutrient, instead of the nutrient itself, is measured. In these cases a higher level of excretion of the metabolite would indicate a greater desaturation of the cells and a greater dietary deficiency of the nutrient.

[1]Krause, R. F.: Laboratory aids in the diagnosis of malnutrition. In *Modern Nutrition in Health and Disease.* 4th ed. Wohl, M. G. and Goodhart, R. S., editors. Lea and Febiger, Philadelphia, 1968.

If a nutrient is one which is stored in the tissues, it may be possible to test for the nutrient in the storage sites. For example, there is no excretion route for iron and one of the places where it is stored is the bone marrow. A test sample of the bone marrow, usually the marrow of the sternum (breast bone), can be taken and will reveal the amount of iron present in storage form. Nutritional surveys, however, would probably favor using a simpler technique for discovering iron status, such as finding the level of hemoglobin, the iron-containing protein in the blood.

Thus it can be seen that the status of a nutrient can be determined by analyzing the nutrient intake and comparing it with the RDA, or by various biochemical tests of the nutrient or its metabolites in the blood, urine, or storage sites, and comparing the results with normal values. These tests can reveal the earliest signs of deficiency and are widely used for this purpose in nutritional surveys.

If a deficiency of a nutrient continues long enough or is very severe, the storage sites will be depleted; eventually, the damage will become evident in the tissues of the skin, eyes, hair, teeth, tongue, and mouth. These are the classical signs of deficiency: signs such as cracks at the corners of the mouth, glossitis, etc., which the trained investigator looks for during the physical examination.

(3) physical examination

"The plan of the Ten-State Nutrition Survey incorporated the following essential basic measurements: clinical assessment including medical history, physical examination, various anthropometric measurements such as height, weight, and subcutaneous fat, and X-ray measurements of bones; biochemical measurements of the levels of various substances in blood and urine; dietary assessment of nutrient and usual patterns of food consumption; dental examinations; and such related data as socio-economic status, food sources, and educational status."[2]

(4) anthropometric measures

The results of this survey called forth protests from groups who believed that their states had been maligned by the reports. Such protests were probably due to a misunderstanding of the purpose of the survey and of the sampling techniques used.

Any survey of a population as large as that of the United States must choose a sample of that population which will provide the data needed to meet the purposes of the survey. In the case of the Ten-State Survey (also called the "National Nutrition Survey"), the purpose was to discover those segments which were malnour-

[2]*Ten-State Nutrition Survey 1968-1970.* U.S. Department of Health, Education and Welfare. DHEW Publication No. (HSM) 72-8130. Center for Disease Control, Atlanta, Georgia.

ished. It was assumed that malnutrition would be more likely to occur among the low income groups. Thus the population of a state as an entirety was not surveyed, but, rather, low income groups within each state. The 1960 U.S. Census was used to identify areas within the state most likely to contain large numbers of people with income below the poverty line.

Whenever the results of a survey are used to make generalizations, they must be interpreted with caution. In the case of the Ten-State Survey, the population studied was a segment selected because it was especially likely to be malnourished.

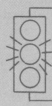

CAUTION WHEN YOU READ!

The Ten-State Survey does not reflect the nutritional status of the *average* American, but of the *unfortunate* American.

The results were given in relation to age, sex, ethnic background, and location (whether the person resided in a low-income or high-income state). The following is a brief summary of the Ten-State Survey findings:

(1) *Clinical*—Few severe deficiencies were established by the clinical examinations. This does not imply that there were no deficiencies present, but, rather, that they were not prolonged or severe enough for the clinical signs to appear.

Deficiencies that have not yet yielded clear-cut clinical signs are **subclinical deficiencies.**

(2) *Anthropometric*—Persons with higher income had greater height, weight, fatness and skeletal weight, larger head circumference, earlier skeletal maturation, and earlier tooth eruption. Blacks were taller than whites and were more advanced in skeletal and dental development. Obesity was more prominent in adult women, especially in Black women (see Figure H12.1). One of the most significant findings was that the trends seen among the children persisted into adulthood, underscoring the effect of early poverty on later development.

(3) *Dental*—Among the children, Spanish Americans were most in need of dental care. Among adults, Spanish Americans and Blacks had the greatest needs. There was a relationship found between the intake of sugar and dental caries among adolescents, and between low income and dental caries in all groups.

(4) *Hemoglobin and related measurements*—Generally, higher dietary iron intakes correlated with higher hemoglobin levels. Black populations particularly showed a prevalence of low hemoglobin in all income groups.

(5) *Protein*—Deficient values for protein were not as wide-

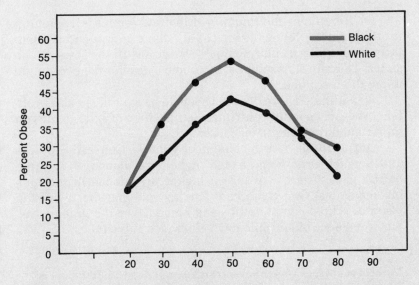

Figure H12.1. Percent Obese of White Female Adults Compared with Black Female Adults by Age for Low and High Income Ratio States—Ten-State Nutrition Survey (1968-1970).

spread as for some of the other parameters. The highest incidence was found among Blacks and Spanish Americans. Protein deficiency correlated with low income level. Pregnant and lactating women exhibited more dietary deficiency and lower serum values, but protein intake seemed to be generally adequate for most groups.

(6) *Vitamin A and carotene*—The data show that vitamin A nutritional status is a major public health concern, particularly among adolescents and Spanish Americans (see Figure H12.2).

(7) *Vitamin C*—There seems to be no cause for concern regarding vitamin C nutriture among the groups studied. There was a greater incidence of low values for Blacks in the low-income states, and also a greater incidence, generally, among males than among females.

Figure H12.2. Percent of Persons Having Deficient or Low Plasma Vitamin A Values by Age, Sex, and Ethnic Group for Low Income Ratio States—Ten-State Nutrition Survey (1968-1970).

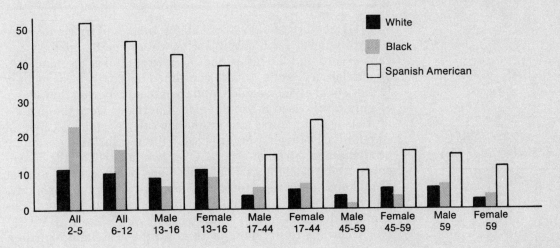

(8) *Riboflavin and thiamin*—Riboflavin status is a potential problem among young persons of all ethnic groups and particularly among Blacks and Spanish Americans in the low-income states. Thiamin status appears to be no cause for concern in the populations studied.

(9) *Iodine*—There does not seem to be a public health problem in regard to iodine nutriture. Iodinization of salt remains an important public health measure.

(10) *Multiple low biochemical values*—Generally, Blacks and Spanish Americans had a higher prevalence of multiple deficiencies. There was also a higher prevalence in the low-income states. One significant finding was that the fewer the years of school completed by the homemaker the greater was the prevalence of multiple low values (see Table H12.1).

Table H12.1
Percent of Persons Under Seventeen Years of Age with Deficient or Low Biochemical Values in Two or More of Six Biochemicals Tested by Years of School Completed by Wife of Head of Family or Female Head of Family for Low Income Ratio States—Ten-State Nutrition Survey (1968-1970)

Years of School Completed	*Number of Persons with Six Bio-chemical Tests*	*Persons with Two or More Deficient or Low Biochemical Tests*	
		Number	*Percent*
TOTAL	2,363	557	23.6
None	122	49	40.2
1-4	369	109	29.5
5-8	896	206	23.0
9-12	899	181	20.1
Post High School	24	4	16.7
College	49	8	16.3
Other	4	0	0.0

(11) *Dietary intake*—In all states, intakes of nutrients were generally lower for Blacks than for whites and Spanish Americans except that the latter had the lowest intakes of vitamin A. Foods rich in vitamin A were consumed on a daily basis by only 15 percent of all households; and 20 percent reported they never or only rarely used them. Spanish Americans were the highest in their use of cereals and grains for calories; they received a substantially lower percentage of their calories from dairy products than did other groups. Over two-thirds of all the households used fresh milk as a beverage daily, while over 80 percent of all households reported *never* using dry skim milk as a beverage. Evidently more education is needed in the use of economical, dry skim milk.

According to the data gathered in the Ten-State Nutrition

Survey, then, target groups in need of help regarding their nutrition are Blacks, Spanish Americans, adolescents, and low income groups. The nutrients in which the largest numbers were deficient were iron, vitamin A, and riboflavin, with protein being a problem for pregnant and lactating women.

There is good reason to believe that the situation for the poor is worse now than it was when the Ten-State Survey was completed in 1970. Inflation and rising food prices have hurt the food buying power of the poor much more than the middle and upper income groups. In the first place, the poor spend a far larger portion of their income on food; it was estimated in March 1973 that the very poorest spend about 61 percent on food. Also, the prices of the foods they eat have risen much faster than those of the foods middle-income and rich people eat. For example, between December 1970 and March 1974 margarine prices increased 63 percent, while butter prices rose only 8.9 percent; pork sausage prices increased 68.8 percent while rib roast prices increased 43.3 percent; dried beans' prices increased 256.3 percent while canned tomato prices increased 20.5 percent; and the price of rice increased 124.3 percent while the price of broccoli increased only 13.3 percent.[3] A meal, then, of rib roast, canned tomatoes, and broccoli with butter increased in price by less than 30 percent; during that same period the meal that a poor family might eat of pork sausage, dried beans and rice with margarine increased in price by more than 100 percent.

Probably one of the reasons for the great increase in prices of the poor person's choices of foods in this period was that middle-income people, caught in inflation and rising prices, were able to lower their food costs by choosing less expensive foods, thereby increasing the demand for these foods and thus increasing their price. But poor people cannot spend much less for food. Therefore, as their utility, transportation, and other costs have gone up, their only choices have been to go hungry or to go into debt.

There are two groups in the United States whose problems of poverty and thus of hunger are unique: the migrant farm workers and the native American Indians. Migrant workers, even though they are essential to the food industry, have been excluded from the protective labor legislation which the rest of America's labor force takes for granted. In 1971, migrant workers' average annual income was $1,580, down from $1,732 in 1969. Since they move constantly with the harvest from state to state, they cannot obtain the social services available to other poor people. Many of these services have a residence require-

[3]*National Nutrition Policy Study—1974.* Hearings before the Select Committee on Nutrition and Human Needs. Part 3—Nutrition and Special Groups, 93rd Congress. U.S. Government Printing Office, Washington, 1974.

ment and their offices are located in the cities. Typically, migrant workers don't even know they are eligible for these services; and if they did know, they would still have to lose a day's pay and find transportation to get to the offices. With their fluctuating pay, they cannot even take advantage of food stamps, since they cannot accumulate the cash to buy them. Their children, since they are rarely in school, cannot participate in school lunch programs.[3] All these circumstances lock the migrant farm worker into a cycle of no education, poor nutrition, poor health, and poverty.

The native Americans, too, are locked into a virtually unbreakable cycle. A total of 543,000 live on reservations. Their annual family income has been estimated as $1,900. Forty percent of Indians living on reservations are below the federal poverty line. They pay 28 percent more for food than people in urban areas. Their median age is 18.4 years as compared to the U.S. median age of 28.1 years. Infant mortality is 22.4 percent higher than the national rate. The postneonatal death rate is 11.2 per 1,000 births compared to the U.S. rate of 4.9. Eight cases of kwashiorkor and nine of marasmus were reported by the Tuba City Hospital on the Navajo Reservation in Arizona between 1969 and 1973. Obesity has been reported in some tribes at a rate of 60 to 90 percent.[3] These statistics point to severe nutrition problems among the Indians.

There are other groups in our society, such as the elderly and infants, that are in need of more and better food, but that are not easily identified because they are scattered throughout the well-nourished population. The elderly poor have multiple difficulties which affect their nutritional status. No transportation to market, inability to cook, no facilities for cooking, ill-fitting dentures, mental depression, and crippling diseases of old age are a few of the obstacles they face.

Infants in poor families are increasingly at risk, nutritionally, because of the trend away from breast feeding. That such a trend does exist is indicated by a study in rural Mississippi which discovered that the majority of mothers did not attempt to breast feed and of those who did only 16 percent nursed the baby for longer than six months.[4] The ingestion of the calories and high quality protein of breast milk during the critical first six months of life (when the brain is completing its development) could make a significant difference in the mental capacity of the child.[5] The sterility of breast milk and the presence of immunoglobulins would be helpful in lowering the incidence of

postneonatal: the period after the infant is one month old. (The **neonatal** period is the first month after birth.)

immunoglobulin: antibody (see page 121, also globulin, page 374).

[4]Brown, R. E.: Breast feeding in modern times. *The American Journal of Clinical Nutrition* 26:556-562, 1973.

[5]Winick, M., Rosso, P. and Waterlow, J.: Cellular growth of cerebrum, cerebellum, and brain stem in normal and marasmic children. *Experimental Neurology* 26:393-400, 1970.

infectious diseases among 4- to 6-month-old infants. In order to use successfully the infant formulas so attractively advertised by the food industry, the mother needs an uncontaminated water supply, education in how to prepare the formula, and knowledge of the importance of sterile bottles and nipples and of refrigeration of the milk. To the very poor mother who is emulating the wealthier mothers in not using the milk provided by nature, the price of the formula may be such a large outlay that she will cut costs by overdiluting the milk.[4] The trend away from breast feeding may be having more of an effect on nutritional status among the poor than can be shown in surveys or from income statistics.

Here again we observe an ugly downward spiral: mothers' poverty, poor nutrition, and poor education lead to poor nutrition of their infants, which leads to the infants' lower mental capacity and poor health, which lead them into a future of more poverty. This spiral was underlined in the Ten-State Survey where an inverse correlation was noted between a mother's educational level and multiple nutritional deficiencies of her children (see Table H12.1).[2]

Is there hunger in America? Yes. Painful as that answer is to face, it is true. There are pockets of hunger, hidden from the mainstream of society. The poor of whatever race, the migrant, the very old, and the very young are in need of nutritional help. The large middle-income group in the United States needs to be educated to the fact that the spiral of poverty—lack of education—more children than can be cared for—lack of good nutrition—ill health—poverty—must be broken, if not for humanitarian reasons, then because it would be good for America to have these people contribute as healthy, mentally alert, productive, tax-paying citizens.

To Explore Further—

An understanding of the part played by a person's culture and the food he/she selects is prerequisite to improving the nutrition of a group:

Knutson, A. L. and Newton, M. E.: Behavioral factors in nutrition education. *Journal of the American Dietetic Association* 37:222-225, 1960.

Wenkaw, N. S.: Cultural determinants of nutritional behavior. Nutrition Program News, U.S. Department of Agriculture, July/ August, 1969.

Tizard's article combines the behavioral sciences and the nutrition sciences to gain an understanding of the role played by nutrition in people's development. Schaefer speaks from the experience of many surveys and in the United States, the Ten-State Survey. Inano conducted one of the well known current surveys. Webb's article points out the dangerous combination of poor nutrition and poor environment.

Inano, M. and Pringle, D. J.: Dietary survey of low income, rural families of Iowa and North Carolina. III Contribution of food groups to nutrients. *Journal of the American Dietetic Association* 66(4):366-370, 1975.

Schaefer, A. E. and Johnson, O. C.: Are we well fed? The search for the answer. *Nutrition Today* 4(1):2, 1969.

Tizard, J.: Early malnutrition, growth and mental development in man. *British Medical Bulletin* 30(2):169-174, 1974.

Webb, T. E. and Oski, F. A.: Iron deficiency anemia and scholastic achievement in young adolescents. *Journal of Pediatrics* 82(5):827-829, 1973.

Volume Two contains an excellent chapter on food habits, taboos, parental attitudes, sociocultural factors, and the role of the educator in effecting change:

Robson, J.R.K., Larkin, F. A., Sandretto, A. M. and Tadayyon, B.: *Malnutrition, Its Causation and Control.* Gordon and Broach, New York, 1972.

Chapter VII, "Fight Against Prevalent Malnutrition," Chapter VIII, "Clinical Approaches to Fight Malnutrition," and Chapter IX, "Nutrition Education," are especially pertinent to the understanding of ways in which the war against hunger can be fought:

Manocha, S. L.: *Malnutrition and Retarded Human Development.* Charles C. Brown, Publisher, Springfield, Illinois, 1972.

Teaching Aid, *Deficiency Disorders—How to Diagnose Nutritional Disorders in Daily Practice* by Sandstead, H. H., Carter, J. P. and Darby, W. J., contains 20 slides which show the clinical signs of nutritional deficiencies. These can be ordered from:

Director, Education Services
Nutrition Today
101 Ridgely Avenue
Annapolis, Maryland 21404

Reprints, *Malnutrition and Hunger in the United States* and *Iron Deficiency in the United States* can be ordered from:

The American Medical Association
Department of Foods and Nutrition
535 N. Dearborn Street
Chicago, Illinois 60610

Film, *Hunger in America* can be ordered from:

A. V. Center
Indiana University
Bloomington, Indiana 47401

Suggested Activities

(1) Study your own diet

Review the record you made in Activity 1 of Chapter 1. Look up each food you ate in Appendix H and record its calcium contributions to your diet.

Which foods made the greatest contribution of calcium?

Compare your intake of this mineral with the RDA for a person your age and sex. What *percent* of the RDA for calcium did you consume? Was this enough? (See page 98).

If your intake was less than 2/3 RDA, find foods or beverages in Appendix H or in Table C12.2 that you would be willing to eat or drink daily that would correct this deficiency.

(Note: The last Highlight in the book invites you to survey your entire diet for adequacy, balance, and economy. You may wish to save this activity until you have read that Highlight, or you may wish to read the Highlight now for a sense of perspective.)

(2) Explode a food fallacy.

A popular writer on nutrition makes the following claims for calcium:

(a) When this mineral is undersupplied, your nerves become tense and you become grouchy.

(b) If you are lacking calcium, you tend to waste energy. You suffer from nervous tension and inability to relax, and so become fatigued out of all proportion to the work you do.

(c) If you are lacking calcium, you are so restless and irritable that people will avoid you; your temper gets out of control, and your popularity declines.

(d) Before you go to the dentist, you should take several calcium tablets with warm milk; then you will suffer no pain when he drills your tooth. Before you bear your baby you should do the same thing, and then you will need no anesthetic during childbirth.

(e) If you have any tendency toward nosebleeds, you should take calcium supplements, and the problem will disappear.

(f) If you suffer from insomnia, take calcium supplements with warm milk, and you will soon be sleeping like a baby.

For each of these claims, explain how the writer is using *logic* rather than *evidence* to come to these conclusions. For each, explain what the real situation probably is.

(3) You know more than you think you do.

From the information on page 386 you can predict what body tissue is tested for accurate information about a given nutrient. For example, knowing where vitamin C is found in the body, what tissue would you expect to reveal a person's vitamin C status?

13

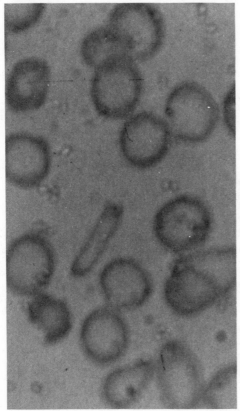

Blood Cells in Anemia

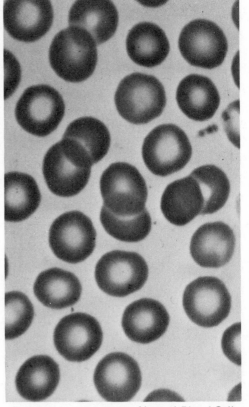

Normal Blood Cells

The Trace Minerals

". . . although erythrocytes occupy less than fifty percent of the volume of the blood fluid, they can adsorb seventy-five times more oxygen than can possibly be dissolved in the plasma itself."

"(Hemoglobin) must be a tricky substance," said Mr. Tompkins thoughtfully.

—GEORGE GAMOW and MARTYNAS YCAS, Mr. Tompkins inside Himself

Iron

Of all the trace minerals, iron deserves the most attention. It is a problem nutrient for many Americans, as the preceding Highlight made clear. Its food sources, absorption, transport, conservation, and roles in the body have been extensively studied and are well understood. A person who wishes to plan and consume a diet adequate in iron must be well informed.

The body's handling of iron (Figure C13.1) shows that this nutrient is as vital as calcium. Every effort is made to conserve it. Only 10 percent of dietary iron is absorbed, on the average, but once it enters the bloodstream it is jealously hoarded, very little being excreted each day. The whole body contains about four grams of iron, less than a teaspoon, and three-fourths of this is found in association with the protein hemoglobin, the oxygen-carrying protein with which the red blood cells are packed. The remainder is attached to other proteins: myoglobin (the oxygen-carrier protein of muscle), and the iron-carrier and storage proteins transferrin, ferritin, and others, which hold iron in reserve, ready for use when new globins are synthesized.

hemoglobin

myoglobin

transferrin, ferritin

The average red blood cell lives about four months. When it has aged and is no longer useful, it is removed from the blood by liver cells, which take it apart and make ready for excretion many of the degradation products. The iron, however, is attached to a protein carrier which returns it to the bone marrow,

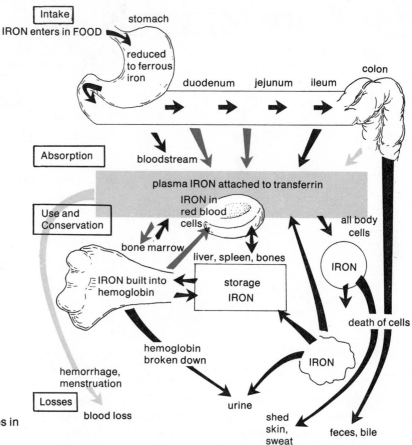

Figure C13.1. Iron Routes in the Body.

where new red blood cells are synthesized. Thus while red blood cells are born, live, and die in the body within a four-month cycle, the iron in the body is repeatedly recycled through each generation of red blood cells. Only tiny amounts are lost, principally in urine, sweat, and shed skin.

Knowing that 75 percent of the iron in the body is in the red blood cells, you can anticipate when iron losses will be greater than those mentioned in the last sentence. When blood is lost, as in menstruation, hemorrhaging, or blood donation, a significant amount of iron goes with it. Since menstruating women obligatorily lose iron every month, their needs for this nutrient are higher than those for men. (See boxed section at end of chapter.)

Iron Deficiency

If iron stores are low, the body cannot make enough hemoglobin to fill its new red blood cells. Without enough hemoglobin, the cells will be small, and since hemoglobin is the bright red pigment of the blood, the skin of a fair person may become noticeably pale. The undersized cells will be unable to carry enough oxygen from the lungs to the tissues, where oxygen is needed to combine with carbon and hydrogen from the energy nutrients as they break down. Hence energy release from these nutrients will be slowed, resulting in fatigue and weakness. A lack of energy supply to the brain can also cause headaches. The symptoms being enumerated here are those of anemia.

As you may recall, a deficiency of certain B vitamins can cause anemia of another kind (see Table C9.1). Iron deficiency, however, is the most common cause.

This is in direct contrast to the situation with respect to calcium. A deficiency of calcium causes withdrawal of the mineral from bones, leaving the blood level constant, since the body's stores of calcium represent 99 percent of the total. The body's stores of iron are at best only a quarter of the total, and a deficiency of iron results directly in a lowered blood concentration of this nutrient. As a result, you feel and see the effects of iron deficiency—weakness, tiredness, headaches, even pallor of the skin—while those of calcium deficiency are insidious and may go unnoticed for years.

The effects of iron-deficiency anemia are being felt today the world over, especially by women and children. This problem, together with that of vitamin A deficiency, ranks second only to PCM as a world health problem; its extent and seriousness even in the United States was summarized in the Highlight which preceded this chapter. Babies are usually born with a stored supply of iron sufficient to carry them through the first three months of life without external sources, but thereafter they must be supplied with iron-rich foods; hence anemia begins to be seen in many children as young as one or two years of age. When they begin to menstruate, girls' need for iron increases, and thus anemia becomes even more common in young women of childbearing age. The stress of repeated pregnancies, which deplete a woman's iron stores, exacerbates the problem.

anemia: the iron-deficiency disease. Properly identified as iron-deficiency anemia, to distinguish it from other less common types of anemia. See pages 284-285.

PCM: protein calorie malnutrition. See Highlight 4.

Iron Overload

Since there is no route of excretion for iron, the problem of iron overload may occur. This is, of course, more likely among men, who both eat more and lose less iron than women. It can also crop up in children whose overzealous mothers feed them too many iron-fortified foods. There is some protection against iron toxicity: iron absorption is decreased when the body's need for iron is being met. The intestinal mucosa prevent absorption by a means not clearly understood. Nevertheless, the risks of

mucosal block to iron
absorption[1]

iron overload complicate the problem of enriching foods since
an upper limit must be set on the amount of iron added to foods.

Food Sources of Iron

In 1973, for the first time, the NAS-NRC published, with
its revision of the RDA, the statement that dietary iron supplements were recommended for women of child-bearing age.
This reflected their recognition of the fact that it was virtually
impossible for a woman to meet her RDA by consuming natural
foods alone without becoming obese. Only with the most dili-
gent application of all nutrition principles is it possible for a
woman to obtain from her diet the necessary amounts of iron
even to meet two-thirds of the RDA.

A look at Table C13.1 and at the recommendations given
below will provide some guidelines for choosing foods that are
rich in iron. Let us assume that a woman balances her diet by
taking two servings of meat, four bread exchanges, two vegetables, two fruits, and two cups of milk, and see whether this
plan alone will ensure iron adequacy. Suppose that she is aim-
ing for 2/3 of her RDA. Since her RDA is 18 milligrams she is
attempting to get 12.

[1]Crosby, W. H.: Intestinal response to the body's requirement for iron. *Journal
of the American Medical Association* 208:347-351, 1969.

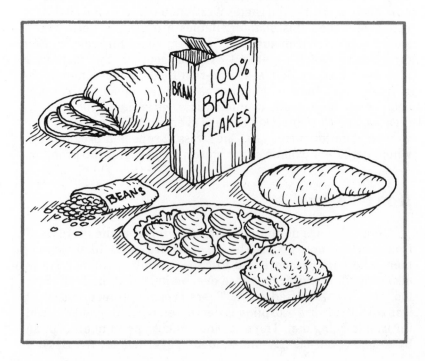

Table C13.1
Fifty Foods Showing Amounts of Iron

The foods listed below are the fifty that rank highest as sources of iron from those which are found on the ADA Exchange Lists and which also have been analyzed for nutrient composition. Serving sizes are the sizes listed in the Exchange Lists except for meat, where 3-ounce servings are shown. The numbers 1 through 6 refer to the numbers of the Exchange Lists: 1 = Milk, 2 = Vegetables, 3 = Fruit, 4 = Bread, 5L = Lean Meat, 5M = Medium-Fat Meat, 5H = High-Fat Meat, 6 = Fats and Oils. Numbers in parentheses are the item numbers on the Table of Food Composition (Appendix H).

Exchange Group	Food (Item Number)	Serving Size	Iron Milligrams
5L	Oysters (140)	¾ cup	10
5M	Beef liver (112)	3 ounces	8
4	Bran flakes (enriched) (338)	½ cup	6.2
5M	Beef heart (104)	3 ounces	5
5L	Chipped beef (92)	3 ounces	4
5L	Lean beef roast (79)	3 ounces	3
5L	Veal roast (132)	3 ounces	2.9
5M	Hamburger (81)	3 ounces	2.7
3	Prune juice (322)	¼ cup	2.6
5L	Sardines (142)	3 ounces	2.5
4	Dried beans (148)	½ cup	2.5
2	Spinach (233)	½ cup	2.4
4	Lima beans (167)	½ cup	2.2
5L	Ham (113)	3 ounces	2.2
	10% of U.S. RDA of 18 milligrams		
5L	Canned tuna (146)	3 ounces	1.6
2	Dandelion greens (201)	½ cup	1.6
4	Green peas (215)	½ cup	1.5
5L	Leg of lamb (108)	3 ounces	1.4
5L	Chicken, meat only (95)	3 ounces	1.4
2	Mustard greens (208)	½ cup	1.3
3	Strawberries (328)	¾ cup	1.1
5M	Egg (73)	1	1.1
2	Tomato juice (244)	½ cup	1.1
4	Rice, enriched (464)	½ cup	.9
2	Brussels sprouts (180)	½ cup	.9
3	Dried apricots (254)	4 halves	.8
4	Winter squash (235)	½ cup	.8
4	Whole wheat bread (372)	1 slice	.8
3	Blackberries (261)	½ cup	.7
4	Pumpkin (229)	¾ cup	.7
5L	Canned salmon (141)	3 ounces	.7
4	Cooked cereal (439)	½ cup	.7
3	Blueberries (262)	½ cup	.7
4	Spaghetti, enriched (474)	½ cup	.7
4	Macaroni, enriched (430)	½ cup	.7
2	Broccoli (179)	½ cup	.7
4	Potato chips (228)	15	.6
3	Raspberries (325)	½ cup	.6
5M	Peanut butter (160)	2 tbsp	.6

Table C13.1 (continued)

Exchange Group	Food (Item Number)	Serving Size	Iron Milligrams
4	White bread (353)	1 slice	.6
3	Dried fig (268)	1	.6
4	Muffin (435)	1	.6
4	Corn muffin (419)	1	.6
3	Applesauce (251)	½ cup	.6
2	Cooked tomatoes (241)	½ cup	.6
4	French fried potatoes (224)	8	.6
4	Popcorn, no fat (456)	3 cups	.6
3	Pear (312)	1	.5
4	Potato (221)	1 small	.5
4	Corn on cob (196)	1 small	.5

The meats are especially rich in iron although meat sources of iron vary in the amounts they contain. By far the most concentrated meat source is liver: two ounces of beef liver supply 5 milligrams. Three ounces of hamburger supply about 2½ milligrams; a half breast of chicken supplies only 1½ milligrams, while two eggs supply 2 milligrams. A generalization then would be that a serving of meat contributes anywhere from 2 to 5 milligrams of iron to the diet. If our woman selects two servings of meat from fair sources such as beef and chicken or eggs, she will obtain about 4 milligrams.

2 servings meat = 4 mg.

Bread exchanges contribute some iron to the diet, provided that the breads or cereals selected are whole-grain or enriched. A serving of enriched or whole-grain bread or cereal provides only about ½ milligram of iron, however. Starchy vegetables, which also appear on the bread exchange list, contribute from 2.5 milligrams per serving (for an iron-rich source such as dried beans) to less than one milligram (for potatoes or winter squash), and average perhaps 1.5 milligrams. If our woman eats three servings of bread or cereal and one starchy vegetable during the day, she will obtain 3 more milligrams of iron.

enriched: see page 288.

3 servings bread/cereal = 1.5 mg.

1 starchy vegetable = 1.5 mg.

Vegetables and fruits are scattered throughout Table C13.1, with spinach near the top and foods such as carrots and apples at the bottom. These foods contribute anywhere from about ½ to 4 milligrams per serving. On the average we can probably expect a serving of vegetables or fruits to contribute about one milligram. Four servings a day from these two groups of foods would add another 4 milligrams to our woman's diet. So far, she has 11 milligrams of iron, and two more exchange groups to go.

4 servings vegetables/fruits = 4 mg.

Milk is a notoriously poor iron source, contributing less than 2/10 of a milligram per cup. The inclusion of two servings of milk in our woman's diet each day, while it makes very important contributions of calcium, riboflavin, and other nutri-

2 cups milk < 0.5 mg.

ents, does nothing to increase her iron intake. Fat adds no iron at all. By the end of the day, then, having made liberal selections from the exchange groups, she falls short of 2/3 RDA, consuming only about 11 milligrams of the recommended 18.

This demonstration shows that the choice of a variety of foods, even of nutritious foods, without some sophistication with respect to individual food values for nutrients does not guarantee iron adequacy. In addition to balancing her diet roughly by using such a guide, a woman needs to be familiar with those foods in each group that are especially rich sources of iron. If she selects a cup of dry beans, like the navy beans listed in Table C13.1, she will obtain 5 milligrams of iron. If she eats a cup of spinach, she gets 4 milligrams. Green peas are another good vegetable source of iron. Among meats, she should probably eat liver often. If she makes the effort to select rich sources from each group often and is familiar with some fair sources as well, she can often come close to meeting at least 2/3 RDA.

Not only rich sources but also variety should be emphasized in the diet of a woman attempting to meet her iron needs from foods. The problem of iron availability from foods has been extensively studied and found to be complex. The binders, phytic acid and oxalic acid, which render calcium unavailable from certain foods, also decrease iron absorption, thus making spinach and whole-grain cereals unreliable as iron sources. A high-fiber meal, by accelerating peristalsis, reduces the length of time in which iron is in contact with the intestinal walls, and thus reduces absorption. An acid environment in the stomach is needed to convert ferric iron to the ferrous form for absorption. Other factors are also involved. Clearly, then, it is important not only to include rich sources of iron in the diet, but also to include many different sources and to use them often.

phytic and oxalic acids: see page 189.

effect of fiber on peristalsis: see page 24.

An IUD (intra-uterine contraceptive device) increases iron losses by increasing menstrual flow, while oral contraceptives decrease the flow, thereby conserving iron.

These awarenesses will, if applied, help people fall into eating patterns that are to be recommended. They are the basis for the advice often offered to women, to (1) eat liver and other organ meats, perhaps every other week, (2) eat dry legumes often, (3) eat greens such as spinach and turnip greens frequently, (4) select only those breads and cereals that are whole-grain or enriched, and (5) snack on dry fruits such as raisins and prunes. Suggested activities at the end of the chapter will help to increase your awareness of the relative iron values of various foods.

The above demonstration, with its heavy emphasis on the problem of a woman's meeting her iron needs, does not reflect a prejudice of the authors in favor of women. We like men and care about maintaining their health. However, in the case of iron, women must be warned that they risk deficiency while men ordinarily do not—for two reasons. First, as already mentioned, women need more. Second, women must obtain this

Example	Iron mg	Kcal
1 egg	1.1	80
3 ounces beef	2.9	245
3 slices bread	1.5	165
½ cup tomatoes	.6	25
½ cup broccoli	.6	40
1 small apple	.4	70
½ small banana	.4	50
1 sweet potato	1.0	155
2 cups milk	.4	320
	8.9	1150

The example shows that selections of a variety of nutritious foods without any added butter, margarine, or sugar uses up 1,150 of a woman's 2,000 kcalories and supplies fewer than 10 mg of iron.

goiter, cretinism (GOY-ter, CREE-tin-ism): iodine deficiency diseases.

goiter belt: the area around the Great Lakes and St. Lawrence seaway, where goiter is endemic in the United States.

endemic (en-DEM-ic): potentially present or native in an area, ready to crop up at any time.

hydroxyapatite

fluorapatite

iron within a smaller calorie allowance: a man can consume 3,000 kcalories a day and so can eat more and larger servings of nutritious foods containing iron; a woman must regulate her calorie intake to about 2,000, and so must make every food serving count.

Other Trace Minerals

Two of the trace minerals, iodine and fluorine, are of interest because they share several important characteristics. They both are found in sea water and are abundant in soil from any part of the world which is near, or was ever under, the sea; they are lacking in soil in glacial areas and freshwater basins such as the St. Lawrence Seaway and the Great Lakes. The distribution of deficiencies of these minerals parallels their availability from the soil and water. For most of the world, there is no problem obtaining enough iodine and fluorine, but for people who suffer deficiencies the consequences are severe.

Iodine, because it forms a structural part of the thyroid hormone which regulates the body's metabolic rate, is conspicuous when absent. A deficiency causes enlargement of the thyroid gland (goiter), a slowed metabolism, and profound disorders in the development of children, including stunted growth and mental retardation (cretinism) so severe as to render a child totally unable to handle life's simplest problems. The inclusion of iodine in the diet in regions where it is not abundant in soil is best guaranteed by the use of iodized salt. People are slow to learn, however. It took a massive educational campaign to eradicate the problem in the U.S. goiter belt. When the publicity was discontinued, and a new generation of young adults grew up in that region who had not been the target of the campaign, the problem crept back and again assumed significance. At present, the use of iodized salt has the problem under control.

People have been slow to learn about *fluorine* as well. Like iodine, it is best supplied in a medium consumed by everybody —in this case, community water—but opposition to the fluoridation of water, based on ignorance and superstition, still persists in many parts of the United States. Fluorine—or more accurately its ionic form, fluoride—is essential to stabilize bones and teeth against destruction by resorption and decay. When calcification occurs, a crystal first is formed from calcium and phosphorus, called hydroxyapatite. Then fluoride replaces the hydroxy (—OH) portion of the crystal, rendering it insoluble in water and resistant to change.

Fluoridation of community water is presently practiced in at least some communities in every state, the total number of people affected numbering over 80 million. As long ago as the

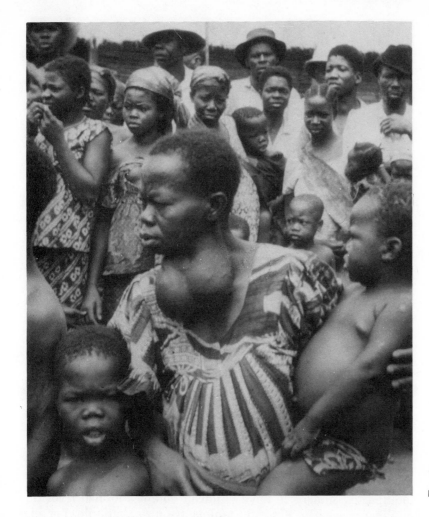

Goiter

FAO Photo.

1940s, the first experiments with adding fluoride to the water were performed. The best known study[2] was performed in the communities of Newburgh, New York, where fluoride was added to the water to the level of one part per million, and in Kingston, New York, a similar town which served as a control. This study showed that over a fifteen-year period fluoridation reduced dental decay by more than 50 percent. Over 26,000 children were examined.

Excess fluoride in the water causes mottling of tooth enamel. This phenomenon has been observed in communities where fluoride occurs naturally in excess but does not occur in communities where fluoride is added to the water supply. Where

[2]Ast, D. B., Smith, D. J., Wachs, B. and Cantwell, K. T.: Newburgh-Kingston caries-fluorine study. XIV. Combined clinical and roentgenographic dental findings after ten years of fluoride experience. *Journal of the American Dental Association* 30:1749, 1956.

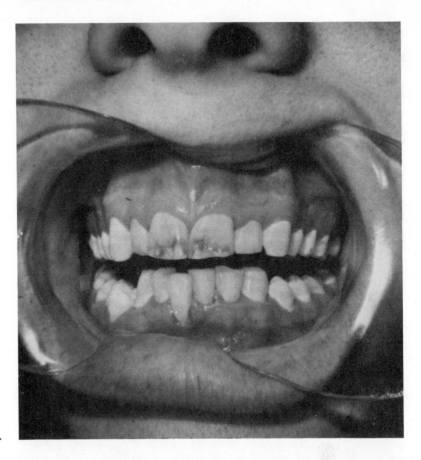

Fluorosis.

fluoridation is not practiced, the best temporary solutions to the problem of preventing dental decay seem to be to use fluoride toothpastes, and/or to have children obtain a topical fluoride application yearly. Fluoride tablets are also available. For infants there are vitamin drops with fluoride, but their effectiveness is limited. Continuous presence of the mineral in body fluids is desirable.

Osteoporosis is significantly lower in communities where the water has been fluoridated,[3] supporting the notion that fluoride protects against this disease.

The list of other trace elements now known to be essential in human nutrition, some in minute amounts, is growing longer. Research into their roles is one of the most active areas in nutrition science today. The element *chromium* is now known to be essential for human beings, and has been shown to remedy impaired carbohydrate metabolism in several groups of Ameri-

[3]Hegsted, D. M.: Calcium, phosphorus and magnesium. In *Modern Nutrition in Health and Disease.* 4th ed. Wohl, M. G. and Goodhart, R. S., editors. Lea and Febiger, Philadelphia, 1968, p. 332.

cans.[4] Experiments on animals have shown that chromium works closely with the hormone insulin, facilitating the uptake of glucose into cells and then the catabolism of glucose. When the mineral is lacking, the effectiveness of insulin alone in these roles is severely impaired.

Like iron, chromium can exist in more than one ionic state; trivalent chromium appears to be most effective in living systems. It also occurs in several different complexes in foods. The one which is best absorbed and most active is a small organic compound which has been named the *glucose tolerance factor*, or GTF. This compound has been purified from brewer's yeast and pork kidney and is believed to be present in many other foods. It may be that when more is known, the GTF, rather than chromium, will be dubbed an essential nutrient and will be classed among the vitamins.

Depleted tissue concentrations of chromium in human beings have been linked to maturity-onset diabetes and growth failure in children with PCM.[4]

Another micronutrient that works with insulin is *zinc*; in fact, this mineral is part of the structure of the hormone, as well as of some twenty enzymes, and cofactor for several others. Dietary deficiencies of zinc have been observed in the Middle East (Egypt and Iran), where the severest effects are felt by adolescent boys. Zinc is concentrated in the male sex glands; a lack of it retards sexual development and severely stunts growth.

trivalent (try-VAY-lent): having three positive charges. See ions, Appendix B.

GTF: glucose tolerance factor, a small organic compound containing chromium.

This of course gives no validity to the faddists' claim that supplementary zinc will improve sexual potency!

[4]Hambidge, K. M.: Chromium nutrition in man. *American Journal of Clinical Nutrition* 27:505-514, 1974.

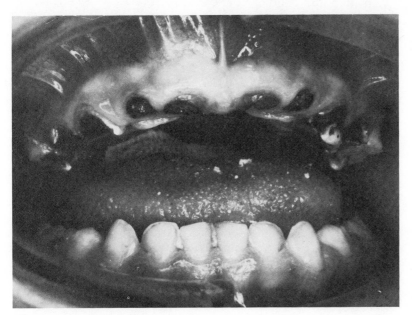

Teeth of a 2½ year old child showing the effect of a mineral-poor diet.

Courtesy of H. Kaplan and V. P. Rabbach.

Perhaps one reason why trace elements, such as these, have recently been uncovered is that our food supply has been increasingly refined. As more and more Americans turn to refined, processed, prepared foods and away from the crude products of the farm, they enjoy a saving in convenience and time but suffer a loss of the richness and variety of nutrients that occur in less pure foods. As a result, deficiencies crop up where the existence of a needed nutrient might never before have been suspected. A case in point is that of chromium. The amounts needed are unbelievably small, but when this mineral is lacking, severe disorders in body physiology occur. Once again, you should be reminded (from page 4) that there may be fringe benefits in obtaining needed nutrients from natural foods rather than from purified nutrient preparations.

halogen (HAL-o-gen): any of the five elements fluorine, chlorine, bromine, iodine, and astatine, whose atoms share the characteristic of having a single electron in their outer shell and so are highly reactive. See Appendix B.

linear relationship: a relationship between two variables in which one increases in direct proportion to the amount the other increases.

nonlinear relationships:

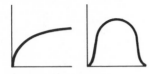

variable: see page 44.

physiological dose: a dose equivalent to the amount of a nutrient (or hormone) normally found in the body.

Many of the minerals share with the fat-soluble vitamins the characteristic of being toxic in excess. The halogens, in particular, are notorious in this respect. The skull and crossbones on the iodine bottle warns the user that this substance is a deadly poison and that it must be kept out of the reach of children. Much of the prejudice against the use of iodized salt and fluoridated water arises from the conclusion that because these minerals are dangerous when used in excess, they must be avoided altogether. This raises a point about all the nutrients and many other substances that it is important to understand: they may work one way at a high concentration and another at a low concentration. There is not a simple linear relationship between the dose level and its effects.

To show that this generalization applies in many situations, let us take three examples—one of a hormone, one of a vitamin, and one of a drug. The hormone insulin, at physiological doses, lowers blood glucose concentrations by facilitating the transport of glucose into cells. At a much higher dose (100 or 1,000 times more than is normally found in the body), insulin seems to *raise* blood glucose concentrations. On closer study it turns out that when the insulin dose exceeds a certain threshold level, the body responds by secreting an antagonistic hormone (glucagon) in such large amounts that a backlash occurs and the reverse effects are seen.

In Highlight 10, in the discussion of the effects of massive doses of vitamin C, the distinction was made between a pharmacological dose and a physiological dose. At the high level used in some experiments, the vitamin acts as a drug, overwhelming body systems which at normal concentrations are impervious to it. It is as if a different compound altogether were acting in the body.

Drugs are similar. The antibiotic streptomycin works by interfering with protein synthesis in growing cells. Since protein synthesis must occur for growth to occur, and since bacterial cells grow rapidly, the drug rapidly kills these cells without affecting the more slowly growing cells of the human digestive tract. At a higher dose level, the drug would also kill the cells of the human body.

Thus, if you read or hear of a certain substance having a certain effect on people, you cannot conclude that the substance is necessarily "good" or "bad" from this one report alone. You must ask what dose was used and whether the same effect would be observed if the substance were used at a higher or lower concentration. Two corollaries to this observation might be the following:

pharmacological dose: a much higher dose, at which unexpected effects are often observed.

pharmacology = the study of drugs.

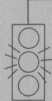

CAUTION WHEN YOU READ!

What is a poison at a high concentration may be an essential nutrient at a low concentration. (What is "bad," high, may be "good," low.)

What is a needed nutrient at a low concentration may be toxic at a high concentration. ("More" is not necessarily "better.")

The laboratory scientists responsible for investigating the effects of additives in foods have discovered these facts over the years. Now, before concluding that an additive in foods is dangerous, for example, they have realized that it is necessary to demonstrate that it causes harm *at the dose level we can realistically expect to find in our foods*. If the general public understood this, many of the scares that appear from time to time in the media would lose their impact. For many reasons, massive doses of many substances have undesirable effects, but in the real world of real people, effects of these kinds are not so often felt.

In the interest of selling a product or an idea, promoters sometimes appeal to our emotions, and a most powerful emotion is fear. "This additive causes cancer, and they are using it in bread." When we feel physically threatened we may not stop to reason and seek out the evidence, we may just do what we are told—in this case avoid the grocery store product and buy the promoter's

Additives proven to cause cancer at any dose are prohibited. See discussion of the Delaney Clause in Highlight 13.

product instead because it makes us feel safe. Yet the additives in our foods are extensively tested before they are approved for general use, and the laws which regulate their use are well enforced. Each additive is there for a reason.

The situation is complex and requires an understanding of many subtleties. The subject of additives is beyond the scope of this book. To be fair, no simple statement can be made about their effects. Each must be investigated individually. Still, it should be clear from this digression that you need not feel fear each time a claim is made that our foods are being contaminated with poisons.

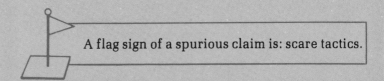

A flag sign of a spurious claim is: scare tactics.

To balance this discussion, remember that sometimes you are right to be scared. An occasional outbreak of food poisoning does occur, for example, showing that the inspection system failed to catch a hazard in time. Occasionally a food product comes on the market only to be later removed when a previously unsuspected side effect of one of its constituents becomes evident. The rarity of these occurrences, however, testifies to the overall effectiveness of our consumer protection agencies. Highlight 13 is devoted to some further aspects of consumer protection and the problems of additives.

The trace minerals iron, iodine, fluorine, chromium, and zinc have been selected for emphasis in this chapter because it seems to be especially important for present-day Americans to be aware of them. Five other trace minerals are itemized in Table C13.2 with a summary of facts about them. These ten do not constitute an exhaustive list; nickel, vanadium, silicon, tin,[5] and others are presently under investigation with the expectation that they, too, will prove to be essential nutrients. Chapter 14 continues the discussion of the minerals, addressing those that are important as electrolytes.

[5]Nielsen, H. and Sandstead, H. H.: Are nickel, vanadium, silicon, fluorine, and tin essential for man? A review. *American Journal of Clinical Nutrition* 27:515-520, 1974.

Table C13.2
Summary of Facts About Trace Minerals

Mineral	Adult RDA	Roles in Body	Deficiency	Major Food Sources
Iron	10 mg (M) 18 mg (F)	blood: part of hemoglobin; muscle: part of myoglobin; found in oxidative enzymes in all cells	anemia	liver, red meat, greens, enriched breads and cereals, dried beans
Zinc	15 mg	enzymes: part of many enzyme systems; insulin: part of this hormone	now known widespread in Middle East; rare in U.S.	many
Selenium	(none)	fat metabolism: plays a part; antioxidant: can substitute for vitamin E in this role but not in others	unknown	many
Manganese	(none)	bone: a minor component; enzymes: part of several enzymes	rare; toxicity more likely	—
Copper	(none)	red blood cell manufacture: needed for proper utilization of iron; part of many enzymes	rare; can cause anemia; toxicity also possible	organ meats, shellfish, many others
Iodine	140 μg (M) 100 μg (F)	energy metabolism: part of thyroid hormone	goiter (enlargement of thyroid gland); cretinism (mental retardation in infants)	unreliable: depends on soil food is grown in; iodized salt
Molybdenum	(none)	part of an essential enzyme; part of proteins involved in oxidation and reduction	unknown	organ meats, greens, green leafy vegetables
Cobalt	(none)	part of vitamin B_{12} (cobalamin)	B_{12} is needed	(see food sources of B_{12}, page 293)
Chromium	(none)	essential for glucose metabolism	rare; causes diabetes-like condition	unrefined foods
Fluorine	(none)	bones and teeth: converts hydroxyapatite (the bony crystal) to fluorapatite, which is harder and more stable	tooth decay, osteoporosis	unreliable; fluoridated water

The Iron RDA for Adults

	Females	Males
Iron	18 mg	10 mg

Like the RDA for many other nutrients already discussed, these numbers represent the amounts of iron that will protect nearly all normal, healthy individuals in the United States from a deficiency of this nutrient.

Since the way in which the iron RDA for women was established gives some insight into the methods used by the NAS-NRC in making recommendations for many nutrients, it will be described briefly here. An adolescent girl's average daily need of iron amounts to:

Losses from urine and shed skin:	½ to 1 milligram
Losses through menstruation:	½ milligram
(about 15 milligrams total, averaged over 30 days)	
Net for growth:	½ milligram
Average daily need:	1½ to 2 milligrams

Since the average person's absorption of iron from foods is about 10 percent of the iron ingested, to obtain 1½ to 2 milligrams a day, an adolescent girl will have to consume 15 to 20 milligrams in food. Hence the RDA is set at 18 milligrams.

CAUTION WHEN YOU READ!

The RDA are recommended *intakes*.

The amount of a nutrient absorbed is taken into account.

These figures are but two of 102 separate recommendations made for mineral intakes for various age-sex groups. A look at Appendix I will show that recommendations are made for five other minerals and that all recommendations vary depending on the age and sex of the groups for whom they are made. In particular, special recommendations are made for pregnant and lactating women, whose needs for certain nutrients (especially calcium) are greatly increased.

Summing Up

Iron is found principally in the red blood cells where it comprises part of the oxygen-carrier protein hemoglobin. When red blood cells die and are dismantled in the liver, the iron is retrieved and transported by iron-carrier proteins back to bone marrow where new red blood cells are synthesized. There is no route of excretion for iron; losses are small except when blood is lost, as in menstruation or hemorrhage. Thus women's needs for iron are greater than men's (RDA = 18 mg a day for women, 10 mg for men).

Iron deficiency anemia, one of the world's most widespread malnutrition problems, is most common in women and children; it causes weakness, fatigue, headaches, and pallor. Food sources of iron for women must be chosen carefully if as much as 2/3 RDA is to be met within a calorie allowance that is not excessive. The enrichment of breads and cereals somewhat improves U.S. women's iron intakes; enrichment or fortification of other foods with iron is complicated by the risk of iron overload in males. Addition of an iron supplement to the diet may be advisable for some women.

Foods relatively rich in iron include (in roughly descending order) liver and other organ meats, dried beans and legumes, red meats, and dark green vegetables. Other significant contributors are enriched breads and cereals, eggs, and dried fruits, such as raisins and prunes. Milk and dairy products are notable for their *lack* of iron. Fiber, phytates, and oxalates interfere with iron absorption, while protein and acid favor it; hence variety and frequency of consumption of good food sources are indicated.

Iodine forms part of the thyroid hormone; deficiency causes goiter (enlargement of the thyroid gland), slowed metabolism, and in children stunted growth and mental retardation. Addition of iodine to salt in minute quantities protects against deficiency, provided the iodized salt is used. Education must accompany this measure to make it effective.

Fluoride ion combines with calcium and phosphorus to stabilize the crystalline structure of bones and teeth against resorption or decay. In communities where the water contains fluoride either naturally or artificially added, dental caries and osteoporosis are less often seen than in communities where the water supply is low in fluoride.

Both *chromium* as part of glucose tolerance factor and *zinc* as part of insulin work with insulin in promoting glucose uptake into cells and normal carbohydrate metabolism. Chromium deficiency is now believed to have a significant incidence among older Americans and to be responsible for some cases of maturity-onset diabetes; it may cause growth failure in children as well. Zinc deficiency, observed in the Middle East, causes retarded sexual development in males and severe growth retardation.

Other trace minerals include *selenium*, important as an

antioxidant and in fat metabolism; *manganese*, important in bone and many enzymes; *copper*, needed for red blood cell manufacture and in many enzymes; *molybdenum*, found in some enzymes and other proteins; and *cobalt*, as part of cobalamin (vitamin B$_{12}$). Trace elements presently under investigation as possibly essential in human nutrition include *nickel, vanadium, silicon, arsenic,* and *tin.*

To Explore Further—

Teaching Aid, *Iron*, by Finch, C. A., contains slides which can be ordered from:

> Director, Education Services
> Nutrition Today
> 101 Ridgely Avenue
> Annapolis, Maryland 21404

Cassette, *Trace Elements in Nutrition* (CAM 2-75) can be ordered from:

> The American Dietetic Association
> 620 North Michigan Avenue
> Chicago, Illinois 60611

Highlight Thirteen ▬▬▬
Consumer Protection Legislation

Would you buy an article of clothing if the merchant would not let you see its size, color, or fabric? Not likely, but you might if you had been attracted by an advertisement of the item. If, after a few such purchases, you became disenchanted with the ads, you would probably demand that you see the item before you paid your money.

This is the situation in which consumers of food products, especially the newer products, found themselves some years ago. They were buying new products on the basis of advertising claims, then continuing to use them if the taste, quality, and price were right. But as consumers became more knowledgeable about nutrition, they realized that taste and price were not satisfactory guidelines and that they needed knowledge about

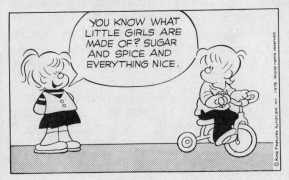

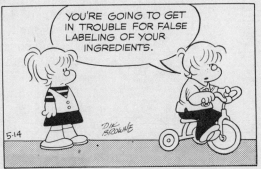

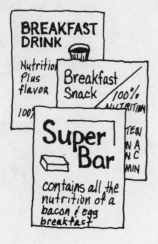

the nutrients contained in the food products *before* they paid their money. Advertising claims that a product was a substitute for breakfast (see Highlight 1) were not satisfactory to the new breed of consumer. The smart consumer read the fine print which listed the ingredients and understood that they were listed in descending order of predominance—but then wanted to know more. If sugar was listed in first place, the buyer then wanted to know, "How much sugar?"

As the new nutrition consumer evolved, the advertisers of food products were quick to respond. They touted the nutritional superiority of their products: high in protein, low in calories, more polyunsaturates, builds bone and teeth, provides energy for active children, a substitute for dairy products, and many other such claims. The advertisers knew that good nutrition had become a salable item. At the same time, many new food products were coming on the market which were not familiar to the consumer—convenience foods and imitations of traditional foods. The consumer was forced to rely on advertising blurbs about these foods because there was no other source of information. Educators in the field of nutrition became concerned over the misinformation that was being promulgated in pseudo-scientific advertisements.

These developments, and others, led to the recognition that today's buyers need to "see inside the package" before they pay their money. In other words, consumers should be protected from fraudulent advertising claims, especially in an area as vital to good health as food purchases. The objections of manufacturers and processors that the revelation of their recipes would be an unfair trade practice (and costly), needed to be resolved.

FDA = Food and Drug Administration

Thus it came about that the White House Conference on Food, Nutrition, and Health of 1969 recommended that the FDA develop nutrition labeling. There followed several years of study by industry, university research, and consumer groups to determine the type of information that would be most meaningful to the consumer. One of these studies found that not many persons would make direct use of nutrition information on labels, but of 4,400 persons interviewed during the study, 88 percent thought such labeling was desirable and 98 percent thought that consumers had a right to know the nutritional value of a food, whether or not they read or used the information to make wiser choices.[1]

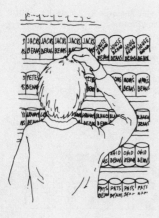

The combined efforts of manufacturers, educators, consumers, and the FDA resulted in the publication of new labeling regulations in 1972, to which the public was asked to respond.

[1]Ross, M. I.: What's happening to food labeling? *Journal of the American Dietetic Association* 64:262-267, 1974.

Then in 1973, the final regulations were published,[2] with full compliance expected in 1976. Three sections dealt with nutrition, a factor that was relatively new to FDA regulations; the three were nutrition labeling, nutritional quality guidelines, and imitation foods.[3]

Nutrition Labeling

Authority for the government to move into the field of nutrition comes from the Food, Drug and Cosmetic Act of 1938 which required that labels state:

Food, Drug and Cosmetic Act, 1938

(1) The common name of the product.
(2) The name and address of the manufacturer, packer, or distributor.
(3) The net contents in terms of weight, measure, or count.
(4) The ingredients listed in order of descending predominance.[1]

However, in conforming to these regulations, manufacturers often printed the information in type too small to be read and in an inconspicuous place on the package. Congress, then, in 1966, passed the Fair Packaging Labeling Act which, in part, required that information for the consumer's use be put in a prominent place on the label, and that words used to convey this information be those ordinarily used. For instance, adjectives such as "economy," or "giant," could not be used to describe the size of the package since they do not ordinarily have a size connotation.[1] With these new regulations, labels are now much more informative than in the past.

Fair Packaging Labeling Act, 1966

A new term is used in the nutritional labeling regulations which needs explanation: U.S. Recommended Daily Allowance (U.S. RDA). U.S. RDA is the term given to the values of the NAS-NRC RDA used on the nutrition labels. As the various interested groups were designing the information to go on the new nutrition label, they discovered that "percentage of RDA" was the most meaningful way to express amounts to consumers. But which value of the RDA should be used? Obviously, to include values for all the ages and both sexes of the RDA would make the label so unwieldy that it probably would not be used by the buyer. It was decided to use "the highest value for each nutrient given in the NAS-NRC RDA tables for males and nonpregnant, nonlactating females, 4 or more years of age, except for calcium, phosphorus, biotin, pantothenic acid, copper, and zinc."[2]

U.S. RDA

The U.S. RDA for calcium and phosphorus are not the highest values in the NAS-NRC RDA tables but were set at one gram each because of their bulk and solubility and the wide variabil-

[2]*Federal Register* 38:2131 (No. 13, January 19), 1973.
[3]Johnson, O. C.: The Food and Drug Administration and labeling. *Journal of the American Dietetic Association* 64:471-475, 1974.

ity in age-based requirements. Biotin, pantothenic acid, copper, and zinc had not been included in the RDA tables of 1968 but were generally recognized as essential for human nutrition. The FDA believed that setting amounts for these nutrients would allow manufacturers to list them, if they wished to do so. It was expected that the values would be amended as more information became available on human nutrition.[2]

You will notice that in the U.S. RDA in the box on page 419, there are two values given for protein. The lower value may be used by the manufacturer for 100 percent RDA *if* the protein in the product has a PER equal to or greater than the PER of casein. If the PER is less than that of casein, the higher value for protein will have to be used for 100 percent U.S. RDA. This rule is an advantage to the consumer who should not be expected to understand the difference between complete and incomplete protein.

As you can see (page 419), there are four different "U.S. RDA's." The set of figures in the third column is the one seen on labels. This set is intended to express the nutrient contents of common foods used by adults and children four years of age and older. "Special Dietary Use" label regulations were intended to go into effect at the same time as the rest of the provisions but at the present have been deferred pending further investigation.[4] These special dietary uses would be for weight control, for infants under twelve months of age, children under four years of age, and pregnant and lactating women. If these provisions are accepted, several types of claims in ads or on labels will be forbidden: (1) that a food is effective as a treatment for a disease, (2) that a balanced diet of ordinary foods cannot supply adequate amounts of nutrients (excepting the iron requirements of infants, children, and pregnant and lactating women), (3) that the soil on which food is grown may be responsible for deficiencies in quality, (4) that storage, transportation, processing, or cooking of a food may be responsible for deficiencies in quality of a food, (5) that a food has particular dietary qualities when such qualities have not been shown to be significant in human nutrition, and (6) that a natural vitamin is superior to a synthetic vitamin.[4]

Vitamin and mineral supplements also come under the jurisdiction of the FDA. On the basis of today's knowledge, our 1940s' idea that there need be no concern for the levels of vitamin and mineral supplements because the excesses are excreted, is "not only obsolete but dangerous."[5] Excessive doses of vitamin D can cause calcification in soft tissues, vitamin C in

PER = protein efficiency ratio. See page 92 and Appendix E.

casein (CAY-seen): the protein of milk.

——— NUTRITION INFORMATION ———

PERCENTAGE OF U.S. RECOMMENDED DAILY ALLOWANCES (U.S. RDA)

	PER SERVING	PER 6 OZ. DAILY
Protein	8	20
Vitamin A	*	*
Vitamin C	*	*
Thiamine (Vitamin B₁)	15	45
Riboflavin (Vitamin B₂)	8	20
Niacin	8	25
Calcium	6	20
Iron	8	25

*Contains less than 2% of the U.S. RDA of these nutrients.

---

[4]Stephenson, M.: Making food labels more informative. *FDA Consumer* 9(8): 13-17, 1975.

[5]*Vitamins, Minerals, and FDA*. Reprint from FDA Consumer. DHEW Publication No. (FDA) 74-2001. U.S. Government Printing Office, Washington, 1973.

very large doses can cause diarrhea, an accumulation of vitamin A can cause serious problems, such as pressure within the skull that mimics a brain tumor, and iron overload is a cause of accidental poisoning of children taking too many vitamin and mineral pills.[5]

In line with this newer evidence, the FDA recommended that high potency vitamins be taken only upon the advice of a physician and that their labels show the amount of vitamin or mineral present as a percentage of the U.S. RDA. Other than vitamins A and D, all vitamin and mineral products in excess of 150 percent of the U.S. RDA were to continue to be sold singly or in combination formulas as nonprescription drugs. "They are, nevertheless, drugs and not dietary supplements."[5] It was recommended that vitamins A and D continue to be sold without prescription in doses up to the U.S. RDA but not above this

dietary supplement: a product containing a physiological dose of a nutrient; it may be sold over the counter.

Table H13.1
U.S. Recommended Daily Allowances (U.S. RDA's) for Essential Nutrients*

	Infants Birth to 12 Months (Tentative)	Children Under 4 Years of Age	Adults and Children 4 or More Years of Age	Pregnant or Lactating Women
Nutrients which MUST be declared on the label:†				
Protein (g), PER ⩾ casein	20	45	45	45
Protein (g), PER < casein	28	65	65	65
Vitamin A (IU)	1,500	2,500	5,000	8,000
Vitamin C (ascorbic acid) (mg)	35	40	60	60
Thiamin (vitamin B_1) (mg)	0.5	0.7	1.5	1.7
Riboflavin (vitamin B_2) (mg)	0.6	0.8	1.7	2.0
Niacin (mg)	8	9	20	20
Calcium (g)	0.6	0.8	1.0	1.3
Iron (mg)	15	10	18	18
Nutrients which MAY be declared on the label:				
Vitamin D (IU)	400	400	400	400
Vitamin E (IU)	5	10	30	30
Vitamin B_6 (mg)	0.4	0.7	2.0	2.5
Folic acid (folacin) (mg)	0.1	0.2	0.4	0.8
Vitamin B_{12} (μg)	2	3	6	8
Phosphorus (g)	0.5	0.8	1.0	1.3
Iodine (μg)	45	70	150	150
Magnesium (mg)	70	200	400	450
Zinc (mg)	5	8	15	15
Copper (mg)	0.6	1	2	2
Biotin (mg)	0.05	0.15	0.3	0.3
Pantothenic acid (mg)	3	5	10	10

*Adapted from *Food Technology* 28(7):5, 1974
†Whenever nutrition labeling is required

drug: a product containing a pharmacological dose of a nutrient or medicine; it must be sold by prescription only.

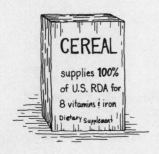

amount. Many groups criticized this action of the FDA and felt it to be an infringement of personal rights.[6] The FDA was taken to court over the recommendation and in 1976, the recommendation was upheld in New York State. Some manufacturers of vitamin and mineral supplements meanwhile have been complying voluntarily with the regulations.

Manufacturers of food products have the freedom to add or not to add nutrients to their products and to advertise or not to advertise the nutritional superiority of the products. However, if they decide in favor of adding the nutrient (for example, adding vitamin C to a breakfast drink) or of advertising its nutritional qualities (for example, advertising orange juice as a source of vitamin C), then they must comply fully with the nutrition labeling section of the law. Without this complete information panel, nutrition claims could deceive the consumer about the true nutritional value of the food.

If any nutrition information or claim is made on the label of a food, it must conform to the following format under the heading of "Nutrition Information:"

(1) A statement of the serving size.
(2) The number of servings per container.
(3) A statement of the caloric content per serving.
(4) A statement of the number of grams of protein in a serving.
(5) A statement of the number of grams of carbohydrate in a serving.
(6) A statement of the number of grams of fat in a serving.
   (a) When fatty acid composition is declared, the information on fatty acids shall be placed on the label immediately adjacent to the statement on fat content.
   (b) When cholesterol content is declared, the information on cholesterol shall immediately follow the statement on fat content (and fatty acid content, if stated).
(7) A statement of the amount per serving of the protein, vitamins, and minerals expressed in percentage of the U.S. RDA. (No claim may be made that a food is a significant source of a nutrient unless that nutrient is present in the food at a level equal to or in excess of 10 percent of the U.S. RDA in a serving. No claim may be made that a food is nutritionally superior to another food unless it contains at least 10 percent more of the U.S. RDA of the claimed nutrient per serving.)[7]

[6]Turner, J. S. and Koch, A. D.: How the FDA's vitamin rules can affect your health. *Organic Gardening and Farming* 21:86/87, 1974.
[7]*Federal Register* 38:6950 (No. 48, March 14), 1973.

Nutritional Quality Guidelines

Guidelines for regulation of nutritional quality have been proposed by the FDA for highly processed foods such as frozen dinners; breakfast cereals; meal replacements; noncarbonated, vitamin C-fortified fruit or vegetable-type beverages; and main dishes such as macaroni and cheese or pizza. If a product complies with the nutritional quality guidelines, it may carry on its label the statement that it "provides nutrients in amounts appropriate for this class of food as determined by the U.S. Government."[8] For frozen dinners, there must be one or more sources of protein from meat, poultry, fish, cheese, or eggs and these must make up at least 70 percent of the total protein; there must be one or more vegetables or vegetable mixtures other than potatoes, rice, or cereal-based products; and the dinner must have a minimum nutrient level for each 100 kcalories, according to the following table:

Table H13.2
Required Nutrient Content of Highly Processed Foods Such as Frozen Dinners*

Nutrient	For Each 100 Calories Required Components	For the Combined Required Components Regardless of Calories
Protein, grams	4.60	16.0
Vitamin A, IU	150.00	520.0
Thiamin, mg	0.05	0.2
Riboflavin, mg	0.06	0.2
Niacin, mg	0.99	3.4
Pantothenic acid, mg	0.32	1.1
Vitamin B_6, mg	0.15	0.5
Vitamin B_{12}, μg	0.33	1.1
Iron, mg	0.62	2.2

*Stephenson, M.: Making food labels more informative. *FDA Consumer* 9(8): 13-17, 1975.

When the Food, Drug, and Cosmetic Act was enacted, some items were given "Standards of Identity" and were excused from the requirement to list ingredients, although many manufacturers did so voluntarily. Standards of Identity were issued for such foods as bread or mayonnaise—common foods often prepared at home, for which the basic recipe was understood by almost everyone. Certain ingredients must be present in a specific percentage before the food may use the standard name; for example, any product called *mayonnaise* must contain 65 percent by weight of vegetable oil, either vinegar or lemon juice, and egg yolk.[4] The FDA does not now have the authority to require that ingredients be listed for foods which have been given

Standard of Identity: a published standard, stating what ingredients must be in the product and in what amounts.

Standards of Identity but it is urging manufacturers to give the consumer more detailed information.

In Standards of Identity, *enriched* is a term which refers to the addition of specific nutrients to a food such as the enrichment of bread. The amounts added generally are moderate and include those commonly present at lower levels. On the other hand, *fortified* is a term which refers to the addition to foods of specific nutrients in which the amounts added are in excess of those normally found in the food. Sometimes the food selected for such fortification is one which is a natural carrier for the nutrient, such as milk being fortified with vitamin D.

enriched

fortified

Imitation Foods

imitation food

A section of the original Food, Drug, and Cosmetic Act of 1938 required that if a food is an imitation of a traditional food, this fact must be stated on its label. With the new food technology, many food products are on the market that may very well be superior to traditional foods; it is misleading to the consumer for these to be called "imitation," since the word implies that the product is inferior. For this reason, the new regulation requires that the word *imitation* must be used on the label only if the product is "a substitute for and resembles another food but is nutritionally inferior to the food imitated. . . . Nutritional inferiority is defined as a reduction in the content of an essential vitamin or mineral or of protein that amounts to 10 percent or more of the U.S. RDA."[2]

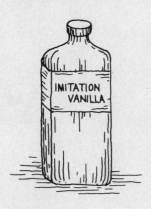

Additives

There is a great deal of controversy today over the additives, both intentional and incidental, which are present in the food supply. On the one hand, articles and books are appearing which tell us that we have the safest food supply in the world and shouldn't be concerned about all this furor raised by various groups; on the other hand, scare stories are constantly in the news about the carcinogens or heavy metals that are being allowed to stay in our food supply because of pressure from big business. Many have found that the more they read, the less clear the issues become. An apparently objective article on the work of the FDA in a reputable journal, for instance, may be suspect if the author is found to have been closely associated with the FDA and is now on the staff of a big food company.[3] Moreover, those who want to know what the pure scientists are finding in their laboratories about pollutants, toxicants, carcinogens, or additives are likely to be overwhelmed by the amount of reading that must be done, because each report is concerned with only ONE additive, and there are thousands to be considered. Furthermore, there are interactions between additives and nutrients which also must be considered. The

carcinogen (car-SIN-oh-gen): an agent that causes cancer.

heavy metal: a metallic element with a high atomic weight, such as mercury or zinc.

reputable journal: see page 76.

pollutant: a substance which pollutes or contaminates.

toxicant: a poison.

reading is never ending. The best that a text in nutrition can do under these circumstances is to define the terminology and to give a brief summary of the laws as they are presently stated.

Intentional food additives are substances purposely put into a food to give it some desirable characteristic: color, flavor, texture, stability, or to retard spoilage.[8] Some additives are nutrients which are added to foods to increase their nutritional value, such as vitamin C added to fruit drinks or potassium iodide added to salt. *Flavoring agents* such as ginger and cinnamon are additives, as well as substances which themselves do not add flavor but bring out the flavor of other ingredients, for example, monosodium glutamate (MSG). *Antioxidants* are used to prevent rancidity of fats during storage and *antimyotic agents* are used to prevent or control spoilage organisms such as mold, bacteria, and yeast; among the most common of the latter additives are salt and sugar. *Emulsifiers* are used to keep oil dispersed in a water medium, such as in salad dressings. *Stabilizers* are used to keep the texture of a product smooth and stable, for instance, keeping the water in ice cream from forming ice crystals and destroying the smoothness of the ice cream. *Coloring compounds* are used to make the product more attractive to the eye. Earlier, these compounds were natural substances, such as beet juice, but today more than 90 percent are synthetic; they are among the most controversial of the additives.[9] There are also many other classes of food additives designed to perform various functions in the processing and manufacture of foods and food products.

It has been pointed out by many writers that the present highly complex food industry could not have developed without the advent of additives to insure stability of the product. Without additives, for instance, it would be impossible to produce food in one part of the world and have it survive processing, packaging, transportation over a great distance, and many months on the store shelf before it is consumed. If, today, these additives were sweepingly eliminated, chaos and widespread starvation would be the result before another system could be evolved. The alternative to eliminating additives, it seems, is to find ways of ensuring that the additives used are safe in the amounts and under the conditions in which they are used. The agency charged with this responsibility is the Food and Drug Administration, and it in turn must depend on an alert and informed public.

It is interesting to note that provisions for adding new substances to the lists of safely-used additives takes into account the responsibility of the public to make its wishes known. The 1958 Food Additives Amendment to the Food, Drug, and Cos-

Food Additives Amendment, 1958

[8]Larkin, T.: Ten fallacies about FDA. *FDA Consumer* 9(9):21, 1975.
[9]Margolius, S.: *Health Food Facts and Fakes.* Walker and Co., New York, 1973.

metic Act requires that if food processors wish to add a substance to a food, they must "submit a petition to FDA, accompanied by extensive information on chemistry, use, function, and safety."[10] There will be public hearings with testimony presented by qualified persons both for and against the substance being added to the food. If such a careful review shows that the substance is safe, the FDA will authorize its use under specified conditions.

When the Additives Amendment was passed, many substances were exempted from complying with this procedure because there were no known hazards in their use at the time, and they were put on what is known as the GRAS (generally recognized as safe) list. Any time there is substantial scientific evidence or public outcry which questions the safety of any of the substances on the GRAS list, a special reevaluation of the substances will be made.[8] FDA is now making reevaluations of all the items on the GRAS list.[11] This investigation will obviously take a number of years to complete.

GRAS list

One of the standards an additive must meet in order to be placed on the GRAS list is that it must not have been found to be a carcinogen in any test on animals or humans. Carcinogens are substances which are cancer-causing either directly or after metabolism in the body. The Delaney Clause of the Additives Amendment of 1958 is very straightforward in speaking to the problem of carcinogens in foods and drugs. It states that "no additive shall be deemed safe if it is found to induce cancer when ingested by man or animal."[11]

Delaney Clause

In recent years, the Delaney Clause has come under fire for not allowing for the difference in effects on the body of varying dose levels. For example, when the artificial sweetener, cyclamate, was banned in 1969, it was estimated that a human would have to drink at least 138 12-ounce bottles a day of soft drinks containing cyclamates in order to ingest an amount of cyclamate comparable to the quantity given animals in the tests which caused the ban.[12] The FDA received criticism for banning the use of cyclamates, but under the law it had no other alternative. Advanced techniques for measuring the quantity of a substance present in a food have made it possible to detect an almost infinitesimal amount of an additive, even lower than the amount of that substance which may be present naturally in a food,[13] yet the application of the Delaney Clause requires that the additive no longer be used in any amount.[12] The FDA does

[10]Consumer Forum. *FDA Consumer* 9(7):3, 1975.
[11]FDA clears some food items, bans others. *Chemical and Engineering News* 52(40):12, 1974.
[12]Middlekauf, R. D.: Legalities concerning food additives. *Food Technology* 28(5):42-49, 1974.
[13]Coon, J. M.: Natural food toxicants—a perspective. *Nutrition Reviews* 32(11): 321-332, 1974.

not have the right to make a judgment on dose levels of carcinogens, or on the applicability of animal research to humans, or even on the reproducibility of an experiment.

One of the tasks of the FDA is to monitor the amounts of pesticides and other pollutants (incidental food additives) actually consumed by Americans. It carries out this assignment by finding the amount and kind of food eaten by a male teenager, buying these foods in the public market, dividing them into categories, and then chemically analyzing the categories for the presence and level of these residues. For example, in 1973, it was found by this method, commonly called the Market Basket Survey, that the level of DDT had declined dramatically from previous years due to its being banned from agricultural use and that the average intake of mercury was down a third from 1972.[14]

Market Basket Survey

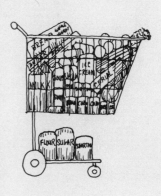

It is one thing to know the level of a pesticide or heavy metal in a Market Basket Survey and an entirely different matter to know the effect of that level on a human. Also, possible interactions among pollutants and between pollutants and nutrients further complicate the picture. For example, inadequate protein in the diet increases the toxicity of most insecticides, as shown in experiments on rats; fat mammals, birds, and fish are more resistant to DDT than their thinner counterparts; DDT depletes the liver of vitamin A so that a vitamin A deficient diet would increase the possibility of damage from this insecticide; cadmium is a toxic substance present in some soils and thus in foods whose toxicity seems to be mitigated by adequate zinc in the diet; and dietary calcium can alter the effect of zinc since excess calcium increases the zinc requirements, especially when there is an abundance of phytic acid.[15] It becomes evident, then, that knowing the level of one chemical or even the interaction of two chemicals is not sufficient knowledge on which to base judgments. There are innumerable interactions between substances which may have an additive or synergistic effect.

synergistic effect: see page 127.

Persons concerned over the levels of various additives and pollutants in the food supply would be well advised to eat as wide a variety of foods as possible so as to dilute the amount of any one substance. "The wider the variety of food intake, the greater is the number of different chemical substances consumed, and the less is the chance that any one chemical will reach a hazardous level in the diet."[13]

To Explore Further—

A good discussion of how food quality is improved by enrichment, restoration, and fortification:

[14]Hopkins, H.: Finding out what else you eat. *FDA Consumer* 9:8-15, 1975.
[15]Shakman, R. A.: Nutritional influences on the toxicity of environmental pollutants. *Archives of Environmental Health* 28:105-113, 1974.

Council on Foods and Nutrition (AMA): Improvement of the nutritive quality of foods. *Journal of the American Medical Association* 225(9):1116-1118, 1973.

Reprint request should be made to:

> AMA Council on Foods and Nutrition
> 535 N. Dearborn St.
> Chicago, Illinois 60610

This review includes an interesting discussion of how the diet influences the toxicity of trace minerals and oxidant air pollutants:

Shakman, R. A.: Nutritional influences on the toxicity of environmental pollutants. *Archives of Environmental Health* 28:105-113, 1974.

The two sides of the question of additives can be viewed in these two books:

Hunter, B. T.: *The Mirage of Safety.* Charles Scribner's Sons, New York, 1975.

Whelan, E. and Stare, F. J.: *Panic in the Pantry.* Atheneum, New York, 1975.

A general review of all color additives and how the FDA regulates them:

Damon, G. E. and Janssen, W. F.: Additives for eye appeal. *FDA Consumer,* July/August:15-18, 1973.

Teaching Aid, *Additives* by Hall, R. L., can be ordered from:

> Director, Education Services
> Nutrition Today
> 101 Ridgely Avenue
> Annapolis, Maryland 21404

Food Labeling is a cassette prepared by Robinson, M. and can be ordered from:

> The American Dietetic Association
> 430 North Michigan Avenue
> Chicago, Illinois 60611

Suggested Activities

(1) Study your own diet.

Review the record you made in Activity 1 of Chapter 1. Look up each food you ate in Appendix H and record its iron contributions to your diet.

Which foods supplied the most iron? What percent of the RDA for iron do you get in a typical day? Is this enough? (See page 98.)

If your intake was less than 2/3 RDA, find foods or beverages in Appendix H or in Table C13.1 that you would be willing to eat or drink daily that would correct this deficiency.

Class the five foods that contributed the most iron to your diet. How many were meats? legumes? greens? Did any of your top five fall outside these classes? If so, what were they?

(2) Learn more about iron sources.

If you have a need to learn more about individual foods and their contributions of iron to the diet, look up some of the following in Appendix H: different kinds of liver; different green leafy vegetables; various breads and cereals (do enriched breads have more, or less, iron than whole-grain breads, or are they about the same?); nuts and legumes; dried fruits; molasses and other sugar sources. Pay particular attention to the foods you eat. Think in terms of percent of RDA: if you are a woman, a food that supplies 1.8 milligrams of iron per serving provides you with 1/10 of your RDA. List your own best possible sources of iron in terms of percent of RDA. Plan several days' menus you would enjoy that provide more than 2/3 RDA.

Note: Knowing where iron is found in the body, can you explain why red meat is a rich iron source? And why liver would be a still better source? Are there any other nutrients for which liver is an excellent source for a similar reason?

(Note: The last Highlight in the book invites you to survey your entire diet for adequacy, balance, and economy. You may wish to save these two activities until you have read that Highlight, or you may wish to read the Highlight now for a sense of perspective.)

(3) Practice reading labels.

Select one nutrient to study. Using the nutritional information on the labels, make a list of several foods, the amount of each, and the calories you would have to eat to obtain 100 percent of the U.S. RDA of that nutrient. Also calculate the cost of a serving of each, then judge which sources were the most economical from the standpoint of (a) calories and (b) cost.

14

Water and Salts ━━━━━━━

It was assuredly not chance that led Thales to found philosophy and science with the assertion that water is the origin of all things.
—*LAWRENCE J. HENDERSON*

The ubiquitous, inconspicuous and often ignored compounds, water and salts, provide the medium in which nearly all of the body's reactions take place as well as participating in many of them and supplying the means of transportation of vital materials *to* cells and of respiration and metabolism end products *away* from cells. Every cell in the body is bathed in water containing the dissolved substances it needs. The fluid found in the eye is composed of materials needed for the best functioning of the rods and cones of the retina; the fluid inside the brain and spinal column is the proper composition for nerve cell function; the fluid at each point along the GI tract is best suited for the cell functions in that part of the tract—and so on.

Each of these fluids is constantly undergoing loss and replacement of its constituent parts as cells withdraw nutrients and oxygen from them and excrete carbon dioxide and other waste materials into them. Yet the composition of the body fluids in each compartment remains remarkably constant at all times. We have examined two examples of this constancy: the regulation of blood glucose concentration (Chapter 1) and that of blood calcium (Chapter 12). On closer examination, it becomes apparent that every important constituent of body fluids is similarly regulated. The interstitial fluid, for example, always has a high concentration of sodium and chloride ions and lower concentrations of about eight other major ions. The intracellular fluid always has high potassium and phosphate concentrations,

interstitial: see page 118.

429

and lower concentrations of other ions. These special fluids regulate the functioning of cells; the cells in turn regulate the composition and amount of the fluids. The entire system of cells and fluids remains in a delicate but firmly maintained state of dynamic equilibrium.

The maintenance of this balance is so important that it is credited with our ability and that of other animals to live on land. Our single-celled ancestors were totally dependent on the surrounding sea water in which they lived to provide nutrients and oxygen and to carry away their waste. We have managed, over the course of our two-billion-year evolutionary history, to internalize the ocean—to continue bathing our cells in a warm, circulating nutritive fluid that keeps each one of them alive.

The purposes of this chapter are threefold: to show you how this regulation works, to show the importance of certain minerals in the maintenance of the water balance, and to give you a sense of the causes and consequences of upsetting the balance.

Body Water and Its Sources

Since water constitutes 55 to 60 percent of your body weight, it is fortunate that the total amount of water remains constant. That it does so is a consequence of two delicate balancing systems, regulating water at both ends—its intake and its excretion. Let us consider each of these in turn.

Water intake: thirst. When you need water, you drink. Everybody knows that, but it takes a thinking physiologist to ask why. The evidence from experiments with thirst points to the possibility that several mechanisms operate in its regulation. One is in the mouth itself: when the blood is too salty (having lost water, but not salts) water is withdrawn from the salivary glands into the blood. The mouth becomes dry as a result, and you drink to wet your mouth. Another is in a brain center where cells sample and monitor the salt concentration in the blood; when they find it too high they initiate impulses that travel to brain centers which, in turn, stimulate drinking behavior. Possibly, the stomach also plays a role; thirsty animals will drink until nerves known as stretch receptors in their stomachs are stimulated enough to turn off the drinking. More is to be learned about these mechanisms, but it is clear from what we know already that thirst is finely adjusted to provide a water intake that exactly meets the need.

Water excretion. This regulation is better understood. The cells of the hypothalamus which monitor salt concentration in the blood stimulate the pituitary gland to release a hormone, ADH, whenever the body's salt concentration is too high. ADH in turn stimulates the kidneys to hold back (actually reabsorb)

dynamic equilibrium: a state of balance in which rapid exchange is taking place. Examples: body fluids, bones, and fat maintain a constant composition but exchange materials continuously with their surroundings. As opposed to a condition of **static equilibrium**, dynamic equilibrium is a condition of **homeostasis**

The salinity (saltiness) of our body fluids, and their temperature, are believed to be the same as in the ocean at the time when our ancestors emerged onto land. The ocean has since become more salty.

"Salt" does not refer only to sodium chloride but to ionic compounds as defined on page 432.

Water follows salt, moving in the direction of higher osmotic pressure (see page 434).

The brain center being described is the **hypothalamus** (hy-po-THAL-a-mus).

(1) the ADH (antidiuretic hormone) mechanism: directly causes water retention by the kidneys.

ADH: a hormone released by the pituitary gland in response to high osmotic pressure of the blood. Target organ: the kidney, which responds by reabsorbing water.

water so that it recirculates in the body rather than being excreted. Thus the more water you need, the less you excrete. There are also cells in the kidney itself that are responsive to the salt concentration in the blood passing through them; when they sense a too-high salt concentration they, too, release a substance that, by a roundabout route, causes the adrenal gland to release a hormone—aldosterone—that in turn causes the kidneys to retain more water. Again, the effect is that when more water is needed, less is excreted.

The renal excretion mechanisms cannot work by themselves to maintain water balance unless you drink enough. This is because there is a minimum amount of water that the body must excrete each day—the amount necessary to carry out of the body the waste products generated by the day's metabolic activities. Above this minimum (about 900 milliliters a day) the amount of water you excrete can be adjusted to balance your intake. Hence drinking plenty of water is never a bad idea.

Water deficiency, or dehydration, occurs whenever there is a massive loss of body water, as in kidney malfunction, blood loss, vomiting, or diarrhea, or when water becomes unavailable. Since the consequences are related to the losses of salts which accompany the water, this phenomenon will be discussed under Salts (below). Water excess in the body is reflected in the symptoms of edema, hypertension, or both; these, too, are related to the body's salt retention.

The constancy of total body water. In addition to the obvious dietary source, water itself, all foods contain water (as a look back at the figures on page 7 will remind you). In addition, water is generated from the energy nutrients in foods (recall that the C's and H's in these nutrients combine with oxygen during metabolism to yield CO_2 and H_2O). Human total daily water intake from these three sources amounts to about 2½ liters.

In addition to the water excreted via the kidneys, some water is lost from the lungs as vapor, some in feces, and some from the skin. The losses of all of these, of course, also total about 2½ liters a day.

Salts

The regulation of body water distribution and transportation is intimately associated with the regulation of salt distribution. A closer look at the way in which the body handles this problem will pave the way for an understanding of the causes and consequences of imbalances.

Interestingly, the very minerals that are most important in regulation of the water balance—sodium, chlorine, phosphorus, and potassium—are those that are abundant in the diet and,

hormone: see page 157.

(2) the aldosterone mechanism: indirectly causes water retention by the kidney.
—kidney releases renin in response to high osmotic pressure of the blood,
—renin converts angiotensinogen (an-gee-o-ten-SIN-o-gen) in the blood to angiotensin (an-gee-o-TEN-sin),
—angiotensin stimulates the adrenal gland to release aldosterone,
—aldosterone stimulates the kidney to reabsorb sodium,
—water follows sodium and is reabsorbed.

aldosterone (al-DOSS-ter-OWN): a hormone released by the adrenal gland in response to the presence of angiotensin. Target organ: the kidney, which responds by reabsorbing sodium.

metabolic wastes: ketones, urea (see pages 211, 212).

But see below (sweating, page 437).

Massive loss of body water through the kidneys is **diuresis** (dye-yoo-REE-sis).

Water intake:

Liquids:	1,200-1,500 ml
Food:	700-1,000 ml
Metabolic water:	200- 300 ml
	2,100-2,800 ml

Water output:

Kidneys:	900-1,400 ml
Lungs:	350 ml
Feces:	150 ml
Skin:	450- 900 ml
	1,850-2,800 ml

Losses from lungs and skin are called **insensible water losses**.

thus, for which deficiencies in humans are virtually unknown (see Table C12.3). This is probably no coincidence. The availability of these elements is guaranteed. The regulation of water balance is so vital that life has had to evolve making use of these elements for this purpose. Any other course would have brought the process of evolution to a dead halt.

To understand how cells regulate the amount of water they contain, it is necessary to take a closer look at the minerals as ions—the form in which cells use minerals for water regulation. Cell membranes are freely permeable to water, which flows back and forth across them all the time. Yet they neither lose all their water, shrinking down and collapsing, nor do they overfill with water, swelling up and bursting like balloons. Along the evolutionary path they have contrived a method of keeping their water constant; they do this beautifully by employing the salts to assist them. They make use of the principle that water follows salt.

Definition of salt. The chemist uses the term *salt* to include many inorganic substances, not just the ordinary table salt with which most of us are familiar. To denote table salt, the chemist refers to *sodium chloride*, NaCl; it is a good example to use in this discussion. In the white crystalline substance the sodium and chlorine atoms are bound to each other by strong electrostatic forces in a rigid crystalline structure. Outwardly they exhibit no electrical charge. However, when dissolved in water, the rigid structure relaxes, and some of the sodium moves about freely as positively charged ions; some of the chlorine too dissociates and moves about as negatively charged ions. The salt thus reveals itself as a compound composed of charged particles. The positive ions are *cations*, the negative, *anions*.

A closer look at ions. The reason sodium ions are positive and chloride ions are negative is made clear in Appendix B (for the student who wishes to review basic chemistry). However, a simplistic description here may help promote an understanding of the fundamental difference between cations and anions. A sodium *atom* has 11 positive particles called protons in its nucleus which do not leave the nucleus under ordinary circumstances; in the vicinity of the nucleus there are 11 fast-moving negative charges called electrons which can travel about and can even attach themselves to other atoms. One electron of the 11 traveling about the sodium nucleus has more energy than the others and is most likely to leave and attach itself to another atom. When this happens, sodium is a positively charged ion. It has 11 positive charges (they are trapped in the nucleus and cannot leave), and it now has only 10 negatively charged particles; thus its net charge is +1.

A chlorine *atom* has 17 protons in its nucleus with 17 electrons surrounding it. Because of the energy requirements of

Na = sodium.

Cl = chlorine.

salt: a compound composed of charged particles (ions). Exception: a compound in which the cations are H + is an acid; a compound in which the anions are OH − is a base. See also Appendix B.

cation (CAT-eye-un): a positively charged ion.

anion (AN-eye-un): a negatively charged ion.

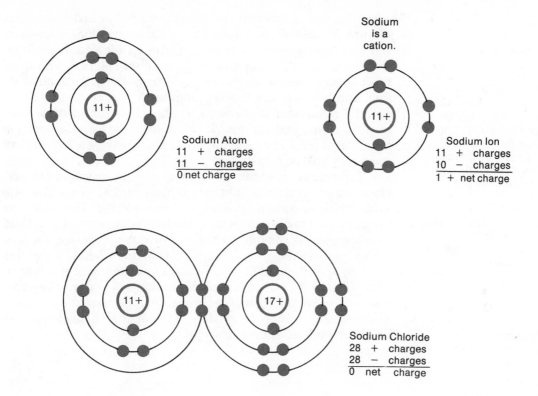

Sodium
is a
cation.

Sodium Atom
11 + charges
11 − charges
0 net charge

Sodium Ion
11 + charges
10 − charges
1 + net charge

Sodium Chloride
28 + charges
28 − charges
0 net charge

these electrons, chlorine is more likely to gain, than to lose, an electron. When this happens, chlorine has one excess negative charge: −1. Table salt is a very stable compound and these peculiarities of sodium and chloride provide insight into the reason for its stability: sodium likes to give up an electron, chlorine likes to gain one, so while they are together, they each supply the other's needs (a good marriage).

An ion can also be a *group* of atoms so bound to each other that the group can have a charge and enter into reactions as if it were a single ion. Many such groups are active in the fluids of the body: the bicarbonate ion is composed of five atoms—1 H, 1 C, and 3 O's—and has a net charge of −1 ($-HCO_3^-$). Another important ion which is composed of several atoms is the phosphate ion: 1 H, 1 P, and 4 O's, with a net charge of −2 ($-HPO_4^{-2}$).

Electrolytes. A salt which partly dissociates in water, as does sodium chloride, is known as an electrolyte. Since the fluids of the body are composed of water and partly dissociated salts, they are electrolyte solutions.

Electrolyte solutions are always electrostatically balanced. There is no such thing as a test tube filled with sodium ions. Sodium ions are always positively charged and cannot exist apart from negatively charged ions. Therefore, in any fluid where there are dissolved electrolytes there will always be the

chloride: the ionic form of chlorine.

phosphate ion: an inorganic chemist would call $-HPO_4^=$ a "biphosphate" ion.

dissociation: physical separation of the ions in an ionic compound.

electrolyte solution: so called because it can conduct electricity.

A **milliequivalent** is a number of ions equal to the number of H$^+$ ions in a milligram of hydrogen. This is a useful measure, because when we are considering ions we are usually interested in the number of positive or negative charges present in a solution, rather than in their weight.

This force is known as the **osmotic pressure** of a solution. Water flows in the direction of the higher osmotic pressure.

Other terms used to describe electrolyte solutions:

isotonic: having the same osmotic pressure as a reference solution. Example: a saline solution may be made isotonic to human blood.

hypertonic: having a higher osmotic pressure than a reference solution.

hypotonic: having a lower osmotic pressure than a reference solution.

same number of positive and negative ions. For instance, in the extracellular fluid, the number of cations and anions each equal 155 milliequivalents per liter (mEq/L). Of the cations, sodium ions make up 142 mEq/L with potassium, calcium, and magnesium ions making up the remainder; of the anions, chloride ions number 104 mEq/L, bicarbonate ions number 27 mEq/L, and the remainder is provided by phosphate ions, sulfate ions, organic acids, and protein. If an anion enters a cell, a cation must accompany it, or another anion must leave, so that electroneutrality will be maintained.

The rule given above was that water follows salt. More precisely, there is a force that moves water into a place where a solute such as sodium chloride is concentrated. The condition for this force to operate is that the divider separating two fluid solutions be permeable to water but not permeable (or less freely permeable) to the solute. The figures below show this force in operation. In the top figure, equal amounts of solute on both sides of the divider cause the amounts of water to be equal also. In the bottom figure, the presence of more solute on side B draws water across the divider so that the *concentration* of solute on both sides becomes equal.

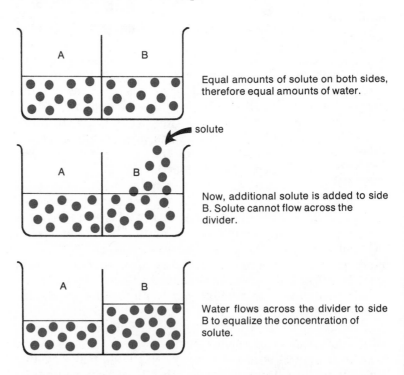

Equal amounts of solute on both sides, therefore equal amounts of water.

solute

Now, additional solute is added to side B. Solute cannot flow across the divider.

Water flows across the divider to side B to equalize the concentration of solute.

You have observed this force pulling water out of *cells* if you have ever salted a lettuce salad an hour before eating it. When you came back to the salad, the lettuce was wilted and there was water in the salad bowl. The high concentration of salt (and therefore low concentration of water) on the outside of the lettuce cells caused water to leave the inside of the cells. They collapsed (the lettuce wilted), and the water puddled in the salad dish. Sugar would have caused the same reaction as the salt. There is one way you could have prevented this occurrence (here's a cooking lesson for the novice): you could have coated the lettuce thoroughly with oil, then salted it or put salad dressing containing salt on it; the oil would have acted as a barrier against the salt, keeping the lettuce crisp.

The divider between the water inside and outside of a cell is the cell membrane. With the above picture in mind, you can see how the living cell manages to move water in and out as it needs to. It cannot pump water directly across its membrane, but it does possess proteins in its membrane which can attach to, and move, sodium ions from one side of the membrane to the other. When these *sodium pumps* in a cell's membrane are active, they pump out sodium faster than it can diffuse into the cell. Water follows the sodium. When *potassium pumps* are active, they pump in potassium, and water follows this ion. Thus by maintaining a certain concentration of sodium outside, and potassium inside, the cell can exactly regulate the amount of water it contains.

Acid-base balance. In addition to regulating the amount of water found in each body compartment, the ions in body fluids regulate the acidity (pH) of the fluids. The major minerals are most important in this regard, since they are present in the highest concentrations. Table C14.1 divides these minerals into the acid- and base-forming classes.

The salty water on the outside of the lettuce cells is hypertonic to the water inside the cells, so attracts water out of the cells.

The cell membrane is **semipermeable:** more permeable to some substances (such as water) than to others. This is the condition necessary for osmotic pressure to operate.

Table C14.1
The Major Minerals

Acid Formers	*Base Formers*
Chlorine	Calcium
Sulfur	Magnesium
Phosphorus	Sodium
	Potassium

NOTE: The task of remembering each of these seven elements as either an acid- or a base-former is somewhat simplified if you are aware that each of these elements forms a common compound that reveals its role. For example, a common compound of calcium is calcium hydroxide. Hydroxides are bases—and calcium is a base former. With phosphorus, a common compound is phosphoric acid; phosphorus is an acid former. The compound of sulfur, sulfuric acid, tells you that sulfur is an acid former. The rule is consistent: for chlorine, remember hydrochloric acid; for magnesium, sodium, and potassium, the hydroxides.

homeostasis: see page 430.

salt intake

There are four kinds of taste receptors on the tongue: those sensitive to salt, sweet, sour, and bitter flavors.

salt excretion

The constancy of total body electrolytes. Predictably, there are several homeostatic mechanisms operating to regulate the body's contents of electrolytes. *Salt hunger* is well known in animals such as cattle, which will go to a salt lick and ingest the amount of sodium chloride they need to balance the losses they experience through sweating on a hot summer day. To retain water, as you have seen, they must have sodium. The tongue, in both animals and humans, is equipped with particular taste receptors that respond only to salt, hence the distinctiveness of the "salty taste" and the animal's ability to seek this stimulus. This mechanism may also work in human beings.

The kidneys also respond sensitively to electrolyte concentrations in the blood passing through them by excreting or retaining the appropriate amounts of each electrolyte to maintain optimal blood concentrations. The result is a constancy of total body electrolytes balanced synchronously with total water in a way that protects the body from all but the most extreme situations.

Fluid and Electrolyte Imbalance

You are thus well protected from imbalance. Your intake and excretion achieve optimal whole-body contents of fluid and electrolytes over a wide range of different conditions. By these mechanisms the body's cells are supplied with the total amounts of sodium, potassium, and other ions that they need in order to maintain their own local balances. However, you may be thrown into situations for which the kidneys, your thirst instinct, and the cell membranes cannot compensate: circumstances over which they have no control and so are overwhelmed. This is the case when large amounts of fluid and electrolytes are lost in an emergency. The most familiar conditions in which this happens are discussed below; it will be helpful in considering these to remember that sodium and chloride are the principal cation and anion *outside* the cell, and that potassium and phosphate are the principal cation and anion *inside* the cell.

Losses of water and salt. When you *vomit*, you lose large amounts of water and hydrochloric acid from your stomach. This leaves you dehydrated, and because of the loss of acid, may initially throw you into alkalosis. If you have a prolonged attack of *diarrhea*, you lose a more alkaline fluid from the lower portion of the GI tract, consisting largely of sodium ions. This, too, can leave you dehydrated, and may throw you into acidosis. Both conditions—vomiting and diarrhea—reflect losses of fluid from one body compartment—the gastrointestinal tract.

When either vomiting or diarrhea occurs, it is astonishing

the amount of fluid involved. One cannot help but wonder where it all comes from. Normally we are not conscious of the large amount of fluid involved in the digestive process because our bodies are so wonderfully made we don't have to drink the fluid necessary for digestion. You will recall from the chapter on digestion that water is added to the GI tract contents at each step along the way—via saliva, gastric, intestinal, and pancreatic juices and bile—but then is normally reabsorbed in the colon and recycled. The amount of digestive secretions put forth each day in the average adult has been estimated at over 9 liters, or more than three times as much as that taken in with food and drink and produced during metabolism. It is obvious that replacement of this fluid is of prime importance in the medical and nutritional management of diarrhea and vomiting. Over half of the deaths in children under four are due to diarrhea.

A liter is a little more than a quart (1.06 quart), so nine liters is about 9½ quarts.

A domino effect operates when the body attempts to maintain water balance: each fluid compartment is affected in turn by a change in the concentration of the fluids of adjacent compartments. For instance, in prolonged diarrhea, when a large amount of sodium has been lost from the GI tract, sodium and water move into the tract from the nearby interstitial and intravascular spaces. These spaces are continuous throughout the body, and their loss of sodium causes cells all over the body to compensate by shifting potassium out into the interstitial space. Meanwhile, since the whole fluid volume of the blood has decreased, the kidneys are experiencing dehydration and are attempting to retrieve needed water. Their principal means of doing this is to retain sodium, because water will travel with sodium. The kidneys thus return sodium from the urine filtrate back to the blood. As the sodium enters, potassium must be exchanged; thus, potassium is lost in the urine. The end result, then, is excretion of potassium which came from cells far removed from the site of the original disturbance. Potassium ion loss severely affects intracellular functions, and if great enough, can lead to cardiac arrest, since potassium ions are needed for the contraction of the heart muscle.

The examples of vomiting and diarrhea illustrate the body's responses to major fluid losses. If you understand the principles, you can predict what will happen in other fluid-loss situations. For example, when you *sweat* excessively, you are losing fluid largely from the interstitial space. The dehydration that results affects not only this space but also the vascular and intracellular spaces; you become dehydrated and other imbalances follow. If you replace the lost water without the salt you may suffer a severe depletion of your body sodium and chloride. Since these are the major electrolytes lost in sweat, the Food and Nutrition Board offers a rule of thumb: if you have drunk more than four quarts of water in a day to replace that lost in heavy sweating,

A gram of sodium chloride = 1/5 teaspoon of salt. Salt tablets are often 1 gram each.

you should take a gram of sodium chloride with each additional quart.

As you have probably anticipated, however, there is a risk of overcompensating. *Excessive salt intake* can be as serious as insufficient intake. To excrete excess sodium, the kidneys must excrete a certain amount of water along with it. Thus too much salt can as readily cause dehydration as too little water. When the kidneys are diseased, a moderate salt intake is especially critical. Unexcreted salt accumulates in extracellular fluids and so may cause either edema or high blood pressure or both.

edema: see also page 119.

high blood pressure = hypertension.

One additional example will illustrate another class of fluid loss: loss from the intracellular space, as when a person is severely *burned*. In this instance, the electrolytes potassium and phosphate and others are lost. Since the salts lost in this case are the chemist's salts, and not the single compound, sodium chloride, the replacement of these must be managed by a physician. The physician's first and most important concern in treating a burn patient is to assess the fluid and electrolyte balance and to plan a careful replacement that will not upset the balance further.

The details of electrolyte balance are among the most important ones that medical students must learn. Mastery of the details is appropriately left to them and to their medical associates. For the layman, and the student of nutrition, it is necessary only to appreciate the importance of this balance and the principles by which it is maintained, and to be aware of the situations which threaten it. When any of these gets out of control, the appropriate action is to consult a physician. The water and salts, which we take for granted and usually ignore, are more vital to life than any of the other nutrients considered in this book.

Putting It All Together

At the end of Chapter 11, it was demonstrated that the inclusion of foods from all six exchange groups was necessary for an adequate diet. This chapter concludes the treatment of the minerals, and some additional pointers on diet adequacy are in order here. For the mineral element iron, some authorities recommend that women take a supplement because so many women fail to get enough from food sources alone. In the case of two other mineral elements—iodine and fluorine—food sources are so unreliable in some geographical locations as to necessitate the inclusion of iodized salt and fluoridated water for protection against deficiencies. Some trace elements, such as chromium, are lost during the refining of foods, so there is some basis for believing that unrefined foods should have a greater place in the diet than they do at present. To cover these needs, some additions must be made to the diagram presented on page 357:

Food Exchange Group	Supplies Substantial Amounts of
Milk	vitamin D
Vegetables	protein, B$_{12}$
Fruits	niacin
Bread, cereal, starchy vegetables	riboflavin
Meat	thiamin
Fat	vitamin C
	vitamin A
	vitamin K
	folacin
(For details, see page 357.)	vitamin E
	linoleic acid
	fiber

Additions:

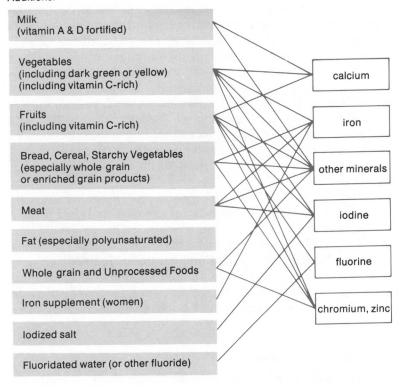

The Highlight following this chapter invites you to put it all together for yourself by studying your own diet with an eye to its adequacy for all the nutrients that have been discussed.

Summing Up

Fluids and electrolytes provide the environment that supports the life of all the body's cells. Their concentration and composition are regulated to remain as constant as possible.

Water comprises 55 to 60 percent of the body weight. Total body water is kept constant by regulating intake and excretion. Intake occurs when the osmotic pressure (solute concentration) of the blood is high, causing withdrawal of water from the salivary glands and the resultant dryness of the mouth, stimulating thirst. High osmotic pressure of the blood also stimulates the kidneys to retain water through two hormonal mechanisms: one regulated by the antidiuretic hormone, the other by aldosterone. Excretion occurs whenever body water exceeds needs.

The principal electrolytes in body fluids are sodium, chlorine, phosphorus, and potassium; each of these is maintained at a constant concentration by means of renal excretion. Sodium and chloride are the major extracellular, and potassium and phosphorus the major intracellular electrolytes.

Fluid and electrolyte imbalances occur when large amounts of fluid are lost, as in vomiting, diarrhea, or sweating. Loss of extracellular fluid occurs in these conditions; intracellular fluid then shifts out of cells to compensate, causing abnormal distribution of electrolytes across cell membranes and consequent cellular malfunction. In the case of sweating, the principal electrolytes lost are sodium and chloride. Replacement is relatively simple (if more than 4 quarts water have been drunk to replace that lost in sweating, take one gram sodium chloride for each additional quart). The imbalances caused by vomiting and diarrhea (and other circumstances such as burns and hemorrhaging) are medical emergencies; replacement should be managed by a physician.

Attention to the mineral needs in diet planning suggests that consumers be aware not only of the need to select a wide variety of nutritious foods from the six exchange groups but also of the following possibilities: that some women may need supplemental iron; that in iodine-poor areas, iodized salt may be needed; and that in unfluoridated counties, supplemental fluoride may be needed. Unrefined, natural foods may provide protection against deficiencies of trace elements, such as chromium and zinc.

To Explore Further—

Both classics in the literature of the history of life on earth, this book and article reveal facets of the intimate relationship between environmental water and the life of cells:

Oparin, A. I.: *Origin of Life.* Dover Publications, Inc., New York, 1938. Paperback.

Wald, George. The origin of life. *Scientific American* 190:44-53, August, 1956. Also Offprint No. 47.

Teaching Aid, *Nutrient Metabolism—Water, the Essential Nutrient* by Robinson, J., can be ordered from:

Director, Education Services
Nutrition Today
101 Ridgely Avenue
Annapolis, Maryland 21404

Highlight Fourteen:
An Extended Activity
Nutritional Self-Study

You have studied the basic facts of nutrition in the chapters of this text, have been exposed to some of the controversy in our science in the Highlights, and have been shown ways to judge nutrition information in the Digressions. However, you may not have been aware of an equally important aspect of nutrition that has been presented in Activity 1 at the end of nearly every chapter. These activities asked you to use the facts you had learned to evaluate your own diet and to improve it. In this Highlight, the authors want to give some additional help in the practical application of nutrition by outlining a way by which you can devise your own unique dietary pattern.

Knowledge of nutrition is worthless if it is not applied. While knowledge and understanding of what nutrients do in our bodies have been stressed throughout this text almost to the exclusion of the discussion of food, it must be remembered that the primary way nutrients get into the body is from foods.

It must also be remembered that food does more for us than nourish our bodies. From our very first experience with food at birth, when we were alone and afraid in a new, strange place, the receiving of food has been associated with emotions. We learned to love that first person who eased our pain by holding us close and giving us warm milk. Throughout our lives many, varied emotions have been tangled up with the act of eating until today we would be hard pressed to untangle more than one or two of them. You probably can recall, however, the event that caused a dislike of a particular food. Perhaps your mother was preparing lamb curry at the same time you were becoming ill with an intestinal virus. To this day when you smell curry a wave of nausea sweeps over you. Not so easy to identify are feelings of—

pride—in an abundant table;

status—eating at the best restaurants;

fear of deprivation—remembering a time when there was never enough food to go around;

lavishing love on someone—"Have another piece of pie, dear;"

need for strokes—"My husband says I'm a wonderful cook;"

nostalgia—liking something "the way Mother used to fix it," even if your mother wasn't a very good cook;

hospitality—"I have plenty; let me share with you."

All these factors and more, in addition to hunger, combine to determine what foods you eat, when, where, and how much you eat. For this reason, dietary regimens imposed by one person on another are often unsuccessful. Even diabetics whose lives depend on eating correct amounts of certain classes of foods at particular times of the day (to correspond with the action of the insulin) very often refuse to follow the doctor's dietary orders if it entails a change in their food habits.[1] Your heritage from your family and culture determines these food habits and makes you the person that is best suited to design your dietary pattern.

A dietary pattern is a guideline by which you can be assured of consuming the nutrients you need. Of necessity it is written in terms of foods, not nutrients. No one says to himself, "I've had no calcium today," and goes to the refrigerator for a glass of calcium. A dietary pattern usually includes the class of food (for example, fruit or bread); the amounts, either in numbers of food exchanges or in kitchen measurements (for example, 2 bread exchanges, 4 lean meat exchanges, or ½ cup vegetable); and how often this amount should be eaten (for example, twice a day, once a week).

A usable dietary pattern is based on an individual's eating habits and makes only those changes which are absolutely necessary. Therefore, your first task in designing your pattern is to discover exactly what you eat, and how much. To do this you will need to keep a record of every bite of food you put in your mouth. This record should be kept for seven consecutive days and should include all snacks and any beverages except water,

[1]Williams, T. F., Anderson, E., Watkins, J. D. and Coyle, V.: Dietary errors made at home by patients with diabetes. *Journal of the American Dietetic Association* 51(7):19-25, 1967.

unsweetened coffee or unsweetened tea, in addition to the regular meals.

It will be difficult to estimate the amounts you eat of some food items. For example, a stew has many ingredients and differs from one cook to another. It is recommended that for foods such as stews, soups, or pizzas you list only the major ingredients with as accurate an estimate of the amounts of the ingredients as possible. Estimating meat servings in ounces presents another difficulty. Figure H14.1 demonstrates one way of estimating the weight of meat servings. The thickness of the fingers represents the thickness of the meat; thus if the meat is twice the thickness of your fingers, the amounts shown in the drawing should be doubled. For the purpose of learning how much of a vegetable is 1/2, 1/3, or 1/4 cup, you could serve a vegetable using a kitchen measuring cup until you have gained skill in estimating amounts.

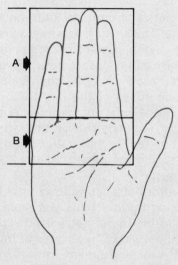

Figure H14.1. A method for making a rough estimate of the weight of a serving of meat, using your hand as a comparative measure: For a serving about the thickness of a finger, a piece of meat the size of the area marked A would approximate three ounces in weight; one the size of the area A plus B would approximate four ounces.

When you have completed the seven-day diet record, choose the three days which you believe are typical of your normal eating pattern. Record each of these days on separate sheets, such as the one in Table H14.1 (page 445). Look up your RDA's in Appendix I; then calculate the nutrient composition of each item of the day's food. (The Table of Food Composition in Appendix H and the Aids to Calculation in Appendix D will prove helpful with these calculations.) Total each day's nutrients and compare with your RDA.

As you make this comparison you will discover that for some of these nutrients your own appetite and normal eating provide you with sufficient amounts. For other nutrients you may be deficient or oversupplied. It is suggested that you keep the three days' results separated while analyzing your diet so that you can notice any day-to-day variations.

Table H14.1
Nutrient Composition of One Day's Food

Food Sources of Nutrients	Amount Eaten in One Day*	Amount of Nutrient in the Amount of Food Eaten in a Day†											
		Food Energy (kcal)	Protein (g)	Total Fat (g)	Linoleic Acid‡ (g)	Carbo-hydrate (g)	Cal-cium (mg)	Iron (mg)	Vita-min A (IU)	Thia-min (mg)	Ribo-flavin (mg)	Ascorbic Acid (mg)
RDA:	✕			✕		✕						

*Amounts should be listed in kitchen measures such as cups, teaspoons, etc., and should include an entire day's intake.
†These amounts should be calculated using the Table of Food Composition, Appendix H. Appendix D offers help in making the calculations.
‡The recommended amount of linoleic acid intake daily is based on the RDA for calories: grams linoleic acid equals the RDA for calories multiplied by 2% and divided by 9 kcalories per gram.

Let us now critically examine the results of comparing your nutrient intake with your RDA. You will want to call on all the principles of nutrition which you have learned and go into more depth in your own analysis than can be done in the following brief outline.

Calories. In considering whether you are consuming a diet which meets your caloric needs, you will want to note if you are presently at a weight which is comfortable for you or if you are gaining or losing weight. Recall that the RDA for calories is based on the average person and that you may not be average. Should you decide that you are consuming too many calories, one of the first revisions to consider is that of your consumption of fats and empty calorie foods, since fats have the highest caloric production and empty calorie foods are often eaten unconsciously. Your use of animal sources of protein may be a cause of excess calories, due to the fat contained in most meats. If you need to have a higher intake of calories you will want to examine nutrient source lists to find foods which will give you, in addition to some extra calories, other beneficial nutrients as well. You might consider selecting your vegetables from the bread list, emphasizing the higher calorie meats, enjoying periodic eggnogs, and eating cereals frequently. These foods would contribute fiber, minerals, and vitamins as well as calories to your diet.

Protein. In addition to being certain that you are meeting at least 2/3 of your RDA for protein, you will want to know that you are obtaining the essential amino acids. Animal sources of protein are the easiest way to meet the amino acid needs but they, particularly the meats (as opposed to the animal products of milk, eggs, and cheese), are also the most expensive items in the food budget. Therefore, if you need to economize you might want to look critically at the amount and source of protein in your diet. You may discover that you will also improve your intake of other nutrients by shifting from meat to plant sources of protein.

Total Fat. The calories from fat should be no higher than 35 or 40 percent of the total calories. If your fat calories are consistently higher on all three days, you may want to ascertain the source of these fat calories and adjust your diet accordingly.

Linoleic Acid. It is usually recommended[2] that calories from linoleic acid be about 2 percent of the total calories. If your intake is lower than this you may want to substitute oils or fats higher in polyunsaturated fatty acids for the ones you currently use.

Carbohydrates. Of particular interest in analyzing the food sources of carbohydrate is the distinction between complex

[2]Krause, M. V. and Hunscher, M. A.: *Food, Nutrition and Diet Therapy.* W. B. Saunders Company, Philadelphia, 1972, p. 64.

and simple carbohydrates. There are no rules for amounts of these that should be in the diet, but it is generally recognized that the consumption of complex carbohydrates offers many side benefits, such as additional fiber, trace elements such as chromium, and perhaps, as yet undiscovered nutrients—which would not be present in highly refined simple carbohydrates, such as sugar and syrups.

Calcium. Absorption of calcium, you will recall, is controlled by physiological mechanisms based on the body's need. Regularity of intake is as important as the amount of calcium since the body can adjust to a low calcium intake but not as well to a fluctuating supply. The effects of a calcium deficiency on the bones are insidious and can go undetected for years, making conscious awareness of daily calcium intake important.

Iron. It is important that iron be supplied daily in the diet. Women have a monthly loss of iron and generally cannot eat enough food to meet their iron RDA, therefore it is recommended that they take an iron supplement. Men do not have such a route of excretion and are usually able to obtain adequate iron from the diet if it includes daily food sources of iron.

Vitamin A. There is no need to have daily sources of vitamin A since it is stored in the adipose tissue. However, you will want to look over the three days of your diet record to see that sometime during those days you have included a major source of this vitamin and on the average are meeting at least 2/3 of your RDA.

Thiamin, Riboflavin, and Ascorbic Acid. Since the B vitamins are not stored in the body, it is necessary to meet your needs for these every day and to see that they are not being destroyed by unwise cooking and handling methods. Most nutritionists recommend that vitamin C be handled similarly.

You will notice the absence of a number of important nutrients from this list. A varied diet which includes the listed nutrients will probably include the ones omitted. For example, niacin is omitted because the RDA table lists it in milligram equivalent units while the nutrient composition tables list it in milligrams, making comparison difficult; however, if protein is adequate in amount and some is from animal sources, niacin intake will probably be adequate. Also, phosphorus will undoubtedly be ingested in a reasonable amount if your protein is adequate; if your protein and vitamin A needs are met, your vitamin D will probably be adequate. Other important nutrients can be included by simple means: iodized salt will take care of iodine needs, and if you do not have sufficient fluorine in your water supply, you will want to discuss this situation with your dentist.

Fiber is the last of the nutrients to be discussed, but not the least important. There is no RDA for fiber and the Table of Food

Composition in Appendix H does not list fiber content; nevertheless, it is important for a healthy GI tract. Have you included plenty of whole-grain cereals, vegetables, and fruits to care for this "forgotten" nutrient?

As you critically analyze this three-day diet record, you will discover that your favorite foods automatically supply, or maybe oversupply, some nutrients while allowing others to be deficient. YOUR APPETITE BECOMES, THEN, A SUFFICIENT GUIDE FOR *SOME* NUTRIENTS, and for these you need no other dietary pattern. List the nutrients for which your appetite can be your guide.

For those nutrients which you have difficulty including in your diet, devise a rule whereby you will remember to include them. For example, "Fish should be eaten three times a week and poultry twice," might be a rule if you find that you have been eating a diet high in saturated fat. Another rule for you might be, "Include highly colored vegetables every day," or, "Don't go to bed until you have had some fresh fruit," if you have a tendency to ignore fruits and vegetables. A colleague, the father of five children, became concerned about the high cholesterol of eggs and wanted also to increase the fiber and fruit in his family's diet. He devised a breakfast pattern which accomplished all these changes. On day one, they had ready-to-eat cereals with milk and canned or fresh fruit; on day two they had cooked cereal with milk and dried fruit; on day three they had eggs and bacon; and on day four they started over again. Every day they had orange juice and whole wheat toast with margarine. Thus at the beginning of the day, the father was assured that his children were well on their way to getting a low-cholesterol, high-fiber diet. Furthermore, the pattern made shopping for and preparing breakfast easier.

In summary, a dietary pattern for yourself will

(1) list those nutrients for which your normal eating pattern is a sufficient guide, and

(2) establish rules which will help you remember to include those nutrients for which your appetite is not a reliable guide.

From time to time you may want to spot check those nutrients which you discovered were a problem for you. Periodically, keep a 24-hour diet record, calculate its nutrient composition, compare with your RDA, then adjust your diet accordingly, making new rules if they are indicated.

For many persons, the overriding determinant of what foods will be eaten is cost, but we have largely ignored that factor in this Highlight. This neglect is a matter of priorities. Good nutrition must be the first objective, then consideration of cost should follow. It is possible within reasonable limits to lower your food costs without denying yourself good nutrition, but it requires careful analysis of the nutrient content of the diet, such as has been detailed here.

There are several points to be considered when discussing the cost of food. First of all, many nonfood items are included in your grocery purchases and should be seen for what they are: cleaning supplies, cosmetics, etc., not food. There are energy costs associated with food: refrigeration, freezing, cooking, and travel to the market, to name a few. Sometimes, also, you are not purchasing nourishment for the body only but also for the soul —love, fun, fellowship, or relaxation—these have a valid claim on your food dollar.

Suppose, however, you do need to economize on food, how can you do it safely? The answers you give to the following questions will alert you to ways in which you can save money and at the same time improve your nutrition.

Do you eat more animal protein than you need?

Do you eat more of any nutrient than you need?

Do you eat the more expensive meats and seafood?

Do you eat the more expensive cuts of meat?

Do you ever substitute cheese, eggs, or legumes and cereal for animal protein?

Have you tried creative ways of incorporating dry skim milk into your diet?

Have you served your family's favorite stew or casserole to guests instead of expensive ham or steak?

Have you investigated the food cooperatives in your town for the purchase of fresh farm vegetables and other groceries at wholesale prices?

Have you comparison-shopped varieties of canned goods, for example, bought three different brands of tomatoes and compared their water content?

Have you tried the meat analogs (textured vegetable protein—TVP—products that taste like meat) and calculated their cost per ounce of protein?

Have you done a cost analysis of snack items? Have you ever substituted fruit for potato chips?

When you eat in a restaurant, do you comparison shop? Do you buy prestige and think you are buying food?

Have you made master-mixes (flour, baking powder, salt, and fat mixed in large quantities for use in making biscuits, pancakes, cakes, etc.) and compared the cost with well-known brands of mixes?

Do you buy hamburger in bulk at lower prices, then freeze in packages of the right size for your needs?

Do you keep a jar in your refrigerator for the surplus liquid from cooking vegetables and juice from cooking meats, then use this liquid for gravies or soups?

Do you boil leftover bones to make soup stock?

How much of your food cost is for convenience foods? Is there enough convenience to justify that cost?

Some nutrients which you have already paid for are lost—

when you buy old vegetables and fruits,

when you buy more meat than you can use in leftovers,

when you buy packages of fruits and vegetables that contain more than you need so that some of them rot,

when you fail to read the nutrition labels so you buy sugar when you wanted to buy cereal,

when you comparison-shop canned goods by looking only at the price, then end up buying water and sugar when you wanted fruit,

when you cook too much food,

when you cook at too high a temperature,

when you leave orange juice exposed to air,

when you pour "pot liquor" down the drain,

when the way you cook food is not appetizing,

when a food is left on the plate,

etc., etc., etc., and etc.

Inherent in these suggestions for lowering food costs is the idea that it is nutrients, not foods, you are purchasing. The body cannot distinguish between a nutrient from an expensive food and a nutrient from a cheap food, nor can the body gain any benefits from a nutrient that was thrown away, no matter how expensive it was.

You have seen in this Highlight that a dietary pattern does not have to be someone else's idea of what food and how much you must eat. However, it does have to be based on the amounts of nutrients you need. Your own food habits can be depended on to provide ample amounts of some of the nutrients and special dietary rules can be devised to care for your problem nutrients. It is possible to economize on food and not lower the nutritional quality of the diet if the less expensive foods donate the required nutrients. Essential to the processes of devising your own dietary pattern and lowering the cost of food is an analysis of the nutrient composition of your food intake. Only when you know the nutrient content of a diet can you make valid decisions about it.

To Explore Further—

A small book that is both entertaining and educational, including a good chapter on food-borne diseases:

Labuza, T. F.: *Food for Thought.* Avi Publishing Company, Inc., Westport, Connecticut, 1974.

This book would be helpful in learning about such things as home preservation, storage, and preparation:

Bradley, H. and Sundberg, C.: *Keeping Food Safe.* Doubleday and Company, Inc., New York, 1975.

This is a good article on care of food after it is bought:

Angelotti, R.: Salmonella and food in your home. *FDA Consumer,* July/August:11-14, 1973.

Nutrient content of brand name products, cookies, snack foods, cookie mixes, canned fruit, TV dinners, condiments, etc., not found in tables of food composition such as Appendix H in this book:

Consumer Guide—Food: the Brand Name Game: Consumer Guide, Skokie, Illinois, 1974.

The three food composition books listed below vary in the number and kinds of foods listed. The first one lists over 600 foods, the second over 2,000 foods. Church's book includes commercially prepared foods and food additives:

Nutritive Value of Foods, Home and Garden Bulletin #72 ($.85), has been largely reprinted as Appendix H in this book.

Agricultural Handbook #8, Composition of Foods, U.S. Department of Agriculture ($2.95), can be ordered from:

> U.S. Government Printing Office
> Washington, D.C.

Church, C. F. and Church, H. N.: *Food Values of Portions Commonly Used.* J. B. Lippincott Company, Philadelphia, 1970. ($5.40)

Composition of Foods Used by Ethnic Groups—Selected References to Sources of Data, can be requested from:

> Dr. Louise Page
> Food and Diet Appraisal Group
> Consumer and Food Economics Institute
> U.S. Dept. of Agriculture
> Agricultural Research Services
> Hyattsville, Maryland 20782

Reprint of an article on Japanese-American food equivalents is available from:

> The American Dietetic Association
> 430 N. Michigan Ave.
> Chicago, Illinois 60611

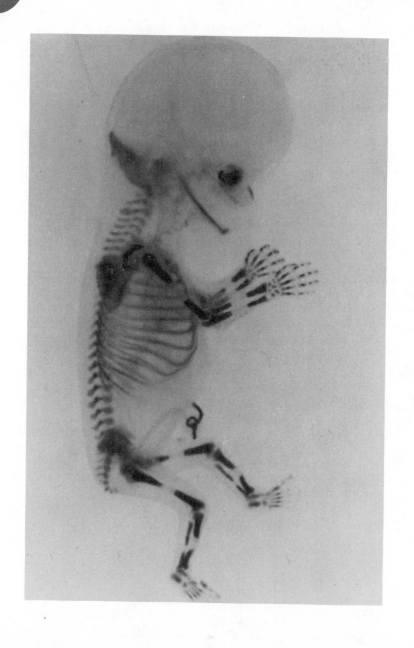

15

Nutrition
Through Life

"I wish you wouldn't squeeze so," said the Dormouse, who was sitting next to her. *"I can hardly breathe."*
"I can't help it," said Alice very meekly: *"I'm growing."*
—LEWIS CARROLL, *Alice's Adventures in Wonderland*

The preceding chapters have been addressed to the young adult. Wherever nutrition information has been relevant to the reader's needs and concerns, examples and illustrations involving adults have been given, with only occasional references to infants, children, and elderly people. The principles of nutrition apply throughout the life span, but there are some changes in emphasis that are appropriate to the various age groups.

Young people, from infancy through the teen years, are growing—a characteristic not shared by adults. In addition to young people's nutritional needs for maintenance, then, they have special needs related to the growth process. Furthermore, people of all ages are growing psychologically. In considering the nutritional needs and the feeding of infants, children, and the aged, it is important to keep both kinds of growth in mind. The following section is devoted to the processes of growth, after which the separate considerations of nourishing people at different ages are unified around these principles.

The Processes of Growth

As has been emphasized before, growth is not a matter of everything simply getting bigger all at once. From conception to adulthood, different organs differentiate, grow, and mature at different rates and times, each with its own characteristic pattern. A few generalizations hold for all growth processes, however, and an understanding of these generalities underlies the knowledge of the special nutritional needs imposed by growth. It is helpful to distinguish three growth levels, that of the whole body, that of the organs and tissues, and that of the cells of each organ or tissue. At each level, different considerations become apparent.

Whole body growth. Between conception and birth, a human organism's weight increases from a fraction of a gram to 3,500 grams. The greatest rate of growth is that between 8 weeks and term—the fetal period—in which the weight increases over 500 times. After birth, babies double their weight from 7 to 14 pounds in four months, then slow down somewhat and add another 7 pounds in the next eight months, reaching about 21 pounds at one year. Thereafter the growth rate slows to 5 pounds a year or less but increases dramatically again during the adolescent growth spurt.

See Figure C15.3 (page 466).

A similar pattern holds for height. From 1/5 of a millimeter at 3 weeks of gestation, the embryo reaches 3 centimeters at 8 weeks, then 50 centimeters at birth. Thereafter the increase in height is greatest during the first year (25 cm), half that much the second year (12-13 cm), and then slower still (6-7 cm a year) until the adolescent growth spurt, when a sudden increase of some 16-20 cm is achieved in a 2 to 2½ year period.

3 intensive growth periods:
  prenatal
  first year
  adolescence

What is important about all this is that growth does not proceed at a steady pace, that the maximal rate of growth is in the prenatal period, and that the two postnatal periods during which growth is fastest are the first year and the teen years.

nonlinear: see page 408.

Growth of organs and tissues. Not only does whole body growth increase nonlinearly, the growth of each organ and tissue type has its own characteristic pattern. In the fetus, for example, the heart and brain are well developed at 16 weeks while the lungs are still nonfunctional 10 weeks later. After birth, the brain doubles in weight during the first year, but increases only about 20 percent thereafter, while the muscles will be more than 30 times heavier at maturity than they are at birth.

Brain and central nervous system are first to reach maturity.

Each organ and tissue, then, has its own unique periods of intensive growth. Whatever nutrients are most important for the growth of a given organ or tissue will be needed most during its intensive growth periods. An interesting example is that of the blood during pregnancy: its volume almost doubles during the formation and growth of the placenta. A pregnant woman's need for the B vitamin, folic acid, which is uniquely involved in the manufacture of red blood cells, doubles during this time.

Growth at the cellular level. A further point of interest emerges when we investigate the cells of a single developing organ—the brain, for example. During development of the fetal brain, there is a period when very little increase in its overall size is observed; nevertheless, remarkable changes are taking place. The cells are increasing dramatically in *number*. Each time a cell divides, it produces two that are half its size. These two do not grow, but divide again, producing four cells that are still smaller. At a later time, the cells begin to grow, and continue dividing, so that their *size and number* are both increasing simultaneously. It is during these first two periods that the total number of cells to be found in the brain is determined for life. Later still, cell division ceases and thereafter the total number of cells is fixed, but they continue to increase in *size*. The development of almost every organ in the body follows a similar three-stage pattern.

The third period, during which increase in cell size alone is taking place, is one in which the most intensive growth may appear to be taking place, but actually the most important developmental events have occurred earlier. This fact has important implications for nutrition. The period of cell division is a *critical period*, critical in the sense that events taking place during that time can occur only at that time and at no other. The needed nutrients and other environmental conditions must be supplied at that time in order for the organ to reach its full potential. Recovery later is impossible. Thus malnutrition at an early period, for example prenatally, can have irreversible effects that may become fully manifest only when the organism reaches maturity.

The effect of malnutrition during critical periods is seen in the shorter stature reached by people who were undernourished in their early years, in the delayed sexual development of those undernourished during early adolescence, and in the smaller brain size and brain cell number of children who have suffered from episodes of marasmus or kwashiorkor. An area of active recent research points strongly to the probability that malnutrition in the perinatal period also affects learning ability and behavior. Clearly, then, it is never too early to try to provide the best of food.

Growth of the person. Interestingly, the concept of critical periods can also be applied to the growth of the person. From the moment of birth (and perhaps even earlier), the human child is learning what to expect from life and how to cope with life's problems. These learning experiences follow one another in a characteristic sequence, and each must reach some degree of completion before the next can proceed. Infants' earliest impressions mold attitudes that in maturity may still affect their behavior. An understanding of what is going on psychologically as well as physically makes it possible for those who nurture children not only to supply the nutrients they need but also to encourage learning and behavior that will help them to develop fully as human beings.

There are many ways of understanding and interpreting

Stages in organ growth:
(1) a period of **hyperplasia** (high-per-PLAY-zee-uh) (increase in cell number)
(2) a period of simultaneous hyperplasia and **hypertrophy** (high-PER-tro-fee) (increase in cell size)
(3) a period of hypertrophy (exception: liver).

critical period: a period of cell division.

See To Explore Further (Chapter 15).

perinatal (perry-NAY-tul): the period immediately before and after birth.

See To Explore Further (Chapter 15).

psychological growth and development. The one we have selected to follow[1] is that of Erik Erikson, whose insightful description of the stages of human growth provides a framework within which to view the whole person at each age. Erikson sees human life as a sequence of eight periods, in each of which the individual has a new learning task. To the extent that individuals master each successfully, they develop a strong foundation from which to proceed to the next. To the extent that they fail, they are handicapped in mastering the task at the next level. The stages in life and their respective learning tasks, as identified by Erikson, are as follows:

Infant	trust vs distrust
Toddler	autonomy vs shame and doubt
Preschooler	initiative vs guilt
School child	industry vs inferiority
Adolescent	identity vs role confusion
Young adult	intimacy vs isolation
Adult	generativity vs stagnation
Older adult	ego integrity vs despair

Whether you, the reader, agree with Erikson's view, or whether you see development in some other light, we hope you agree with the principle that understanding the whole person is important, even in the providing of food.

Each section that follows is devoted to a special stage in life, its physical growth and development, the related nutrient needs, and a feeding pattern that will supply the needed nutrients. Only the adult is omitted, having been the subject of all of the preceding chapters. Each section concludes with an attempt to put these nutrient needs in perspective in relation to the needs of the whole person.

Nutrition in Pregnancy

3 layers:

ectoderm (EK-to-derm): the outer layer (presumptive nervous system and skin).

mesoderm (MEZZ-o-derm): the middle layer (presumptive muscles and internal organs).

endoderm (EN-do-derm): the inner layer (presumptive glands and linings).

ecto = outside
meso = middle
endo = inside
derm = skin

Growth. The state of the mother's nutrition *prior* to pregnancy is important for the *future* health of her infant. Conditions in the uterus at the time of conception determine whether the fertilized egg will successfully implant itself in the uterine wall and begin development as it should. During the two weeks following fertilization, the egg cell divides into many cells and these sort themselves out into three layers. Very little growth in size takes place at this time; as defined above this is a critical period which precedes growth. Adverse influences at this time lead to failure to implant or other disturbances so severe as to

[1]We are indebted to S. R. Williams who, in her book, *Nutrition and Diet Therapy* (The C. V. Mosby Company, St. Louis, 1973), showed how Erikson's scheme could be integrated with nutrition principles.

cause loss of the fertilized egg, possibly even before the woman knows she is pregnant. Many drugs affect the earliest intrauterine events and later cross the placenta freely. Most health professionals agree that, if possible, a potential mother should be taking no drugs at all, not even aspirin. Nutrition should be, and should have been, continuously optimal.

The next five weeks, the period of embryonic development, register astonishing physical changes. From the outermost layer of cells, the nervous system and skin begin to develop; from

implantation: 0-2 weeks.

embryo: 2-8 weeks.

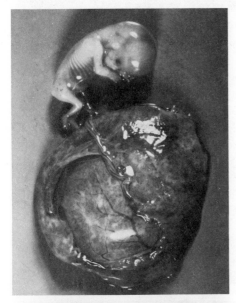

Ten-week-old fetus attached to the placenta. The blood vessels in the umbilical cord are clearly visible.

Courtesy of Dr. Roberts Rugh.

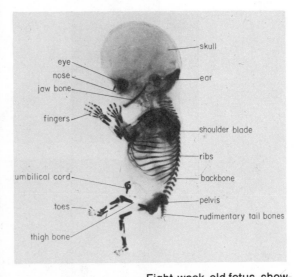

Eight-week-old fetus, showing development of the skeleton. The other tissues were treated so as to be transparent.

Courtesy of Dr. Roberts Rugh.

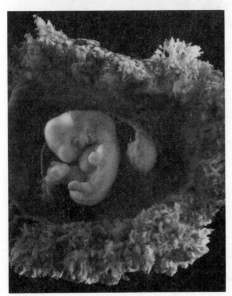

Six-week-old fetus attached to the placenta. At this time the fetus is less than one half inch long.

Courtesy of Dr. Roberts Rugh.

the middle layer, the muscles and internal organ systems; and from the innermost layer, the glands and linings of the digestive, respiratory, and excretory systems. At eight weeks, the three-centimeter-long embryo has a complete central nervous system, a beating heart, a fully formed digestive system, and the beginnings of facial features; already the "tail" has formed and almost completely disappeared again, and the fingers and toes are well formed.

Human embroyo, 3 days

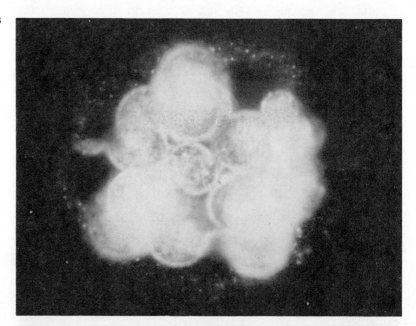

4 days

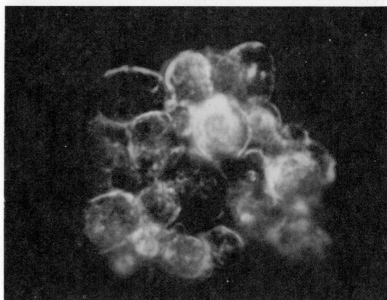

Photos courtesy of Landrum B. Shettles, M.D., F.A.C.S., F.A.C.O.G.

The last seven months of pregnancy, the fetal period, bring about the tremendous increase in size and further periods of cell division in organ after organ.

Meanwhile, the mother's body is undergoing changes. She grows a whole new organ, the placenta; her uterus and its supporting muscles increase greatly in size, her breasts change and

fetus: 2-9 months.

placenta (pla-SEN-tuh): the organ inside the uterus in which the mother's and fetus' circulatory systems mingle. Exchange of materials between mother's and fetal blood takes place here, the maternal blood supplying nutrients and oxygen and carrying away waste products.

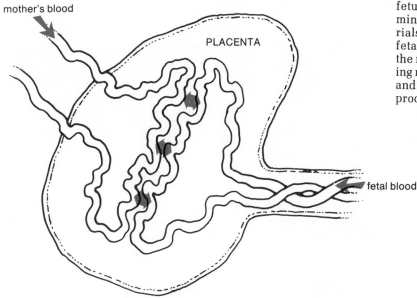

mother's blood

PLACENTA

fetal blood

grow in preparation for lactation, and her blood volume almost doubles. Thus the overall gain in weight of mother and child during pregnancy amounts to about 24 pounds:

Infant at birth:	7½ pounds
Placenta	1
Increase in mother's blood volume to supply placenta	4
Increase in size of mother's uterus and muscles to support it	2½
Increase in size of mother's breasts in preparation for lactation	3
Fluid to surround baby in amniotic sac	2
Mother's stores	4
	24 pounds

Nutrient needs during periods of intensive growth are greater than at any other time, and are greater for certain nutrients than for others, as shown in Figure C15.1.

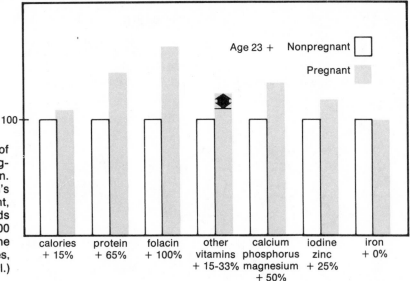

Figure C15.1. Comparison of nutrient needs of nonpregnant and pregnant woman. The nonpregnant woman's needs are set at 100 percent, the pregnant woman's needs shown as increases over 100 percent. (Calculated from the NAS-NRC RDA tables, Appendix I.)

Chart labels: calories + 15%; protein + 65%; folacin + 100%; other vitamins + 15-33%; calcium phosphorus magnesium + 50%; iodine zinc + 25%; iron + 0%. Legend: Age 23 + Nonpregnant / Pregnant. 100.

How transferrin increases iron absorption: see page 189.

Oral contraceptives mimic the hormones of pregnancy; see To Explore Further (Chapter 15).

The **growth nutrients:**
  protein
  calcium
  phosphorus
  magnesium

Whenever intensive growth is going on, the nutrients, protein, calcium, phosphorus, and magnesium, are of greatest concern because of their roles in the structure and functions of rapidly dividing or growing cells and growing bones. The extraordinary need for folacin in the pregnant woman has already been explained (page 454); as you might expect, the vitamin needed in the next highest amount is the other B vitamin associated with red blood cell manufacture: B_{12}.

Interestingly, the recommendation for iron is only slightly increased for the pregnant woman. Some thought may reveal one reason why this is so: the major route of excretion for iron is menstruation, which ceases during pregnancy. Some of the iron a woman needs to increase her blood stores is saved by reducing the losses ordinarily incurred in this way. As her blood volume increases so do all its constituents, including transferrin, which increases absorption. An additional adjustment is accomplished by the hormones of pregnancy which act to raise the concentration of iron in the blood, either by increasing absorption still further, by mobilizing iron stores, or both, as research with oral contraceptives has shown. Since, however, many women enter pregnancy with inadequate stores, physicians often recommend the use of an iron supplement during this time, as a kind of insurance.

Eating pattern. Whatever dietary pattern a person has adopted, it can be adjusted to meet changing nutrient needs by selecting and increasing the serving sizes or frequency of eating of those foods that supply the most needed nutrients. Since, as shown above, the greatest nutrient increases needed during pregnancy are in protein, calcium, phosphorus, magnesium, and folacin, the foods selected for the greatest increases might well be those in the Milk, Meat, and Vegetable Exchange Lists. Since calorie needs are less greatly increased, the selection of foods to be added should, for the average woman, be low-calorie, nutritious foods such as skimmed milk, cottage cheese, dark green vegetables, and liver. Regarding vitamin C, if a woman's routine has been to include one serving of a C-rich food such as a citrus juice or fruit each day, she should, during pregnancy, either increase the serving size of this food or add a second fair C source, such as tomatoes.

The pregnant woman must gain weight. Ideally she will begin her pregnancy at the "ideal" weight for her height, and will gain about 25 pounds, mostly in the second half of the pregnancy's nine-month course. This sounds like a lot, but a look back at the components of the pregnant woman's weight gain (page 459) will show that all these pounds—in nutritious calories—are needed to provide for healthy placental, uterine, blood, and breast growth of the mother, as well as for a strong 7½ pound baby. There is little place in her diet, however, for calories from foods such as sugar, which cannot support the growth of these tissues and will only contribute to excessive fat accumulation. Much of the weight gained is lost immediately at delivery; the remainder is generally lost within a few weeks as the mother's blood volume returns to normal and she loses the fluids she has accumulated.

ideal weight: see page 239.

To avoid the most common problems encountered by women in pregnancy, some additional pointers are helpful. Edema is not uncommon. It often appears to be due to a lack of protein and/or salts (see pages 118-119). When the blood concentration of these water-attracting constituents becomes too low, the water balance is disturbed and fluid leaves the bloodstream to accumulate in the tissues. A recent recommendation is that the pregnant woman's salt intake should be about 25 grams (5 teaspoons) a day, about 7 grams above the usual intake.[2] This means that there is rarely justification for restricting salt in the diet during pregnancy. However, this increased need will normally be met by the increased food intake, and no special efforts to increase salt intake need to be made.

The edema that occurs in pregnancy is often part of a larger cluster of symptoms known as **toxemia**, which has variable causes. Toxemia, once started, is a medical problem; a physician should be consulted.

Another common problem in pregnant women, revealed by the Ten-State Survey (see Highlight 12), is iron-deficiency anemia. Attention should be paid to getting enough iron during this important time. At birth a baby is supposed to have been able to store enough iron to last three to six months; this iron must come from the mother's iron stores which therefore ought to be adequate and to have been adequate even before pregnancy.

[2]Pitkin, R. M., Kaminetsky, H. A., Newton, M. and Pritchard, J. A.: Maternal nutrition. A selective review of clinical topics. *Journal of Obstetrics and Gynecology* 40:773-785, 1972.

Morning sickness in the early stages disappears of its own accord, but a hint found helpful by the expectant mother is to start the day with a few sips of water and a few nibbles of a soda cracker or other bland carbohydrate food. Later, as the thriving infant crowds her intestinal organs, she may complain of constipation; a high-fiber diet and a plentiful water intake then will help to alleviate this condition.

For causes and remedies of constipation, see Highlight 5.

Calcification of the baby teeth begins in the fifth month after conception; for this and for the bones, fluoride is needed. The woman in a county without fluoridated water needs to get a supplement that includes fluoride from her physician.

What a lot for a woman to remember! And this is only the briefest summary of the nutrient needs in pregnancy. With all of this to worry about, can a woman relax and enjoy her baby?

Psychological needs of the pregnant woman. The developing fetus cannot be said to have many psychological needs (although even this is debatable), but pregnancy for many women is a time of adjustment to major changes. The woman who is expecting to bear a baby is a growing person in more ways than one. Not only physically, but also emotionally, her needs are changing. If it is her first baby, she knows her life style will have to change as she takes on the new responsibility

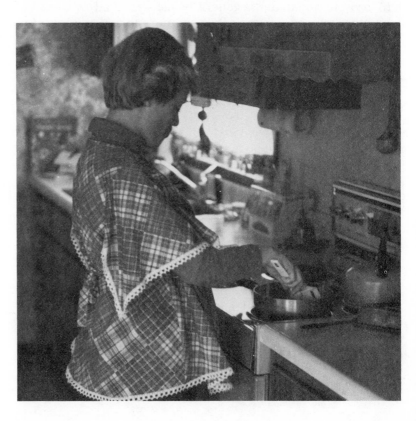

of caring for a child. Ideally, she will be encouraged to develop this sense of responsibility beginning with caring for herself during pregnancy. According to Erikson, the psychological events of adolescence culminate in the formation of an identity; experts from many schools of thought agree that one's self-image begins to form early, and ideally is strongly positive: "I'm OK!" The expectant mother needs encouragement in thinking of herself as a thoroughly worthwhile and important person with a new and challenging task that she can and will perform well.

A question commonly asked is whether the so-called cravings of the pregnant woman reflect physiological needs. The evidence says no: if a woman wakes up at 2:00 A.M. and begs her husband to go to the nearest all-night grocery to buy her some pickles and chocolate sauce, this is probably *not* because she lacks a combination of nutrients uniquely supplied by these foods. The only real physiological cravings are for water, possibly salt, and food. She is expressing a need, however, perhaps as real and as important as her need for nutrients—for support, understanding, and love.

Nutrition in Lactation

Growth and nutrient needs. A nursing mother's needs for some nutrients increase further during lactation because she is feeding a larger infant now. A comparison between her RDA's during pregnancy (second half) and lactation is shown in Figure C15.2.

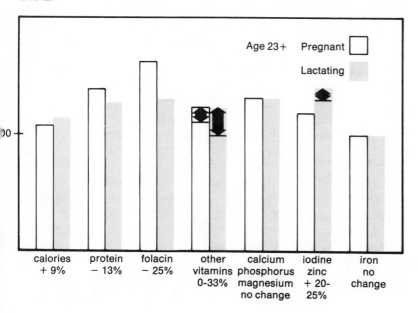

Figure C 15.2. Comparison of RDAs of pregnant and lactating women. The nonpregnant woman's RDA's are set at 100 percent. (Calculated from the NAS-NRC RDA tables, Appendix I.)

Inspection of the figure reveals that her needs for several nutrients are down, while for others they increase only slightly. A significant increase is needed in calories, both for those that go into her milk and for the energy needed to make the milk. Calcium, phosphorus, magnesium, and protein needs continue to be high. They were going into the baby in the womb; now they are flowing into the baby through the mother's milk. Since little iron is secreted in milk, no increase in iron intake is needed, provided, of course, that the mother's iron nutrition has been good all along. The folacin requirement goes down as the mother's blood volume declines.

The secretion of milk by a nursing mother is a beautiful illustration of the ways in which nature provides for its own. To give but a few examples: the amount of milk she produces depends on how much the infant needs. If the baby sucks until the breast is empty, a hormone is released which stimulates the mammary glands to produce more milk the next time around; if the baby leaves milk in the breast the amount secreted is reduced. If a mother is nursing twins, reserving one breast for each, the breasts can even adjust separately to the different infants' demands! This same hormone causes the uterus to contract, helping it to return to normal size. The infant's crying stimulates a conditioned mother to "let down" her milk: in anticipation of feeding, the milk moves to the front of the breast and, as the infant begins to suck, flows so freely that the infant may be hard put to keep up with the flow. Like many other designs of living systems, the lactation system is a marvel.

Eating pattern. For once, the logical statement is true: since mother is making milk, she needs to drink milk. The composition of cow's milk, being quite similar to human milk, makes it the most efficient means of supplying exactly those nutrients needed for lactation. As before, nutritious foods should make up the remainder of the calorie increase. Since breast milk is a fluid, the mother's fluid intake should be liberal; a busy new mother often forgets this.

For nonmilk drinkers: alternative sources of calcium and riboflavin are dark green leafy vegetables (see pages 291, 377).

The question is often raised whether a mother's milk may lack a nutrient if she is not getting enough in her diet. The answer is complex (it depends on the nutrient), but in general the effect of nutritional deprivation of the mother is to reduce the quantity, not the quality of her milk. For most nutrients, the milk has a constant composition; if one nutrient is in short supply, correspondingly less milk of the proper composition will be produced. The reminder should be repeated here: water is the major ingredient of milk, and a nursing mother's fluid intake should be ample.

While there need be no concern about the nutritional composition of breast milk, a warning is in order for the nursing mother. Chemicals other than nutrients readily enter the milk.

The list of drugs, both medical and other, known to be secreted in significant amounts in human milk now numbers over 100 items. Notable among them are nicotine, caffeine, marijuana, morphine, and alcohol. The time during which a woman is nursing her baby is a good time for abstinence from these and all other drugs.

Psychological needs of the nursing mother. To nurse successfully, a woman needs rest and freedom from stress and anxiety. The supportive care of her husband, family, and friends can provide this for her. Many resources are also available to provide her with the information and advice she needs; some are listed in the references at the end of this chapter.

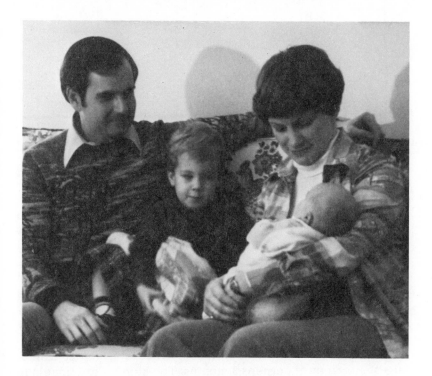

Nutrition in the First Year

Growth and development. Babies grow faster during their first year than ever again in their lives, as is shown in Figure C15.3. As mentioned before, babies double their birth weight in four months, from 7 to 14 pounds, and add another 7 pounds in the next eight months. (If ten-year-old children were to do this, their weight would increase from 70 to 210 pounds in a single year.) By the end of the first year the growth rate has slowed down, and the weight gained between the first and second birthdays amounts to only about five pounds.

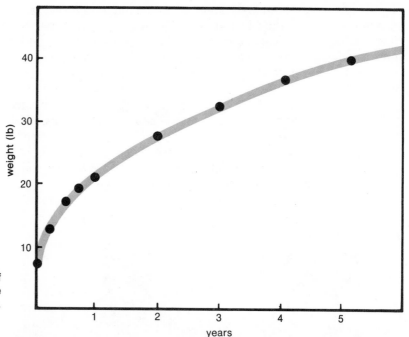

Figure C15.3. Weight gain of human infants (boys) in the first five years.

This tremendous whole-body growth reflects a composite of the differing growth patterns of all the internal organs. The generalization holds that many critical periods occur early.

critical period: see page 455.

Changes in body organs during the first year affect the babies' readiness to accept solid foods. At first, all they can do is suck (though they can do that powerfully), then (at 6 weeks) they can smile, later (at 2 months or so) they can move the tongue against the palate in such a way as to swallow semisolid food. Still later the first teeth erupt, but it is not until sometime during the second year that babies can begin to handle chewy food. The stomach and intestines are also immature at first; they can digest milk sugar (lactose), but cannot manufacture significant quantities of amylase until somewhat later and so cannot digest starch until perhaps 3 months. The kidneys are unable to concentrate waste efficiently, so babies must excrete relatively more water than adults to carry off a comparable solute load. Their metabolism is fast (their hearts beat 120-140 times a minute and they breathe 20 times a minute as compared with an adult's 70-80 and 12-14, respectively), so their energy needs are high.

Developmental events in the GI tract determine babies' readiness to accept solid foods: their developmental readiness.

Nutrient needs. The rapid whole-body growth and rapid metabolism of the infant demand ample supplies of the growth and energy nutrients—protein, carbohydrate, fat, calcium, phosphorus, and magnesium—and, for their utilization, the B vitamins and vitamins A, C, and D. While babies, because they are small, need smaller total amounts of these nutrients than

growth nutrients: see page 460.

energy nutrients: see page 6.

adults do, as percentages of body weight, they need over twice as much of most nutrients. Figure C15.4 compares a 3-month-old baby's needs with those of an adult man; as you can see, some of the differences are extraordinary.

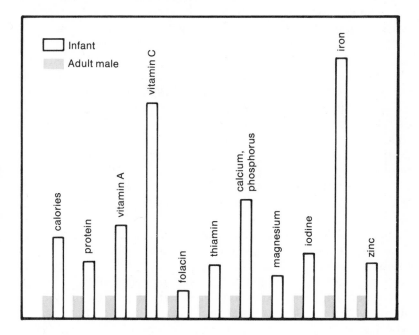

Figure C15.4. Comparison of RDAs of three-month old infant with those of an adult male (age 23+) per pound of body weight. The adult male's RDAs are set at 100 percent. (Calculated from the NAS-NRC RDA tables, Appendix I.)

Feeding pattern. The obvious food to supply the nutrients most needed by the young infant is milk. On this everyone agrees, though to determine which milk is best raises issues too numerous to settle in a book of this size. Everyone seems to have a strong opinion on the matter. Breast milk advocates argue that nursing is the better way—that breast milk is more nutritious than cow's milk and provides antibodies to protect the infant against disease; that breast feeding is safer, more sanitary, and more economical than formula feeding, and that it promotes a closeness between mother and child that is denied to the bottle-fed baby.

breast vs bottle

Actually, for the middle-class American today, these arguments may not hold. The comparison of the nutrient composition of human and cow's milk shows that they do indeed differ (cow's milk is significantly *higher* in protein, calcium, and phosphorus, for example, reflecting the design of the milk to support the calf's faster growth rate), but a formula can be made from cow's milk that does not differ significantly from human milk in these ways. Antibodies are secreted from the breast in colostrum, and are absorbed into the infant's bloodstream, providing temporary immunity against diseases to which the

colostrum (co-LAHS-trum): a milklike secretion from the breast which precedes milk during the first day or so after delivery.

mother has been exposed, but the high level of preventive medical care (vaccinations) and public health measures achieved in the developed countries, and especially in the United States, make these considerations less important than they used to be. Safety and sanitation can be achieved with either mode of feeding. The economy argument is not entirely valid; extra money must be spent to feed a baby, whether directly for formula or indirectly for the added food needed by the nursing mother, although the formula costs somewhat more. As for closeness, clearly that is important. Infants' first impressions of the world relate to the way they are handled during feeding, but holding them with love and a bottle will do more for their psychological development than with resentment at the breast; and bottle-feeding gives the *father* and other family members, as well as mothers, a chance to develop a warm, affectionate relationship with the baby.

The equal value of the two modes of feeding holds only for the healthy baby of the middle-class, well-educated mother in a country such as the United States. If the baby shows any tendency towards allergy or sickness, breast feeding may confer a great advantage. Many doctors recommend that all mothers breast feed their infants at least for two weeks, so that they will have a chance to detect sickness or allergy before bottle feeding has become the only possible choice. In an unclean environment, where the educational level of the mother is poor, or where poverty or ignorance makes the buying and mixing of a sanitary, nutritious formula unlikely, breast feeding also has all the advantages.

Once the mother has made her choice, she should be supported. Especially with her first infant, she may be experiencing some trials and tribulations, and heavy pressure against her decision constitutes an avoidable stress.

Whichever is chosen, there are nutrients that must be supplied in addition to those in milk, notably vitamin C and iron. The first nonmilk food usually added to a baby's diet is orange juice, diluted to half strength with water at first. Addition of iron-containing foods can wait, since the baby is born with a 3-month supply of iron stored in the liver. Supplements of the three vitamins A, D, and C (with the addition of fluoride, if necessary) provide, with milk, all the needed nutrients at first. There are variations in the need for these nutrients depending on whether the baby is fed breast milk or formula.

The addition of foods to babies' diets should be governed by two considerations: first, to supply the nutrients they need, and second, to supply the nutrients in a form the babies are physically ready to handle. A suggested pattern of additions of foods to a baby's diet up to the age of a year, based on these two considerations, might read as follows:

Principles guiding the addition of foods to a baby's diet during the first year:

nutrient needs
developmental readiness

0-1 month   ADC (+ fluoride) supplement (A and D not needed if formula is fortified)

1-2 months   diluted orange juice—for vitamin C

2-3 months   strained enriched cereal, fruit, egg yolk—for iron (they can begin to digest starch now)

3-4 months   strained, cooked vegetables and meats (they can swallow better now)

5-7 months   teething crackers (teeth are erupting; they can begin to chew, can hold these, and start to feed themselves)

7-9 months   finely chopped meat (they can chew and swallow lumps now)

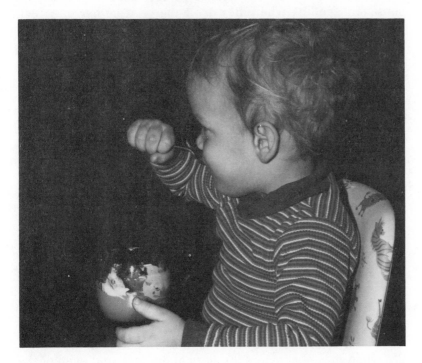

At a year, the obvious food to supply most of the nutrients the baby needs is still milk; two to three cups a day are now sufficient. The other foods — meat, cereal, bread, fruit, and vegetables — should be supplied in variety and in amounts sufficient to round out total calorie needs. A meal plan that meets these requirements for the one-year-old is shown below.

Breakfast: 1 cup milk
              2-3 tbsp cereal
              2-3 tbsp strained fruit
              teething crackers

Lunch:	1 cup milk
	2-3 tbsp vegetables
	chopped meat
	2-3 tbsp pudding
Snack:	teething crackers
	½ cup milk
Supper:	1 cup milk
	1 egg
	2 tbsp cereal or potato
	2-3 tbsp cooked fruit
	teething crackers

Psychological needs. At birth, babies' needs are simple: warmth, affection, relief when they feel pain; and constant, consistent feeding when they are hungry. A mother may feel, quite rightly, that her major task at the start is to "keep putting it in one end, and keep removing it from the other." But by the time babies have reached the age of one, mothers often realize with consternation that they are no longer the malleable, accepting little creatures they used to be. They are becoming individuals, and the ways they express this new development can be exasperating. In recent months they have been "getting into everything;" now that they are just learning to walk, their range is greatly expanding, and nothing below adult waist level in the house is safe. Toddlers explore and experiment endlessly, twisting the knobs on the television set, poking fingers into wall sockets, tugging on lamp cords and curtains, pulling all the toilet paper off the roll, stirring the soil in potted plants, and scattering the contents of mother's purse.

· They used to be receptive and eager to please; now they are contrary and willful. Whatever mother suggests, they refuse, even if it's something they normally like to do. When a mother tells her child to stop hitting the cat with the car keys, the child casts an appraising eye at her, hesitates only a moment — and continues hitting the cat.

The wise mother is aware that this is a period in her child's life when these behaviors are normal, natural, and even desirable. The child is developing a sense of *autonomy* which, if allowed to flower, will provide the foundation for later security and effectiveness as an individual. Wise mothers use their toddlers' short attention span to distract them away from the television set. They absolutely forbid — by force, if necessary — their children to poke into wall sockets or to eat matches. But they also avoid coming down on the children too hard. A child's urge to explore and experiment, if consistently denied, can turn to shame and self-doubt.

One-year-olds behave the same way at the table as in other settings. They display their urge to experiment by dipping bananas into spaghetti, by fingerpainting with chocolate pudding, or by pouring milk over the tabletop and watching, fascinated, as it drips onto the floor. Children's sense of autonomy is strengthened when they refuse to eat their cereal and insist on more applesauce instead. The dilemma mothers face, knowing how important it is for their children to eat a balanced diet, can be resolved if they are prepared for these developments and know how to handle them to the best advantage of them both. While mothers attempt to feed their children all the necessary nutrients in good balance and in amounts sufficient to promote optimal growth and health, they will, at the same time, want to encourage those behaviors that make children feel secure, confident, and independent, and to avoid shaming them and limiting their psychological growth.

In the light of these developmental and nutritional needs, and in the face of the often contrary and willful behavior of the one-year-old, mothers might find a few feeding guidelines helpful. The most typical problem behaviors are listed below, with suggestions for how to handle them.

(1) Some one-year-olds stand and play at the table instead of eating. Don't let them. This is unacceptable behavior and should be firmly discouraged. Put them down and let them wait until the next feeding to eat again. Be consistent and firm, not punitive. If they are really hungry, children will soon learn to sit still while eating. Be aware that babies' appetites are less keen now than at eight months, and that their calorie needs are relatively lower. One-year-olds will get enough to eat if they let their own hunger be their guide.

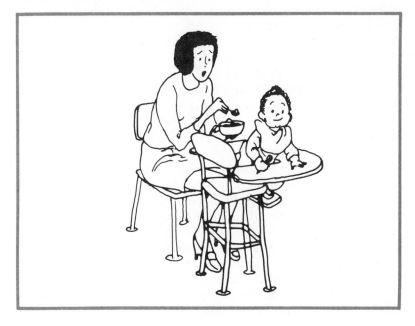

(2) One-year-olds often want to poke their fingers into their food. Let them. They have much to learn from feeling the texture of their food. When they know all about it they'll naturally graduate to the use of a spoon.

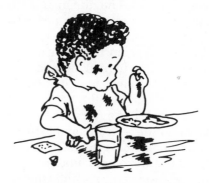

(3) One-year-olds want to manage the spoon themselves but can't handle it. Let them try. As they master it, withdraw gradually until they are feeding themselves competently. This is the age at which most babies can and do learn to feed themselves and are most strongly motivated to do so. They will spill, of course. Mother's best attitude probably is that "one-year-olds don't last forever;" they all grow out of it in time.

(4) They refuse food that their mothers know is good for them. This way of demonstrating autonomy is most satisfying to one-year-olds. Don't force. The one- to two-year-old stage is the age when most of the feeding problems develop that can last throughout life. As long as they are getting enough milk and are offered a variety of nutritious foods from which to choose, they can and will gradually acquire a taste for different additional foods—provided that they feel *they* are making the choice. *This year is the most important year of children's lives in establishing future food preferences.*

If they refuse milk, an alternative source of the bone- and muscle-building nutrients it supplies must be provided. Milk-based puddings and custards and cheese are often successful substitutes. For the baby who is allergic to milk, soy milk and other formulas are available.

(5) They prefer sweets — candy and sugary confections — to foods containing more nutrients. Human beings of all races and cultures have a natural inborn preference for sweet-tasting foods. Limit them strictly. There is no room in a baby's daily 1,000 kcalories for the calories from sweets, except occasionally. The meal plan shown above provides more than 500 kcalories from milk; one or two servings of each of the other types of food provide the other 500. If a candy bar were substituted for these foods, the baby would lose out on valuable nutrients; if it were added daily, the child would gradually become obese.

Setting the pattern for life. If babies spend two hours a day eating, they total over 700 hours a year in this activity — as much time as a college student spends in classes in two years. The potential value of this time is enormous. Not only are children obtaining needed nutrients for their growth and development, they are also learning — about food, about themselves, about the behaviors that win approval, and about those that do not. Properly handled, eating times can make a tremendous contribution to a child's future well being, both physical and psychological.

The Middle Years of Childhood

Growth. After the age of one, a child's growth rate slows, as shown in Figure C15.3. During the next year, the body changes dramatically. At one, children have just learned to stand erect and toddle, often losing their balance and abruptly sitting down. By two, they can take long strides with solid confidence and are learning to run, jump, and climb. The internal changes that make these new accomplishments possible are the accumulations of a larger mass and greater density of bone and muscle tissue. The changes are obvious in the figure below: two-year-olds have lost much of their body fat; their muscles (especially in the back, buttocks, and legs) have firmed and strengthened, and the leg bones have lengthened and increased in density.

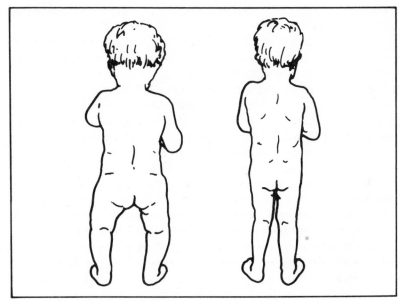

one   two

Figure C15.5. One-year-old child and two-year-old child reduced to same height.

Thereafter the same trend—lengthening of the long bones and an increase in musculature—continues, unevenly and still more slowly, until adolescence. Growth comes in spurts; a six-year-old child may wear the same pair of shoes for a year, then need new shoes twice in the next four months.

A factor of importance is that there seems to be a period of rapid cell division in the adipose tissue before the age of one or two. As with other critical periods, this is limited in time; later, cell division slows down and the proportion of adipose cells becomes fixed. If a child is overfed during this time, the fat cell number may increase beyond the normal limit, leaving the baby with too many adipose cells for life. If (and this is only theoretical) the number of fat cells is involved in hunger regulation in the adult, this may mean that the fat baby is destined to be fat for life.

While the above hypothesis is not clearly established for human beings, it is known that the obesity of childhood differs from adult-onset obesity in several respects. Excess weight in the early years places a demand on the skeletal and muscular tissue so that they, too, hypertrophy. Obese children become adults whose fat tissues, skeleton, and muscles are all denser than those of their slimmer counterparts. The excess weight is less often successfully and permanently lost in such an adult.

As adolescence begins, the growth patterns of girls and boys become distinct. In girls, fat becomes a larger percentage of the total body weight, while in boys the lean body mass—muscle and bone—becomes much greater. Around this time, growth in height may seem to stop altogether for a while, as if the child were settling into a countdown before takeoff. This is the calm before the storm.

Nutritional needs and feeding. One-year-old children need perhaps 1,000 kcalories a day; three-year-olds need only 300-500 kcalories more. Appetites decrease markedly around the age of one year, in line with the great reduction in growth rate. Thereafter, appetite fluctuates; children will need and demand much more food during periods of rapid growth than during periods of quiescence. The nutrients that need emphasis continue to be protein, calcium, and phosphorus, and the food best suited to supply them continues to be milk.

The gradually increasing needs for all nutrients during the growing years are evident from the RDA tables (Appendix I) which list separate averages for each span of three years. A scrutiny of the tables reveals that, while milk is certainly an important food for children, its overemphasis can indirectly deprive the child of other needed nutrients; a balance and variety of foods are needed.

Little children like to eat at little tables and be served little portions of foods. An easy way to maintain a balanced diet for a

newborn: 12% fat

one-year-old: 24% fat

the "fat baby syndrome"

juvenile-onset, or **developmental obesity**

Adult-onset, or **reactive obesity** often starts in response to an emotional trauma.

hypertrophy: see page 455.

milk anemia: see page 380.

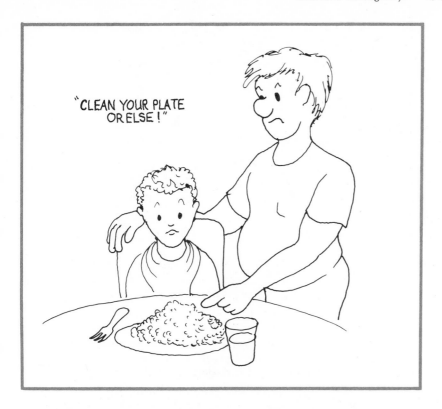

child is to begin at the age of one with a pattern such as that presented above (pages 469-70), and to increase the serving sizes of each food gradually. In this way, by about four years of age a serving of vegetables, fruit, or meats is four tablespoons. Thereafter, the serving size can be increased a tablespoon a year, without changing the pattern.

One problem in the feeding of young children deserves a moment's thought: they frequently dislike and refuse vegetables. Even a tiny serving of spinach, cooked carrots, or squash may elicit an expression that registers the utmost in negative feelings (as well as great pride in the ability to make a super ugly face). How to get around this response? If you put yourself in the child's place, you may remember how you yourself felt about certain foods at that age. For one thing, you hated mixtures; before you could eat peas-and-carrots or lima beans-and-corn, you felt compelled to sort them out until the peas were on one side of the plate and the carrots on the other, and then to separate, into a reject pile, all those that got mashed in the process or contaminated with gravy from the mashed potatoes. After that, you were willing to eat the intact, clean peas and carrots one by one. An understanding parent might do well to encourage this behavior and suggest making a game of it—combined with eating the peas and carrots after they are sorted.

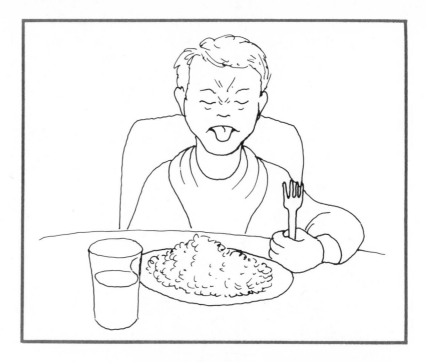

Why children respond this way to foods that look "off" or "messy" to them is a matter for conjecture. The parent need only be aware that this is how many children feel and then honor those feelings. Children prefer vegetables that are slightly undercooked and crunchy, bright in color, and served separately. You may also recall that if you ever burned your tongue on a food such as soup you were very reluctant to try it again. Foods served to children should be warm, not hot. Children's mouths are more sensitive than adults'.

Since they enjoy helping in the kitchen, their participation in preparing foods may provide an opportunity to adopt a ploy. Children who help their mothers shell peas may eat so many raw peas before the meal that their rejection of the cooked equivalent at the dinner table is a matter for no concern.

Experimentation with food patterns for children shows that candy, cola beverages, and other sugar foods must be limited in a child's diet if the needed nutrients are to be supplied. If such foods are permitted in large quantities, there are only two possible outcomes: nutrient deficiencies or obesity. The possibility that overfeeding at critical times in children's lives can predispose them to lifelong obesity makes this especially important. On the other hand, an active child can enjoy the higher-calorie *nutritious* foods in each category: ice cream or pudding in the milk group, cake and cookies in the bread group. These foods made from milk and grain carry valuable nutrients and encourage a child to learn, appropriately, that eating is fun.

Children sometimes seem to lose their appetites for awhile; this is nothing to worry about. The perfection of appetite regulation in children of normal weight guarantees that their calorie intake will be right for each. Children who want to eat less are probably in a quiescent stage of growth. As long as the calories they do consume are from nutritious foods, they are well provided for during this time. (One caution, however: wandering school-aged children may be spending pocket money at the nearby candy store.) Many overzealous mothers, unaware that one-year-olds are supposed to slow down, begin a life-long conflict over food by trying to force more food on their children than the children feel like eating.

Many boys, beginning in early adolescence, are striving to excel in athletics, sometimes too hard. When competing for an

The accuracy of appetite regulation is described on page 238.

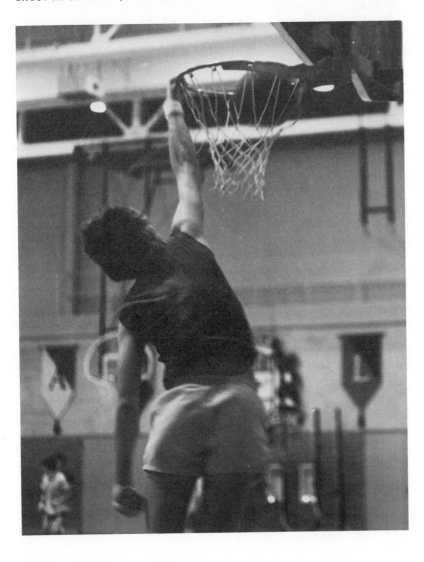

important prize, pushed on by cheerleaders, alumnae, and anxious parents, boys may over-extend themselves, attempting to run so hard and tackle with such abandon that they may damage the ends of their growing bones which have not yet hardened into maturity. While excelling at sports is a source of pride in boys, they can alternatively be encouraged to excel at non-contact sports such as tennis, touch football, swimming, and track, and to play for the fun of it—for the companionship with peers, for release from the tension of sitting in the classroom, for the sheer pleasure of physical activity. Noncontact sports are less likely to damage the bones; in fact, pushing against a bone makes it grow, as the use of a broken bone helps it to heal.

The preadolescent period is the last one in which parental food choices have much influence. As children gather their forces for the adolescent growth spurt, they are accumulating stores of nutrients that will be needed in the coming years. When they take off on that growth spurt, there will be a period during which their nutrient intakes, especially of calcium, cannot meet the demands of rapidly growing bones; then they will be drawing on those stores. The denser their bones are before this occurs, the better prepared they will be.

Psychological growth. The key word (at one year) is *trust*; the parental behavior best suited to promote it is affectionate holding. At two years, the word is *autonomy*; parents should allow children to make their own choices, including giving them the right to say their favorite word ("No!") to offered foods —at the same time providing, of course, other nutritious foods to choose from. (A child may also take great pride in saying, "No," to toilet training by withholding a bowel movement for several days; this is not dangerous.) At four, when the development of *initiative* is their proudest achievement, children can be encouraged to participate in the planning and preparation of meals. At each age, food can be given and enjoyed in the context of growth in its largest, most inclusive sense. If the beginnings are right, children will grow without the kind of conflict and confusion over food which can lead to nutritional problems.

constipation: see pages 166-169.

At every age, there is a negative counterpart to the desired development: *distrust, shame, guilt, inferiority.* These, too, can be promoted by unaware parents even if they have the best of intentions. Mealtimes can be nightmarish for the child who is struggling with these issues. If, as he sits down to the table, he is confronted with a barrage of accusations—"Johnny, your hands are filthy . . . get your elbows off the table . . . your report card . . . and clean your plate! Your mother cooked that food . . ."— mealtimes may be unbearable. His stomach may recoil, for his body as well as his mind reacts to stress of this kind.

In the interest of promoting both a positive self-concept and a positive attitude toward good food, it is important for mother and father to help Johnny or Susie remember that they are good kids. Their behavior may need correcting; what they do may be unacceptable; but on the inside they are normal, healthy, growing, fine human beings.

The Teen Years

Growth and nutrient needs. At twelve, Lynn was a stocky, solid, straight-legged child; at fifteen she is a tall, curvaceous, glowing woman. Most of the boys in her class are shorter than she is; Mike is just beginning to shoot up, but still has a boy's interests and the high-pitched voice of a girl. Just you wait, Lynn: two years from now Mike will have reached and passed your height and may have become the man of your dreams. Keep your eye on him!

The adolescent growth spurt, which begins in girls at ten or eleven and in boys at twelve or thirteen, brings not only a dramatic increase in height but hormonal changes that profoundly affect every organ of the body (including the brain), and which culminate in the emergence of physically mature adults within two or three years after onset. The same nutrition principles apply to this period as to the growth periods previously discussed: the growth nutrients are needed in increased quantities, and for girls the onset of menstruation brings an added need for iron. These changes, which are taking place in nearly-adult-sized people, make adolescence the time in life when nutrient needs may be higher than at any other time. A rapidly growing, active boy of fifteen may need 4,000 kcalories or more a day, just to maintain his weight. An inactive girl of the same age, however, whose growth is nearly at a standstill, may need fewer than 2,000 if she is to avoid becoming obese. It is hard to generalize about the nutrient needs of adolescents.

Teenagers as a group do have nutritional problems, however. Nearly every nutrient can be found lacking in one or another group: iron in the girls, calories in young men (especially Blacks), vitamin A in girls (especially Spanish Americans), calcium, riboflavin, vitamin C, even protein. The insidious problem of obesity begins to become more apparent, mostly in girls, especially in Blacks.

For further information on these findings, see references pertaining to the Ten-State Survey at the end of Highlight 12.

The teenager with the greatest nutritional problems of all is the pregnant teenaged girl. Even under the best of circumstances, she will be hard put to meet her nutrient needs at a time of maximal growth of her own body as well as that of her baby. The comparison below (Figure C15.6) shows that her needs for many nutrients double, while her calorie allowance increases by only a few percent. In the case of a girl who begins pregnancy with inadequate nutrient stores, or who lacks the education she needs in order to provide for herself, these problems are compounded.

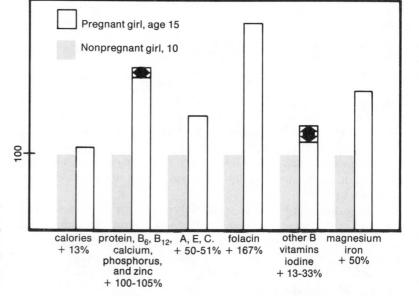

Figure C15.6. Comparison of RDAs of a ten-year-old girl with those of a pregnant, fifteen-year-old girl. Calculated by adding the difference between the RDA for a ten-year-old and a fourteen-year-old to the difference between the RDA for a fourteen-year-old and that for a pregnant woman (Appendix I).

Feeding the person: facilitation. Teenaged boys and girls are not fed; they eat. The time is past when mother or school can make decisions for them. "Feeding" adolescents is no longer a matter of putting food into them; they come and go as they choose, when they choose, and eat what they want when they have time. The adult gatekeeper, concerned with making sure their nutrient needs are met, cannot nag, scold, or pressure them into eating as they should. Teenagers turn a deaf ear to coercion and often to persuasion. To "feed" effectively, the gatekeeper must make every effort to allow these young people independence while providing a physical environment that favors healthy development and an emotional climate that encourages adaptive choices.

In the home, a wise maneuver is to provide access to nutritious and economical energy foods low in sugar and fat and discouraging to tooth decay. Many parents have discovered independently the wisdom of welcoming their teenaged sons and daughters and their friends into the kitchen with an invitation to "Help yourselves! There's plenty of food in the refrigerator (cooked chicken, raw vegetables, milk, fruit juice) and more on the table (fruit, nuts, raisins, popcorn)." The snacker—and a well-established characteristic of teenagers is that they are snackers—who finds only nutritious foods to snack on is well provided for.

Outside the home, teachers and educators can forward the same objectives by several means. One, perhaps the most important, is by example. When nutrition teachers are moralists who fail to practice what they preach, their words of wisdom may fall on deaf ears. The coach and the gym teacher, the friendly young French teacher, the admired city recreation director—those who enthusiastically maintain their own health can have a great impact on teenagers who seek to emulate those they admire. Remember, this is the period of *identity* formation, the time of seeking and emulating models.

Inevitably, teenagers will do a lot of eating away from home, at snack bars, hamburger stands, and corner stores. There, as well as at home, their nutritional welfare can be favored or hindered by the choices they make. A lunch of hamburgers, shake, and French fries[3] supplies nutrients in the following amounts, at a kcalorie cost of 950:

Nutrient	% of U.S. RDA	
Protein	91	U.S. RDA: see Highlight 13.
Calcium	53	
Iron	25	
Vitamin A	24	
Thiamin	25	
Riboflavin	58	
Niacin	39	
Vitamin C	28	

These are substantial percentages of the RDA. Depending on how they adjust their breakfast and dinner choices, teenagers may serve their needs more than adequately with this sort of lunch. (Fruits and vegetables for vitamins A and C, a good fiber source, and more good iron sources are needed.)

If a teaching approach is to be effective, it must *not* teach content alone. Students in a nutrition class can get A's on test after test, without undertaking any improvement in their own eating habits. Habit change occurs only when we *choose* to change it; we choose only when we *want* to change, and we want to change only when we *feel the need*. The way to begin to teach teenagers is to abandon all methods of pushing ideas at them, of forcing information into their heads, and to try instead to facilitate learning. Real learning takes place when the connection is made between what students feel is important—between what they want to know and the information being offered to them.

---

[3] A 3 oz hamburger on a roll with one tablespoon of catsup; a milkshake made with 1 cup milk and 1 cup ice cream; and 10 pieces of French fries fried in deep fat—calculated from Appendix H. Similar conclusions are drawn by Appledorf, H.: Nutritional analysis of foods from fast-food chains. *Food Technology* 28:50-55, 1974.

With teenagers, the key word here seems to be *image*. As they seek to discover who they are and what they want, they strive to develop a positive self-concept.

While most teenaged boys strive to become "manly," and many engage enthusiastically in sports, our society has unconsciously, perhaps, encouraged teenaged girls to be less physically active. Even with today's emphasis on new freedom for girls to enjoy "masculine" activities, many girls become sedentary during their teens. They sit in the public schools from 8:00 to 3:00, then sit some more with their homework. Boredom may result—and a bored girl may turn to food. If she chooses high-calorie snacks, she may start on the road to obesity.

Many girls are aware of this, and nearly all are strongly motivated to control their weight. The accumulation of additional body fat that occurs naturally in early adolescence, is an unwelcome development to the girl who is unaware that women are *supposed* to have more body fat than men. Instead of turning to increased physical activity to strengthen her body and improve her coordination, the girl is likely to diet. This often means skipping breakfast and lunch, only to reach a point where she is so "starving" that she gorges herself on cookies, cake, or potato chips after school. With spending money in her pocket and the invitation of her friends to join them for a Coke and some junk food at the favorite hangout, she eats the wrong foods to satisfy her hunger.

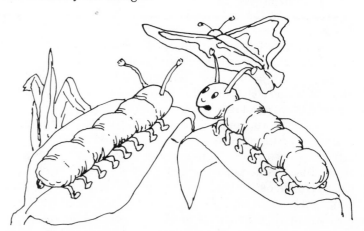

"You'll never get me up in one of those things."

Not all teenaged girls eat this way, of course; many are already on the road to excellent physical health (and many teenaged boys also fall into bad eating and exercise habits). For those who need guidance, the rule remains: good food and the information needed to apply nutrition principles can be provided, but the choice of what and how to eat is up to the teenagers themselves. Leave it to them. They will ultimately make the choice anyway.

Old Age

Aging. The biological course of aging entails processes that are as irrevocable as those of growth, and are programmed, like the growth process, into the genes of each individual. Like growth, too, the processes can be modified by environmental factors such as nutrition, so that their rate or extent may be altered, but they will occur, predictably and inevitably.

As the body ages, its metabolic rate slows, due to a reduction in the number of cells in many organs. The capacity of the lungs to hold air, and that of the heart to pump blood gradually decrease; the kidneys filter waste less efficiently. Body secretions, notably saliva and the digestive juices, decrease in amount. The taste buds become less sensitive. In many individuals, atherosclerosis advances with age, narrowing the arteries, while the collagen in connective tissues undergoes

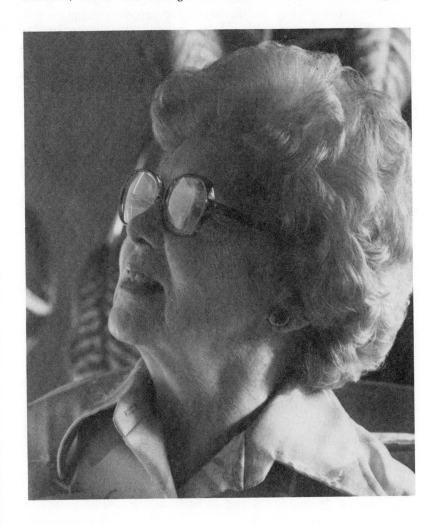

chemical changes that make it inelastic and inflexible. Balding, the whitening of the hair, and the wrinkling of the skin are visible changes that occur in parallel with these internal processes.

As the body ages it becomes more susceptible to disease than before. Among diseases whose incidence is higher in the aged than in the young are diabetes, hypertension, renal and liver disease, osteoporosis, arthritis, and many others. Tooth and gum diseases become common, necessitating the use of dentures by many. Many oldsters become too lame or crippled to walk, so that they are confined to a wheelchair or to bed.

With these handicaps to contend with, older persons not surprisingly have major needs of many kinds that to them may overshadow their nutritional needs.

Nutrient needs and eating pattern. The slowing of the metabolic rate during aging reduces energy needs by about 5 to 8 percent per decade after the age of twenty. However, while calorie needs decrease, the needs for protein, vitamins, and minerals remain approximately the same for the older person as for the twenty-year-old, according to the Food and Nutrition Board (see Appendix I). This means that men and women of eighty are advised to consume as many nutrients as they did sixty years earlier but within a calorie allowance that may be reduced some 30 percent or more. Succinctly stated, the *nutrient density* of the older person's diet must increase.

To accommodate this requirement, persons in their thirties and forties are advised to cut down gradually on their food intake, especially if their life styles become more sedentary, while retaining the more nutritious foods (such as vegetables, fruits, whole-grain cereals and breads, low-calorie meats, and milk), and slowly eliminating the less nutritious or higher calorie foods such as sugar in beverages, candies, cakes, and confections. In actuality, what often happens is either that obesity gradually sets in or that people eliminate their least-preferred foods, returning gradually to their childhood food preferences. The habits of a lifetime are firmly established and are very resistant to change. Depending on the choices made, nutritional as well as other health problems may be compounded as aging occurs.

The choices for the elderly person may also not be entirely free. Wheelchair-bound or bedridden persons must depend on others to supply their needs. Poverty may complicate the problem still further. If the stove or refrigerator is broken, it takes effort and money to get them repaired; sometimes the job does not get done. If elderly people must walk to the store for food, they must carry their groceries home; if the store is too far away they must either depend on others for transportation or be able to drive and maintain a car.

Related needs. According to Erikson, the challenge to old

persons is to maintain their ego integrity. In the face of the problems that may confront them, this is a challenge indeed.

One of the problems many old people face is that of financial security. The widow or widower on a pension or on social security must struggle to meet mounting food and medical costs on an income that is either fixed or that does not keep pace with rising prices in times of inflation. For many, a primary need is to maintain "a home of my own": this cherished independence may have to be won at considerable sacrifice.

There is also the problem of loneliness. Many old people living alone find that they lose interest in food, that it is no fun to cook and eat alone. Add to this the facts that food does not taste as good as it used to, that eating with dentures limits the choices, and that digestive problems are common, and it is not hard to see that undernutrition becomes as serious a problem for some elderly people as obesity does for others.

A major need is for a sense of self-worth and usefulness—the feeling that one has something to give and is making a valuable contribution to family, friends, and society. Instead of this, many old people experience a feeling of dependency and of being a burden, which is degrading and demoralizing.

People and agencies who work with the elderly have found that all the needs mentioned above must be taken into account. In particular, in the realm of nutrition, programs such as congregate meal programs (in which retired people can be brought together for meals and for some social interaction), have been found to favor the enthusiastic partaking of food. Help for the financially needy can be provided by means of food stamps, for which recipients pay on a sliding scale according to ability to pay, thus not having to feel that they are receiving a free handout. For the homebound elderly in some areas, Meals on Wheels programs provide a home-delivered hot meal once a day. Living centers where many older people can form a community, where shopping, laundry facilities, and social activities are nearby, help to remediate the problems of transportation and isolation for some.

It should be emphasized that not all old people face all of these problems. With an awareness of the social, psychological, and health needs that may arise, many people can plan and prepare for old age so that they can adjust to it with dignity and self-respect as well as with a minimum of health and other problems.

Conclusion

Whoever you are, and whatever your walk of life, you will be engaged in feeding. Even as a person whose food is prepared by others, you are the one best suited to determine what your own needs are and to select from what is offered those foods that will best meet your needs. If you are responsible for feeding a family, your decisions and choices will have a greater impact: you are the gatekeeper, the person through whom flow the nutrients that sustain the life and support the health of those you feed.

But people are more than just living machines designed for metabolizing food, and in feeding them you are providing more than mere nutrients. Doctors recognize this when they prescribe *TLC* for the babies on the pediatric ward; they are instructing the nurses to take time out from their more formal duties to serve up some *tender loving care.* They know that this prescription may do more to bring a sick child back to health than any bottled medicine. So, too, with all people. An awareness of the psychological and social needs of people, and some skill in meeting those needs, is an important part of the equipment of the nutritionist, the gatekeeper, and you yourself.

Much of this final chapter has been devoted to psychology. The reader may have felt like objecting at times, "This book is supposed to be about nutrition. Give us the facts, let us develop our own philosophy of life." But what failures we have been when we have tried to dish out doses of straight nutrition! We make no apologies for our choice of emphasis. There is a movement afoot among professional nutritionists, currently, to stress *recipients* of nutrition information. They will not use that information unless they feel it applies to them. Whether we are dealing with our own food patterns, with a two-year-old child, or with an underdeveloped country receiving surplus foods, we cannot expect to achieve the goal of better nutrition without showing full and insightful understanding of all of the characteristics of the receiver. Like the sections of this chapter, the references that follow give equal time to the considerations of psychology, sociology, and anthropology that are indispensable to the effective serving of good nutrition.

To Explore Further—

A collection of important research articles documenting the theory that malnutrition in animals and humans influences learning ability and behavior:

Scrimshaw, N.S. and Gordon, J. E., editors: *Malnutrition, Learning and Behavior.* MIT Press, Cambridge, Massachusetts, 1968.

This article presents and documents the theory that adipose cell number is increased by overfeeding early in life and predisposes to obesity:

Hirsch, J. and Knittle, J. L.: The cellularity of obese and nonobese human adipose tissue. *Federation Proceedings* 29(4):1516-1521, 1970.

The beautiful picture essay from which the photographs of pre-natal development in this book were reprinted:

Rugh, R. and Shettles, L. B.: *From Conception to Birth, The Drama of Life's Beginnings.* Harper and Row, Publishers, Inc., New York, 1971.

The tolerance with which we recommend contending with the antics of the young child originated with:

Erikson, E.: *Childhood and Society.* 2nd ed. W. W. Norton and Company, Inc., New York, 1963.

Clinical test standards must be changed for women taking the pill:

Weindling, H. and Henry, J. B.: Laboratory test results altered by "the pill." *Journal of the American Medical Association* 229(13):1762-1768, 1974.

A description of two of the most common diseases afflicting the elderly:

Varrick, M.: Serum cholesterol concentration and atherosclerotic cardiovascular disease in the aged. *Journal of the American Geriatric Society* 22(2):56-61, 1974.

Helpful in adapting a reduced budget to nutritional needs:

For Older People, Eating Right for Less. Consumer's Union, Orangeburg, New York 10962, 1975.

A solution to one of the problems of the elderly:

Pelcovitz, J. and Wolgamot, I. H.: Nutrition programs for the elderly: selecting a meal delivery system. *Journal of Home Economics* 66(1): 43-45, 1974.

Two examples of the approach to feeding people that takes their culture into account:

Simoons, F. J.: The geographic approach to food prejudices. *Food Technology* 20:42, 1966.

Mead, M.: Understanding cultural patterns. *Nursing Outlook* 4: 260, 1956.

Teaching Aids, *Infant Nutrition, Nutrition in Pregnancy,* and *Nutrition and Aging,* can be ordered from:

> Director, Education Services
> Nutrition Today
> 101 Ridgely Avenue
> Annapolis, Maryland 21404

Pregnancy (CAM 6-75) can be ordered from:

> The American Dietetic Association
> 620 North Michigan Avenue
> Chicago, Illinois 60611

Afterword

While the chapter titles in this book have been the names of nutrients, the subject throughout has been you: your body and mind and experience. You may have learned more than you realize. You need not read further chapters entitled "Making the Diet Adequate," or "Feeding a Family;" the information is all here, in one place or another. It remains only for you to put it together and use it. What you do with it depends on how important you feel it is, and what you choose to do. And on who you are.

Who are you, anyway? Are you a young male college student responsible only for your own food, which you sometimes cook at home but more often eat in the hamburger chains that cluster near the campus? Or are you a young wife and graduate student, just starting back to college after the birth of your baby, struggling with coursework, housework, baby tending, and grocery shopping? Are you Black, White, Spanish, Oriental? Are you rich or poor? Do you get hungry for rice and black beans or for a plate heaped high with turnip greens and cornbread?

Whoever you are, whatever your taste in food, however many others you must feed—daily you must make decisions about food. The choices you make affect your health, your future, your pocketbook, and through it the entire business community. The choices are yours; we have given you no prescriptions. No one food pattern is required for you to achieve good nutrition, nor do you have to give up your favorite foods. Your own proper subject of study is yourself: you can adapt your own food pattern to meet your nutrient needs.

The story is told of a pair of teachers who visited a cafeteria one day and observed, to their distress, that many of the student patrons made extraordinarily poor food choices. In the hope of remedying this problem, the teachers hit upon the idea of offering a nutrition course. A class of students was rounded up and for half a year was taught nutrition principles and applications. The teaching was good, all the best methods were used, and the students were enthusiastic about the course; they smiled brightly in class, nodded their heads enthusiastically, and made A's on all their tests.

After the course was over, the teachers returned to the cafeteria to see the results of their teaching. With bated breath, they watched as their students approached the cafeteria line. The outcome? No change! The students' food choices were the same as before.

Why are we telling you this? You can answer that. Your story is still unfinished. You can finish it yourself.

Appendix A ━━━━━
History of Discoveries
in Biochemistry
and Nutrition

As early as 1500 B.C., *scurvy* was described by the Egyptians in the Ebers papyrus, discovered at Thebes. Attempts at diagnosis and treatment of diseases have been made by all peoples since that time (and perhaps before). Understanding of the scientific principles underlying health and the life process followed speculation by Leonardo da Vinci (1452-1510) and Van Helmont (1648) that animal nutrition was in some way similar to the burning of a candle. Real progress in the history of biochemistry and nutrition began to be made in the latter half of the eighteenth century and has been accelerating ever since.[1] The following are a few selected major events in that history, up to 1953. Since then, significant events have become too numerous to mention.

1753	Lind used limes to prevent *scurvy* in British sailors.
1770-1774	Priestley discovered *oxygen* and showed that it was produced by plants and consumed by animals.
1770-1786	Scheele first *isolated an organic compound*, glycerol, from natural sources, as well as citric, malic, lactic, and uric acids.
1773	Rouelle *isolated urea* from urine.
1780-1789	Lavoisier demonstrated that animal life depends on oxygen, showed that *respiration is oxidation*, and

[1]Dates and events are as given in Lehninger, A. L.: *Biochemistry*, Worth Publishers, Inc., New York, 1970; and in Wohl, M. G. and Goodhart, R. S., editors: *Modern Nutrition in Health and Disease*. 4th ed. Lea and Febiger, Philadelphia, 1968.

491

	first measured oxygen consumption in a human being.
1783	Spallanzani proposed that gastric *digestion of proteins is a chemical process*.
1806	Vauquelin and Robiquet *first isolated an amino acid*, asparagine.
1807	Bardsley reported that *cod liver oil* was effective against *osteomalacia*.
1811	Courtois discovered *iodine* while preparing saltpeter from seaweed for Napoleon's army.
1820	Coindet reported *curing goiter with iodine*.
1828	Wohler *synthesized the first organic compound*, urea.
1833	Payen and Persoz purified the *enzyme* diastase (amylase) from wheat.
1838	Schleiden and Schwann theorized that the basic unit of life was the *cell*.
1838	Mulder initiated systematic study of *proteins*.
1850-1855	Bernard *isolated glycogen* from the liver and showed that it is a source of *blood glucose*.
1862	Sachs showed that *photosynthesis* results in the production of *starch*.
1864	Hoppe-Seyler *crystallized a protein*, hemoglobin.
1867	Huber *purified nicotinic acid* (niacin).
1872	Pfluger proved *oxygen* is used in all animal tissues, not only blood or lungs.
1877	Kühne proposed the term *enzyme*.
1882	Takaki cured *beriberi* in the Japanese army by substituting natural and whole-grain foods for polished rice.
1890	Lam suggested that sunlight was effective against *rickets*.
1893	Ostwald proved that *enzymes are catalysts*.
1894	Emil Fischer showed the *specificity of enzymes* and enunciated the lock-and-key model as the way enzymes fit their substrates.
1897	Eijkman reported *causing polyneuritis* (beriberi) in hens by feeding them polished rice.
1901	Grijns originated the idea of a *deficiency disease*, suggesting that polyneuritis was due to the lack of something.
1902	Emil Fischer and Hofmeister showed that proteins are *polypeptides*.
1905	Harden and Young *isolated the first coenzyme* (NAD).
1905	Knoop reported details of the *oxidation of fatty acids*.
1906	Eijkman showed that a water-soluble extract from rice polishings can *cure beriberi*.

1911	Casimir Funk *isolated niacin* from rice polishings and coined the word "*vitamine.*"
1912	Warburg showed that *iron* is required for respiration.
1916	McCollum and Kennedy further purified "*water-soluble B*" from rice polishings which contained the antiberiberi substance.
1917	McCollum and Simmonds demonstrated that *xerophthalmia* was due specifically to lack of a *fat-soluble vitamin.*
1917-1918	Marine confirmed that *iodine deficiency caused goiter.*
1919	Huldchinsky *cured rickets* with *ultraviolet rays* from a mercury vapor lamp.
1920	Rosenheim and Drummond showed that *carotene* in plants had a biological activity similar to that of vitamin A.
1922	McCollum proved that cod liver oil contains two vitamins (A and D), and showed that *vitamin D deficiency causes rickets.*
1923-1924	Evans, Bishop, and others showed a dietary fat-soluble factor (*vitamin E*) to be essential for reproduction in the rat.
1926	Smith and Hendrick divided "water-soluble B" into antiberiberi and antipellagra fractions; Jansen and Donath *isolated vitamin B_1* (thiamin).
1927	Windaus showed that *ergosterol* is a *vitamin D precursor.*
1928	Euler *isolated carotene.*
1928	Szent-Györgi isolated *hexuronic acid* from orange juice, cabbage juice, and the adrenal glands of oxen. In the same year, Waugh and King showed that it was identical to the antiscorbutic substance, *vitamin C,* which they had isolated from lemon juice. Haworth determined its *structure* and Reichstein *synthesized* it.
1929	Dam described a *hemorrhagic* disease in chicks fed a fat-free diet, later showed this to be due to *vitamin K deficiency.*
1930	Moore showed that *carotene is converted to vitamin A* in animal tissues.
1930-1933	Northrup *crystallized pepsin and trypsin* and showed they were proteins.
1932	Warburg and Christian identified a *yellow enzyme needed for respiration.*
1935	Williams and his colleagues determined the *structure of vitamin B_1.*
1935	Rose *discovered the last amino acid,* threonine.

1935	Best showed choline *essential in animals.*
1935	Kuhn discovered that riboflavin (vitamin B_2) *is part of the yellow* enzyme discovered by Warburg and Christian.
1936	Evans, Emerson, and Emerson *isolated pure vitamin E* from wheat germ oil.
1937	Krebs reported details of the citric acid cycle (*Krebs Cycle*).
1938	Elvehjem, Madden, Strong, and Woolley's work led to recognition that *nicotinic acid* (niacin) *is a vitamin* and cures the deficiency disease, blacktongue, in dogs. Soon after, niacin was confirmed as the human *antipellagra vitamin.*
1938	Karrer, Fritzsche, Ringier, and Salomon reported the *structure and synthesis of vitamin E.*
1938	Braunstein and Kritzmann discovered *transamination* reactions.
1938	Williams isolated *pantothenic acid.*
1939-1941	Lipmann suggested that ATP *plays a central role in energy metabolism.*
1940	Williams and Major *synthesized pantothenic acid* and showed it cures the deficiency disease dermatitis in chicks.
1943	Tucker and Eckstein showed *choline and methionine* are methyl donors in transmethylation reactions.
1945	Angier and his associates *synthesized folacin.*
1947-1950	Lipmann and Kaplan isolated and characterized coenzyme *A.*
1951	Lehninger showed that *ATP is generated from the electron transport chain.*
1951	Pauling and Corey postulated the alpha-helical *structure of proteins.*
1953	Sanger deduced the *amino acid sequence of a protein,* insulin.
1953	Watson and Crick published the *structure of DNA.*

Appendix B
Summary of
Basic Chemistry
Concepts

Chemistry is the branch of natural science that is concerned with the description and classification of *matter*, with the changes which matter undergoes, and with the *energy* associated with each of these changes.

Matter is anything which takes up space and has mass. *Energy* is the ability to do work.

Matter: the Properties of Atoms

Description of matter. Every substance has a set of characteristics or properties which distinguishes it from all other substances and thus gives it a unique identity. These properties are both physical and chemical in nature. The *physical properties* include such characteristics as color, taste, texture, and odor, as well as the particular temperature at which a substance changes its state (changes from a solid to a liquid or from a liquid to a gas), and the weight of a unit volume (its density). The *chemical properties* of a substance describe the manner in which it reacts with other substances or responds to a change in its environment so that new substances with different sets of properties are produced.

A *physical change*, such as a change in state from ice to liquid water to steam, is one that does not change a substance's chemical composition: in this case, two hydrogen atoms and one

495

oxygen atom bound together to form water. However, if an electric current is passed through water, a *chemical change* will result; the water will disappear and two different substances will be formed: hydrogen gas, which is flammable, and oxygen gas, which supports life. Chemical changes are also referred to as *chemical reactions*.

Classes of matter. Single pure substances were early classified as either elements or compounds. *Elements* are described as substances that cannot be decomposed by simple chemical change into two or more different substances (see Table B.1). *Compounds* are described as substances of definite composition that can be decomposed by a simple chemical change into two or more different substances. Common salt is an example of a compound. It can be decomposed into a shiny, active metal (sodium) and a poisonous, greenish yellow gas (chlorine). Today, just over 100 elements are known, but there are over one million compounds; some familiar compounds are water, sugar, alcohol, carbon dioxide, and ammonia. *A pure compound is always composed of the same elements combined in a definite proportion by weight.* For example, carbon dioxide always contains one atom of carbon which weighs 12 atomic weight units and two atoms of oxygen, each of which weighs 16 atomic weight units. Thus the carbon-to-oxygen ratio by weight of carbon dioxide is always 12:32. If there is a compound which has a carbon-to-oxygen weight ratio different from this it is not carbon dioxide.

The nature of atoms. The first modern theory of the atom was stated by John Dalton (1803). He described *atoms* as the smallest particles of elements, and *molecules* as the smallest particles of compounds. Additional assumptions were that: (1) The atoms of a given element are all alike. (2) The molecules of a given compound are all alike. (3) During chemical reactions atoms may combine, or combinations of atoms may break down, but the atoms themselves are unchanged. (4) When atoms form molecules, they unite in small whole-numbered ratios, such as 1:1, 1:2, 1:3, 2:3.

However, the simple definitions of the atoms and molecules by Dalton have undergone change. Today, molecules are thought of as the smallest particles of a substance, compound or element, which retain all the properties of that substance. In the case of a compound, the molecule does consist of two or more atoms; in the case of elements, the molecule may consist of single atoms such as carbon (C) or iron (Fe), or of two or more atoms, such as the diatomic molecules of oxygen (O_2) or iodine (I_2).

It is now known that atoms are divisible; they consist of smaller particles. The atomic nucleus contains *protons* (positively charged subatomic particles) and *neutrons* (neutral sub-

Table B.1
Chemical Symbols for the Elements

Atomic Number	Element	Symbol	Atomic Weight	Electrons in Outer Shell
1	Hydrogen	H	1	1
2	Helium	He	4	2
3	Lithium	Li	7	1
4	Beryllium	Be	9	2
5	Boron	B	11	3
6	Carbon	C	12	4
7	Nitrogen	N	14	5
8	Oxygen	O	16	6
9	Fluorine	F	19	7
10	Neon	Ne	20	8
11	Sodium	Na	23	1
12	Magnesium	Mg	24	2
13	Aluminum	Al	27	3
14	Silicon	Si	28	4
15	Phosphorus	P	31	5
16	Sulfur	S	32	6
17	Chlorine	Cl	35.5	7
18	Argon	Ar	40	8
19	Potassium	K	39	1
20	Calcium	Ca	40	2
21	Scandium	Sc	45	2
22	Titanium	Ti	48	2
23	Vanadium	V	51	2
24	Chromium	Cr	52	1
25	Manganese	Mn	55	2
26	Iron	Fe	56	2
27	Cobalt	Co	59	2
28	Nickel	Ni	59	2
29	Copper	Cu	63.5	1
30	Zinc	Zn	65	2
31	Gallium	Ga	70	3
32	Germanium	Ge	73	4
33	Arsenic	As	75	5
34	Selenium	Se	79	6
35	Bromine	Br	80	7
36	Krypton	Kr	84	8
37	Rubidium	Rb	85	1
38	Strontium	Sr	88	2
39	Yttrium	Y	89	2
40	Zirconium	Zr	91	2
41	Niobium	Nb	93	1
42	Molybdenum	Mo	96	1
43	Technetium	Tc	—	1
44	Ruthenium	Ru	101	1
45	Rhodium	Rh	103	1
46	Palladium	Pd	106	—
47	Silver	Ag	108	1
48	Cadmium	Cd	112	2
49	Indium	In	115	3
50	Tin	Sn	119	4

Table B.1 (continued)

Atomic Number	Element	Symbol	Atomic Weight	Electrons in Outer Shell
51	Antimony	Sb	122	5
52	Tellurium	Te	128	6
53	Iodine	I	127	7
54	Xenon	Xe	131	8
55	Cesium	Cs	133	1
56	Barium	Ba	137	2
57	Lanthanum	La	139	2
58	Cerium	Ce	140	2
59	Praseodymium	Pr	141	2
60	Neodymium	Nd	144	2
61	Promethium	Pm	—	2
62	Samarium	Sm	150	2
63	Europium	Eu	152	2
64	Gadolinium	Gd	157	2
65	Terbium	Tb	159	2
66	Dysprosium	Dy	163	2
67	Holmium	Ho	165	2
68	Erbium	Er	167	2
69	Thulium	Tm	169	2
70	Ytterbium	Yb	173	2
71	Lutetium	Lu	175	2
72	Hafnium	Hf	179	2
73	Tantalum	Ta	181	2
74	Tungsten	W	184	2
75	Rhenium	Re	186	2
76	Osmium	Os	190	2
77	Iridium	Ir	192	2
78	Platinum	Pt	195	1
79	Gold	Au	197	1
80	Mercury	Hg	201	2
81	Thallium	Tl	204	3
82	Lead	Pb	207	4
83	Bismuth	Bi	209	5
84	Polonium	Po	—	6
85	Astatine	At	—	7
86	Radon	Rn	—	8
87	Francium	Fr	—	1
88	Radium	Ra	—	2
89	Actinium	Ac	—	2
90	Thorium	Th	232	2
91	Protactinium	Pa	—	2
92	Uranium	U	238	2
93	Neptunium	Np	—	2
94	Plutonium	Pu	—	2
95	Americium	Am	—	2
96	Curium	Cm	—	2
97	Berkelium	Bk	—	2
98	Californium	Cf	—	2
99	Einsteinium	Es	—	2
100	Fermium	Fm	—	2
101	Mendelevium	Md	—	2
102	Nobelium	No	—	2

atomic particles); around the nucleus circulate *electrons* (negatively charged particles) equal in number to the protons. Protons and neutrons are of equal mass and give an atom its weight. Protons and electrons, having charge, determine the arrangement of the atom. Electrons are of negligible mass.

The hydrogen atom (symbol H) is the simplest of all atoms. It possesses a single proton, with a single electron in orbit around it:

Hydrogen Atom (H)

The proton and the electron have equal charges, so that they cancel each other out. If the hydrogen atom loses its single orbiting electron, it will have a charge of +1, becoming H^+. Such charged atoms or groups of atoms are referred to as *ions*. (A hydrogen ion consists of a single proton and is often referred to simply as a proton.)

Each type of atom has a characteristic number of protons in its nucleus: hydrogen has one, helium 2, lithium 3, etc. Helium also has 2 neutrons in its nucleus and thus has an atomic weight of 4. All atoms, except hydrogen, have neutrons in their nuclei, contributing to the atomic weight (see Table B.1). Chemists have given an *atomic number* to each type of atom, corresponding to the number of protons in its nucleus, as shown in Table B.1.

The atomic elements found in living things are shown in Table B.2. "All cells, regardless of origin (animal, plant, or microbial) contain the same elements in approximately the same proportions."[1]

Besides hydrogen, the atoms most common in living things are carbon (C), nitrogen (N), and oxygen (O), whose atomic numbers are 6, 7, and 8 respectively. Their structures are more complicated than that of hydrogen. Each possesses a number of electrons equal to the number of protons in its nucleus. These electrons have two energy levels symbolized in the following diagrams as two orbits, or shells:

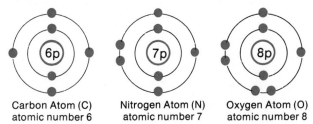

| Carbon Atom (C) | Nitrogen Atom (N) | Oxygen Atom (O) |
| atomic number 6 | atomic number 7 | atomic number 8 |

[1]Rodwell, Victor, Ph.D.: Appendix: Organic Chemistry (A Brief Review), in Harper, H.: *Review of Physiological Chemistry.* Lange Medical Publications, Los Altos, California, 1971, p. 499.

Table B.2
The Elemental Composition of Living Cells

Element	Chemical Symbol	Composition by Weight
Oxygen	O	65
Carbon	C	18
Hydrogen	H	10
Nitrogen	N	3
Calcium	Ca	1.5
Phosphorus	P	1.0
Sulfur	S	0.25
Sodium	Na	0.15
Magnesium	Mg	0.05
		99.30

Trace elements, comprising the remaining 0.70 percent by weight are: copper (Cu), zinc (Zn), selenium (Se), molybdenum (Mo), fluorine (F), chlorine (Cl), iodine (I), manganese (Mn), cobalt (Co), iron (Fe). There are also variable traces of some of the following in cells: lithium (Li), strontium (Sr), aluminum (Al), silicon (Si), lead (Pb), vanadium (V), arsenic (As), bromium (Br), and others.

The shells shown as closer to the nucleus are occupied by electrons of lesser energy. Thus the two electrons in the first shells of carbon, nitrogen, and oxygen have less energy than the electrons in their second or outer shells. Also, the first shell can only hold two electrons; when it is full, it is in a very stable energy state or state of lowest energy.

The most important structural feature of an atom in determining its chemical behavior is the number of electrons in its outer shell. Since the first shell is full when it is occupied by two electrons, an atom which has 3 protons will have 2 electrons in the first shell; its third electron will possess greater energy and will have a greater probability of being further from the nucleus. In other words, the third electron will not be as tightly bound as the first two and has a high probability of flying off to join other substances in chemical reactions. As a matter of fact, lithium, atomic number 3, is such a highly reactive element.

If the second shell is completely full (eight electrons), the

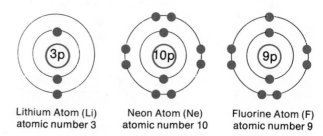

Lithium Atom (Li)   Neon Atom (Ne)   Fluorine Atom (F)
atomic number 3   atomic number 10   atomic number 9

tendency is for the substance possessing such an outer shell to enter into no chemical reactions. Atomic number 10, neon, is a chemically inert substance since its outer shell is complete. On the other hand, fluorine, atomic number 9, has a great tendency to draw an electron in from other substances to complete its outer shell and thus is highly reactive. Carbon has a half-full outer shell, which offers some understanding of its great versatility; it can join with other elements in a variety of ways to form a large number of compounds.

Chemical Bonding

Atoms seek to reach a state of maximum stability or of lowest energy in the same way that a ball will roll down a hill until it reaches the lowest place. An atom achieves a state of maximum stability by two means:

(1) by having an outer shell occupied by the maximum number of electrons it can hold, and

(2) by being electrically neutral.

In order to achieve this stability, an atom may become bonded to other atoms. There are three important ways by which atoms undergo chemical bonding: covalent, ionic, and hydrogen bonding.

Covalent Bonding

Atoms often complete their outer shells by *sharing* electrons with other atoms. In order to complete its outer shell, a carbon atom requires four electrons. A hydrogen atom requires one. Thus when one carbon atom shares electrons with four hydrogen atoms, each completes its outer shell:

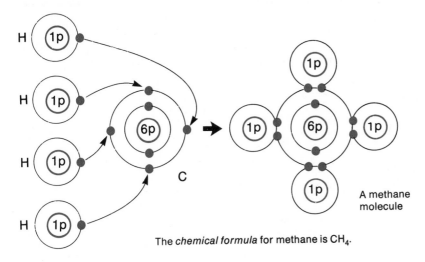

A methane molecule

The *chemical formula* for methane is CH_4.

This electron-sharing binds the atoms together and satisfies the conditions of maximum stability for the molecule: (1) the outer shell of each atom is complete, since hydrogen effectively has the required 2 electrons in its first and outer shell and carbon has 8 electrons in its second and outer shell; and (2) the molecule is electrically neutral, with a total of 10 protons and 10 electrons.

Bonds like this which involve the sharing of electrons are called covalent. A single *pair* of shared electrons forms a *single bond*. A simplified means of representing such a bond is with a single line. Thus the structure of methane could be represented (ignoring the electrons which do not participate in bonding):

$$
\begin{array}{c}
\text{H} \\
| \\
\text{H} - \text{C} - \text{H} \\
| \\
\text{H}
\end{array}
$$

Methane (*chemical structure*)

Similarly, one nitrogen atom and three hydrogen atoms can share electrons to form one molecule of ammonia:

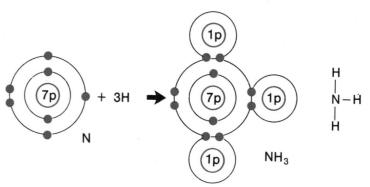

$$
\begin{array}{c}
\text{H} \\
| \\
\text{N} - \text{H} \\
| \\
\text{H}
\end{array}
$$

NH_3

An ammonia molecule

Similarly, one oxygen atom may be covalently bonded to two hydrogen atoms to form one molecule of water:

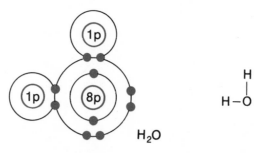

$$
\begin{array}{c}
\text{H} \\
| \\
\text{H} - \text{O}
\end{array}
$$

H_2O

A water molecule

When two oxygen atoms form a molecule of oxygen, they must share two pairs of electrons. This *double bond* may be represented as two single lines:

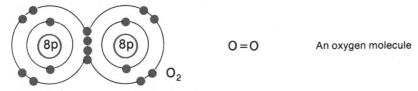

$O = O$ An oxygen molecule

Small atoms form the tightest, most stable bonds. H, O, N, and C are the smallest atoms capable of forming 1-, 2-, 3-, and 4-electron bonds respectively.

Ionic Bonding

An atom such as sodium (Na, atomic number 11) is more likely to lose an electron than to share electrons. Sodium possesses a filled inner shell of 2 electrons and a filled second shell of 8; there is one electron in its outermost shell:

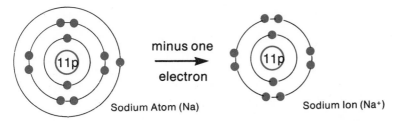

minus one electron

Sodium Atom (Na)   Sodium Ion (Na$^+$)

If sodium loses this electron it satisfies one condition for stability: a filled outer shell. However, it is not electrically neutral. It has 11 protons (positive) and only 10 electrons (negative). It therefore is positively charged. Such a structure is called an ion, that is, an atom or molecule that has lost or gained one or more electrons and so is electrically charged.

An atom such as chlorine (Cl, atomic number 17) is likely to gain an electron for a similar reason. It possesses filled inner shells of 2 and 8 electrons, and 7 electrons in its outermost shell. Gaining one electron makes its outer shell complete and makes it a negatively charged ion:

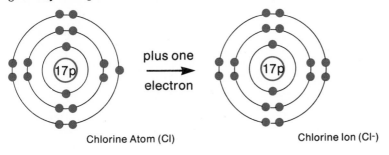

plus one electron

Chlorine Atom (Cl)   Chlorine Ion (Cl$^-$)

A positively charged ion such as Na^+ is a cation; a negatively charged ion such as Cl^- is an anion. Cations and anions attract one another, and form *salts* such as sodium chloride, Na^+Cl^-. The wide distribution of salt (NaCl) in nature attests to the stability of this union; also, the rarity of finding the metal sodium or the gas chlorine shows they must be highly reactive.

(For a description of the behavior of salts in water, electrolytes, and osmosis, which follows from this, see Chapter 14.)

Ionic states of iron. Whereas many elements have only one configuration in the outer shell and thus only one way they can bond with other elements, some elements have the possibility of varied configurations. Iron is such an element. Under some conditions, iron has two electrons in its outer shell and under other circumstances it has three:

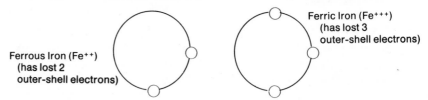

Ferrous Iron (Fe^{++}) (has lost 2 outer-shell electrons)

Ferric Iron (Fe^{+++}) (has lost 3 outer-shell electrons)

If iron has two electrons to donate, we say it has a valence of +2 and call it "ferrous": if it has three electrons to donate, we say it has a valence of +3 and call it "ferric" iron. Chapter 6 discusses the physiological need for iron to be in the reduced or ferrous state for absorption to take place, meaning that conditions in the GI tract must be such that most of the iron has lost only 2 electrons.

Hydrogen Bonding

The water molecule is electrically neutral, having an equal number of protons and electrons. However, if the hydrogen atom is to *share* its one electron with oxygen, that electron will necessarily tend to be located on the oxygen side of the hydrogen atom; this leaves the positive proton exposed on the outer part of the water molecule. We know, too, that the two hydrogens bond to the oxygen at an angle of 105° to each other. These two ideas explain the fact that water molecules are *polar*, that is, they have regions of more positive and more negative charge:

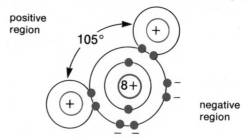

positive region

105°

negative region

Polar molecules such as water are drawn to each other in a weak bond named a hydrogen bond. The negative side of the molecule associates with the positive side of another molecule:

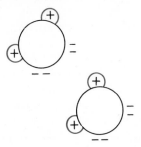

Hydrogen bonds are weak and shortlived in comparison with covalent and ionic bonds but are exceedingly important, particularly in determining protein structure.

Acids and Bases

Water molecules have a slight tendency to ionize, separating into H^+ and OH^- ions. In any given amount of pure water, a small but constant number of these ions is present, and the number of H^+ ions exactly equals the number of OH^- ions. A solution becomes an acid when the H^+ ions outnumber the OH^- ions; it becomes a base when the OH^- ions outnumber the H^+ ions.

The compound HCl (hydrochloric acid) is an *acid* because in water solution it dissociates into H^+ and Cl^- ions, thus releasing additional H^+ ions into the solution. The compound NaOH (sodium hydroxide) is a *base* because in water solution it dissociates into Na^+ and OH^- ions, thus releasing additional OH^- ions into the solution.

Chemists define degrees of acidity by means of the pH scale. At pH 7, the concentrations of free H^+ and OH^- ions are exactly the same, 1/10,000,000 moles per liter (10^{-7} moles per liter).[2] At pH 4, the concentration of free H^+ ions is one-ten thousandth (10^{-4}) moles per liter. This is a higher concentration of H^+ ions and the solution is therefore acidic. Any pH below 7 is acidic, and any pH above 7 is basic.

Chemical Reactions: Oxidation and Reduction

A chemical reaction or chemical change is one which results in the disappearance of substances and the formation of

[2]A mole is a certain number (about 6×10^{23}) molecules.

new ones. Every chemical reaction involves a change in energy. Either the reaction takes place and energy is liberated to the adjacent surroundings or the reaction takes place and energy is absorbed from the adjacent surroundings. The first type of reaction is called *exothermic* and the second type is termed *endothermic*.

Energy conversions in chemical systems involve the movement of electrons from one energy level to another. An atom's electrons have a high probability of being found at certain distances from its nucleus, the lower energy electrons being held closer to the nucleus. An input of energy can raise an electron to a higher level. For example, photosynthesis is a way of using light energy to push electrons to a higher level ("uphill").

The movement "uphill" or "downhill" of an electron often involves transferring the electron from one atom or molecule to another atom or molecule. The transfer of an electron from one molecule to another is known as an *oxidation-reduction reaction*. The loss of an electron is known as *oxidation*, and the compound that loses the electron is said to be *oxidized*. The reason electron loss is called oxidation is that many substances—such as carbohydrates—will lose electrons only when oxygen is available to accept them.

Reduction is the gain of an electron. Oxidation and reduction take place simultaneously because an electron that is lost by one atom is accepted by another.

Often an electron travels in company with a proton as part of a hydrogen atom. In that case, oxidation involves the removal of the hydrogen ion (proton) and its electron from one substance; reduction involves the transfer of both a hydrogen ion and an electron to another substance. The reduction of oxygen—the addition of hydrogen atoms—thus results in the formation of water. The oxidation of carbohydrate yields carbon dioxide and water.

If a reaction results in a net increase in chemical bond energy, it is referred to as a reduction reaction; for example, the chief result of photosynthesis is the reduction of carbon. Conversely, if there is a net decrease in chemical bond energy (with a release of energy as heat or light), the reaction is often referred to as an oxidation process. For example, sugar is oxidized to carbon dioxide and water.

Appendix C
Biochemical Structures

Fatty Acids Found in Natural Fats

Saturated Fatty Acids	Chemical Formula	Found in
Butyric	C_3H_7COOH	butter fat
Caproic	$C_5H_{11}COOH$	butter fat
Caprylic	$C_7H_{15}COOH$	coconut oil
Capric	$C_9H_{19}COOH$	palm oil
Lauric	$C_{11}H_{23}COOH$	coconut oil
Myristic	$C_{13}H_{27}COOH$	nutmeg oil
*Palmitic	$C_{15}H_{31}COOH$	animal and vegetable fat
*Stearic	$C_{17}H_{35}COOH$	animal and vegetable fat
Arachidic	$C_{19}H_{39}COOH$	peanut oil

Structural formulae:

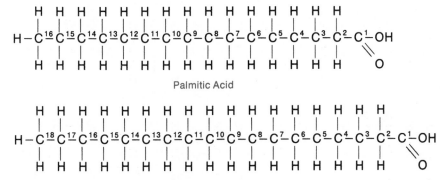

Palmitic Acid

Stearic Acid

*Most common saturated fatty acids.

507

Unsaturated Fatty Acids	Chemical Formula	Position of Double Bonds	Found In
Palmitoleic	$C_{15}H_{29}COOH$	between C9-C10	butter fat
Oleic	$C_{17}H_{33}COOH$	between C9-C10	olive oil
Linoleic	$C_{17}H_{31}COOH$	between C9-C10 and C12-C13	linseed oil
Linolenic	$C_{17}H_{29}COOH$	between C9-C10 and C12-C13 and C15-C16	linseed oil
Arachidonic	$C_{19}H_{31}COOH$	between C5-C6 and C8-C9 and C11-C12 and C14-C15	lecithin

Structural Formulae of the Unsaturated Fatty Acids

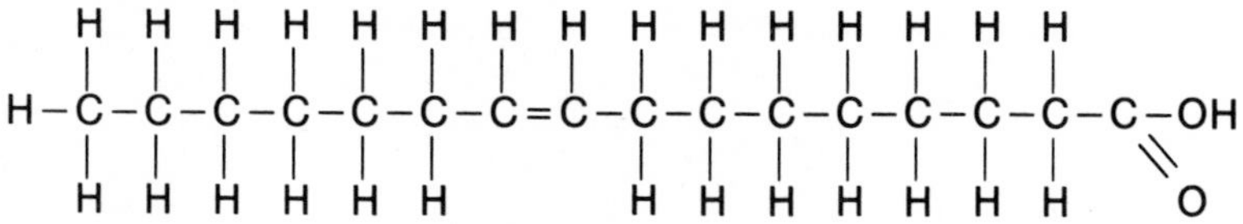

Palmitoleic Acid

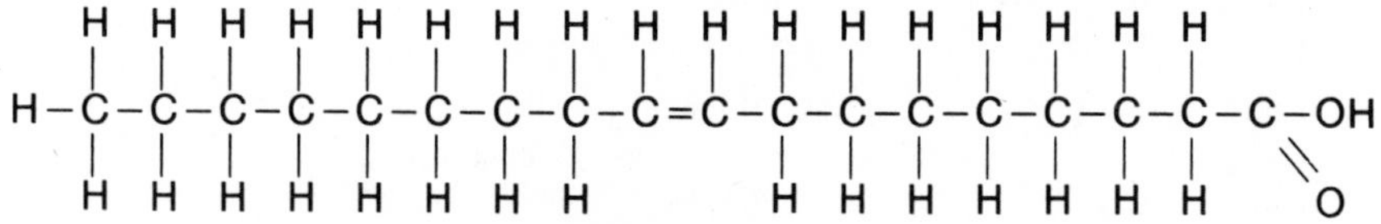

Oleic Acid

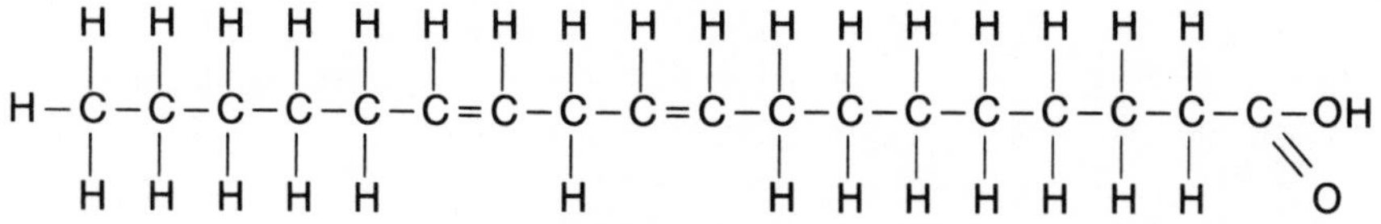

Linoleic Acid

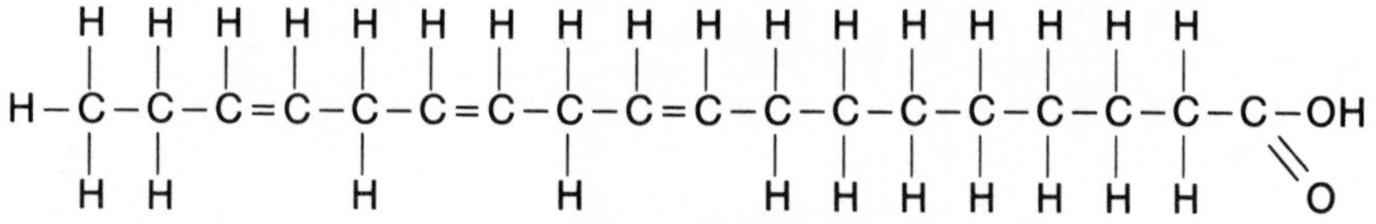

Linolenic Acid

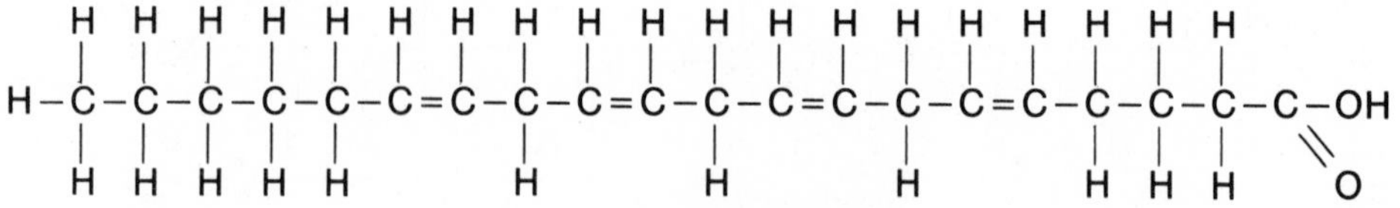

Arachidonic Acid

Amino Acids

Glycine
Gly

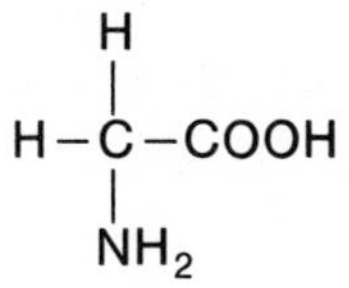

$$H-\underset{\underset{NH_2}{|}}{\overset{\overset{H}{|}}{C}}-COOH$$

Alanine
Ala

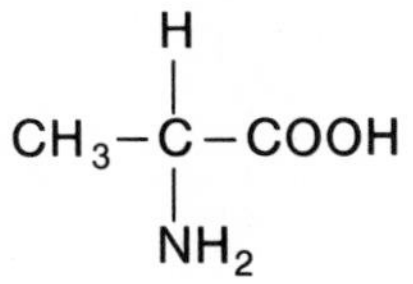

$$CH_3-\underset{\underset{NH_2}{|}}{\overset{\overset{H}{|}}{C}}-COOH$$

*Valine
Val

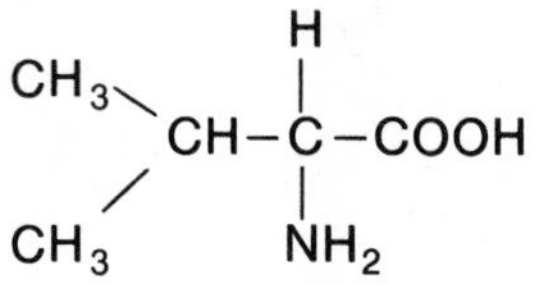

$$\underset{CH_3}{\overset{CH_3}{\diagdown}}CH-\underset{\underset{NH_2}{|}}{\overset{\overset{H}{|}}{C}}-COOH$$

*Leucine
Leu

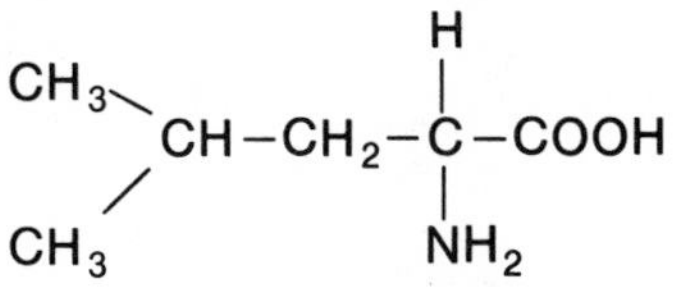

$$\underset{CH_3}{\overset{CH_3}{\diagdown}}CH-CH_2-\underset{\underset{NH_2}{|}}{\overset{\overset{H}{|}}{C}}-COOH$$

*Isoleucine
Ile

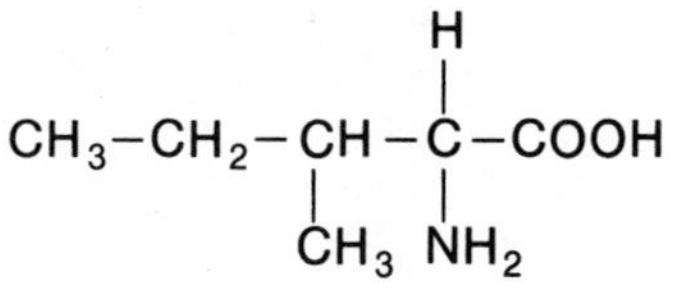

$$CH_3-CH_2-\underset{\underset{CH_3}{|}}{CH}-\underset{\underset{NH_2}{|}}{\overset{\overset{H}{|}}{C}}-COOH$$

Serine
Ser

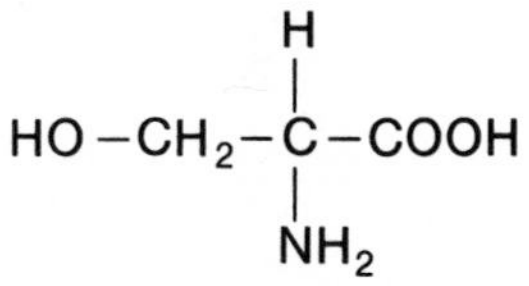

$$HO-CH_2-\underset{\underset{NH_2}{|}}{\overset{\overset{H}{|}}{C}}-COOH$$

*Threonine
Thr

$$CH_3-\underset{\underset{OH}{|}}{CH}-\underset{\underset{NH_2}{|}}{\overset{\overset{H}{|}}{C}}-COOH$$

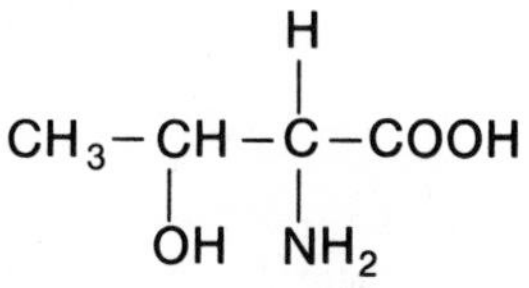

*Essential, since human beings cannot synthesize

Aspartic Acid
Asp

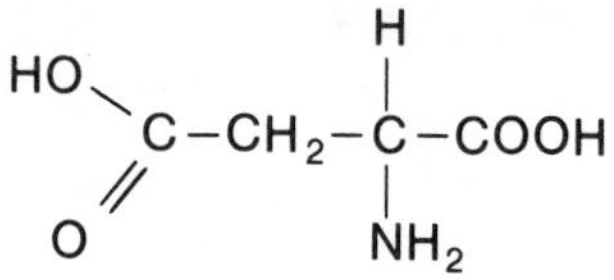

$$HO-\underset{\underset{O}{\|}}{C}-CH_2-\underset{\underset{NH_2}{|}}{\overset{\overset{H}{|}}{C}}-COOH$$

Glutamic Acid
Glu

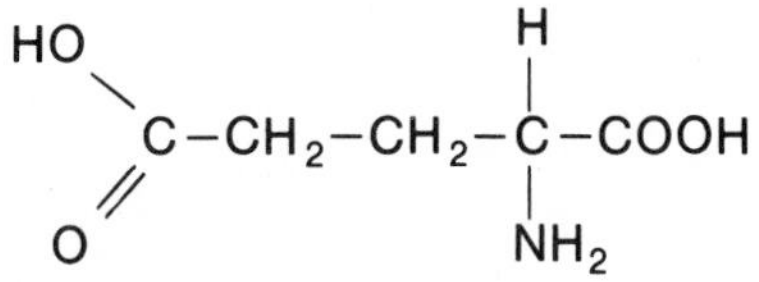

$$HO-\underset{\underset{O}{\|}}{C}-CH_2-CH_2-\underset{\underset{NH_2}{|}}{\overset{\overset{H}{|}}{C}}-COOH$$

*Lysine
Lys

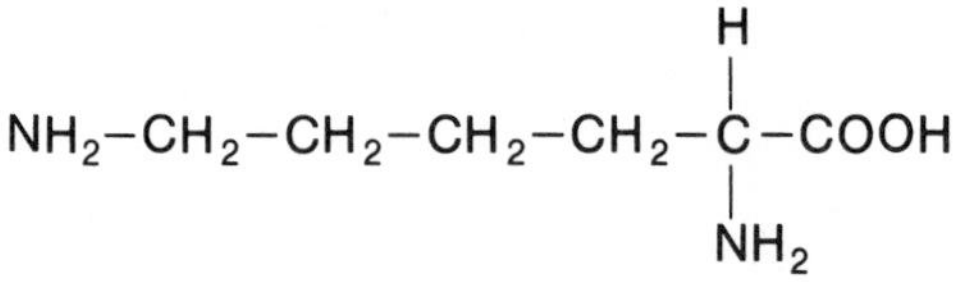

$$NH_2-CH_2-CH_2-CH_2-CH_2-\underset{\underset{NH_2}{|}}{\overset{\overset{H}{|}}{C}}-COOH$$

*Arginine
Arg

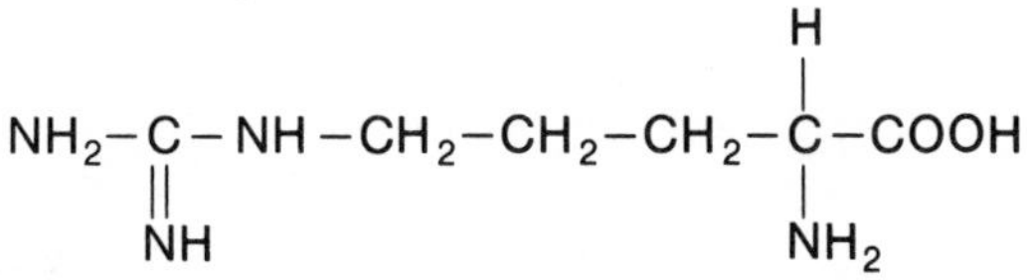

$$NH_2-\underset{\underset{NH}{\|}}{C}-NH-CH_2-CH_2-CH_2-\underset{\underset{NH_2}{|}}{\overset{\overset{H}{|}}{C}}-COOH$$

Cysteine
Cys

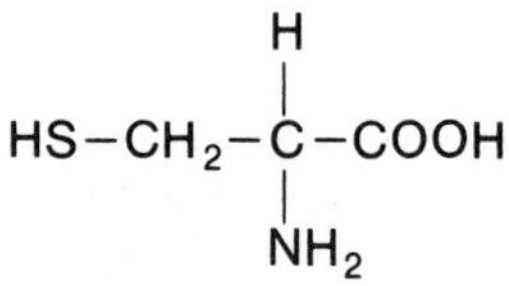

$$HS-CH_2-\underset{\underset{NH_2}{|}}{\overset{\overset{H}{|}}{C}}-COOH$$

Cystine
Cys-Cys

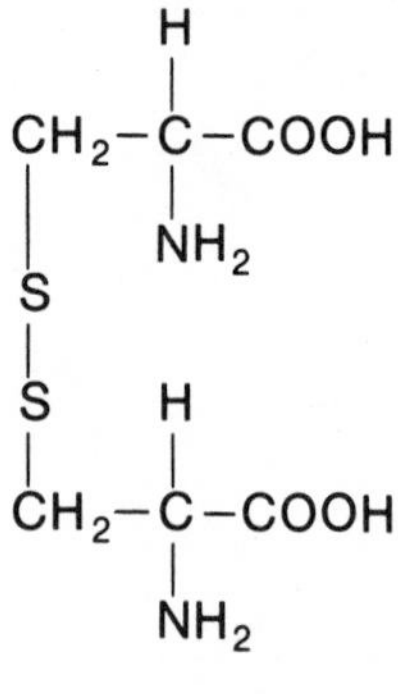

$$CH_2-\underset{\underset{NH_2}{|}}{\overset{\overset{H}{|}}{C}}-COOH$$
$$\underset{\underset{\underset{\underset{CH_2-\underset{\underset{NH_2}{|}}{\overset{\overset{H}{|}}{C}}-COOH}{|}}{S}}{|}}{S}$$

*Methionine
Met

$$CH_3-S-CH_2-CH_2-\underset{\underset{NH_2}{|}}{\overset{\overset{H}{|}}{C}}-COOH$$

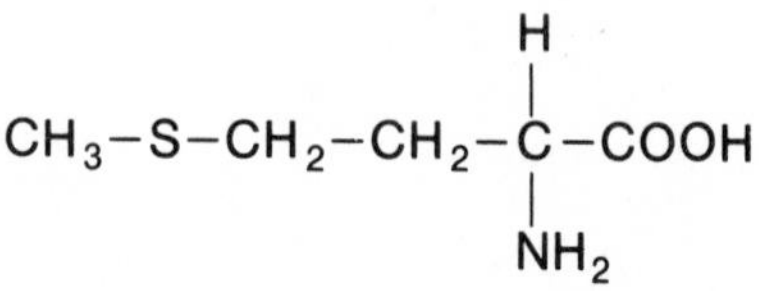

*Essential, since human beings cannot synthesize

Tyrosine
Tyr

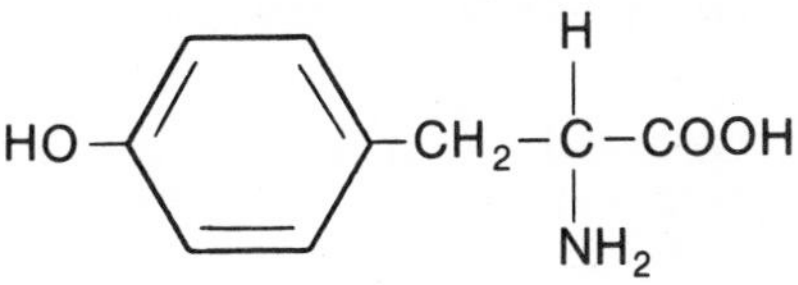

$$HO-\bigcirc-CH_2-\underset{\underset{NH_2}{|}}{\overset{\overset{H}{|}}{C}}-COOH$$

*Phenylalanine
Phe

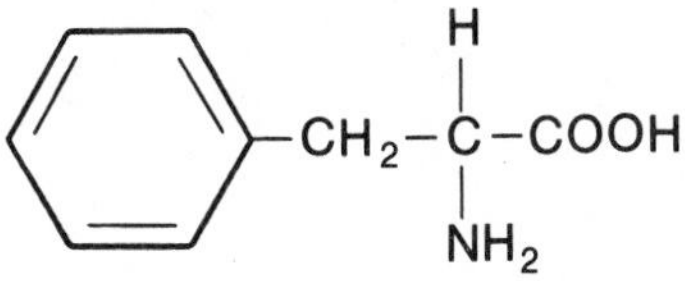

$$\bigcirc-CH_2-\underset{\underset{NH_2}{|}}{\overset{\overset{H}{|}}{C}}-COOH$$

*Tryptophan
Try

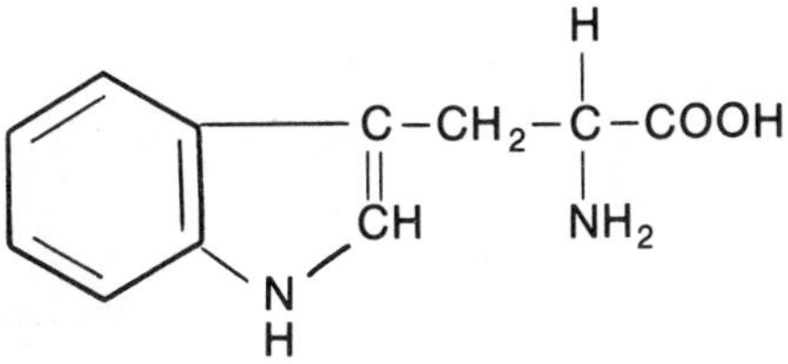

$$\underset{\substack{N\\H}}{\overset{}{\bigcirc}}\overset{}{\underset{CH}{C}}-CH_2-\underset{\underset{NH_2}{|}}{\overset{\overset{H}{|}}{C}}-COOH$$

Proline
Pro

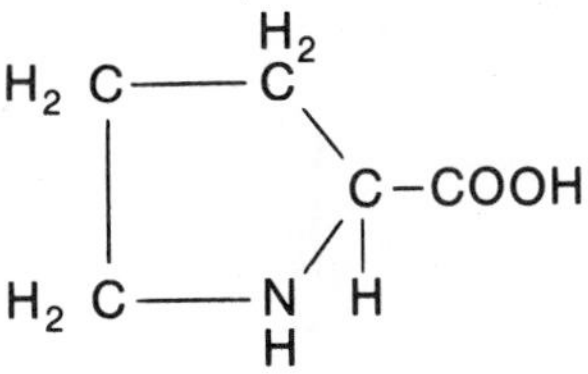

$$\begin{array}{c} H_2C-\overset{H_2}{C}\\ |\qquad\qquad C-COOH\\ H_2C-\underset{H}{N}\;H \end{array}$$

*Histidine
His

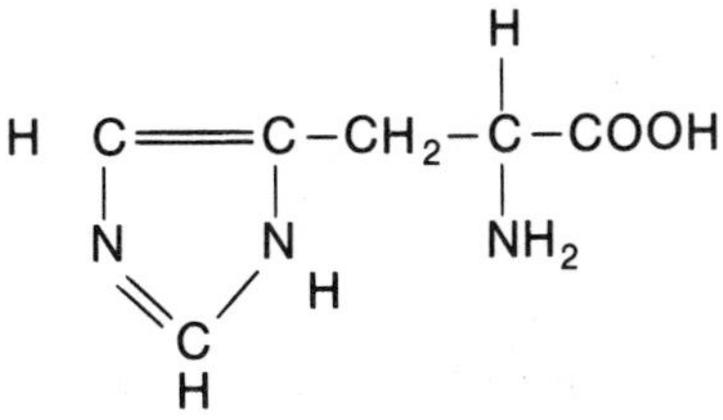

$$\underset{\substack{N\\\;\;\searrow\\C\\H}}{\overset{H}{C}}=\overset{}{\underset{\substack{N\\H}}{C}}-CH_2-\underset{\underset{NH_2}{|}}{\overset{\overset{H}{|}}{C}}-COOH$$

Asparagine
Asn

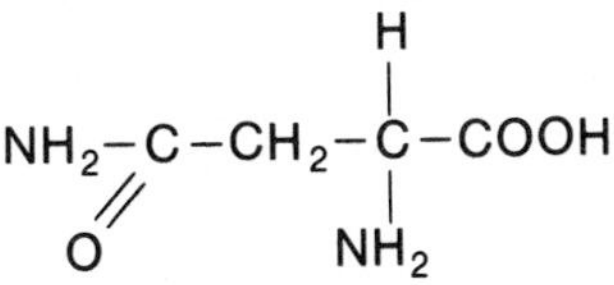

$$\underset{O}{\overset{}{NH_2-C}}-CH_2-\underset{\underset{NH_2}{|}}{\overset{\overset{H}{|}}{C}}-COOH$$

Glutamine
Gln

$$\underset{O}{\overset{NH_2}{C}}-CH_2-CH_2-\underset{\underset{NH_2}{|}}{\overset{\overset{H}{|}}{C}}-COOH$$

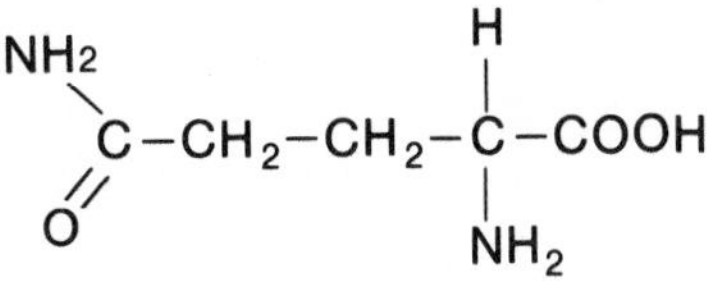

*Essential, since human beings cannot synthesize

Vitamins and Coenzymes

Vitamin A_1 (retinol): predominant form in most higher animals.

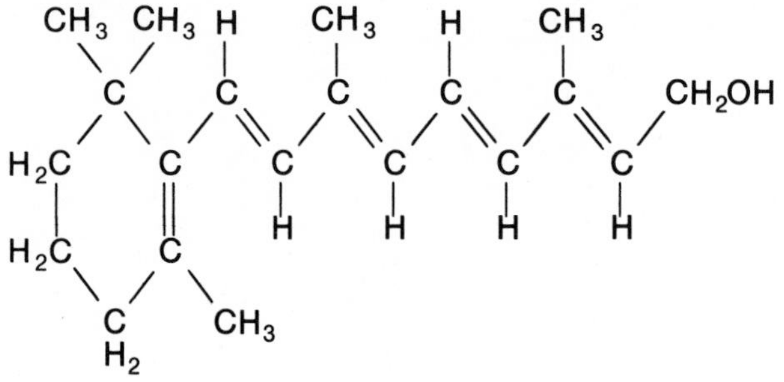

Vitamin A_2: predominant form in fish liver oils.

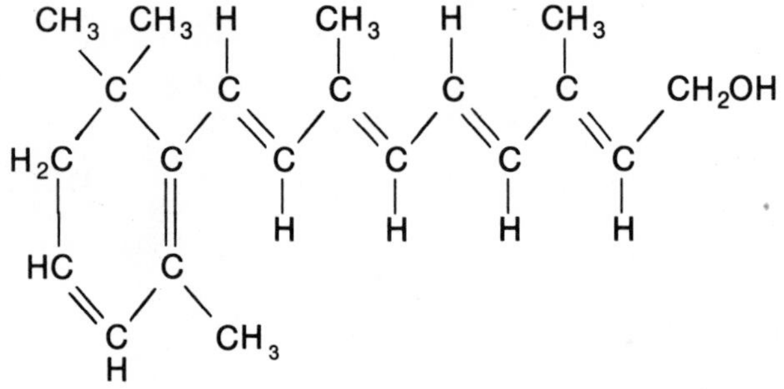

B-Carotene: carotenoid pigment in plants yields vitamin A in animals.

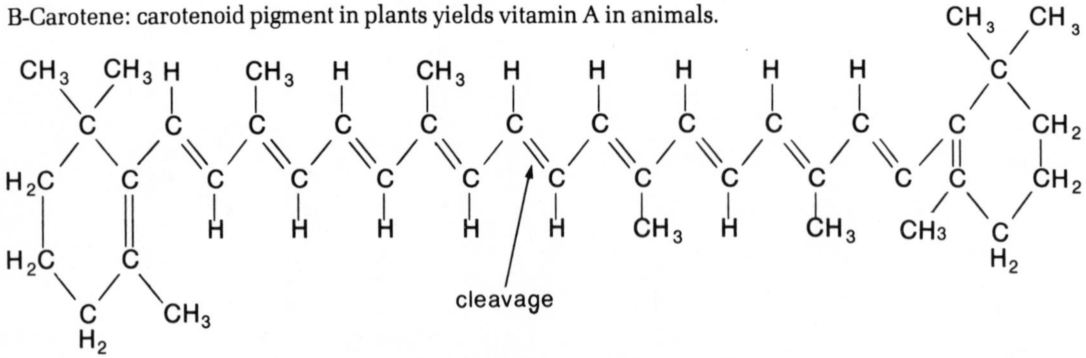

cleavage

Thiamin (vitamin B$_1$), and the coenzyme of which it is a part, thiamin pyrophosphate (TPP).

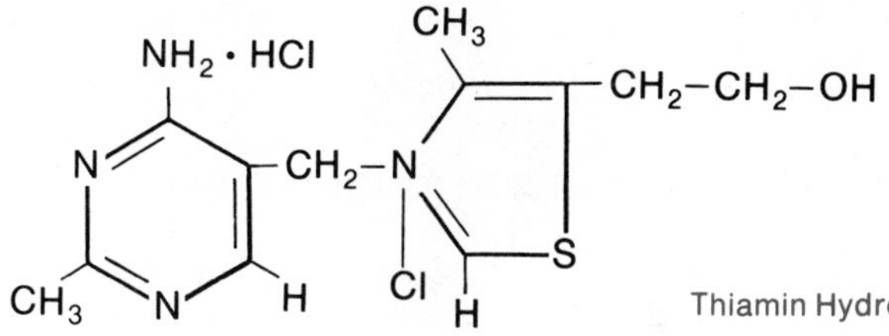

Thiamin Hydrochloride (vitamin B$_1$)

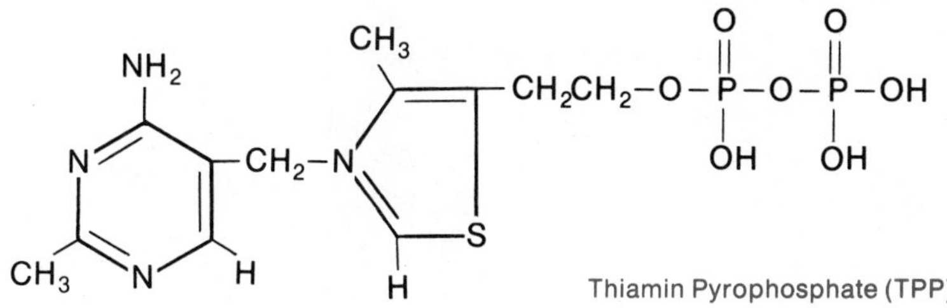

Thiamin Pyrophosphate (TPP)

Riboflavin (vitamin B$_2$) and the two coenzymes of which it is a part, flavin mononucleotide (FMN) and flavin adenine dinucleotide (FAD).

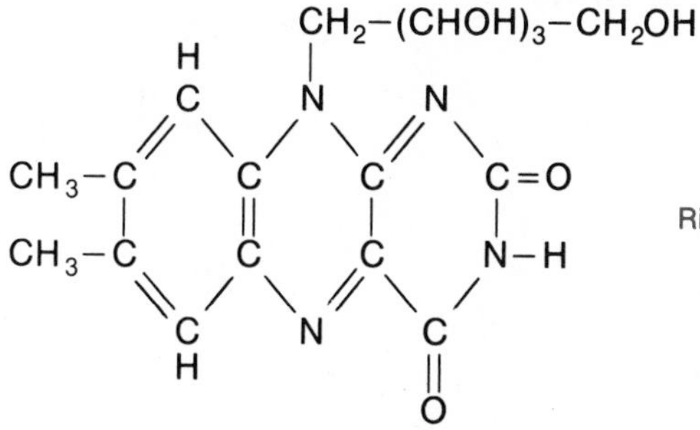

Riboflavin

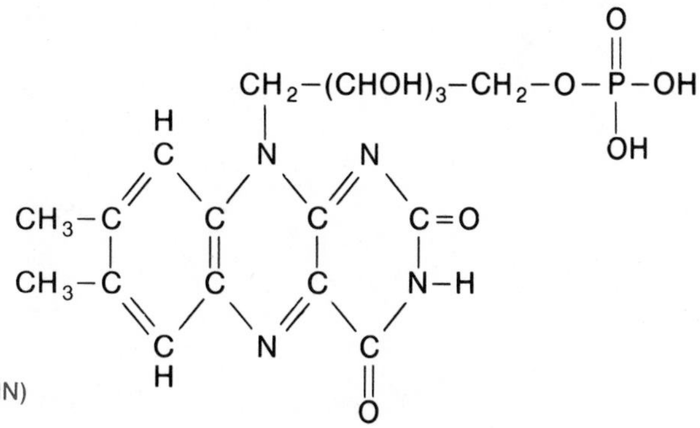

Flavin Mononucleotide (FMN)

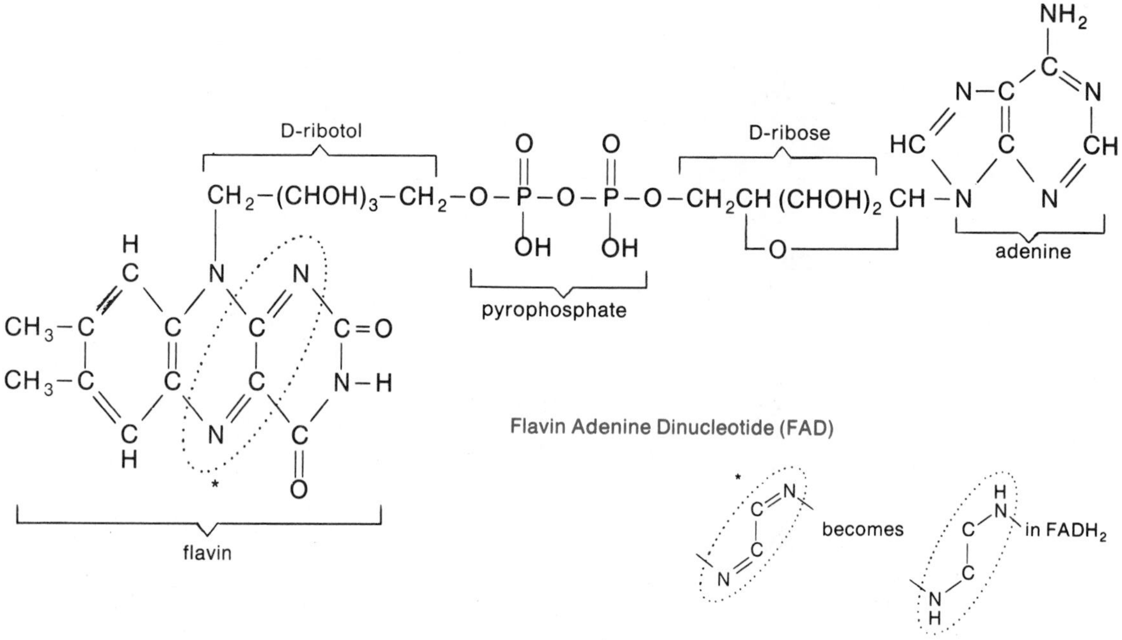

D-ribotol

$CH_2-(CHOH)_3-CH_2-O-P-O-P-O-CH_2CH(CHOH)_2 CH-N$

D-ribose

adenine

pyrophosphate

flavin

Flavin Adenine Dinucleotide (FAD)

becomes ... in FADH$_2$

Niacin (nicotinic acid and nicotinamide) and the two coenzymes of which it is a part, nicotinamide adenine dinucleotide (NAD*) and nicotinamide adenine dinucleotide phosphate (NADP†)

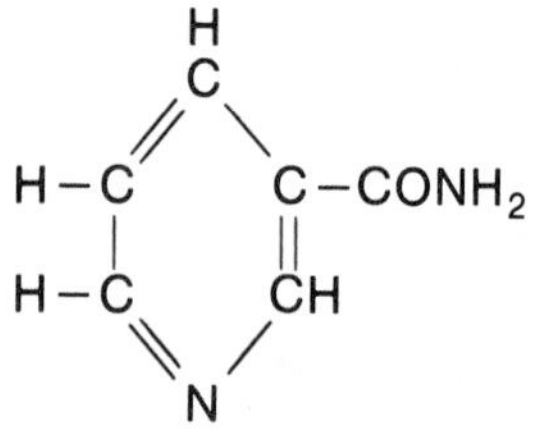

Nicotinamide

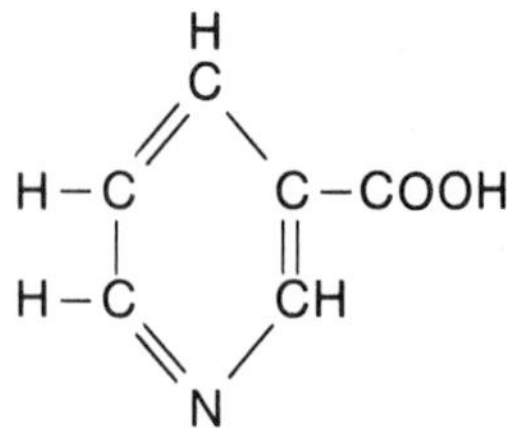

nicotinamide

adenine

D-ribose

D-ribose

Nicotinic Acid

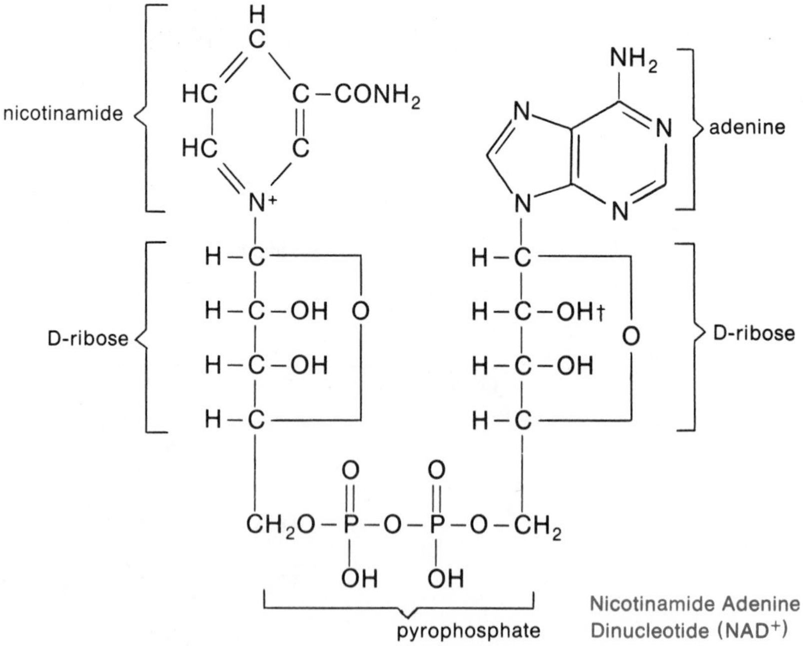

pyrophosphate

Nicotinamide Adenine Dinucleotide (NAD$^+$)

* NAD has been called coenzyme I and DPN; NADP has been called coenzyme II and TPN.

† NADP has the same structure as NAD with a phosphate group attached here.

NAD+ when reduced becomes NADH.

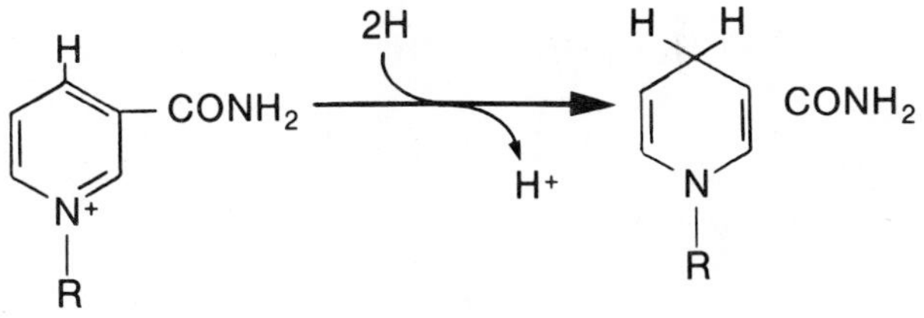

Pyridoxine (vitamin B_6) is a general name for three compounds, pyridoxine, pyridoxal, and pyridoxamine. Pyridoxal phosphate and pyridoxamine phosphates are the coenzymes necessary for transamination and other important processes.

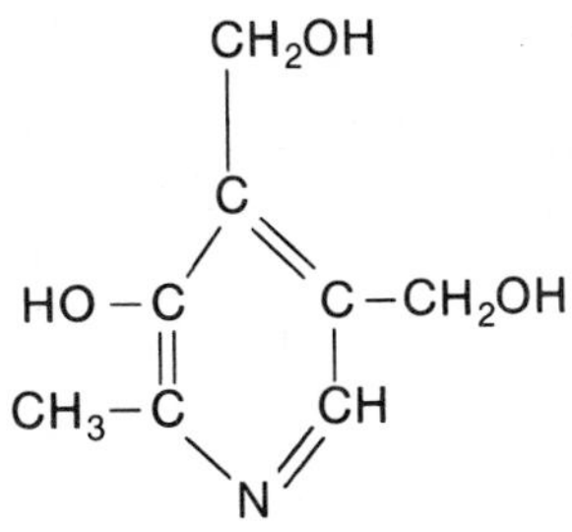

Pyridoxine

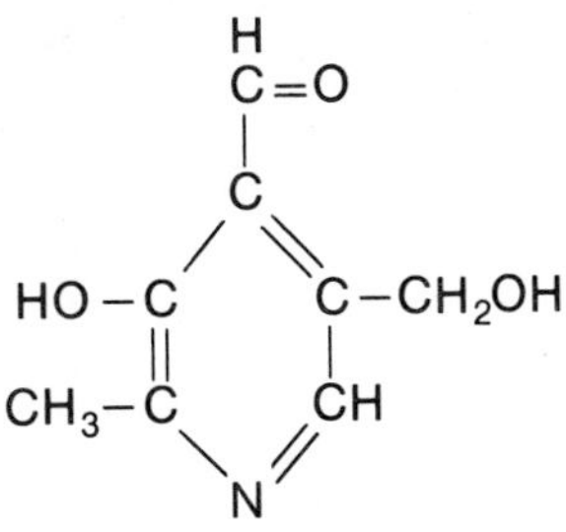

Pyridoxal

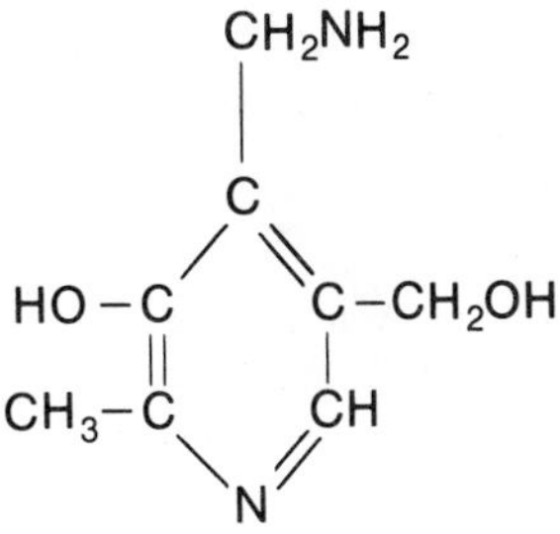

Pyridoxamine

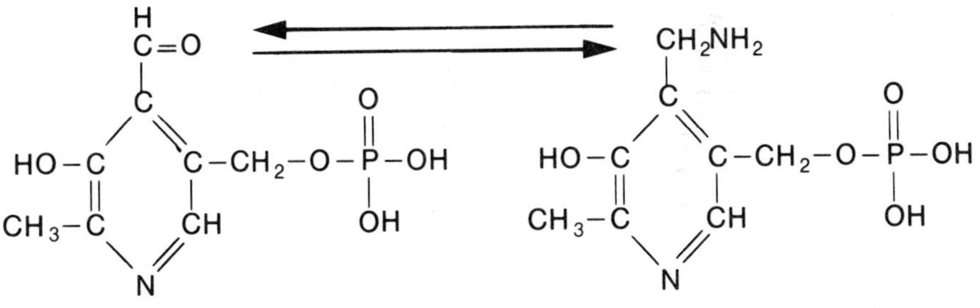

Pyridoxal Phosphate

Pyridoxamine Phosphate

Vitamin B$_{12}$ (cyanocobalamin).

Vitamin B$_{12}$

Vitamin C (ascorbic acid) and its oxidized form, dehydroascorbic acid.

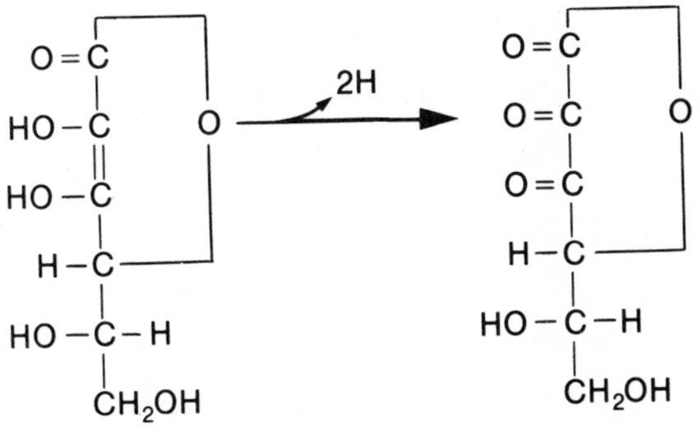

Ascorbic Acid
(reduced form)

Dehydroascorbic Acid
(oxidized form)

Vitamins D_2 and D_3 and their precursors.

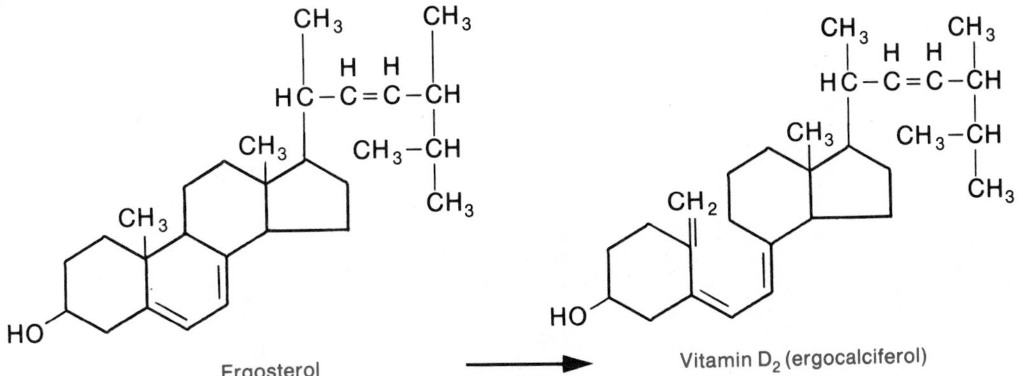

Ergosterol

irradiation

Vitamin D_2 (ergocalciferol)

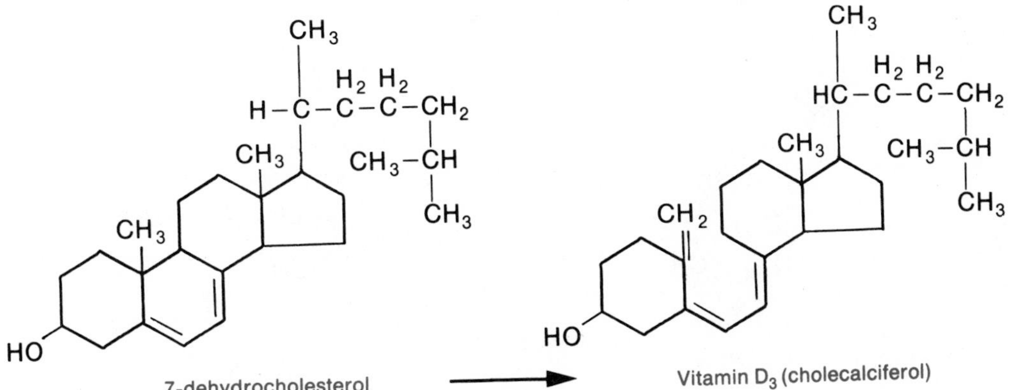

7-dehydrocholesterol

irradiation

Vitamin D_3 (cholecalciferol)

Vitamin E (∝-tocopherol).

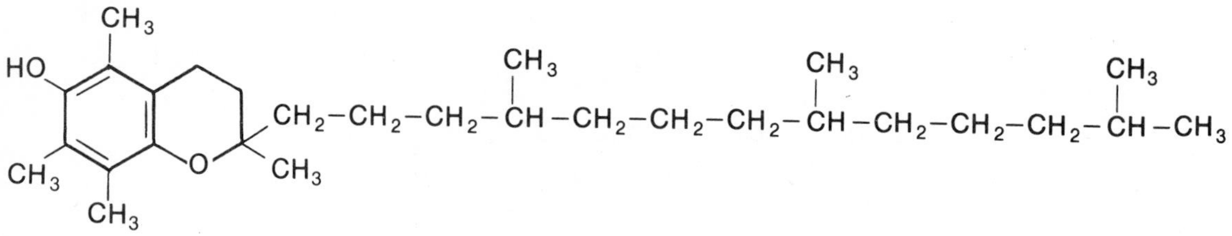

Vitamin K$_1$, a naturally occurring compound, and menadione, a synthetic compound which exhibits vitamin K activity.

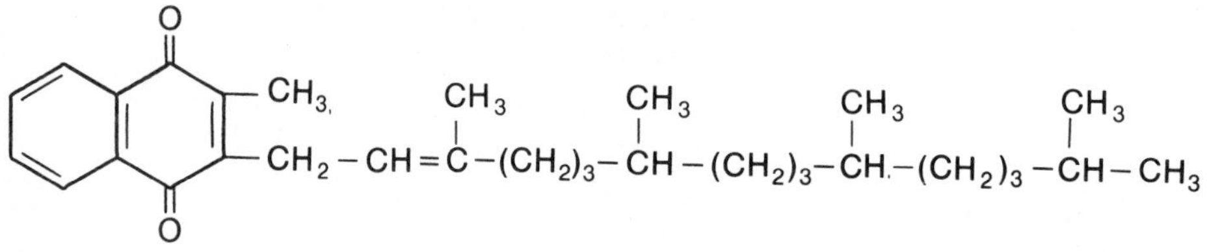

Vitamin K

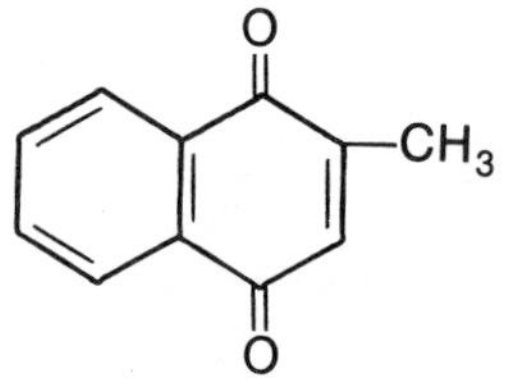

Menadione

Folic acid (folacin) and its active coenzyme form, tetrahydrofolic acid.

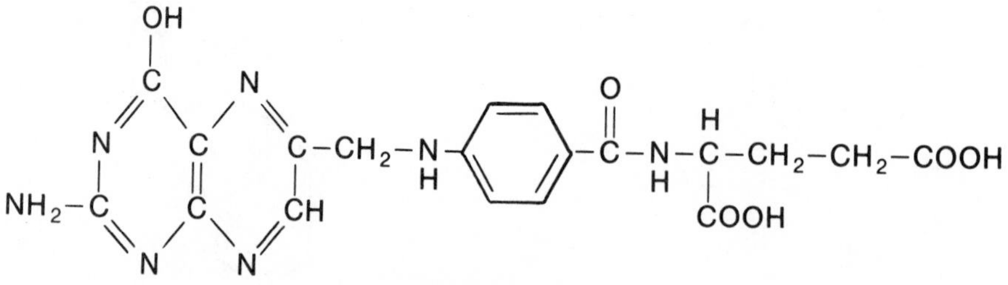

Folic Acid

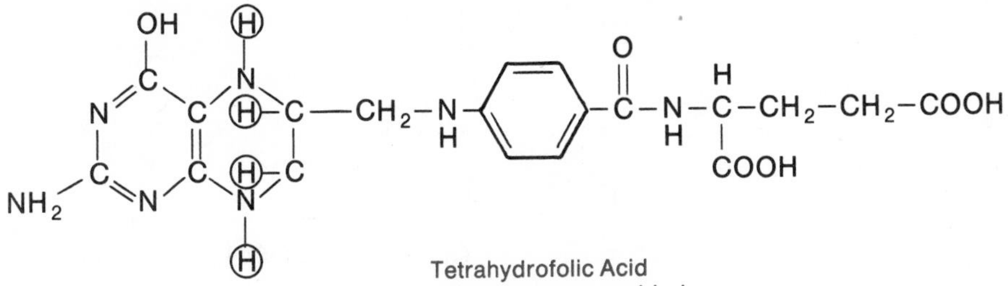

Tetrahydrofolic Acid
(The four hydrogens added
to folic acid are circled.)

Pantothenic acid and the coenzyme of which it is a part, coenzyme A (Co-A).

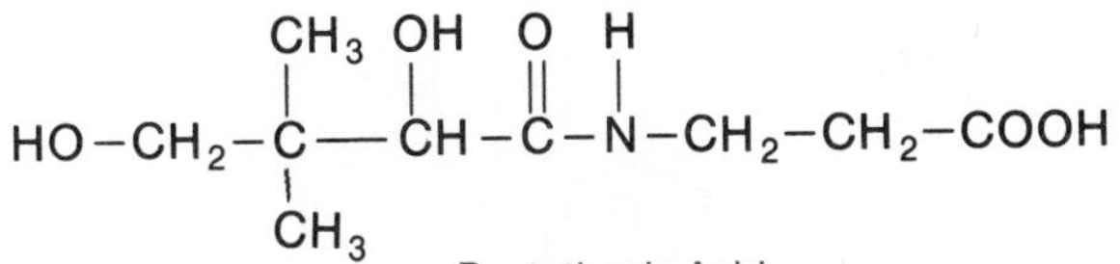

Pantothenic Acid

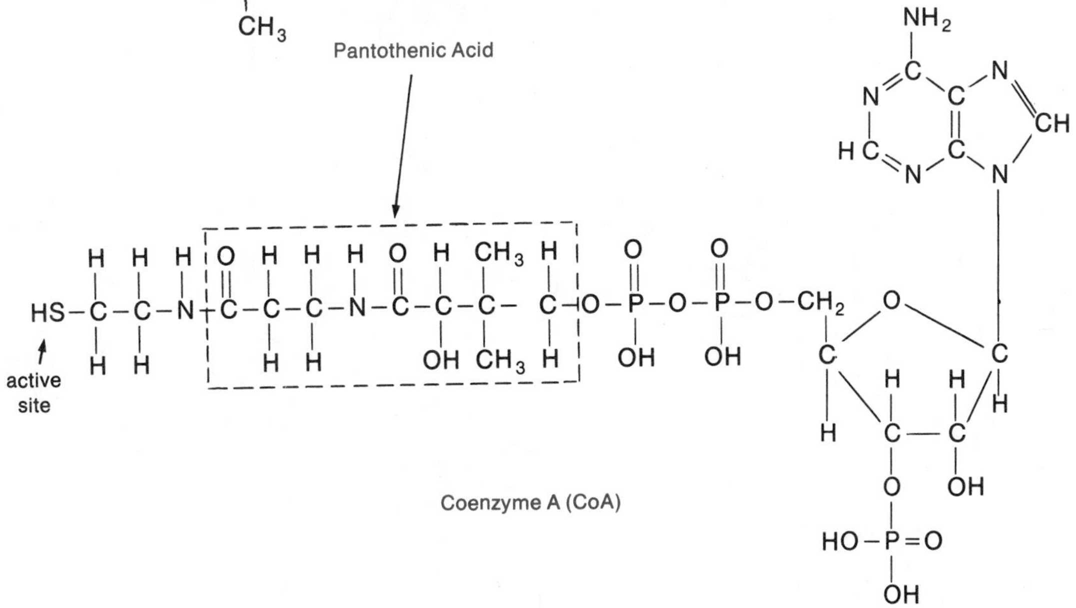

Coenzyme A (CoA)

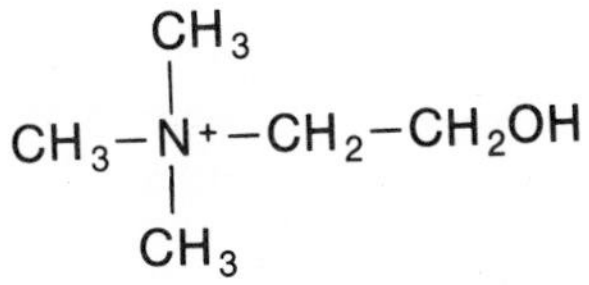

active site

Choline

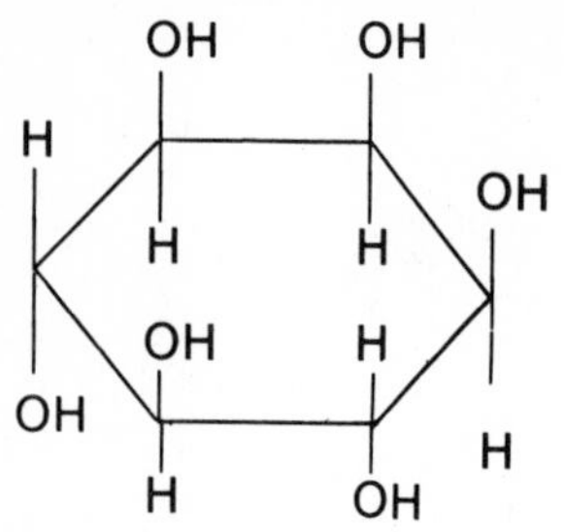

Inositol

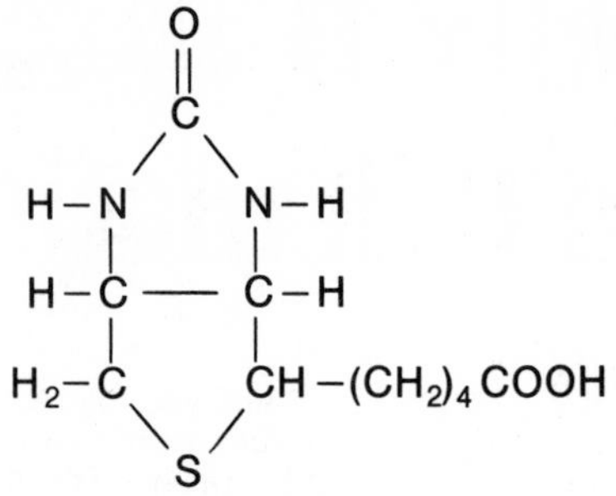

Biotin

ADP (adenosine diphosphate) and ATP (adenosine triphosphate), the energy carriers.

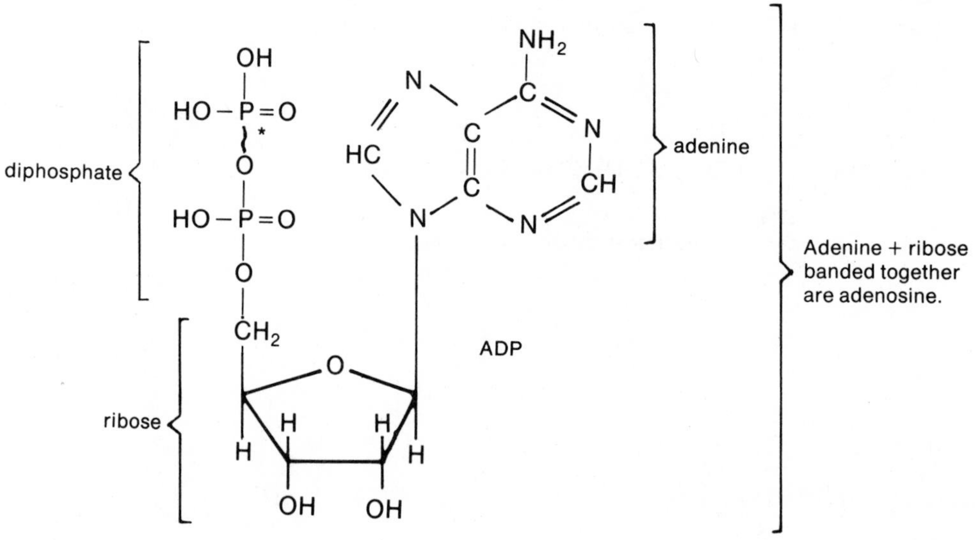

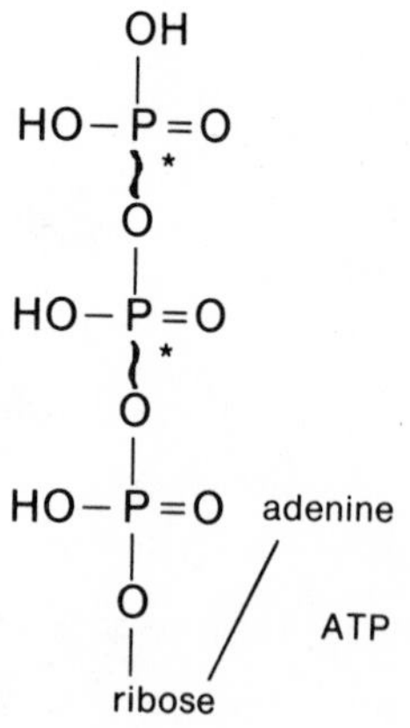

ADP

diphosphate

ribose

adenine

Adenine + ribose banded together are adenosine.

ATP

adenine

ribose

* ⟨ represents a high-energy bond

Appendix D ▬▬▬
Aids to Calculation

In this appendix examples will be given of solutions to each type of mathematical problem encountered in the text. Two general methods of solving problems are first reviewed: the use of conversion factors with cancellation of units, and ratio and proportion. The steps toward the solutions are especially adapted for use with pocket calculators.

General Review

Conversion Factors and Cancellation of Units. Conversion factors are useful mathematical tools in everyday calculations, such as the ones encountered in a nutrition course. Skill in the use of conversion factors and employment of cancellation of units is especially desirable currently as the United States moves from the British system of measurements to the Metric system. Pages 527-528 in this appendix list both systems and British-Metric equivalents.

A *conversion factor* is a fraction in which the numerator and the denominator have different units for the same quantity. For example, 4 cups and 1 quart are equivalent amounts of a substance. The conversion factor for 4 cups and 1 quart would be either $\frac{4 \text{ cups}}{1 \text{ quart}}$ or $\frac{1 \text{ quart}}{4 \text{ cups}}$. Since both fractions equal one, measurements can be multiplied by the factor without changing the value of the measurement. Conversion factors are used to convert measurements expressed in one unit to another unit in the following manner:

Example: 2 quarts are how many cups?

Facts you know: conversion factor, either $\dfrac{1 \text{ quart}}{4 \text{ cups}}$ or $\dfrac{4 \text{ cups}}{1 \text{ quart}}$

Statement: 2 quarts $\times$ $\dfrac{4 \text{ cups}}{1 \text{ quart}} = 8$ cups

In the above example, the choice of the form, $\dfrac{4 \text{ cups}}{1 \text{ quart}}$, was made because the answer sought was to be in "cups," thus cups must be in the numerator of the factor. A way of confirming that the problem is stated correctly is to cancel the units in the same manner that numerals are cancelled in a problem involving multiplication of fractions. The unit which cannot be cancelled is the one in which the answer will be stated. For example:

$$\cancel{\text{quarts}} \times \frac{\text{cups}}{\cancel{\text{quarts}}} = \text{cups}$$

Following are two examples of problems commonly encountered in a nutrition course; they illustrate the use of conversion factors and cancellation of units in their solutions.

EXAMPLE 1. Convert your weight in pounds (lb) to kilograms (kg).
(See page 528 for conversions.)

Facts you know: conversion factor; either $\dfrac{2.2 \text{ lb}}{1 \text{ kg}}$ or $\dfrac{1 \text{ kg}}{2.2 \text{ lb}}$

You weigh, for example, 130 lb.

Statement: 130 $\cancel{\text{lb}} \times \dfrac{1 \text{ kg}}{2.2 \cancel{\text{lb}}} = \boxed{}$

Note: The answer you are seeking should carry the unit kilograms; therefore, kilograms must remain uncancelled and in the numerator.

Calculation: $\dfrac{130}{2.2} = \boxed{}$

Note: This would be fed into a calculator as $130 \div 2.2$.

Answer: 59.09 is the number obtained on the calculator and kg is the unit, but this answer is unacceptable because 59.09 denotes an accuracy of measurement not present in the original measurement, 130 lb. A more acceptable answer is either 59 kg or 60 kg.[1]

EXAMPLE 2: Determine the grams protein per day which you should consume in order to meet 2/3 your RDA for protein.
(See Appendix I.)

Facts you know: conversion factor, either $\dfrac{.8 \text{ g protein}}{1 \text{ kg ideal body weight}}$

$$\text{or } \dfrac{1 \text{ kg ideal body weight}}{.8 \text{ g protein}}$$

Your ideal body weight (Appendix F) is, for example, 115 lb.

Statement:

$$115 \text{ lb ideal weight} \times \frac{1 \text{ kg}}{2.2 \text{ lb}} \times \frac{.8 \text{ g protein}}{1 \text{ kg ideal weight}} \times \frac{2}{3} = \boxed{}$$

Note: cancellation of units "kg," "lb," "ideal weight," leaves "grams protein" uncancelled and in the numerator.

Calculation: $\dfrac{115 \times .8 \times 2}{2.2 \times 3} = \boxed{}$

Answer: 28 grams protein per day to meet 2/3 RDA for a 115 lb adult.

Ratio and Proportion. Some students find the ratio and proportion method convenient to use in many calculations in nutrition courses (such as seeking the amount of saturated fat in a 4-ounce broiled hamburger when Appendix H gives the amount in a 3-ounce hamburger). A ratio and proportion is a statement that a ratio, for example 2:3, is equal to another ratio, say 4:6. The usefulness of this statement is that if one of the four num-

---

[1]The degree of accuracy of a measurement is reflected in the recording of that measurement and is not altered by any subsequent calculations. The measurement "130 lb" denotes to the reader that the person's weight is *about* 130 lb; if the person's weight had been very accurately determined, and if that degree of accuracy had been considered necessary, the weight would have been recorded as "130.0" signifying that the weight was *exactly* 130.0 lb, correct to a tenth of a pound. Any mathematical calculation with a measurement does not improve the accuracy of the original measurement and the recording of answers should reflect this. In this example, "59.09 kg" would indicate that the weight is correct to a hundredth of a kilogram, which is impossible given the fact that the original measurement was not that accurate. Either 59 kg or 60 kg would more properly reflect the truth.

bers is unknown and the other three are known, the unknown number can be calculated using simple algebra.

As an illustration of the above, suppose that the number 6 is unknown in the above proportion but 2, 3, and 4 are known. You would think, "2 is to 3 as 4 is to what number?" This would be written: $\dfrac{2}{3} = \dfrac{4}{x}$.

The simple algebra involved would be: $2x = 3 \times 4$

$$x = \frac{3 \times 4}{2}$$

$$x = 6$$

Care must be taken when stating a problem using ratio and proportion that the *units* of measurement are the same on both sides of the equation.

EXAMPLE 3: How many grams saturated fat are contained in a 4-ounce broiled hamburger?

Facts you know: By consulting Appendix H you will learn that a 3-ounce broiled hamburger contains 8 grams saturated fat.

Statement: $\dfrac{3 \text{ oz hamburger}}{8 \text{ g saturated fat}} = \dfrac{4 \text{ oz hamburger}}{x \text{ g saturated fat}}$

$$3x = 4 \times 8$$

$$x = \frac{4 \times 8}{3}$$

Note: $\dfrac{\text{oz}}{\text{g}} = \dfrac{\text{oz}}{\text{g}}$. The units of measurement are the same on both sides of equation. Proceed with the calculation.

Calculation: $\dfrac{4 \times 8}{3} = \boxed{}$

Answer: 11 grams saturated fat in a 4-ounce broiled hamburger.

Specific Problems

Finding Percent. To find what percent a part is of a whole, express the relationship of the part to the whole as a fraction, multiply by 100 and reduce to simplest terms. In the fraction, the figure which represents the whole amount goes into the denominator and the figure which represents that part of the whole with which you are concerned becomes the numerator.

EXAMPLE 4: Calculate the percentage of your carbohydrate calories which is derived from sweets.

Facts you know: kcalories from carbohydrate, for example, 850.

kcalories from sweets, for example, 175.

Statement: $\dfrac{175 \text{ kcalories from sweets}}{850 \text{ kcalories from all carbohydrates}} \times 100 =$ ☐

Calculation: $\dfrac{175 \times 100}{850} =$ ☐

Answer: 21 percent of kcalories from carbohydrate derived from sweets.

P:S Ratio. The ratio of the number of grams of polyunsaturated fatty acid (linoleic acid) in the diet to the number of grams of saturated fatty acid in the diet is called the P:S ratio. To calculate, determine the number of grams of linoleic acid and of total saturated fatty acid in the diet, using Appendix H. (The value for the monounsaturated fatty acid, oleic acid, given in Appendix H, is not used in this calculation.) Divide the grams of linoleic acid by the grams of saturated fatty acid. The answer is usually expressed as correct to a tenth of a whole number; for example, 0.7 to 2.5 is the range of the P:S ratios usually recommended for heart patients.[2]

EXAMPLE 5: Calculate the P:S ratio of a diet which contains 80 grams of saturated fatty acid and 32 grams of linoleic acid.

Statement: $\dfrac{32 \text{ grams polyunsaturated fatty acid}}{80 \text{ grams saturated fatty acid}} =$ ☐

Calculation: $\dfrac{32}{80} =$ ☐

Answer: 0.4 is the P:S ratio. (This denotes a diet high in saturated fat.) This means 0.4:1.0.

Basal Metabolic Rate (BMR) Estimate. The basal metabolic rate is the number of kilocalories per unit of time used by an individual to maintain basal functions of the body. BMR is described in Chapter 8.

One kilocalorie per kilogram of body weight per hour is a "ball-park" figure for a quick estimate of the BMR.

EXAMPLE 6: Find the kilocalories needed to maintain the basal functions of a person who weighs 110 pounds.

[2]Bennett, I.: *The Prudent Diet.* David White Publishers, New York, 1973.

Facts you know: Ball-park figure for estimating BMR: 1-kcal/kg/hr

$$110\,\cancel{lb}\times\frac{1\text{ kg}}{2.2\,\cancel{lb}}=50\text{ kg}$$

Statement: $50\,\cancel{\text{kg}}\times\dfrac{1\text{ kcal}}{\cancel{\text{kg/hr}}}\times\dfrac{24\,\cancel{\text{hr}}}{\text{day}}=\boxed{}$

Calculation: $50\times24=\boxed{}$

Answer: 1,200 kilocalories/day for basal functions (BMR).

BMR Calculated from Surface Area. A means of calculating BMR from height and weight is to calculate the surface area in square meters using the nomogram (Figure D.1) on page 530, then to find the kilocalories per square meter per hour for the age and sex by using Table D.1 on page 529, as illustrated in the following example.

EXAMPLE 7: Find the kilocalories needed to maintain for 24 hours the basal functions of a female who is 20 years old, five feet three inches tall, and weighs 110 pounds.

Facts you know: From Figure D.1, the surface area of a 5 ft 3 in, 110 lb person: 1.5 sq m. From Table D.1, the kcal per sq m per hr for a 20 yr old female: 35.3 kcal/sq m/hr.

Statement: $\dfrac{35.3\text{ kcal}}{\cancel{\text{sq m/hr}}}\times1.5\,\cancel{\text{sq m}}\times\dfrac{24\,\cancel{\text{hr}}}{\text{day}}=\boxed{}$

Calculation: $35.3\times1.5\times24=\boxed{}$

Answer: 1,270 kcal/day needed to maintain basal functions of a 20-yr-old female who is 5-ft 3-in tall and weighs 110 lb.

Energy Costs of Activities. Physical activities use varying amounts of kilocalories depending on the muscular effort involved in the activity as well as on the amount of body weight which must be moved during the activity. Table D.2 lists the costs of activities exclusive of basal metabolism and the influence of food.

To calculate the number of kilocalories expended in a day on physical activity, an exact record of the time in minutes spent on each activity must be kept, converted to hours, and multiplied by the kilocalories per kilogram per hour, as shown in Example 8. The column on the right, kcal per kg, after being totaled for the day, is then multiplied by the person's weight in kilograms, giving the kilocalories spent on physical activity in a day.

EXAMPLE 8: The following is a suggested format for recording activities and shows the calculations that need to be made in order to discover the number of kilocalories spent on physical activity in a day.

Activity	Minutes Engaged in Activity (min)	÷ 60 = (min/hr)	Hours Engaged in Activity (hr)	×	Energy Cost of Activity* (kcal/kg/hr)	=	Energy Cost per Weight (kcal/kg)
Running	10	÷ 60 =	.17	×	7.0	=	1.19
Dressing	40	÷ 60 =	.67	×	.7	=	.47
etc.	etc.		etc.		etc.		etc.

Total kcal/kg for the day 6.5

(Weight of person: 110 lb × $\frac{1\ kg}{2.2\ lb}$ = 50 kg) TOTAL $\frac{\times\ 50}{325.0}\frac{kcal}{day}$

*From Table D.2. If activity engaged in is not listed, choose one that is comparable in the amount of muscular effort needed.

Systems of Measurement

The Metric System. The metric system is a uniform, international system of units of measure. It is simple to use since, like the United States' monetary system, it is a decimal system.

Length units: 1 meter (m) = 100 centimeters (cm)
                  1,000 meters =   1 kilometer (km)

Weight units: 1 kilogram (kg) = 1,000 grams (gm or g)
                         1 gm = 1,000 milligrams (mg)
                         1 mg = 1,000 micrograms (μg)

Volume units: 1 liter (l) = 1,000 milliliters (ml)
                  1 milliliter = 1 cubic centimeter (cc)

Temperature units: The Celsius thermometer scale is based on 100 equal divisions between the point at which pure water will turn to ice (0° C) and the point at which it will boil (100° C) at standard atmospheric pressure. Temperatures recorded in this system are recorded as degrees Celsius (° C). This scale, also known as the centigrade scale, is used for all scientific work.

Energy units: The Committee on Nomenclature of the American Institute of Nutrition in 1970 recommended that the term kilojoule (kJ) replace the kilocalorie (kcal) as soon as practicable. 1 kilocalorie is the amount of energy required to raise a kilogram of pure water one degree on the Celsius scale.

1 kilocalorie = 4.184 kilojoules

To Explore Further—

Further information on the metric system can be obtained by writing to:

Metric Information Office
National Bureau of Standards
Washington, D.C. 20234

The British System. The British system is not a decimal system.

Length units:	1 foot (ft) = 12 inches (in)
	1 yard (yd) = 3 feet
Weight units:	1 pound (lb) = 16 ounces (oz)
Volume units:	3 teaspoons (tsp) = 1 tablespoon (tbsp)
	16 tablespoons = 1 cup (c)
	1 cup = 8 fluid ounces (fl oz)
	4 cups = 1 quart (qt)

Temperature units: The Fahrenheit thermometer scale is based on 180 divisions between the point at which pure water will turn to ice (32° F) and the point at which pure water will boil (212° F) at standard atmospheric pressure. This scale is commonly used in the United States for everyday household use but is not used for scientific measurements.

Conversion Between Metric and British Systems of Measurement

Length:	1 inch = 2.54 centimeters
	1 foot = 30.48 centimeters
	39.37 inches = 1 meter
Weight:	1 ounce = 28.35 grams (nutritionists usually use either 28 or 30 grams)
	2.2 pounds = 1 kilogram
Volume:	1.06 quarts = 1 liter

Temperature:

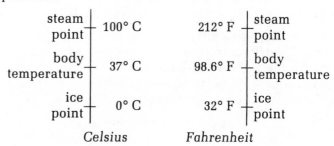

Celsius	Fahrenheit
steam point — 100° C	212° F — steam point
body temperature — 37° C	98.6° F — body temperature
ice point — 0° C	32° F — ice point

The symbol t_F in the following conversion equations represents the numerical value of a temperature on the Fahrenheit scale; t_C represents that of the Celsius scale.

$$t_F = 9/5\ t_C + 32$$
$$t_C = 5/9\ (t_F - 32)$$

Table D.1
Basal metabolic rate in kilocalories
per square meter per hour by sex and age.*

Age (yr)	Males (kcal/sq m/hr)	Females (kcal/sq m/hr)	Age (yr)	Males (kcal/sq m/hr)	Females (kcal/sq m/hr)
3	60.1	54.5	26	38.2	35.0
4	57.9	53.9	27	38.0	35.0
5	56.3	53.0			
6	54.0	51.2	28	37.8	35.0
7	52.3	49.7	29	37.7	35.0
			30	37.6	35.0
8	50.8	48.0	31	37.4	35.0
9	49.5	46.2	32	37.2	34.9
10	47.7	44.9			
11	46.5	43.5	33	37.1	34.9
12	45.3	42.0	34	37.0	34.9
			35	36.9	34.8
13	44.5	40.5	36	36.8	34.7
14	43.8	39.2	37	36.7	34.6
15	42.9	38.3			
16	42.0	37.2	38	36.7	34.5
17	41.5	36.4	39	36.6	34.4
			40-44	36.4	34.1
18	40.8	35.8	45-49	36.2	33.8
19	40.5	35.4	50-54	35.8	33.1
20	39.9	35.3			
21	39.5	35.2	55-59	35.1	32.8
22	39.2	35.2	60-64	34.5	32.0
			65-69	33.5	31.6
23	39.0	35.2	70-74	32.7	31.1
24	38.7	35.1	75+	31.8	
25	38.4	35.1			

*From Boothby, W. M.: In *Handbook of Biological Data*. W. S. Spector, editor, 1956. Reprinted courtesy W. B. Saunders Company, Philadelphia.

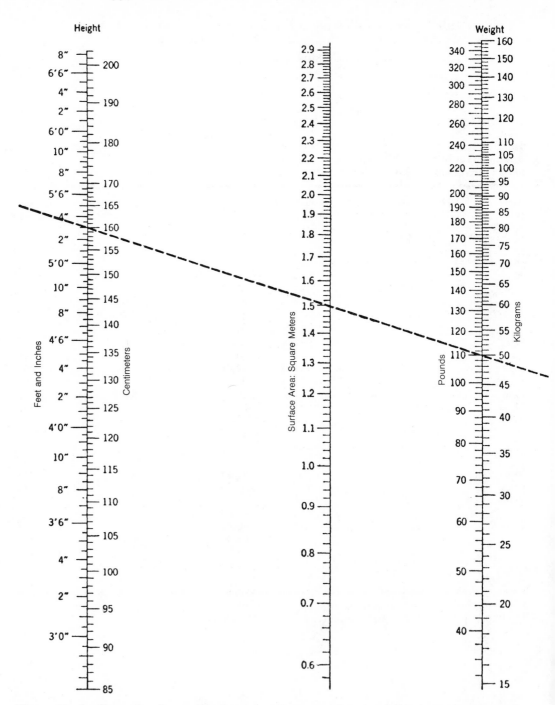

Figure D. 1. Chart for determination of surface area.* Dotted line is drawn between height (5 feet 3 inches) and weight (110 pounds), showing 1.5 square meters as the surface area.

*From Boothby, W. M. Berkson, J. and Dunn, H. L.: Studies of the energy of normal individuals: a standard for basal metabolism, with a nomogram for clinical application. *American Journal of Physiology* 116: 468–484, 1936. Courtesy of the publisher.

Table D.2
Costs of activities in kilocalories per kilogram per hour
exclusive of basal metabolism and the influence of food.*

Activity	kcal/ kg/hr	Activity	kcal/ kg/hr
Bicycling (century run)	7.6	Piano playing (Liszt's "Tarantella")	2.0
Bicycling (moderate speed)	2.5	Reading aloud	0.4
Bookbinding	0.8	Rowing in race	16.0
Boxing	11.4	Running	7.0
Carpentry (heavy)	2.3	Sawing wood	5.7
Cello playing	1.3	Sewing, hand	0.4
Crocheting	0.4	Sewing, foot-driven machine	0.6
Dancing, foxtrot	3.8	Sewing, motor-driven machine	0.4
Dancing, waltz	3.0	Shoemaking	1.0
Dishwashing	1.0	Singing in loud voice	0.8
Dressing and undressing	0.7	Sitting quietly	0.4
Driving automobile	0.9	Skating	3.5
Eating	0.4	Standing at attention	0.6
Fencing	7.3	Standing relaxed	0.5
Horseback riding, walk	1.4	Stone masonry	4.7
Horseback riding, trot	4.3	Sweeping w/broom, bare floor	1.4
Horseback riding, gallop	6.7	Sweeping with carpet sweeper	1.6
Ironing (5-pound iron)	1.0	Sweeping w/vacuum sweeper	2.7
Knitting sweater	0.7	Swimming (2 mph)	7.9
Laundry, light	1.3	Tailoring	0.9
Lying still, awake	0.1	Typewriting rapidly	1.0
Organ playing (30% to 40% of energy hand work)	1.5	Violin playing	0.6
		Walking (3 mph)	2.0
Painting furniture	1.5	Walking rapidly (4 mph)	3.4
Paring potatoes	0.6	Walking at high speed (5.3 mph)	9.3
Playing Ping-Pong	4.4		
Piano playing (Mendelssohn's songs)	0.8	Walking downstairs	†
		Walking upstairs	‡
Piano playing (Beethoven's "Apassionata")	1.4	Washing floors	1.2
		Writing	0.4

*From Taylor, C. M. and McLeod, G.: Rose's Laboratory Handbook for Dietetics.
  5th ed. New York, The Macmillan Company, 1949, p. 18.
†Allow 0.012 kcal per kilogram for an ordinary staircase with 15 steps without
  regard to time.
‡Allow 0.036 kcal per kilogram for an ordinary staircase with 15 steps without
  regard to time.

Appendix E
Measures of
Protein Quality

PER is the protein efficiency ratio. It is designed especially for feeding experiments with small animals and gives the ratio between the weight gain of a growing animal (new tissue formed) and the amount of protein consumed.

BV is the ratio of nitrogen retained to nitrogen absorbed. It is best expressed by this formula:

$$\frac{\text{food N} - (\text{fecal N} - \text{metabolic N}) - (\text{urinary N} - \text{endogenous N})}{\text{food N} - (\text{fecal N} - \text{metabolic N})} \times 100$$

NPU is the net protein utilization and represents the proportion of food protein which is retained. The formula $P = \dfrac{BW \times N}{1,000}$ is used where P is protein utilization, BW is body weight change in gm per day, and N is nitrogen retention in mg per kg per day. The coefficient of the products being tested such as infant formula then can be expressed as the ratio $\dfrac{\text{P of the test infant formula}}{\text{P of evaporated milk formula}}$.

Appendix F
"Ideal" Weights

Rule of Thumb Method of Estimating "Ideal" Weight

To estimate a female's ideal weight by a quick method, give the height of five feet an ideal weight of 100 pounds. For every inch above five feet, add five pounds. Thus a woman who is five feet four inches tall would add 20 pounds (4 inches x 5 pounds/inch) to 100 pounds making her ideal weight 120 pounds.

To estimate a male's ideal weight by this quick method, the same procedure holds except that a five foot man's ideal weight is considered to be 110 pounds. Thus a six foot man would have an ideal weight of 170 pounds, 110 + (12 x 5).

Ideal weights are to be taken with a grain of salt; see discussion on pages 239-240.

Approximation of Frame Size

Although the tables below give ideal weights for three different frame sizes, at the time they were published no means of estimating frame size was supplied.[1] A simple rule is to compare the wristbones of several women or several men and to make an arbitrary judgment as to which are small, medium, or large.

[1]Wohl, M. G. and Goodhart, R. S., editors: *Modern Nutrition in Health and Disease.* 4th ed. Lea and Febiger, Philadelphia, 1968, p. 6.

Ideal Weights Derived from Life Insurance Statistics

Desirable weights for women aged 25 and over

Height with Shoes 2-inch Heels		Small Frame	Medium Frame	Large Frame
Feet	Inches			
4	10	92- 98	96-107	104-119
4	11	94-101	98-110	106-122
5	0	96-104	101-113	109-125
5	1	99-107	104-116	112-128
5	2	102-110	107-119	115-131
5	3	105-113	110-122	118-134
5	4	108-116	113-126	121-138
5	5	111-119	116-130	125-142
5	6	114-123	120-135	129-146
5	7	118-127	124-139	133-150
5	8	122-131	128-143	137-154
5	9	126-135	132-147	141-158
5	10	130-140	136-151	145-163
5	11	134-144	140-155	149-168
6	0	138-148	144-159	153-173

For nude weight, deduct 2 to 4 lbs.
Prepared by Metropolitan Life Insurance Company. Derived primarily from data of the Build and Blood Pressure Study, 1959, Society of Actuaries.

Desirable weights for men aged 25 and over

Height with Shoes 1-inch Heels		Small Frame	Medium Frame	Large Frame
Feet	Inches			
5	2	112-120	118-129	126-141
5	3	115-123	121-133	129-144
5	4	118-126	124-136	132-148
5	5	121-129	127-139	135-152
5	6	124-133	130-143	138-156
5	7	128-137	134-147	142-161
5	8	132-141	138-152	147-166
5	9	136-145	142-156	151-170
5	10	140-150	146-160	155-174
5	11	144-154	150-165	159-179
6	0	148-158	154-170	164-184
6	1	152-162	158-175	168-189
6	2	156-167	162-180	173-194
6	3	160-171	167-185	178-199
6	4	164-175	172-190	182-204

For nude weight, deduct 5 to 7 lbs.
Prepared by Metropolitan Life Insurance Company. Derived primarily from data of the Build and Blood Pressure Study, 1959, Society of Actuaries.

Appendix G
Cholesterol Content of Foods

This table is intended to provide a *rough estimate* of the cholesterol content of foods in typical portion sizes. Values were calculated from Table 4, Cholesterol Content of Foods, USDA Handbook No. 8,[1] in which the amounts of cholesterol per 100 grams edible portion, usually of raw food, are presented. The amount of cholesterol in 3 ounces of lean cooked beef, for example, was estimated as follows:

1 lb raw beef without the bone has 320 mg cholesterol
(from Handbook No. 8)

16 oz as purchased yields 9-12 oz cooked lean beef, so it is possible that 9 oz cooked lean beef has 320 mg cholesterol

3 oz might then have 107 mg cholesterol.

Thus the estimates are high and are to be used only as ball-park figures.

Foods are organized by Exchange Lists (pages 33-38).

[1]Watt, B. K. and Merrill, A. L.: *Composition of Foods, Raw, Processed, Prepared.* United States Department of Agriculture Handbook No. 8. United States Government Printing Office, Washington, D.C., 1963.

List 1: Milk Exchanges

(One exchange of milk is calculated for cholesterol content.)

		Cholesterol (mg)
Skim milk	1 cup	7
Whole milk	1 cup	25
Ice cream (not on milk exchange lists)	¼ cup	50

List 5: Meat Exchanges

(Three exchanges of meat are calculated for cholesterol content since three ounces are considered to be more nearly an average serving. One exchange of eggs and cheeses is calculated for cholesterol content since one exchange of these foods is considered more nearly an average serving.)

Beef, lean, cooked	3 oz	110
Chicken, flesh only, cooked	3 oz	90
Egg, whole (50 g)	1	255
white (33 g)	1	0
yolk (17 g)	1	255
Fish, fillet, cooked	3 oz	60
Heart, cooked	3 oz	130
Kidney, cooked	3 oz	320
Lamb, lean, cooked	3 oz	110
Liver, cooked	3 oz	260
Lobster, cooked	3 oz	170
Mutton, lean, cooked	3 oz	130
Oysters, raw	3 oz (15)	165
Pork, lean, cooked	3 oz	140
Shrimp, flesh only, cooked	3 oz	105
Veal, lean, cooked	3 oz	180
Caviar (not on exchange list)	1 oz	85
Cheddar cheese	1 oz	30
Creamed cottage cheese	¼ cup	9
Cream cheese	1 oz	35

List 6: Fat Exchanges

(One exchange of fat is calculated for cholesterol content.)

Butter	1 tsp	12
Margarine, all vegetable	1 tsp	0
Margarine, 2/3 animal fat, 1/3 vegetable fat	1 tsp	3
Lard or other animal fat	1 tsp	5

Appendix H Table of Food Composition*

[Dashes in the columns for nutrients show that no suitable value could be found although there is reason to believe that a measurable amount of the nutrient may be present]

Food, approximate measure, and weight (in grams)		Water	Food energy	Protein	Fat	Fatty acids			Carbohydrate	Calcium	Iron	Vitamin A value	Thiamin	Riboflavin	Niacin	Ascorbic acid
						Saturated (total)	Unsaturated									
							Oleic	Linoleic								
	Grams	Percent	Calories	Grams	Grams	Grams	Grams	Grams	Grams	Milligrams	Milligrams	International units	Milligrams	Milligrams	Milligrams	Milligrams
MILK, CHEESE, CREAM, IMITATION CREAM; RELATED PRODUCTS																
Milk:																
Fluid:																
1 Whole, 3.5% fat---- 1 cup----	244	87	160	9	9	5	3	Trace	12	288	0.1	350	0.07	0.41	0.2	2
2 Nonfat (skim)---- 1 cup----	245	90	90	9	Trace				12	296	.1	10	.09	.44	.2	2
3 Partly skimmed, 2% 1 cup---- nonfat milk solids added.	246	87	145	10	5	3	2	Trace	15	352	.1	200	.10	.52	.2	2
Canned, concentrated, undiluted:																
4 Evaporated, unsweetened. 1 cup----	252	74	345	18	20	11	7	1	24	635	.3	810	.10	.86	.5	3
5 Condensed, sweetened. 1 cup----	306	27	980	25	27	15	9	1	166	802	.3	1,100	.24	1.16	.6	3
Dry, nonfat instant:																
6 Low-density (1⅓ cups needed for reconstitution to 1 qt.). 1 cup----	68	4	245	24	Trace				35	879	.4	[1]20	.24	1.21	.6	5
7 High-density (⅞ cup needed for reconstitution to 1 qt.). 1 cup----	104	4	375	37	1				54	1,345	.6	[1]30	.36	1.85	.9	7
Buttermilk:																
8 Fluid, cultured, made 1 cup---- from skim milk.	245	90	90	9	Trace				12	296	.1	10	.10	.44	.2	2
9 Dried, packaged---- 1 cup----	120	3	465	41	6	3	-	2	Trace	60	1,498	.7	260	.31	2.06	1.1	----
Cheese:																
Natural:																
Blue or Roquefort type:																
10 Ounce---- 1 oz.----	28	40	105	6	9	5	3	Trace	1	89	.1	350	.01	.17	.3	0
11 Cubic inch---- 1 cu. in.----	17	40	65	4	5	3	2	Trace	Trace	54	.1	210	.01	.11	.2	0

[1] Value applies to unfortified product; value for fortified low-density product would be 1500 I.U., and the fortified high-density product would be 2290 I.U.

*Table 1, Nutritive Values of the Edible Parts of Foods, in Nutritive Value of Foods, Home and Garden Bulletin No. 72. United States Department of Agriculture, United States Government Printing Office, Washington, D.C., 1971.

Table of Food Composition (continued)

[Dashes in the columns for nutrients show that no suitable value could be found although there is reason to believe that a measurable amount of the nutrient may be present]

MILK, CHEESE, CREAM, IMITATION CREAM; RELATED PRODUCTS—Con.

	Food, approximate measure, and weight (in grams)		Water	Food energy	Protein	Fat	Fatty acids Saturated (total)	Fatty acids Unsaturated Oleic	Fatty acids Linoleic	Carbohydrate	Calcium	Iron	Vitamin A value	Thiamin	Riboflavin	Niacin	Ascorbic acid
		Grams	Percent	Calories	Grams	Grams	Grams	Grams	Grams	Grams	Milligrams	Milligrams	International units	Milligrams	Milligrams	Milligrams	Milligrams
	Cheese—Continued																
	Natural—Continued																
12	Camembert, packaged in 4-oz. pkg. with 3 wedges per pkg. 1 wedge	38	52	115	7	9	5	3	Trace	1	40	0.2	380	0.02	0.29	0.3	0
	Cheddar:																
13	Ounce 1 oz.	28	37	115	7	9	5	3	Trace	1	213	.3	370	.01	.13	Trace	0
14	Cubic inch 1 cu. in.	17	37	70	4	6	3	2	Trace	Trace	129	.2	230	.01	.08	Trace	0
	Cottage, large or small curd:																
	Creamed:																
15	Package of 12-oz., net wt. 1 pkg.	340	78	360	46	14	8	5	Trace	10	320	1.0	580	.10	.85	.3	0
16	Cup, curd pressed down. 1 cup	245	78	260	33	10	6	3	Trace	7	230	.7	420	.07	.61	.2	0
	Uncreamed:																
17	Package of 12-oz., net wt. 1 pkg.	340	79	290	58	1	1	Trace	Trace	9	306	1.4	30	.10	.95	.3	0
18	Cup, curd pressed down. 1 cup	200	79	170	34	1	Trace	Trace	Trace	5	180	.8	20	.06	.56	.2	0
	Cream:																
19	Package of 8-oz., net wt. 1 pkg.	227	51	850	18	86	48	28	3	5	141	.5	3,500	.05	.54	.2	0
20	Package of 3-oz., net wt. 1 pkg.	85	51	320	7	32	18	11	1	2	53	.2	1,310	.02	.20	.1	0
21	Cubic inch 1 cu. in.	16	51	60	1	6	3	2	Trace	Trace	10	Trace	250	Trace	.04	Trace	0
	Parmesan, grated:																
22	Cup, pressed down 1 cup	140	17	655	60	43	24	14	1	5	1,893	.7	1,760	.03	1.22	.3	0
23	Tablespoon 1 tbsp.	5	17	25	2	2	1	Trace	Trace	Trace	68	Trace	60	Trace	.04	Trace	0
24	Ounce 1 oz.	28	17	130	12	9	5	3	Trace	1	383	.1	360	.01	.25	.1	0
	Swiss:																
25	Ounce 1 oz.	28	39	105	8	8	4	3	Trace	1	262	.3	320	Trace	.11	Trace	0
26	Cubic inch 1 cu. in.	15	39	55	4	4	2	1	Trace	Trace	139	.1	170	Trace	.06	Trace	0

Dairy products — continued (values per indicated measure)

No.	Food	Measure	Grams	Water (%)	Food energy (cal.)	Protein (g)	Fat (g)	Saturated fat (g)	Oleic (g)	Linoleic (g)	Carbohydrate (g)	Calcium (mg)	Iron (mg)	Vitamin A (I.U.)	Thiamine (mg)	Riboflavin (mg)	Niacin (mg)	Ascorbic acid (mg)
	Pasteurized processed cheese:																	
	American:																	
27	Ounce	1 oz	28	40	105	7	9	5	3	Trace	1	198	.3	350	.01	.12	Trace	0
28	Cubic inch	1 cu. in.	18	40	65	4	5	3	2	Trace	Trace	122	.2	210	Trace	.07	Trace	0
	Swiss:																	
29	Ounce	1 oz	28	40	100	8	8	4	3	Trace	1	251	.3	310	Trace	.11	Trace	0
30	Cubic inch	1 cu. in.	18	40	65	5	5	3	2	Trace	Trace	159	.2	200	Trace	.07	Trace	0
	Pasteurized process cheese food, American:																	
31	Tablespoon	1 tbsp	14	43	45	3	3	2	1	Trace	1	80	.1	140	Trace	.08	Trace	0
32	Cubic inch	1 cu. in.	18	43	60	4	4	2	1	Trace	1	100	.1	170	Trace	.10	Trace	0
33	Pasteurized process cheese spread, American	1 oz	28	49	80	6	6	3	2	Trace	2	160	.2	250	Trace	.15	Trace	0
	Cream:																	
34	Half-and-half (cream and milk)	1 cup	242	80	325	8	28	15	9	1	11	261	.1	1,160	.07	.39	.1	2
35	Light, coffee or table	1 tbsp	15	80	20	1	2	1	1	Trace	1	16	Trace	70	Trace	.02	Trace	Trace
36		1 cup	240	72	505	7	49	27	16	1	10	245	.1	2,020	.07	.36	.1	2
37		1 tbsp	15	72	30	Trace	3	2	1	Trace	1	15	Trace	130	Trace	.02	Trace	Trace
38	Sour	1 cup	230	72	485	7	47	26	16	1	10	235	.1	1,930	.07	.35	.1	2
39		1 tbsp	12	72	25	Trace	2	1	1	Trace	1	12	Trace	100	Trace	.02	Trace	Trace
40	Whipped topping (pressurized)	1 cup	60	62	155	2	14	8	5	Trace	6	67	Trace	570	Trace	.04	Trace	Trace
41		1 tbsp	3	62	10	Trace	1	Trace	Trace	---	Trace	3	---	30	---	Trace	---	---
	Whipping, unwhipped (volume about double when whipped):																	
42	Light	1 cup	239	62	715	6	75	41	25	2	9	203	.1	3,060	.05	.29	.1	2
43		1 tbsp	15	62	45	Trace	5	3	2	Trace	1	13	Trace	190	Trace	.02	Trace	Trace
44	Heavy	1 cup	238	57	840	5	90	50	30	3	7	179	.1	3,670	.05	.26	.1	2
45		1 tbsp	15	57	55	Trace	6	3	2	Trace	1	11	Trace	230	Trace	.02	Trace	Trace
	Imitation cream products (made with vegetable fat):																	
	Creamers:																	
46	Powdered	1 cup	94	2	505	4	33	31	1	0	52	21	.6	²200	---	---	---	---
47		1 tsp	2	2	10	Trace	1	Trace	Trace	0	1	1	Trace	²Trace	---	---	---	---
48	Liquid (frozen)	1 cup	245	77	345	3	27	25	1	0	25	29	---	²100	0	0	0	0
49		1 tbsp	15	77	20	Trace	2	Trace	Trace	0	2	2	---	²10	0	0	0	0
50	Sour dressing (imitation sour cream) made with nonfat dry milk	1 cup	235	72	440	9	38	35	1	Trace	17	277	.1	10	.07	.38	Trace	1
51		1 tbsp	12	72	20	Trace	2	2	Trace	Trace	1	14	---	Trace	Trace	Trace	---	Trace
	Whipped topping:																	
52	Pressurized	1 cup	70	61	190	1	17	15	1	0	9	5	Trace	²340	0	0	0	0
53		1 tbsp	4	61	10	Trace	1	1	Trace	0	Trace	Trace	---	²20	0	0	0	0

² Contributed largely from beta-carotene used for coloring.

Table of Food Composition (continued)

[Dashes in the columns for nutrients show that no suitable value could be found although there is reason to believe that a measurable amount of the nutrient may be present]

MILK, CHEESE, CREAM, IMITATION CREAM; RELATED PRODUCTS—Con.

	Food, approximate measure, and weight (in grams)	Water	Food energy	Protein	Fat	Fatty acids Saturated (total)	Fatty acids Unsaturated Oleic	Fatty acids Unsaturated Linoleic	Carbohydrate	Calcium	Iron	Vitamin A value	Thiamin	Riboflavin	Niacin	Ascorbic acid
		Percent	Calories	Grams	Grams	Grams	Grams	Grams	Grams	Milligrams	Milligrams	International units	Milligrams	Milligrams	Milligrams	Milligrams
	Whipped topping—Continued															
54	Frozen 1 cup — 75	52	230	1	20	18	Trace	0	15	5	---	[2]560	0	0	0	0
55	1 tbsp — 4	52	10	Trace	1	1	Trace	0	1	Trace	---	[2]30	0	0	---	---
56	Powdered, made with whole milk. 1 cup — 75	58	175	3	12	10	1	Trace	15	62	Trace	[2]330	.02	.08	.1	Trace
57	1 tbsp — 4	58	10	Trace	1	1	Trace	Trace	1	3	Trace	[2]20	Trace	Trace	Trace	Trace
	Milk beverages:															
58	Cocoa, homemade 1 cup — 250	79	245	10	12	7	4	Trace	27	295	1.0	400	.10	.45	.5	3
59	Chocolate-flavored drink made with skim milk and 2% added butterfat. 1 cup — 250	83	190	8	6	3	2	Trace	27	270	.5	210	.10	.40	.3	3
	Malted milk:															
60	Dry powder, approx. 1 oz. 3 heaping teaspoons per ounce. — 28	3	115	4	2				20	82	.6	290	.09	.15	.1	0
61	Beverage 1 cup — 235	78	245	11	10				28	317	.7	590	.14	.49	.2	2
	Milk desserts:															
62	Custard, baked 1 cup — 265	77	305	14	15	7	5	1	29	297	1.1	930	.11	.50	.3	1
	Ice cream:															
63	Regular (approx. 10% fat). 1/2 gal. — 1,064	63	2,055	48	113	62	37	3	221	1,553	.5	4,680	.43	2.23	1.1	11
64	1 cup — 133	63	255	6	14	8	5	Trace	28	194	.1	590	.05	.28	.1	1
65	3 fl. oz. cup — 50	63	95	2	5	3	2	Trace	10	73	Trace	220	.02	.11	.1	1
66	Rich (approx. 16% fat). 1/2 gal. — 1,188	63	2,635	31	191	105	63	6	214	927	.2	7,840	.24	1.31	1.2	12
67	1 cup — 148	63	330	4	24	13	8	1	27	115	Trace	980	.03	.16	.1	1
	Ice milk:															
68	Hardened 1/2 gal. — 1,048	67	1,595	50	53	29	17	2	235	1,635	1.0	2,200	.52	2.31	1.0	10
69	1 cup — 131	67	200	6	7	4	2	Trace	29	204	.1	280	.07	.29	.1	1
70	Soft-serve 1 cup — 175	67	265	8	9	5	3	Trace	39	273	.2	370	.09	.39	.2	2

No.	Food, approximate measure, and weight (grams)	Water (%)	Food energy (calories)	Protein (g)	Fat (g)	Saturated (total) (g)	Oleic (g)	Linoleic (g)	Carbohydrate (g)	Calcium (mg)	Iron (mg)	Vitamin A (I.U.)	Thiamine (mg)	Riboflavin (mg)	Niacin (mg)	Ascorbic acid (mg)
	Yoghurt:															
71	Made from partially skimmed milk. 1 cup — 245	89	125	8	4	2	1	Trace	13	294	.1	170	.10	.44	.2	2
72	Made from whole milk. 1 cup — 245	88	150	7	8	5	3	Trace	12	272	.1	340	.07	.39	.2	2
	EGGS															
	Eggs, large, 24 ounces per dozen:															
	Raw or cooked in shell or with nothing added:															
73	Whole, without shell. 1 egg — 50	74	80	6	6	2	3	Trace	Trace	27	1.1	590	.05	.15	Trace	0
74	White of egg. 1 white — 33	88	15	4	Trace	---	---	---	Trace	3	Trace	0	Trace	.09	Trace	0
75	Yolk of egg. 1 yolk — 17	51	60	3	5	2	2	Trace	Trace	24	.9	580	.04	.07	Trace	0
76	Scrambled with milk and fat. 1 egg — 64	72	110	7	8	3	3	Trace	1	51	1.1	690	.05	.18	Trace	0
	MEAT, POULTRY, FISH, SHELLFISH; RELATED PRODUCTS															
77	Bacon, (20 slices per lb. raw), broiled or fried, crisp. 2 slices — 15	8	90	5	8	3	4	1	1	2	.5	0	.08	.05	.8	---
	Beef,[3] cooked:															
	Cuts braised, simmered, or pot-roasted:															
78	Lean and fat. 3 ounces — 85	53	245	23	16	8	7	Trace	0	10	2.9	30	.04	.18	3.5	---
79	Lean only. 2.5 ounces — 72	62	140	22	5	2	2	Trace	0	10	2.7	10	.04	.16	3.3	---
	Hamburger (ground beef), broiled:															
80	Lean. 3 ounces — 85	60	185	23	10	5	4	Trace	0	10	3.0	20	.08	.20	5.1	---
81	Regular. 3 ounces — 85	54	245	21	17	8	8	Trace	0	9	2.7	30	.07	.18	4.6	---
	Roast, oven-cooked, no liquid added:															
	Relatively fat, such as rib:															
82	Lean and fat. 3 ounces — 85	40	375	17	34	16	15	1	0	8	2.2	70	.05	.13	3.1	---
83	Lean only. 1.8 ounces — 51	57	125	14	7	3	3	Trace	0	6	1.8	10	.04	.11	2.6	---
	Relatively lean, such as heel of round:															
84	Lean and fat. 3 ounces — 85	62	165	25	7	3	3	Trace	0	11	3.2	10	.06	.19	4.5	---
85	Lean only. 2.7 ounces — 78	65	125	24	3	1	1	Trace	0	10	3.0	Trace	.06	.18	4.3	---
	Steak, broiled:															
	Relatively fat, such as sirloin:															
86	Lean and fat. 3 ounces — 85	44	330	20	27	13	12	1	0	9	2.5	50	.05	.16	4.0	---
87	Lean only. 2.0 ounces — 56	59	115	18	4	2	2	Trace	0	7	2.2	10	.05	.14	3.6	---
	Relatively lean, such as round:															
88	Lean and fat. 3 ounces — 85	55	220	24	13	6	6	Trace	0	10	3.0	20	.07	.19	4.8	---
89	Lean only. 2.4 ounces — 68	61	130	21	4	2	2	Trace	0	9	2.5	10	.06	.16	4.1	---
	Beef, canned:															
90	Corned beef. 3 ounces — 85	59	185	22	10	5	4	Trace	0	17	3.7	20	.01	.20	2.9	---
91	Corned beef hash. 3 ounces — 85	67	155	7	10	5	4	Trace	9	11	1.7	---	.01	.08	1.8	---
92	Beef, dried or chipped. 2 ounces — 57	48	115	19	4	2	2	Trace	0	11	2.9	---	.04	.18	2.2	---
93	Beef and vegetable stew. 1 cup — 235	82	210	15	10	5	4	Trace	15	28	2.8	2,310	.13	.17	4.4	15

[2] Contributed largely from beta-carotene used for coloring.

[3] Outer layer of fat on the cut was removed to within approximately ½-inch of the lean. Deposits of fat within the cut were not removed.

Table of Food Composition (continued)

[Dashes in the columns for nutrients show that no suitable value could be found although there is reason to believe that a measurable amount of the nutrient may be present]

	Food, approximate measure, and weight (in grams)		Water	Food energy	Protein	Fat	Fatty acids			Carbo-hy-drate	Cal-cium	Iron	Vita-min A value	Thia-min	Ribo-flavin	Niacin	Ascor-bic acid
							Satu-rated (total)	Unsaturated									
								Oleic	Lin-oleic								
		Grams	Per-cent	Calo-ries	Grams	Grams	Grams	Grams	Grams	Grams	Milli-grams	Milli-grams	Inter-national units	Milli-grams	Milli-grams	Milli-grams	Milli-grams
	MEAT, POULTRY, FISH, SHELLFISH; RELATED PRODUCTS—Continued																
94	Beef potpie, baked, 4¼-inch diam., weight before baking about 8 ounces. — 1 pie	227	55	560	23	33	9	20	2	43	32	4.1	1,860	0.25	0.27	4.5	7
	Chicken, cooked:																
95	Flesh only, broiled — 3 ounces	85	71	115	20	3	1	1	1	0	8	1.4	80	.05	.16	7.4	---
	Breast, fried, ½ breast:																
96	With bone — 3.3 ounces	94	58	155	25	5	1	2	1	1	9	1.3	70	.04	.17	11.2	---
97	Flesh and skin only — 2.7 ounces	76	58	155	25	5	1	2	1	1	9	1.3	70	.04	.17	11.2	---
	Drumstick, fried:																
98	With bone — 2.1 ounces	59	55	90	12	4	1	2	1	Trace	6	.9	50	.03	.15	2.7	---
99	Flesh and skin only — 1.3 ounces	38	55	90	12	4	1	2	1	Trace	6	.9	50	.03	.15	2.7	---
100	Chicken, canned, boneless — 3 ounces	85	65	170	18	10	3	4	2	0	18	1.3	200	.03	.11	3.7	3
101	Chicken potpie, baked 4¼-inch diam., weight before baking about 8 ounces. — 1 pie	227	57	535	23	31	10	15	3	42	68	3.0	3,020	.25	.26	4.1	5
	Chili con carne, canned:																
102	With beans — 1 cup	250	72	335	19	15	7	7	Trace	30	80	4.2	150	.08	.18	3.2	---
103	Without beans — 1 cup	255	67	510	26	38	18	17	1	15	97	3.6	380	.05	.31	5.6	---
104	Heart, beef, lean, braised — 3 ounces	85	61	160	27	5	---	---	---	1	5	5.0	20	.21	1.04	6.5	1
	Lamb,[3] cooked:																
	Chop, thick, with bone, broiled:																
105	— 1 chop, 4.8 ounces.	137	47	400	25	33	18	12	1	0	10	1.5	---	.14	.25	5.6	---
106	Lean and fat — 4.0 ounces	112	47	400	25	33	18	12	1	0	10	1.5	---	.14	.25	5.6	---
107	Lean only — 2.6 ounces	74	62	140	21	6	3	2	Trace	0	9	1.5	---	.11	.20	4.5	---
	Leg, roasted:																
108	Lean and fat — 3 ounces	85	54	235	22	16	9	6	Trace	0	9	1.4	---	.13	.23	4.7	---
109	Lean only — 2.5 ounces	71	62	130	20	5	3	2	Trace	0	9	1.4	---	.12	.21	4.4	---
	Shoulder, roasted:																
110	Lean and fat — 3 ounces	85	50	285	18	23	13	8	1	0	9	1.0	---	.11	.20	4.0	---
111	Lean only — 2.3 ounces	64	61	130	17	6	3	2	Trace	0	8	1.0	---	.10	.18	3.7	---

No.	Food, approximate measure	Measure	Grams	Water (pct.)	Food energy (Cal.)	Protein (g)	Fat (g)	Saturated (g)	Oleic (g)	Linoleic (g)	Carbohydrate (g)	Calcium (mg)	Iron (mg)	Vitamin A (I.U.)	Thiamine (mg)	Riboflavin (mg)	Niacin (mg)	Ascorbic acid (mg)
112	Liver, beef, fried	2 ounces	57	57	130	15	6	------	------	------	3	6	5.0	30,280	.15	2.37	9.4	15
113	Pork, cured, cooked: Ham, light cure, lean and fat, roasted.	3 ounces	85	54	245	18	19	7	8	2	0	8	2.2	0	.40	.16	3.1	------
114	Luncheon meat: Boiled ham, sliced	2 ounces	57	59	135	11	10	4	4	1	0	6	1.6	0	.25	.09	1.5	------
115	Canned, spiced or unspiced.	2 ounces	57	55	165	8	14	5	6	1	1	5	1.2	0	.18	.12	1.6	------
116	Pork, fresh,[3] cooked: Chop, thick, with bone.	1 chop, 3.5 ounces.	98	42	260	16	21	8	9	2	0	8	2.2	0	.63	.18	3.8	------
117	Lean and fat	2.3 ounces	66	42	260	16	21	8	9	2	0	8	2.2	0	.63	.18	3.8	------
118	Lean only	1.7 ounces	48	53	130	15	7	2	3	1	0	7	1.9	0	.54	.16	3.3	------
119	Roast, oven-cooked, no liquid added: Lean and fat	3 ounces	85	46	310	21	24	9	10	2	0	9	2.7	0	.78	.22	4.7	------
120	Lean only	2.4 ounces	68	55	175	20	10	3	4	1	0	9	2.6	0	.73	.21	4.4	------
121	Cuts, simmered: Lean and fat	3 ounces	85	46	320	20	26	9	11	2	0	8	2.5	0	.46	.21	4.1	------
122	Lean only	2.2 ounces	63	60	135	18	6	2	3	1	0	8	2.3	0	.42	.19	3.7	------
123	Sausage: Bologna, slice, 3-in. diam. by ⅛ inch.	2 slices	26	56	80	3	7	------	------	------	Trace	2	.5	------	.04	.06	.7	------
124	Braunschweiger, slice 2-in. diam. by ¼ inch.	2 slices	20	53	65	3	5	------	------	------	Trace	2	1.2	1,310	.03	.29	1.6	------
125	Deviled ham, canned	1 tbsp.	13	51	45	2	4	2	2	Trace	0	1	.3	------	.02	.01	.2	------
126	Frankfurter, heated (8 per lb. purchased pkg.).	1 frank	56	57	170	7	15	------	------	------	1	3	.8	------	.08	.11	1.4	------
127	Pork links, cooked (16 links per lb. raw).	2 links	26	35	125	5	11	4	5	1	Trace	2	.6	0	.21	.09	1.0	------
128	Salami, dry type	1 oz.	28	30	130	7	11	------	------	------	Trace	4	1.0	------	.10	.07	1.5	------
129	Salami, cooked	1 oz.	28	51	90	5	7	------	------	------	Trace	3	.7	------	.07	.07	1.2	------
130	Vienna, canned (7 sausages per 5-oz. can).	1 sausage	16	63	40	2	3	------	------	------	Trace	1	.3	------	.01	.02	.4	------
131	Veal, medium fat, cooked, bone removed: Cutlet.	3 oz.	85	60	185	23	9	5	4	Trace	------	9	2.7	------	.06	.21	4.6	------
132	Roast	3 oz.	85	55	230	23	14	7	6	Trace	0	10	2.9	0	.11	.26	6.6	------
133	Fish and shellfish: Bluefish, baked with table fat.	3 oz.	85	68	135	22	4	------	------	------	0	25	.6	40	.09	.08	1.6	------
134	Clams: Raw, meat only	3 oz.	85	82	65	11	1	------	------	------	2	59	5.2	90	.08	.15	1.1	8
135	Canned, solids and liquid.	3 oz.	85	86	45	7	1	------	------	------	2	47	3.5	------	.01	.09	.9	------
136	Crabmeat, canned	3 oz.	85	77	85	15	2	------	------	------	1	38	.7	------	.07	.07	1.6	------

[3] Outer layer of fat on the cut was removed to within approximately ½-inch of the lean. Deposits of fat within the cut were not removed.

Table of Food Composition (continued)

[Dashes in the columns for nutrients show that no suitable value could be found although there is reason to believe that a measurable amount of the nutrient may be present]

	Food, approximate measure, and weight (in grams)		Water	Food energy	Protein	Fat	Fatty acids			Carbohydrate	Calcium	Iron	Vitamin A value	Thiamin	Riboflavin	Niacin	Ascorbic acid
							Saturated (total)	Unsaturated Oleic	Unsaturated Linoleic								
		Grams	Percent	Calories	Grams	Grams	Grams	Grams	Grams	Grams	Milligrams	Milligrams	International units	Milligrams	Milligrams	Milligrams	Milligrams
	MEAT, POULTRY, FISH, SHELLFISH; RELATED PRODUCTS—Continued																
	Fish and shellfish—Continued																
137	Fish sticks, breaded, cooked, frozen; stick 3¾ by 1 by ½ inch. 10 sticks or 8 oz. pkg.	227	66	400	38	20	5	4	10	15	25	0.9	---	0.09	0.16	3.6	---
138	Haddock, breaded, fried 3 oz.	85	66	140	17	5	1	3	Trace	5	34	1.0	---	.03	.06	2.7	---
139	Ocean perch, breaded, fried. 3 oz.	85	59	195	16	11	---	---	---	6	28	1.1	---	.08	.09	1.5	2
140	Oysters, raw, meat only (13–19 med. selects). 1 cup	240	85	160	20	4	---	---	---	8	226	13.2	740	.33	.43	6.0	---
141	Salmon, pink, canned 3 oz.	85	71	120	17	5	1	1	Trace	0	4167	.7	60	.03	.16	6.8	---
142	Sardines, Atlantic, canned in oil, drained solids. 3 oz.	85	62	175	20	9	---	---	---	0	372	2.5	190	.02	.17	4.6	---
143	Shad, baked with table fat and bacon. 3 oz.	85	64	170	20	10	---	---	---	0	20	.5	20	.11	.22	7.3	---
144	Shrimp, canned, meat. 3 oz.	85	70	100	21	1	---	---	---	1	98	2.6	50	.01	.03	1.5	---
145	Swordfish, broiled with butter or margarine. 3 oz.	85	65	150	24	5	---	---	---	0	23	1.1	1,750	.03	.04	9.3	---
146	Tuna, canned in oil, drained solids. 3 oz.	85	61	170	24	7	2	1	1	0	7	1.6	70	.04	.10	10.1	---
	MATURE DRY BEANS AND PEAS, NUTS, PEANUTS; RELATED PRODUCTS																
147	Almonds, shelled, whole kernels. 1 cup	142	5	850	26	77	6	52	15	28	332	6.7	0	.34	1.31	5.0	Trace
	Beans, dry: Common varieties as Great Northern, navy, and others: Cooked, drained:																
148	Great Northern. 1 cup	180	69	210	14	1	---	---	---	38	90	4.9	0	.25	.13	1.3	0

No.	Food and approximate measure	Grams	Water (%)	Food energy (cal.)	Protein (g)	Fat (g)	Saturated (g)	Oleic (g)	Linoleic (g)	Carbohydrate (g)	Calcium (mg)	Iron (mg)	Vitamin A (I.U.)	Thiamine (mg)	Riboflavin (mg)	Niacin (mg)	Ascorbic acid (mg)
149	Navy (pea) _____ 1 cup	190	69	225	15	1	—	—	—	40	95	5.1	0	.27	.13	1.3	0
	Canned, solids and liquid: White with—																
150	Frankfurters (sliced). 1 cup	255	71	365	19	18	—	—	—	32	94	4.8	330	.18	.15	3.3	Trace
151	Pork and tomato sauce. 1 cup	255	71	310	16	7	2	3	1	49	138	4.6	330	.20	.08	1.5	5
152	Pork and sweet sauce. 1 cup	255	66	385	16	12	4	5	1	54	161	5.9	10	.15	.10	1.3	—
153	Red kidney _____ 1 cup	255	76	230	15	1	—	—	—	42	74	4.6	—	.13	.10	1.5	—
154	Lima, cooked, drained. 1 cup	190	64	260	16	1	—	—	—	49	55	5.9	—	.25	.11	1.3	—
155	Cashew nuts, roasted 1 cup	140	5	785	24	64	11	45	4	41	53	5.3	140	.60	.35	2.5	—
156	Coconut, fresh, meat only: Pieces, approx. 2 by 2 by ½ inch. 1 piece	45	51	155	2	16	14	1	Trace	4	6	.8	0	.02	.01	.2	1
157	Shredded or grated, firmly packed. 1 cup	130	51	450	5	46	39	3	Trace	12	17	2.2	0	.07	.03	.7	4
158	Cowpeas or blackeye peas, dry, cooked. 1 cup	248	80	190	13	1	—	—	—	34	42	3.2	20	.41	.11	1.1	—
159	Peanuts, roasted, salted, halves. 1 cup	144	2	840	37	72	16	31	21	27	107	3.0	—	.46	.19	24.7	Trace
160	Peanut butter _____ 1 tbsp.	16	2	95	4	8	2	4	2	3	9	.3	—	.02	.02	2.4	0
161	Peas, split, dry, cooked 1 cup	250	70	290	20	1	—	—	—	52	28	4.2	100	.37	.22	2.2	0
162	Pecans, halves _____ 1 cup	108	3	740	10	77	5	48	15	16	79	2.6	140	.93	.14	1.0	2
163	Walnuts, black or native, chopped. 1 cup	126	3	790	26	75	4	26	36	19	Trace	7.6	380	.28	.14	.9	—

VEGETABLES AND VEGETABLE PRODUCTS

No.	Food and approximate measure	Grams	Water (%)	Food energy (cal.)	Protein (g)	Fat (g)	Saturated (g)	Oleic (g)	Linoleic (g)	Carbohydrate (g)	Calcium (mg)	Iron (mg)	Vitamin A (I.U.)	Thiamine (mg)	Riboflavin (mg)	Niacin (mg)	Ascorbic acid (mg)
	Asparagus, green: Cooked, drained:																
164	Spears, ½-in. diam. at base. 4 spears	60	94	10	1	Trace	—	—	—	2	13	.4	540	.10	.11	.8	16
165	Pieces, 1½ to 2-in. lengths. 1 cup	145	94	30	3	Trace	—	—	—	5	30	.9	1,310	.23	.26	2.0	38
166	Canned, solids and liquid. 1 cup	244	94	45	5	1	—	—	—	7	44	4.1	1,240	.15	.22	2.0	37
	Beans:																
167	Lima, immature seeds, cooked, drained. 1 cup	170	71	190	13	1	—	—	—	34	80	4.3	480	.31	.17	2.2	29
	Snap: Green:																
168	Cooked, drained __ 1 cup	125	92	30	2	Trace	—	—	—	7	63	.8	680	.09	.11	.6	15
169	Canned, solids and liquid. 1 cup	239	94	45	2	Trace	—	—	—	10	81	2.9	690	.07	.10	.7	10

[4] If bones are discarded, value will be greatly reduced.

Table of Food Composition (continued)

[Dashes in the columns for nutrients show that no suitable value could be found although there is reason to believe that a measurable amount of the nutrient may be present]

	Food, approximate measure, and weight (in grams)		Water	Food energy	Protein	Fat	Fatty acids Saturated (total)	Unsaturated Oleic	Unsaturated Linoleic	Carbohydrate	Calcium	Iron	Vitamin A value	Thiamin	Riboflavin	Niacin	Ascorbic acid
		Grams	Percent	Calories	Grams	Grams	Grams	Grams	Grams	Grams	Milligrams	Milligrams	International units	Milligrams	Milligrams	Milligrams	Milligrams
	VEGETABLES AND VEGETABLE PRODUCTS—Continued																
	Beans—Continued																
	Snap—Continued																
	Yellow or wax:																
170	Cooked, drained -- 1 cup	125	93	30	2	Trace	------	------	------	6	63	0.8	290	0.09	0.11	0.6	16
171	Canned, solids and liquid. 1 cup	239	94	45	2	1	------	------	------	10	81	2.9	140	.07	.10	.7	12
172	Sprouted mung beans, cooked, drained. 1 cup	125	91	35	4	Trace	------	------	------	7	21	1.1	30	.11	.13	.9	8
	Beets:																
	Cooked, drained, peeled:																
173	Whole beets, 2-in. diam. 2 beets	100	91	30	1	Trace	------	------	------	7	14	.5	20	.03	.04	.3	6
174	Diced or sliced. 1 cup	170	91	55	2	Trace	------	------	------	12	24	.9	30	.05	.07	.5	10
175	Canned, solids and liquid. 1 cup	246	90	85	2	Trace	------	------	------	19	34	1.5	20	.02	.05	.2	7
176	Beet greens, leaves and stems, cooked, drained. 1 cup	145	94	25	3	Trace	------	------	------	5	144	2.8	7,400	.10	.22	.4	22
	Blackeye peas. See Cowpeas.																
	Broccoli, cooked, drained:																
177	Whole stalks, medium size. 1 stalk	180	91	45	6	1	------	------	------	8	158	1.4	4,500	.16	.36	1.4	162
178	Stalks cut into ½-in. pieces. 1 cup	155	91	40	5	1	------	------	------	7	136	1.2	3,880	.14	.31	1.2	140
179	Chopped, yield from 10-oz. frozen pkg. 1⅜ cups	250	92	65	7	1	------	------	------	12	135	1.8	6,500	.15	.30	1.3	143
180	Brussels sprouts, 7-8 sprouts (1¼ to 1½ in. diam.) per cup, cooked. 1 cup	155	88	55	7	1	------	------	------	10	50	1.7	810	.12	.22	1.2	135
	Cabbage:																
	Common varieties:																

No.	Food	Measure	Weight (g)	Water (%)	Food energy (cal.)	Protein (g)	Fat (g)	Saturated fatty acids	Oleic	Linoleic	Carbohydrate (g)	Calcium (mg)	Iron (mg)	Vitamin A (I.U.)	Thiamine (mg)	Riboflavin (mg)	Niacin (mg)	Ascorbic acid (mg)
	Raw:																	
181	Coarsely shredded or sliced.	1 cup	70	92	15	1	Trace	---	---	---	4	34	.3	90	.04	.04	.2	33
182	Finely shredded or chopped.	1 cup	90	92	20	1	Trace	---	---	---	5	44	.4	120	.05	.05	.3	42
183	Cooked	1 cup	145	94	30	2	Trace	---	---	---	6	64	.4	190	.06	.06	.4	48
184	Red, raw, coarsely shredded.	1 cup	70	90	20	1	Trace	---	---	---	5	29	.6	30	.06	.04	.3	43
185	Savoy, raw, coarsely shredded.	1 cup	70	92	15	2	Trace	---	---	---	3	47	.6	140	.04	.06	.2	39
186	Cabbage, celery or Chinese, raw, cut in 1-in. pieces.	1 cup	75	95	10	1	Trace	---	---	---	2	32	.5	110	.04	.03	.5	19
187	Cabbage, spoon (or pakchoy), cooked.	1 cup	170	95	25	2	Trace	---	---	---	4	252	1.0	5,270	.07	.14	1.2	26
	Carrots: Raw:																	
188	Whole, 5½ by 1 inch (25 thin strips).	1 carrot	50	88	20	1	Trace	---	---	---	5	18	.4	5,500	.03	.03	.3	4
189	Grated	1 cup	110	88	45	1	Trace	---	---	---	11	41	.8	12,100	.06	.06	.7	9
190	Cooked, diced	1 cup	145	91	45	1	Trace	---	---	---	10	48	.9	15,220	.08	.07	.7	9
191	Canned, strained or chopped (baby food).	1 ounce	28	92	10	Trace	Trace	---	---	---	2	7	.1	3,690	.01	.01	.1	1
192	Cauliflower, cooked, flowerbuds.	1 cup	120	93	25	3	Trace	---	---	---	5	25	.8	70	.11	.10	.7	66
	Celery, raw:																	
193	Stalk, large outer, 8 by about 1½ inches, at root end.	1 stalk	40	94	5	Trace	Trace	---	---	---	2	16	.1	100	.01	.01	.1	4
194	Pieces, diced	1 cup	100	94	15	1	Trace	---	---	---	4	39	.3	240	.03	.03	.3	9
195	Collards, cooked	1 cup	190	91	55	5	1	---	---	---	9	289	1.1	10,260	.27	.37	2.4	87
	Corn, sweet:																	
196	Cooked, ear 5 by 1¾ inches.[5]	1 ear	140	74	70	3	1	---	---	---	16	2	.5	[6]310	.09	.08	1.0	7
197	Canned, solids and liquid.	1 cup	256	81	170	5	2	---	---	---	40	10	1.0	[6]690	.07	.12	2.3	13
198	Cowpeas, cooked, immature seeds.	1 cup	160	72	175	13	1	---	---	---	29	38	3.4	560	.49	.18	2.3	28
	Cucumbers, 10-ounce; 7½ by about 2 inches:																	
199	Raw, pared	1 cucumber	207	96	30	1	Trace	---	---	---	7	35	.6	Trace	.07	.09	.4	23
200	Raw, pared, center slice ⅛-inch thick.	6 slices	50	96	5	Trace	Trace	---	---	---	2	8	.2	Trace	.02	.02	.1	6
201	Dandelion greens, cooked.	1 cup	180	90	60	4	1	---	---	---	12	252	3.2	21,060	.24	.29		32

[5] Measure and weight apply to entire vegetable or fruit including parts not usually eaten.

[6] Based on yellow varieties; white varieties contain only a trace of cryptoxanthin and carotenes, the pigments in corn that have biological activity.

Table of Food Composition (continued)

[Dashes in the columns for nutrients show that no suitable value could be found although there is reason to believe that a measurable amount of the nutrient may be present]

	Food, approximate measure, and weight (in grams)	Weight	Water	Food energy	Protein	Fat	Fatty acids — Saturated (total)	Fatty acids — Unsaturated Oleic	Fatty acids — Unsaturated Linoleic	Carbohydrate	Calcium	Iron	Vitamin A value	Thiamin	Riboflavin	Niacin	Ascorbic acid
		Grams	Percent	Calories	Grams	Grams	Grams	Grams	Grams	Grams	Milligrams	Milligrams	International units	Milligrams	Milligrams	Milligrams	Milligrams
	VEGETABLES AND VEGETABLE PRODUCTS—Continued																
202	Endive, curly (including escarole). 2 ounces	57	93	10	1	Trace	---	---	---	2	46	1.0	1,870	0.04	0.08	0.3	6
203	Kale, leaves including stems, cooked. 1 cup	110	91	30	4	1	---	---	---	4	147	1.3	8,140	---	---	---	68
	Lettuce, raw:																
204	Butterhead, as Boston types; head, 4-inch diameter. 1 head	220	95	30	3	Trace	---	---	---	6	77	4.4	2,130	.14	.13	.6	18
205	Crisphead, as Iceberg; head, 4¾-inch diameter. 1 head	454	96	60	4	Trace	---	---	---	13	91	2.3	1,500	.29	.27	1.3	29
206	Looseleaf, or bunching varieties, leaves. 2 large	50	94	10	1	Trace	---	---	---	2	34	.7	950	.03	.04	.2	9
207	Mushrooms, canned, solids and liquid. 1 cup	244	93	40	5	Trace	---	---	---	6	15	1.2	Trace	.04	.60	4.8	4
208	Mustard greens, cooked. 1 cup	140	93	35	3	1	---	---	---	6	193	2.5	8,120	.11	.19	.9	68
209	Okra, cooked, pod 3 by ⅝ inch. 8 pods	85	91	25	2	Trace	---	---	---	5	78	.4	420	.11	.15	.8	17
	Onions:																
	Mature:																
210	Raw, onion 2½-inch diameter. 1 onion	110	89	40	2	Trace	---	---	---	10	30	.6	40	.04	.04	.2	11
211	Cooked. 1 cup	210	92	60	3	Trace	---	---	---	14	50	.8	80	.06	.06	.4	14
212	Young green, small, without tops. 6 onions	50	88	20	1	Trace	---	---	---	5	20	.3	Trace	.02	.02	.2	12
213	Parsley, raw, chopped. 1 tablespoon	4	85	Trace	Trace	Trace	---	---	---	Trace	8	.2	340	Trace	.01	Trace	7
214	Parsnips, cooked. 1 cup	155	82	100	2	1	---	---	---	23	70	.9	50	.11	.12	.2	16
	Peas, green:																
215	Cooked. 1 cup	160	82	115	9	1	---	---	---	19	37	2.9	860	.44	.17	3.7	33
216	Canned, solids and liquid. 1 cup	249	83	165	9	1	---	---	---	31	50	4.2	1,120	.23	.13	2.2	22

No.	Food, approximate measure, and weight	Measure	Grams	Water (%)	Food energy (cal)	Protein (g)	Fat (g)	Saturated (g)	Unsat. oleic (g)	Unsat. linoleic (g)	Carbohydrate (g)	Calcium (mg)	Iron (mg)	Vitamin A (IU)	Thiamine (mg)	Riboflavin (mg)	Niacin (mg)	Ascorbic acid (mg)
217	Canned, strained (baby food)	1 ounce	28	86	15	1	Trace				3	3	.4	140	.02	.02	.4	3
218	Peppers, hot, red, without seeds, dried (ground chili powder, added seasonings).	1 tablespoon	15	8	50	2	2				8	40	2.3	9,750	.03	.17	2.3	2
	Peppers, sweet: Raw, about 5 per pound:																	
219	Green pod without stem and seeds.	1 pod	74	93	15	1	Trace				4	7	.5	310	.06	.06	.4	94
220	Cooked, boiled, drained	1 pod	73	95	15	1	Trace				3	7	.4	310	.05	.05	.4	70
	Potatoes, medium (about 3 per pound raw):																	
221	Baked, peeled after baking.	1 potato	99	75	90	3	Trace				21	9	.7	Trace	.10	.04	1.7	20
	Boiled:																	
222	Peeled after boiling	1 potato	136	80	105	3	Trace				23	10	.8	Trace	.13	.05	2.0	22
223	Peeled before boiling	1 potato	122	83	80	2	Trace				18	7	.6	Trace	.11	.04	1.4	20
	French-fried, piece 2 by ½ by ½ inch:																	
224	Cooked in deep fat	10 pieces	57	45	155	2	7	2	2	4	20	9	.7	Trace	.07	.04	1.8	12
225	Frozen, heated	10 pieces	57	53	125	2	5	1	1	2	19	5	1.0	Trace	.08	.01	1.5	12
	Mashed:																	
226	Milk added	1 cup	195	83	125	4	1				25	47	.8	50	.16	.10	2.0	19
227	Milk and butter added.	1 cup	195	80	185	4	8	4	3	Trace	24	47	.8	330	.16	.10	1.9	18
228	Potato chips, medium, 2-inch diameter.	10 chips	20	2	115	1	8	2	2	4	10	8	.4	Trace	.04	.01	1.0	3
229	Pumpkin, canned	1 cup	228	90	75	2	1				18	57	.9	14,590	.07	.12	1.3	12
230	Radishes, raw, small, without tops.	4 radishes	40	94	5	Trace	Trace				1	12	.4	Trace	.01	.01	.1	10
231	Sauerkraut, canned, solids and liquid.	1 cup	235	93	45	2	Trace				9	85	1.2	120	.07	.09	.4	33
	Spinach:																	
232	Cooked	1 cup	180	92	40	5	1				6	167	4.0	14,580	.13	.25	1.0	50
233	Canned, drained solids.	1 cup	180	91	45	5	1				6	212	4.7	14,400	.03	.21	.6	24
	Squash: Cooked:																	
234	Summer, diced	1 cup	210	96	30	2	Trace				7	52	.8	820	.10	.16	1.6	21
235	Winter, baked, mashed.	1 cup	205	81	130	4	1				32	57	1.6	8,610	.10	.27	1.4	27
	Sweetpotatoes: Cooked, medium, 5 by 2 inches, weight raw about 6 ounces:																	
236	Baked, peeled after baking.	1 sweet- potato	110	64	155	2	1				36	44	1.0	8,910	.10	.07	.7	24
237	Boiled, peeled after boiling.	1 sweet- potato	147	71	170	2	1				39	47	1.0	11,610	.13	.09	.9	25

Table of Food Composition (continued)

[Dashes in the columns for nutrients show that no suitable value could be found although there is reason to believe that a measurable amount of the nutrient may be present]

	Food, approximate measure, and weight (in grams)	Water	Food energy	Pro-tein	Fat	Fatty acids Satu-rated (total)	Unsaturated Oleic	Unsaturated Lin-oleic	Carbo-hy-drate	Cal-cium	Iron	Vita-min A value	Thia-min	Ribo-flavin	Niacin	Ascor-bic acid
		Per-cent	Calo-ries	Grams	Grams	Grams	Grams	Grams	Grams	Milli-grams	Milli-grams	Inter-national units	Milli-grams	Milli-grams	Milli-grams	Milli-grams
	VEGETABLES AND VEGETABLE PRODUCTS—Continued															
	Sweetpotatoes—Continued															
238	Candied, 3½ by 2¼ inches. 1 sweetpotato.	60	295	2	6	2	3	1	60	65	1.6	11,030	0.10	0.08	0.8	17
239	Canned, vacuum or solid pack. 1 cup	72	235	4	Trace				54	54	1.7	17,000	.10	.10	1.4	30
	Tomatoes:															
240	Raw, approx. 3-in. diam. 2⅛ in. high; wt. 7 oz. 1 tomato	94	40	2	Trace				9	24	.9	1,640	.11	.07	1.3	[7] 42
241	Canned, solids and liquid. 1 cup	94	50	2	1				10	14	1.2	2,170	.12	.07	1.7	41
	Tomato catsup:															
242	Cup	69	290	6	1				69	60	2.2	3,820	.25	.19	4.4	41
243	Tablespoon	69	15	Trace	Trace				4	3	.1	210	.01	.01	.2	2
	Tomato juice, canned:															
244	Cup	94	45	2	Trace				10	17	2.2	1,940	.12	.07	1.9	39
245	Glass (6 fl. oz.)	94	35	2	Trace				8	13	1.6	1,460	.09	.05	1.5	29
246	Turnips, cooked, diced. 1 cup	94	35	1	Trace				8	54	.6	Trace	.06	.08	.5	34
247	Turnip greens, cooked. 1 cup	94	30	3	Trace				5	252	1.5	8,270	.15	.33	.7	68
	FRUITS AND FRUIT PRODUCTS															
248	Apples, raw (about 3 per lb.).[5] 1 apple	85	70	Trace	Trace				18	8	.4	50	.04	.02	.1	3
249	Apple juice, bottled or canned. 1 cup	88	120	Trace	Trace				30	15	1.5	--------	.02	.05	.2	2
	Applesauce, canned:															
250	Sweetened. 1 cup	76	230	1	Trace				61	10	1.3	100	.05	.03	.1	[8] 3
251	Unsweetened or artificially sweetened. 1 cup	88	100	1	Trace				26	10	1.2	100	.05	.02	.1	[8] 2

No.	Food, approximate measure	Grams	Water (%)	Food energy (cal.)	Protein (g)	Fat (g)	Saturated (g)	Oleic (g)	Linoleic (g)	Carbohydrate (g)	Calcium (mg)	Iron (mg)	Vitamin A (I.U.)	Thiamin (mg)	Riboflavin (mg)	Niacin (mg)	Ascorbic acid (mg)
	Apricots:																
252	Raw (about 12 per lb.)[5] 3 apricots	114	85	55	1	Trace	---	---	---	14	18	.5	2,890	.03	.04	.7	10
253	Canned in heavy sirup 1 cup	259	77	220	2	Trace	---	---	---	57	28	.8	4,510	.05	.06	.9	10
254	Dried, uncooked (40 halves per cup) 1 cup	150	25	390	8	1	---	---	---	100	100	8.2	16,350	.02	.23	4.9	19
255	Cooked, unsweetened, fruit and liquid 1 cup	285	76	240	5	1	---	---	---	62	63	5.1	8,550	.01	.13	2.8	8
256	Apricot nectar, canned 1 cup	251	85	140	1	Trace	---	---	---	37	23	.5	2,380	.03	.03	.5	8[8]
	Avocados, whole fruit, raw:[5]																
257	California (mid- and late-winter; diam. 3⅛ in.) 1 avocado	284	74	370	5	37	7	17	5	13	22	1.3	630	.24	.43	3.5	30
258	Florida (late summer, fall; diam. 3⅝ in.) 1 avocado	454	78	390	4	33	7	15	4	27	30	1.8	880	.33	.61	4.9	43
259	Bananas, raw, medium size[5] 1 banana	175	76	100	1	Trace	---	---	---	26	10	.8	230	.06	.07	.8	12
260	Banana flakes 1 cup	100	3	340	4	1	---	---	---	89	32	2.8	760	.18	.24	2.8	7
261	Blackberries, raw 1 cup	144	84	85	2	1	---	---	---	19	46	1.3	290	.05	.06	.5	30
262	Blueberries, raw 1 cup	140	83	85	1	1	---	---	---	21	21	1.4	140	.04	.08	.6	20
263	Cantaloupes, raw; medium; 5-inch diameter about 1⅔ pounds[5] ½ melon	385	91	60	1	Trace	---	---	---	14	27	.8	6,540[9]	.08	.06	1.2	63
264	Cherries, canned, red, sour, pitted, water pack 1 cup	244	88	105	2	Trace	---	---	---	26	37	.7	1,660	.07	.05	.5	12
265	Cranberry juice cocktail, canned 1 cup	250	83	165	Trace	Trace	---	---	---	42	13	.8	Trace	.03	.03	.1	40[10]
266	Cranberry sauce, sweetened, canned, strained 1 cup	277	62	405	Trace	Trace	---	---	---	104	17	.6	60	.03	.03	.1	6
267	Dates, pitted, cut 1 cup	178	22	490	4	1	---	---	---	130	105	5.3	90	.16	.17	3.9	0
268	Figs, dried, large, 2 by 1 in. 1 fig	21	23	60	1	Trace	---	---	---	15	26	.6	20	.02	.02	.1	0
269	Fruit cocktail, canned, in heavy sirup 1 cup	256	80	195	1	Trace	---	---	---	50	23	1.0	360	.05	.03	1.3	5

[5] Measure and weight apply to entire vegetable or fruit including parts not usually eaten.

[7] Year-round average. Samples marketed from November through May, average 20 milligrams per 200-gram tomato; from June through October, around 52 milligrams.

[8] This is the amount from the fruit. Additional ascorbic acid may be added by the manufacturer. Refer to the label for this information.

[9] Value for varieties with orange-colored flesh; value for varieties with green flesh would be about 540 I.U.

[10] Value listed is based on products with label stating 30 milligrams per 6 fl. oz. serving.

Table of Food Composition (continued)

[Dashes in the columns for nutrients show that no suitable value could be found although there is reason to believe that a measurable amount of the nutrient may be present]

	Food, approximate measure, and weight (in grams)	Water	Food energy	Protein	Fat	Fatty acids Saturated (total)	Fatty acids Unsaturated Oleic	Fatty acids Unsaturated Linoleic	Carbohydrate	Calcium	Iron	Vitamin A value	Thiamin	Riboflavin	Niacin	Ascorbic acid
		Percent	Calories	Grams	Grams	Grams	Grams	Grams	Grams	Milligrams	Milligrams	International units	Milligrams	Milligrams	Milligrams	Milligrams
	FRUITS AND FRUIT PRODUCTS—Con.															
	Grapefruit:															
	Raw, medium, 3¾-in. diam.[5]															
270	White ½ grapefruit.	89	45	1	Trace				12	19	0.5	10	0.05	0.02	0.2	44
271	Pink or red ½ grapefruit.	89	50	1	Trace				13	20	0.5	540	0.05	0.02	0.2	44
272	Canned, sirup pack 1 cup	81	180	2	Trace				45	33	.8	30	.08	.05	.5	76
	Grapefruit juice:															
273	Fresh 1 cup	90	95	1	Trace				23	22	.5	[11]	.09	.04	.4	92
	Canned, white:															
274	Unsweetened 1 cup	89	100	1	Trace				24	20	1.0	20	.07	.04	.4	84
275	Sweetened 1 cup	86	130	1	Trace				32	20	1.0	20	.07	.04	.4	78
	Frozen, concentrate, unsweetened:															
276	Undiluted, can, 6 fluid ounces. 1 can	62	300	4	1				72	70	.8	60	.29	.12	1.4	286
277	Diluted with 3 parts water, by volume. 1 cup	89	100	1	Trace				24	25	.2	20	.10	.04	.5	96
278	Dehydrated crystals 4 oz.	1	410	6	1				102	100	1.2	80	.40	.20	2.0	396
279	Prepared with water 1 cup (1 pound yields about 1 gallon).	90	100	1	Trace				24	22	.2	20	.10	.05	.5	91
	Grapes, raw:[5]															
280	American type (slip skin). 1 cup	82	65	1	1				15	15	.4	100	.05	.03	.2	3
281	European type (adherent skin). 1 cup	81	95	1	Trace				25	17	.6	140	.07	.04	.4	6
	Grapejuice:															
282	Canned or bottled 1 cup	83	165	1	Trace				42	28	.8		.10	.05	.5	Trace
	Frozen concentrate, sweetened:															
283	Undiluted, can, 6 fluid ounces. 1 can	53	395	1	Trace				100	22	.9	40	.13	.22	1.5	[12]

No.	Food, approximate measure, and weight	Measure	Weight (g)	Water (%)	Food energy (cal)	Protein (g)	Fat (g)	Saturated fatty acids	Oleic	Linoleic	Carbohydrate (g)	Calcium (mg)	Iron (mg)	Vitamin A (I.U.)	Thiamine (mg)	Riboflavin (mg)	Niacin (mg)	Ascorbic acid (mg)
284	Diluted with 3 parts water, by volume.	1 cup	250	86	135	1	Trace	---	---	---	33	8	.3	10	.05	.08	.5	(12)
285	Grapejuice drink, canned	1 cup	250	86	135	Trace	Trace	---	---	---	35	8	.3	---	.03	.03	.3	(12)
286	Lemons, raw, 2⅛-in. diam., size 165.⁵ Used for juice.	1 lemon	110	90	20	1	Trace	---	---	---	6	19	.4	10	.03	.01	.1	39
287	Lemon juice, raw	1 cup	244	91	60	1	Trace	---	---	---	20	17	.5	50	.07	.02	.2	112
	Lemonade concentrate:																	
288	Frozen, 6 fl. oz. per can	1 can	219	48	430	Trace	Trace	---	---	---	112	9	.4	40	.04	.07	.7	66
289	Diluted with 4⅓ parts water, by volume.	1 cup	248	88	110	Trace	Trace	---	---	---	28	2	Trace	Trace	Trace	.02	.2	17
	Lime juice:																	
290	Fresh	1 cup	246	90	65	1	Trace	---	---	---	22	22	.5	20	.05	.02	.2	79
291	Canned, unsweetened	1 cup	246	90	65	1	Trace	---	---	---	22	22	.5	20	.05	.02	.2	52
	Limeade concentrate, frozen:																	
292	Undiluted, can, 6 fluid ounces.	1 can	218	50	410	Trace	Trace	---	---	---	108	11	.2	Trace	.02	.02	.2	26
293	Diluted with 4⅓ parts water, by volume.	1 cup	247	90	100	Trace	Trace	---	---	---	27	2	Trace	Trace	Trace	Trace	Trace	5
294	Oranges, raw, 2⅝-in. diam., all commercial varieties.⁵	1 orange	180	86	65	1	Trace	---	---	---	16	54	.5	260	.13	.05	.5	66
295	Orange juice, fresh, all varieties.	1 cup	248	88	110	2	1	---	---	---	26	27	.5	500	.22	.07	1.0	124
296	Canned, unsweetened	1 cup	249	87	120	2	Trace	---	---	---	28	25	1.0	500	.17	.05	.7	100
	Frozen concentrate:																	
297	Undiluted, can, 6 fluid ounces.	1 can	213	55	360	5	Trace	---	---	---	87	75	.9	1,620	.68	.11	2.8	360
298	Diluted with 3 parts water, by volume.	1 cup	249	87	120	2	Trace	---	---	---	29	25	.2	550	.22	.02	1.0	120
299	Dehydrated crystals	4 oz.	113	1	430	6	2	---	---	---	100	95	1.9	1,900	.76	.24	3.3	408
300	Prepared with water (1 pound yields about 1 gallon).	1 cup	248	88	115	2	1	---	---	---	27	25	.5	500	.20	.07	1.0	109
301	Orange-apricot juice drink	1 cup	249	87	125	1	Trace	---	---	---	32	12	.2	1,440	.05	.02	.5	¹⁰40

⁵ Measure and weight apply to entire vegetable or fruit including parts not usually eaten.

¹⁰ Value listed is based on product with label stating 30 milligrams per 6 fl. oz. serving.

¹¹ For white-fleshed varieties value is about 20 I.U. per cup; for red-fleshed varieties, 1,080 I.U. per cup.

¹² Present only if added by the manufacturer. Refer to the label for this information.

Table of Food Composition (continued)

[Dashes in the columns for nutrients show that no suitable value could be found although there is reason to believe that a measurable amount of the nutrient may be present]

	Food, approximate measure, and weight (in grams)		Water	Food energy	Pro-tein	Fat	Fatty acids			Carbo-hy-drate	Cal-cium	Iron	Vita-min A value	Thia-min	Ribo-flavin	Niacin	Ascor-bic acid
							Satu-rated (total)	Unsaturated									
								Oleic	Lin-oleic								
		Grams	Per-cent	Calo-ries	Grams	Grams	Grams	Grams	Grams	Grams	Milli-grams	Milli-grams	Inter-national units	Milli-grams	Milli-grams	Milli-grams	Milli-grams
	FRUITS AND FRUIT PRODUCTS—Con.																
	Orange and grapefruit juice:																
	Frozen concentrate:																
302	Undiluted, can, 6 fluid ounces.	1 can ------ 210	59	330	4	1	---	---	---	78	61	0.8	800	0.48	0.06	2.3	302
303	Diluted with 3 parts water, by volume.	1 cup ------ 248	88	110	1	Trace	---	---	---	26	20	.2	270	.16	.02	.8	102
304	Papayas, raw, ½-inch cubes.	1 cup ------ 182	89	70	1	Trace	---	---	---	18	36	.5	3,190	.07	.08	.5	102
	Peaches:																
	Raw:																
305	Whole, medium, 2-inch diameter, about 4 per pound.[5]	1 peach ---- 114	89	35	1	Trace	---	---	---	10	9	.5	[13]1,320	.02	.05	1.0	7
306	Sliced.	1 cup ------ 168	89	65	1	Trace	---	---	---	16	15	.8	[13]2,230	.03	.08	1.6	12
	Canned, yellow-fleshed, solids and liquid:																
	Sirup pack, heavy:																
307	Halves or slices.	1 cup ------ 257	79	200	1	Trace	---	---	---	52	10	.8	1,100	.02	.06	1.4	7
308	Water pack.	1 cup ------ 245	91	75	1	Trace	---	---	---	20	10	.7	1,100	.02	.06	1.4	7
309	Dried, uncooked.	1 cup ------ 160	25	420	5	1	---	---	---	109	77	9.6	6,240	.02	.31	8.5	28
310	Cooked, unsweet-ened, 10-12 halves and juice.	1 cup ------ 270	77	220	3	1	---	---	---	58	41	5.1	3,290	.01	.15	4.2	6
	Frozen:																
311	Carton, 12 ounces, not thawed.	1 carton ---- 340	76	300	1	Trace	---	---	---	77	14	1.7	2,210	.03	.14	2.4	[14]135
	Pears:																
312	Raw, 3 by 2½-inch diameter.[5]	1 pear ------ 182	83	100	1	1	---	---	---	25	13	.5	30	.04	.07	.2	7
	Canned, solids and liquid:																
	Sirup pack, heavy:																
313	Halves or slices.	1 cup ------ 255	80	195	1	1	---	---	---	50	13	.5	Trace	.03	.05	.3	4

No.	Food, approximate measure, and weight		Grams	Water (%)	Food energy (cal.)	Protein (g)	Fat (g)	Carbohydrate (g)	Calcium (mg)	Iron (mg)	Vitamin A (I.U.)	Thiamin (mg)	Riboflavin (mg)	Niacin (mg)	Ascorbic acid (mg)
	Pineapple:														
314	Raw, diced	1 cup	140	85	75	1	Trace	19	24	.7	100	.12	.04	.3	24
	Canned, heavy sirup pack, solids and liquid:														
315	Crushed	1 cup	260	80	195	1	Trace	50	29	.8	120	.20	.06	.5	17
316	Sliced, slices and juice.	2 small or 1 large.	122	80	90	Trace	Trace	24	13	.4	50	.09	.03	.2	8
317	Pineapple juice, canned	1 cup	249	86	135	1	Trace	34	37	.7	120	.12	.04	.5	[8]22
	Plums, all except prunes:														
318	Raw, 2-inch diameter, 1 plum about 2 ounces.[5]	1 plum	60	87	25	Trace	Trace	7	7	.3	140	.02	.02	.3	3
319	Canned, sirup pack (Italian prunes): Plums (with pits) and juice.[5]	1 cup	256	77	205	1	Trace	53	22	2.2	2,970	.05	.05	.9	4
	Prunes, dried, "softenized", medium:														
320	Uncooked[5]	4 prunes	32	28	70	1	Trace	18	14	1.1	440	.02	.04	.4	1
321	Cooked, unsweetened, 17–18 prunes and ⅓ cup liquid.[5]	1 cup	270	66	295	2	1	78	60	4.5	1,860	.08	.18	1.7	2
322	Prune juice, canned or bottled.	1 cup	256	80	200	1	Trace	49	36	10.5	------	.03	.03	1.0	[8]5
	Raisins, seedless:														
323	Packaged, ½ oz. or 1½ tbsp. per pkg.	1 pkg.	14	18	40	Trace	Trace	11	9	.5	Trace	.02	.01	.1	Trace
324	Cup, pressed down	1 cup	165	18	480	4	Trace	128	102	5.8	30	.18	.13	.8	2
	Raspberries, red:														
325	Raw	1 cup	123	84	70	1	1	17	27	1.1	160	.04	.11	1.1	31
326	Frozen, 10-ounce carton, not thawed.	1 carton	284	74	275	2	1	70	37	1.7	200	.06	.17	1.7	59
327	Rhubarb, cooked, sugar added.	1 cup	272	63	385	1	Trace	98	212	1.6	220	.06	.15	.7	17
	Strawberries:														
328	Raw, capped	1 cup	149	90	55	1	1	13	31	1.5	90	.04	.10	1.0	88
329	Frozen, 10-ounce carton, not thawed.	1 carton	284	71	310	1	1	79	40	2.0	90	.06	.17	1.5	150
330	Tangerines, raw, medium, 2⅜-in. diam., size 176.[5]	1 tangerine	116	87	40	1	Trace	10	34	.3	360	.05	.02	.1	27
331	Tangerine juice, canned, sweetened.	1 cup	249	87	125	1	1	30	45	.5	1,050	.15	.05	.2	55
332	Watermelon, raw, wedge, 4 by 8 inches (1⁄16 of 10 by 16-inch melon, about 2 pounds with rind).[5]	1 wedge	925	93	115	2	1	27	30	2.1	2,510	.13	.13	.7	30

[5] Measure and weight apply to entire vegetable or fruit including parts not usually eaten.

[8] This is the amount from the fruit. Additional ascorbic acid may be added by the manufacturer. Refer to the label for this information.

[13] Based on yellow-fleshed varieties; for white-fleshed varieties value is about 50 I.U. per 114-gram peach and 80 I.U. per cup of sliced peaches.

[14] This value includes ascorbic acid added by manufacturer.

Table of Food Composition (continued)

[Dashes in the columns for nutrients show that no suitable value could be found although there is reason to believe that a measurable amount of the nutrient may be present]

	Food, approximate measure, and weight (in grams)		Water	Food energy	Protein	Fat	Fatty acids Saturated (total)	Fatty acids Unsaturated Oleic	Fatty acids Unsaturated Linoleic	Carbohydrate	Calcium	Iron	Vitamin A value	Thiamin	Riboflavin	Niacin	Ascorbic acid
		Grams	Percent	Calories	Grams	Grams	Grams	Grams	Grams	Grams	Milligrams	Milligrams	International units	Milligrams	Milligrams	Milligrams	Milligrams
	GRAIN PRODUCTS																
	Bagel, 3-in. diam.:																
333	Egg, 1 bagel	55	32	165	6	2				28	9	1.2	30	0.14	0.10	1.2	0
334	Water, 1 bagel	55	29	165	6	2				30	8	1.2	0	.15	.11	1.4	0
335	Barley, pearled, light, uncooked, 1 cup	200	11	700	16	2	Trace	1	1	158	32	4.0	0	.24	.10	6.2	0
336	Biscuits, baking powder from home recipe with enriched flour, 2-in. diam., 1 biscuit	28	27	105	2	5	1	2	1	13	34	.4	Trace	.06	.06	.1	Trace
337	Biscuits, baking powder from mix, 2-in. diam., 1 biscuit	28	28	90	2	3	1	1	1	15	19	.6	Trace	.08	.07	.6	Trace
338	Bran flakes (40% bran), added thiamin and iron, 1 cup	35	3	105	4	1				28	25	12.3	0	.14	.06	2.2	0
339	Bran flakes with raisins, added thiamin and iron, 1 cup	50	7	145	4	1				40	28	13.5	Trace	.16	.07	2.7	0
	Breads:																
340	Boston brown bread, slice 3 by ¾ in., 1 slice	48	45	100	3	1				22	43	.9	0	.05	.03	.6	0
	Cracked-wheat bread:																
341	Loaf, 1 lb., 1 loaf	454	35	1,190	40	10	2	5	2	236	399	5.0	Trace	.53	.41	5.9	Trace
342	Slice, 18 slices per loaf, 1 slice	25	35	65	2	1				13	22	.3	Trace	.03	.02	.3	Trace
	French or vienna bread:																
343	Enriched, 1 lb. loaf, 1 loaf	454	31	1,315	41	14	3	8	2	251	195	10.0	Trace	1.27	1.00	11.3	Trace
344	Unenriched, 1 lb. loaf, 1 loaf	454	31	1,315	41	14	3	8	2	251	195	3.2	Trace	.36	.36	3.6	Trace
	Italian bread:																
345	Enriched, 1 lb. loaf, 1 loaf	454	32	1,250	41	4	Trace	1	2	256	77	10.0	0	1.32	.91	11.8	0
346	Unenriched, 1 lb. loaf, 1 loaf	454	32	1,250	41	4	Trace	1	2	256	77	3.2	0	.41	.27	3.6	0
	Raisin bread:																
347	Loaf, 1 lb., 1 loaf	454	35	1,190	30	13	3	8	2	243	322	5.9	Trace	.23	.41	3.2	Trace

Rye bread:

White bread, enriched:[15]

Soft-crumb type:

Firm-crumb type:

Whole-wheat bread, soft-crumb type:

No.	Food and measure	Grams	Water (%)	Food energy (cal.)	Protein (g)	Fat (g)	Saturated fat (g)	Oleic (g)	Linoleic (g)	Carbohydrate (g)	Calcium (mg)	Iron (mg)	Vitamin A (I.U.)	Thiamin (mg)	Riboflavin (mg)	Niacin (mg)	Ascorbic acid (mg)
348	Slice, 18 slices per loaf — 1 slice	25	35	65	2	1	—	—	—	13	18	.3	Trace	.01	.02	.2	Trace
349	American, light (⅓ rye, ⅔ wheat): Loaf, 1 lb. — 1 loaf	454	36	1,100	41	5	—	—	—	236	340	7.3	0	.82	.32	6.4	0
350	Slice, 18 slices per loaf — 1 slice	25	36	60	2	Trace	—	—	—	13	19	.4	0	.05	.02	.4	0
351	Pumpernickel, loaf, 1 lb. — 1 loaf	454	34	1,115	41	5	—	—	—	241	381	10.9	0	1.04	.64	5.4	0
352	Loaf, 1 lb. — 1 loaf	454	36	1,225	39	15	3	8	2	229	381	11.3	Trace	1.13	.95	10.9	Trace
353	Slice, 18 slices per loaf — 1 slice	25	36	70	2	1	—	—	—	13	21	.6	Trace	.06	.05	.6	Trace
354	Slice, toasted — 1 slice	22	25	70	2	1	—	—	—	13	21	.6	Trace	.06	.05	.6	Trace
355	Slice, 22 slices per loaf — 1 slice	20	36	55	2	1	—	—	—	10	17	.5	Trace	.05	.04	.5	Trace
356	Slice, toasted — 1 slice	17	25	55	2	1	—	—	—	10	17	.5	Trace	.05	.04	.5	Trace
357	Loaf, 1½ lbs. — 1 loaf	680	36	1,835	59	22	5	12	3	343	571	17.0	Trace	1.70	1.43	16.3	Trace
358	Slice, 24 slices per loaf — 1 slice	28	36	75	2	1	—	—	—	14	24	.7	Trace	.07	.06	.7	Trace
359	Slice, toasted — 1 slice	24	25	75	2	1	—	—	—	14	24	.7	Trace	.07	.06	.7	Trace
360	Slice, 28 slices per loaf — 1 slice	24	36	65	2	1	—	—	—	12	20	.6	Trace	.06	.05	.6	Trace
361	Slice, toasted — 1 slice	21	25	65	2	1	—	—	—	12	20	.6	Trace	.06	.05	.6	Trace
362	Loaf, 1 lb. — 1 loaf	454	35	1,245	41	17	4	10	2	228	435	11.3	Trace	1.22	.91	10.9	Trace
363	Slice, 20 slices per loaf — 1 slice	23	35	65	2	1	—	—	—	12	22	.6	Trace	.06	.05	.6	Trace
364	Slice, toasted — 1 slice	20	24	65	2	1	—	—	—	12	22	.6	Trace	.06	.05	.6	Trace
365	Loaf, 2 lbs. — 1 loaf	907	35	2,495	82	34	8	20	4	455	871	22.7	Trace	2.45	1.81	21.8	Trace
366	Slice, 34 slices per loaf — 1 slice	27	35	75	2	1	—	—	—	14	26	.7	Trace	.07	.05	.6	Trace
367	Slice, toasted — 1 slice	23	24	75	2	1	—	—	—	14	26	.7	Trace	.07	.05	.6	Trace
368	Loaf, 1 lb. — 1 loaf	454	36	1,095	41	12	2	6	2	224	381	13.6	Trace	1.36	.45	12.7	Trace
369	Slice, 16 slices per loaf — 1 slice	28	36	65	3	1	—	—	—	14	24	.8	Trace	.09	.03	.8	Trace
370	Slice, toasted — 1 slice	24	24	65	3	1	—	—	—	14	24	.8	Trace	.09	.03	.8	Trace

[15] Values for iron, thiamin, riboflavin, and niacin per pound of unenriched white bread would be as follows:

	Iron (Milligrams)	Thiamin (Milligrams)	Riboflavin (Milligrams)	Niacin (Milligrams)
Soft crumb	3.2	.31	.39	5.0
Firm crumb	3.2	.32	.59	4.1

Table of Food Composition (continued)

[Dashes in the columns for nutrients show that no suitable value could be found although there is reason to believe that a measurable amount of the nutrient may be present]

	Food, approximate measure, and weight (in grams)		Water	Food energy	Protein	Fat	Fatty acids Saturated (total)	Unsaturated Oleic	Unsaturated Linoleic	Carbohydrate	Calcium	Iron	Vitamin A value	Thiamin	Riboflavin	Niacin	Ascorbic acid
		Grams	Percent	Calories	Grams	Grams	Grams	Grams	Grams	Grams	Milligrams	Milligrams	International units	Milligrams	Milligrams	Milligrams	Milligrams
	GRAIN PRODUCTS—Continued																
	Bread—Continued																
	Whole-wheat bread, firm-crumb type:																
371	Loaf, 1 lb. 1 loaf	454	36	1,100	48	14	3	6	3	216	449	13.6	Trace	1.18	0.54	12.7	Trace
372	Slice, 18 slices per loaf. 1 slice	25	36	60	3	1				12	25	.8	Trace	.06	.03	.7	Trace
373	Slice, toasted 1 slice	21	24	60	3	1				12	25	.8	Trace	.06	.03	.7	Trace
374	Breadcrumbs, dry, grated. 1 cup	100	6	390	13	5	1	2	1	73	122	3.6	Trace	.22	.30	3.5	Trace
375	Buckwheat flour, light, sifted. 1 cup	98	12	340	6	1				78	11	1.0	0	.08	.04	.4	0
376	Bulgur, canned, seasoned. 1 cup	135	56	245	8	4				44	27	1.9	0	.08	.05	4.1	0
	Cakes made from cake mixes:																
	Angelfood:																
377	Whole cake 1 cake	635	34	1,645	36	1				377	603	1.9	0	.03	.70	.6	0
378	Piece, 1/12 of 10-in. diam. cake. 1 piece	53	34	135	3	Trace				32	50	.2	0	Trace	.06	.1	0
	Cupcakes, small, 2½ in. diam.:																
379	Without icing 1 cupcake	25	26	90	1	3	1	1	1	14	40	.1	40	.01	.03	.1	Trace
380	With chocolate icing. 1 cupcake	36	22	130	2	5	2	2	1	21	47	.3	60	.01	.04	.1	Trace
	Devil's food, 2-layer, with chocolate icing:																
381	Whole cake 1 cake	1,107	24	3,755	49	136	54	58	16	645	653	8.9	1,660	.33	.89	3.3	1
382	Piece, 1/16 of 9-in. diam. cake. 1 piece	69	24	235	3	9	3	4	1	40	41	.6	100	.02	.06	.2	Trace
383	Cupcake, small, 2½ in. diam. 1 cupcake	35	24	120	2	4	1	2	Trace	20	21	.3	50	.01	.03	.1	Trace
	Gingerbread:																
384	Whole cake 1 cake	570	37	1,575	18	39	10	19	9	291	513	9.1	Trace	.17	.51	4.6	2
385	Piece, 1/9 of 8-in. square cake. 1 piece	63	37	175	2	4	1	2	1	32	57	1.0	Trace	.02	.06	.5	Trace
	White, 2-layer, with chocolate icing:																
386	Whole cake 1 cake	1,140	21	4,000	45	122	45	54	17	716	1,129	5.7	680	.23	.91	2.3	2

560

No.	Food, approximate measure, and weight (in grams)		Grams															
387	Piece, 1/16 of 9-in. diam. cake.	1 piece	71	21	250	3	8	3	3	1	45	70	.4	40	.01	.06	.1	Trace
	Cakes made from home recipes: [16]																	
388	Boston cream pie; piece 1/12 of 8-in. diam.	1 piece	69	35	210	4	6	2	3	1	34	46	.3	140	.02	.08	.1	Trace
	Fruitcake, dark, made with enriched flour:																	
389	Loaf, 1-lb.	1 loaf	454	18	1,720	22	69	15	37	13	271	327	11.8	540	.59	.64	3.6	2
390	Slice, 1/30 of 8-in. loaf.	1 slice	15	18	55	1	2	Trace	1	Trace	9	11	.4	20	.02	.02	.1	Trace
	Plain sheet cake:																	
	Without icing:																	
391	Whole cake.	1 cake	777	25	2,830	35	108	30	52	21	434	497	3.1	1,320	.16	.70	1.6	2
392	Piece, 1/9 of 9-in. square cake.	1 piece	86	25	315	4	12	3	6	2	48	55	.3	150	.02	.08	.2	Trace
393	With boiled white icing, piece, 1/9 of 9-in. square cake.	1 piece	114	23	400	4	12	3	6	2	71	56	.3	150	.02	.08	.2	Trace
	Pound:																	
394	Loaf, 8½ by 3½ by 3 in.	1 loaf	514	17	2,430	29	152	34	68	17	242	108	4.1	1,440	.15	.46	1.0	0
395	Slice, 1/2-in. thick.	1 slice	30	17	140	2	9	2	4	1	14	6	.2	80	.01	.03	.1	0
	Sponge:																	
396	Whole cake.	1 cake	790	32	2,345	60	45	14	20	4	427	237	9.5	3,560	.40	1.11	1.6	Trace
397	Piece, 1/12 of 10-in. diam. cake.	1 piece	66	32	195	5	4	1	2	Trace	36	20	.8	300	.03	.09	.1	Trace
	Yellow, 2-layer, without icing:																	
398	Whole cake.	1 cake	870	24	3,160	39	111	31	53	22	506	618	3.5	1,310	.17	.70	1.7	2
399	Piece, 1/16 of 9-in. diam. cake.	1 piece	54	24	200	2	7	2	3	1	32	39	.2	80	.01	.04	.1	Trace
	Yellow, 2-layer, with chocolate icing:																	
400	Whole cake.	1 cake	1,203	21	4,390	51	156	55	69	23	727	818	7.2	1,920	.24	.96	2.4	Trace
401	Piece, 1/16 of 9-in. diam. cake.	1 piece	75	21	275	3	10	3	4	1	45	51	.5	120	.02	.06	.2	Trace
	Cake icings. See Sugars, Sweets.																	
	Cookies:																	
	Brownies with nuts:																	
402	Made from home recipe with enriched flour.	1 brownie	20	10	95	1	6	1	3	1	10	8	.4	40	.04	.02	.1	Trace
403	Made from mix.	1 brownie	20	11	85	1	4	1	2	1	13	9	.4	20	.03	.02	.1	Trace

[16] Unenriched cake flour used unless otherwise specified.

561

Table of Food Composition (continued)

[Dashes in the columns for nutrients show that no suitable value could be found although there is reason to believe that a measurable amount of the nutrient may be present]

	Food, approximate measure, and weight (in grams)	Water	Food energy	Protein	Fat	Fatty acids Saturated (total)	Unsaturated Oleic	Unsaturated Linoleic	Carbohydrate	Calcium	Iron	Vitamin A value	Thiamin	Riboflavin	Niacin	Ascorbic acid
		Grams	Percent	Calories	Grams	Grams	Grams	Grams	Grams	Grams	Milligrams	Milligrams	International units	Milligrams	Milligrams	Milligrams	Milligrams
	GRAIN PRODUCTS—Continued																
	Cookies—Continued																
	Chocolate chip:																
404	Made from home recipe with enriched flour. 1 cookie	10	3	50	1	3	1	1	1	6	4	0.2	10	0.01	0.01	0.1	Trace
405	Commercial 1 cookie	10	3	50	1	2	1	1	Trace	7	4	.2	10	Trace	Trace	Trace	Trace
406	Fig bars, commercial 1 cookie	14	14	50	1	1	1	1		11	11	.2	20	Trace	.01	.1	Trace
407	Sandwich, chocolate or vanilla, commercial. 1 cookie	10	2	50	1	2	1	1	Trace	7	2	.1	0	Trace	Trace	.1	0
	Corn flakes, added nutrients:																
408	Plain 1 cup	25	4	100	2	Trace				21	4	.4	0	.11	.02	.5	0
409	Sugar-covered 1 cup	40	2	155	2	Trace				36	5	.4	0	.16	.02	.8	0
	Corn (hominy) grits, degermed, cooked:																
410	Enriched 1 cup	245	87	125	3	Trace				27	2	.7	[17] 150	.10	.07	1.0	0
411	Unenriched 1 cup	245	87	125	3	Trace				27	2	.2	[17] 150	.05	.02	.5	0
	Cornmeal:																
412	Whole-ground, unbolted, dry. 1 cup	122	12	435	11	5	1	2	2	90	24	2.9	[17] 620	.46	.13	2.4	0
413	Bolted (nearly whole-grain) dry. 1 cup	122	12	440	11	4	Trace	1	2	91	21	2.2	[17] 590	.37	.10	2.3	0
	Degermed, enriched:																
414	Dry form 1 cup	138	12	500	11	2				108	8	4.0	[17] 610	.61	.36	4.8	0
415	Cooked 1 cup	240	88	120	3	1				26	2	1.0	[17] 140	.14	.10	1.2	0
	Degermed, unenriched:																
416	Dry form 1 cup	138	12	500	11	2				108	8	1.5	[17] 610	.19	.07	1.4	0
417	Cooked 1 cup	240	88	120	3	1				26	2	.5	[17] 140	.05	.02	.2	0
418	Corn muffins, made with enriched degermed cornmeal and enriched flour; muffin 2⅜-in. diam. 1 muffin	40	33	125	3	4	2	2	Trace	19	42	.7	[17] 120	.08	.09	.6	Trace

No.	Food	Measure	Grams	Water (%)	Food energy (cal)	Protein (g)	Fat (g)	Saturated (g)	Oleic (g)	Linoleic (g)	Carbohydrate (g)	Calcium (mg)	Iron (mg)	Vitamin A (I.U.)	Thiamin (mg)	Riboflavin (mg)	Niacin (mg)	Ascorbic acid (mg)
419	Corn muffins, made with mix, egg, and milk; muffin 2⅜-in. diam.	1 muffin	40	30	130	3	4	1	2	1	20	96	.6	100	.07	.08	.6	Trace
420	Corn, puffed, presweetened, added nutrients.	1 cup	30	2	115	1	Trace	—	—	—	27	3	.5	0	.13	.05	.6	0
421	Corn, shredded, added nutrients.	1 cup	25	3	100	2	Trace	—	—	—	22	1	.6	0	.11	.05	.5	0
	Crackers:																	
422	Graham, 2½-in. square	4 crackers	28	6	110	2	3	—	—	—	21	11	.4	0	.01	.06	.4	0
423	Saltines	4 crackers	11	4	50	1	1	—	1	—	8	2	.1	0	Trace	Trace	.1	0
	Danish pastry, plain (without fruit or nuts):																	
424	Packaged ring, 12 ounces.	1 ring	340	22	1,435	25	80	24	37	15	155	170	3.1	1,050	.24	.51	2.7	Trace
425	Round piece, approx. 4¼-in. diam. by 1 in.	1 pastry	65	22	275	5	15	5	7	3	30	33	.6	200	.05	.10	.5	Trace
426	Ounce	1 oz	28	22	120	2	7	2	3	1	13	14	.3	90	.02	.04	.2	Trace
427	Doughnuts, cake type	1 doughnut	32	24	125	1	6	1	4	Trace	16	13	[18].4	30	[18].05	[18].05	[18].4	Trace
428	Farina, quick-cooking, enriched, cooked.	1 cup	245	89	105	3	Trace	—	—	—	22	147	[19].7	0	[19].12	[19].07	[19]1.0	0
	Macaroni, cooked: Enriched:																	
429	Cooked, firm stage (undergoes additional cooking in a food mixture).	1 cup	130	64	190	6	1	—	—	—	39	14	[19]1.4	0	[19].23	[19].14	[19]1.8	0
430	Cooked until tender	1 cup	140	72	155	5	1	—	—	—	32	8	[19]1.3	0	[19].20	[19].11	[19]1.5	0
	Unenriched:																	
431	Cooked, firm stage (undergoes additional cooking in a food mixture).	1 cup	130	64	190	6	1	—	—	—	39	14	.7	0	.03	.03	.5	0
432	Cooked until tender	1 cup	140	72	155	5	1	—	—	—	32	11	.6	0	.01	.01	.4	0
433	Macaroni (enriched) and cheese, baked.	1 cup	200	58	430	17	22	10	9	2	40	362	1.8	860	.20	.40	1.8	Trace
434	Canned	1 cup	240	80	230	9	10	4	3	1	26	199	1.0	260	.12	.24	1.0	Trace
435	Muffins, with enriched white flour; muffin, 3-inch diam.	1 muffin	40	38	120	3	4	1	2	1	17	42	.6	40	.07	.09	.6	Trace
	Noodles (egg noodles), cooked:																	
436	Enriched	1 cup	160	70	200	7	2	—	1	Trace	37	16	[19]1.4	110	[19].22	[19].13	[19]1.9	0
437	Unenriched	1 cup	160	70	200	7	2	—	1	Trace	37	16	1.0	110	.05	.03	.6	0

[17] This value is based on product made from yellow varieties of corn; white varieties contain only a trace.

[18] Based on product made with enriched flour. With unenriched flour, approximate values per doughnut are: Iron, 0.2 milligram; thiamin, 0.01 milligram; riboflavin, 0.03 milligram; niacin, 0.2 milligram.

[19] Iron, thiamin, riboflavin, and niacin are based on the minimum levels of enrichment specified in standards of identity promulgated under the Federal Food, Drug, and Cosmetic Act.

Table of Food Composition (continued)

[Dashes in the columns for nutrients show that no suitable value could be found although there is reason to believe that a measurable amount of the nutrient may be present]

	Food, approximate measure, and weight (in grams)	Water	Food energy	Protein	Fat	Fatty acids Saturated (total)	Unsaturated Oleic	Unsaturated Linoleic	Carbohydrate	Calcium	Iron	Vitamin A value	Thiamin	Riboflavin	Niacin	Ascorbic acid
		Percent	Calories	Grams	Grams	Grams	Grams	Grams	Grams	Milligrams	Milligrams	International units	Milligrams	Milligrams	Milligrams	Milligrams
	GRAIN PRODUCTS—Continued															
438	Oats (with or without corn) puffed, added nutrients. 1 cup — 25 Grams	3	100	3	1	---	---	---	19	44	1.2	0	0.24	0.04	0.5	0
439	Oatmeal or rolled oats, cooked. 1 cup — 240	87	130	5	2	---	---	1	23	22	1.4	0	.19	.05	.2	0
	Pancakes, 4-inch diam.:															
440	Wheat, enriched flour (home recipe). 1 cake — 27	50	60	2	2	Trace	1	Trace	9	27	.4	30	.05	.06	.4	Trace
441	Buckwheat (made from mix with egg and milk). 1 cake — 27	58	55	2	2	1	1	Trace	6	59	.4	60	.03	.04	.2	Trace
442	Plain or buttermilk (made from mix with egg and milk). 1 cake — 27	51	60	2	2	1	1	Trace	9	58	.3	70	.04	.06	.2	Trace
	Pie (piecrust made with unenriched flour): Sector, 4-in., ⅟₇ of 9-in. diam. pie:															
443	Apple (2-crust). 1 sector — 135	48	350	3	15	4	7	3	51	11	.4	40	.03	.03	.5	1
444	Butterscotch (1-crust). 1 sector — 130	45	350	6	14	5	6	2	50	98	1.2	340	.04	.13	.3	Trace
445	Cherry (2-crust). 1 sector — 135	47	350	4	15	4	7	3	52	19	.4	590	.03	.03	.7	Trace
446	Custard (1-crust). 1 sector — 130	58	285	8	14	5	6	2	30	125	.8	300	.07	.21	.4	0
447	Lemon meringue (1-crust). 1 sector — 120	47	305	4	12	4	6	2	45	17	.6	200	.04	.10	.2	4
448	Mince (2-crust). 1 sector — 135	43	365	3	16	4	8	3	56	38	1.4	Trace	.09	.05	.5	1
449	Pecan (1-crust). 1 sector — 118	20	490	6	27	4	16	5	60	55	3.3	190	.19	.08	.4	Trace
450	Pineapple chiffon (1-crust). 1 sector — 93	41	265	6	11	3	5	2	36	22	.8	320	.04	.08	.4	1
451	Pumpkin (1-crust). 1 sector — 130	59	275	5	15	5	6	2	32	66	.7	3,210	.04	.13	.7	Trace
	Piecrust, baked shell for pie made with:															
452	Enriched flour. 1 shell — 180	15	900	11	60	16	28	12	79	25	3.1	0	.36	.25	3.2	0
453	Unenriched flour. 1 shell — 180	15	900	11	60	16	28	12	79	25	.9	0	.05	.05	.9	0

No.	Food, approximate measure, and weight	Grams	Water (percent)	Food energy (calories)	Protein (grams)	Fat (grams)	Saturated (grams)	Oleic (grams)	Linoleic (grams)	Carbohydrate (grams)	Calcium (mg)	Iron (mg)	Vitamin A (I.U.)	Thiamine (mg)	Riboflavin (mg)	Niacin (mg)	Ascorbic acid (mg)
	Piecrust mix including stick form:																
454	Package, 10-oz., for double crust. — 1 pkg	284	9	1,480	20	93	23	46	21	141	131	1.4	0	.11	.11	2.0	0
455	Pizza (cheese) 5½-in. sector; ⅛ of 14-in. diam. pie. — 1 sector	75	45	185	7	6	2	3	Trace	27	107	.7	290	.04	.12	.7	4
	Popcorn, popped:																
456	Plain, large kernel — 1 cup	6	4	25	1	Trace	---	---	Trace	5	1	.2	---	---	.01	.1	0
457	With oil and salt — 1 cup	9	3	40	1	2	---	Trace	1	5	1	.2	---	---	.01	.2	0
458	Sugar coated — 1 cup	35	4	135	2	1	---	---	1	30	2	.5	---	---	.02	.4	0
	Pretzels:																
459	Dutch, twisted — 1 pretzel	16	5	60	2	1	---	---	Trace	12	4	.2	0	Trace	Trace	.1	0
460	Thin, twisted — 1 pretzel	6	5	25	1	Trace	---	---	Trace	5	1	.1	0	Trace	Trace	Trace	0
461	Stick, small, 2¼ inches — 10 sticks	3	5	10	Trace	Trace	---	Trace	Trace	2	1	Trace	0	Trace	Trace	Trace	0
462	Stick, regular, 3⅛ inches. — 5 sticks	3	5	10	Trace	Trace	---	Trace	Trace	2	1	Trace	0	Trace	Trace	Trace	0
	Rice, white:																
	Enriched:																
463	Raw — 1 cup	185	12	670	12	1	---	---	---	149	44	[20]5.4	0	[20].81	[20].06	[20]6.5	0
464	Cooked — 1 cup	205	73	225	4	Trace	---	---	---	50	21	[20]1.8	0	[20].23	[20].02	[20]2.1	0
465	Instant, ready-to-serve. — 1 cup	165	73	180	4	Trace	---	---	---	40	5	[20]1.3	0	[20].21	[20]---	[20]1.7	0
466	Unenriched, cooked — 1 cup	205	73	225	4	Trace	---	---	---	50	21	.4	0	.04	.02	.8	0
467	Parboiled, cooked — 1 cup	175	73	185	4	Trace	---	---	---	41	33	[20]1.4	0	[20].19	[20]---	[20]2.1	0
468	Rice, puffed, added nutrients. — 1 cup	15	4	60	1	Trace	---	---	---	13	3	.3	0	.07	.01	.7	0
	Rolls, enriched:																
	Cloverleaf or pan:																
469	Home recipe — 1 roll	35	26	120	3	3	1	1	1	20	16	.7	30	.09	.09	.8	Trace
470	Commercial — 1 roll	28	31	85	2	2	Trace	1	Trace	15	21	.5	Trace	.08	.05	.6	Trace
471	Frankfurter or hamburger. — 1 roll	40	31	120	3	2	1	1	1	21	30	.8	Trace	.11	.07	.9	Trace
472	Hard, round or rectangular. — 1 roll	50	25	155	5	2	Trace	1	Trace	30	24	1.2	Trace	.13	.12	1.4	Trace
473	Rye wafers, whole-grain, 1⅞ by 3½ inches. — 2 wafers	13	6	45	2	Trace	---	---	---	10	7	.5	0	.04	.03	.2	0
474	Spaghetti, cooked, tender stage, enriched. — 1 cup	140	72	155	5	1	---	---	---	32	11	[19]1.3	0	[19].20	[19].11	[19]1.5	0

[19] Iron, thiamin, riboflavin, and niacin are based on the minimum levels of enrichment specified in standards of identity promulgated under the Federal Food, Drug, and Cosmetic Act.

[20] Iron, thiamin, and niacin are based on the minimum levels of enrichment specified in standards of identity promulgated under the Federal Food, Drug, and Cosmetic Act. Riboflavin is based on unenriched rice. When the minimum level of enrichment for riboflavin specified in the standards of identity becomes effective the value will be 0.12 milligram per cup of parboiled rice and of white rice.

Table of Food Composition (continued)

[Dashes show that no basis could be found for imputing a value although there was some reason to believe that a measurable amount of the constituent might be present]

	Food, approximate measure, and weight (in grams)	Water	Food energy	Protein	Fat	Fatty acids Saturated (total)	Fatty acids Unsaturated Oleic	Fatty acids Unsaturated Linoleic	Carbohydrate	Calcium	Iron	Vitamin A value	Thiamin	Riboflavin	Niacin	Ascorbic acid
		Percent	Calories	Grams	Grams	Grams	Grams	Grams	Grams	Milligrams	Milligrams	International units	Milligrams	Milligrams	Milligrams	Milligrams
	GRAIN PRODUCTS—Continued															
	Spaghetti with meat balls, and tomato sauce:															
475	Home recipe — 1 cup — 248	70	330	19	12	4	6	1	39	124	3.7	1,590	0.25	0.30	4.0	22
476	Canned — 1 cup — 250	78	260	12	10	2	3	4	28	53	3.3	1,000	.15	.18	2.3	5
	Spaghetti in tomato sauce with cheese:															
477	Home recipe — 1 cup — 250	77	260	9	9	2	5	1	37	80	2.3	1,080	.25	.18	2.3	13
478	Canned — 1 cup — 250	80	190	6	2	1	1	1	38	40	2.8	930	.35	.28	4.5	10
479	Waffles, with enriched flour, 7-in. diam. — 1 waffle — 75	41	210	7	7	2	4	1	28	85	1.3	250	.13	.19	1.0	Trace
480	Waffles, made from mix, enriched, egg and milk added, 7-in. diam. — 1 waffle — 75	42	205	7	8	3	3	1	27	179	1.0	170	.11	.17	.7	Trace
481	Wheat, puffed, added nutrients. — 1 cup — 15	3	55	2	Trace	---	---	---	12	4	.6	0	.08	.03	1.2	0
482	Wheat, shredded, plain — 1 biscuit — 25	7	90	2	1	---	---	---	20	11	.9	0	.06	.03	1.1	0
483	Wheat flakes, added nutrients. — 1 cup — 30	4	105	3	Trace	---	---	---	24	12	1.3	0	.19	.04	1.5	0
	Wheat flours:															
484	Whole-wheat, from hard wheats, stirred. — 1 cup — 120	12	400	16	2	Trace	1	1	85	49	4.0	0	.66	.14	5.2	0
	All-purpose or family flour, enriched:															
485	Sifted — 1 cup — 115	12	420	12	1	---	---	---	88	18	[19]3.3	0	[19].51	[19].30	[19]4.0	0
486	Unsifted — 1 cup — 125	12	455	13	1	---	---	---	95	20	[19]3.6	0	[19].55	[19].33	[19]4.4	0
487	Self-rising, enriched — 1 cup — 125	12	440	12	1	---	---	---	93	331	[19]3.6	0	[19].55	[19].33	[19]4.4	0
488	Cake or pastry flour, sifted. — 1 cup — 96	12	350	7	1	---	---	---	76	16	.5	0	.03	.03	.7	0
	FATS, OILS															
	Butter:															
	Regular, 4 sticks per pound:															
489	Stick — ½ cup — 113	16	810	1	92	51	30	3	1	23	0	[21]3,750	0	---	---	0

No.	Food, approximate measure, and weight	Grams	Water (percent)	Food energy	Protein (grams)	Fat (grams)	Saturated (total) (grams)	Oleic (grams)	Linoleic (grams)	Carbohydrate (grams)	Calcium (mg)	Iron (mg)	Vitamin A value (I.U.)	Thiamin (mg)	Riboflavin (mg)	Niacin (mg)	Ascorbic acid (mg)
490	Tablespoon (approx. 1 tbsp. ⅛ stick)	14	16	100	Trace	12	6	4	Trace	Trace	3	0	[21]470	—	—	—	0
491	Pat (1-in. sq. ⅓-in. high; 90 per lb.), 1 pat	5	16	35	Trace	4	2	1	Trace	Trace	1	0	[21]170	—	—	—	0
	Whipped, 6 sticks or 2, 8-oz. containers per pound:																
492	Stick, ½ cup	76	16	540	1	61	34	20	2	Trace	15	0	[21]2,500	0	0	0	0
493	Tablespoon (approx. 1 tbsp. ⅛ stick)	9	16	65	Trace	8	4	3	Trace	Trace	2	0	[21]310	0	0	0	0
494	Pat (1¼-in. sq. ⅓-in. high; 120 per lb.), 1 pat	4	16	25	Trace	3	2	1	Trace	Trace	1	0	[21]130	0	0	0	0
	Fats, cooking:																
495	Lard, 1 cup	205	0	1,850	0	205	78	94	20	0	0	0	0	0	0	0	0
496	Lard, 1 tbsp.	13	0	115	0	13	5	6	1	0	0	0	0	0	0	0	0
497	Vegetable fats, 1 cup	200	0	1,770	0	200	50	100	44	0	0	0	—	0	0	0	0
498	Vegetable fats, 1 tbsp.	13	0	110	0	13	3	6	3	0	0	0	—	0	0	0	0
	Margarine:																
	Regular, 4 sticks per pound:																
499	Stick, ½ cup	113	16	815	1	92	17	46	25	1	23	0	[22]3,750	0	0	1	0
500	Tablespoon (approx. 1 tbsp. ⅛ stick)	14	16	100	Trace	12	2	6	3	Trace	3	0	[22]470	0	0	Trace	0
501	Pat (1-in. sq. ⅓-in. high; 90 per lb.), 1 pat	5	16	35	Trace	4	1	2	1	Trace	1	0	[22]170	0	0	Trace	0
	Whipped, 6 sticks per pound:																
502	Stick, ½ cup	76	16	545	1	61	11	31	17	Trace	15	0	[22]2,500	0	0	Trace	0
	Soft, 2 8-oz. tubs per pound:																
503	Tub, 1 tub	227	16	1,635	1	184	34	68	68	1	45	0	[22]7,500	0	0	1	0
504	Tablespoon, 1 tbsp.	14	16	100	Trace	11	2	4	4	Trace	3	0	[22]470	0	0	Trace	0
	Oils, salad or cooking:																
505	Corn, 1 cup	220	0	1,945	0	220	22	62	117	0	0	0	—	0	0	0	0
506	Corn, 1 tbsp.	14	0	125	0	14	1	4	7	0	0	0	—	0	0	0	0
507	Cottonseed, 1 cup	220	0	1,945	0	220	55	46	110	0	0	0	—	0	0	0	0
508	Cottonseed, 1 tbsp.	14	0	125	0	14	4	3	7	0	0	0	—	0	0	0	0
509	Olive, 1 cup	220	0	1,945	0	220	24	167	15	0	0	0	—	0	0	0	0
510	Olive, 1 tbsp.	14	0	125	0	14	2	11	1	0	0	0	—	0	0	0	0
511	Peanut, 1 cup	220	0	1,945	0	220	40	103	64	0	0	0	—	0	0	0	0
512	Peanut, 1 tbsp.	14	0	125	0	14	3	7	4	0	0	0	—	0	0	0	0
513	Safflower, 1 cup	220	0	1,945	0	220	18	37	165	0	0	0	—	0	0	0	0
514	Safflower, 1 tbsp.	14	0	125	0	14	1	2	10	0	0	0	—	0	0	0	0
515	Soybean, 1 cup	220	0	1,945	0	220	33	44	114	0	0	0	—	0	0	0	0
516	Soybean, 1 tbsp.	14	0	125	0	14	2	3	7	0	0	0	—	0	0	0	0

[19] Iron, thiamin, riboflavin, and niacin are based on the minimum levels of enrichment specified in standards of identity promulgated under the Federal Food, Drug, and Cosmetic Act.

[21] Year-round average.

[22] Based on the average vitamin A content of fortified margarine. Federal specifications for fortified margarine require a minimum of 15,000 I.U. of vitamin A per pound.

Table of Food Composition (continued)

[Dashes in the columns for nutrients show that no suitable value could be found although there is reason to believe that a measurable amount of the nutrient may be present]

	Food, approximate measure, and weight (in grams)	Water	Food energy	Protein	Fat	Fatty acids Saturated (total)	Fatty acids Unsaturated Oleic	Fatty acids Unsaturated Linoleic	Carbohydrate	Calcium	Iron	Vitamin A value	Thiamin	Riboflavin	Niacin	Ascorbic acid
		Grams	Percent	Calories	Grams	Grams	Grams	Grams	Grams	Grams	Milligrams	Milligrams	International units	Milligrams	Milligrams	Milligrams	Milligrams

FATS, OILS—Continued

	Food, approximate measure, and weight	Grams	Water Percent	Food energy Calories	Protein Grams	Fat Grams	Saturated (total) Grams	Oleic Grams	Linoleic Grams	Carbohydrate Grams	Calcium Milligrams	Iron Milligrams	Vitamin A International units	Thiamin Milligrams	Riboflavin Milligrams	Niacin Milligrams	Ascorbic acid Milligrams
	Salad dressings:																
517	Blue cheese 1 tbsp	15	32	75	1	8	2	2	4	1	12	Trace	30	Trace	0.02	Trace	Trace
	Commercial, mayonnaise type:																
518	Regular 1 tbsp	15	41	65	Trace	6	1	1	3	2	2	Trace	30	Trace	Trace	Trace	---
519	Special dietary, low-calorie 1 tbsp	16	81	20	Trace	2	Trace	Trace	1	1	3	Trace	40	Trace	Trace	Trace	---
	French:																
520	Regular 1 tbsp	16	39	65	Trace	6	1	1	3	3	2	.1	---	---	---	---	---
521	Special dietary, low-fat with artificial sweeteners 1 tbsp	15	95	Trace	Trace	Trace	---	---	---	Trace	2	.1	---	---	---	---	---
522	Home cooked, boiled 1 tbsp	16	68	25	1	2	1	1	Trace	2	14	.1	80	.01	.03	Trace	Trace
523	Mayonnaise 1 tbsp	14	15	100	Trace	11	2	2	6	Trace	3	.1	40	Trace	.01	Trace	Trace
524	Thousand island 1 tbsp	16	32	80	Trace	8	1	2	4	3	2	.1	50	Trace	Trace	Trace	Trace
	SUGARS, SWEETS																
	Cake icings:																
525	Chocolate made with milk and table fat. 1 cup	275	14	1,035	9	38	21	14	1	185	165	3.3	580	.06	.28	.6	1
526	Coconut (with boiled icing). 1 cup	166	15	605	3	13	11	1	Trace	124	10	.8	0	.02	.07	.3	0
527	Creamy fudge from mix with water only. 1 cup	245	15	830	7	16	5	8	3	183	96	2.7	Trace	.05	.20	.7	Trace
528	White, boiled 1 cup	94	18	300	1	0	---	---	---	76	2	Trace	0	Trace	.03	Trace	0
	Candy:																
529	Caramels, plain or chocolate. 1 oz	28	8	115	1	3	2	1	Trace	22	42	.4	Trace	.01	.05	.1	Trace
530	Chocolate, milk, plain. 1 oz	28	1	145	2	9	5	3	Trace	16	65	.3	80	.02	.10	.1	Trace
531	Chocolate-coated peanuts. 1 oz	28	1	160	5	12	3	6	2	11	33	.4	Trace	.10	.05	2.1	Trace

No.	Food, approximate measure, and weight	Grams	Water (%)	Food energy (cal.)	Protein (g)	Fat (g)	Saturated (g)	Oleic (g)	Linoleic (g)	Carbo- hydrate (g)	Calcium (mg)	Iron (mg)	Vit. A (I.U.)	Thiamine (mg)	Ribo- flavin (mg)	Niacin (mg)	Ascorbic acid (mg)
532	Fondant; mints, uncoated; candy corn. 1 oz.	28	8	105	Trace	1	Trace	--	--	25	4	.3	0	Trace	Trace	Trace	0
533	Fudge, plain. 1 oz.	28	8	115	1	3	2	1	Trace	21	22	.3	Trace	.01	.03	.1	Trace
534	Gum drops. 1 oz.	28	12	100	Trace	Trace	--	--	--	25	2	.1	0	0	Trace	Trace	0
535	Hard. 1 oz.	28	1	110	0	Trace	--	--	--	28	6	.5	0	0	0	0	0
536	Marshmallows. 1 oz.	28	17	90	1	Trace	--	--	--	23	5	.5	0	0	Trace	Trace	0
	Chocolate-flavored sirup or topping:																
537	Thin type. 1 fl. oz.	38	32	90	1	1	Trace	Trace	Trace	24	6	.6	Trace	.01	.03	.2	0
538	Fudge type. 1 fl. oz.	38	25	125	2	5	3	2	Trace	20	48	.5	60	.02	.08	.2	Trace
	Chocolate-flavored beverage powder (approx. 4 heaping teaspoons per oz.):																
539	With nonfat dry milk. 1 oz.	28	2	100	5	1	--	--	--	20	167	.5	10	.04	.21	.2	1
540	Without nonfat dry milk. 1 oz.	28	1	100	1	1	--	--	--	25	9	.6	0	.01	.03	.1	0
541	Honey, strained or extracted. 1 tbsp.	21	17	65	Trace	0	--	--	--	17	1	.1	0	Trace	.01	.1	Trace
542	Jams and preserves. 1 tbsp.	20	29	55	Trace	Trace	--	--	--	14	4	.2	Trace	Trace	.01	Trace	Trace
543	Jellies. 1 tbsp.	18	29	50	Trace	Trace	--	--	--	13	4	.3	Trace	Trace	.01	Trace	1
	Molasses, cane:																
544	Light (first extraction). 1 tbsp.	20	24	50	--	--	--	--	--	13	33	.9	--	.01	.01	Trace	--
545	Blackstrap (third extraction). 1 tbsp.	20	24	45	--	--	--	--	--	11	137	3.2	--	.02	.04	.4	--
	Sirups:																
546	Sorghum. 1 tbsp.	21	23	55	--	0	--	--	--	14	35	2.6	0	--	.02	Trace	0
547	Table blends, chiefly corn, light and dark. 1 tbsp.	21	24	60	0	0	--	--	--	15	9	.8	0	0	0	0	0
	Sugars:																
548	Brown, firm packed. 1 cup.	220	2	820	0	0	--	--	--	212	187	7.5	0	.02	.07	.4	0
	White:																
549	Granulated. 1 cup.	200	Trace	770	0	0	--	--	--	199	0	.2	0	0	0	0	0
550	Granulated. 1 tbsp.	11	Trace	40	0	0	--	--	--	11	0	Trace	0	0	0	0	0
551	Powdered, stirred before measuring. 1 cup.	120	Trace	460	0	0	--	--	--	119	0	.1	0	0	0	0	0
	MISCELLANEOUS ITEMS																
552	Barbecue sauce. 1 cup.	250	81	230	4	17	2	5	9	20	53	2.0	900	.03	.03	.8	13
	Beverages, alcoholic:																
553	Beer. 12 fl. oz.	360	92	150	1	0	--	--	--	14	18	Trace	--	.01	.11	2.2	--
	Gin, rum, vodka, whiskey:																
554	80-proof. 1½ fl. oz. jigger.	42	67	100	--	--	--	--	--	Trace	--	--	--	--	--	--	--
555	86-proof. 1½ fl. oz. jigger.	42	64	105	--	--	--	--	--	Trace	--	--	--	--	--	--	--
556	90-proof. 1½ fl. oz. jigger.	42	62	110	--	--	--	--	--	Trace	--	--	--	--	--	--	--

Table of Food Composition (continued)

[Dashes in the columns for nutrients show that no suitable value could be found although there is reason to believe that a measurable amount of the nutrient may be present]

	Food, approximate measure, and weight (in grams)		Water	Food energy	Pro-tein	Fat	Fatty acids Satu-rated (total)	Fatty acids Unsaturated Oleic	Fatty acids Unsaturated Lin-oleic	Carbo-hy-drate	Cal-cium	Iron	Vita-min A value	Thia-min	Ribo-flavin	Niacin	Ascor-bic acid
		Grams	Per-cent	Calo-ries	Grams	Grams	Grams	Grams	Grams	Grams	Milli-grams	Milli-grams	Inter-national units	Milli-grams	Milli-gram	Milli-grams	Milli-grams
	MISCELLANEOUS ITEMS—Continued																
	Beverages, alcoholic—Continued																
	Gin, rum, vodka, whiskey—Con.																
557	94-proof	1½ fl. oz. jigger.	42	60	115						Trace						
558	100-proof	1½ fl. oz. jigger.	42	58	125						Trace						
	Wines:																
559	Dessert	3½ fl. oz. glass.	103	77	140	Trace	0				8	8			.01	.02	.2	
560	Table	3½ fl. oz. glass.	102	86	85	Trace	0				4	9	.4		Trace	.01	.1	
	Beverages, carbonated, sweetened, nonalcoholic:																
561	Carbonated water	12 fl. oz.	366	92	115	0	0				29			0	0	0	0	
562	Cola type	12 fl. oz.	369	90	145	0	0				37			0	0	0	0	
563	Fruit-flavored sodas and Tom Collins mixes.	12 fl. oz.	372	88	170	0	0				45			0	0	0	0	
564	Ginger ale	12 fl. oz.	366	92	115	0	0				29			0	0	0		
565	Root beer	12 fl. oz.	370	90	150	0	0				39			0	0	0		
566	Bouillon cubes, approx. ½ in.	1 cube	4	4	5	1	Trace				Trace							
	Chocolate:																
567	Bitter or baking	1 oz.	28	2	145	3	15	8	6	Trace	8	22	1.9	20	.01	.07	.4	0
568	Semi-sweet, small pieces.	1 cup	170	1	860	7	61	34	22	1	97	51	4.4	30	.02	.14	.9	0
	Gelatin:																
569	Plain, dry powder in envelope.	1 envelope	7	13	25	6	Trace				0							
570	Dessert powder, 3-oz. package.	1 pkg.	85	2	315	8	0				75							
571	Gelatin dessert, prepared with water.	1 cup	240	84	140	4	0				34							

Table — foods items 572–592 (nutrient values). Column order: food and measure, weight (g), water (%), food energy (cal.), protein (g), fat (g), saturated fat (g), oleic (g), linoleic (g), carbohydrate (g), calcium (mg), iron (mg), vitamin A (I.U.), thiamine (mg), riboflavin (mg), niacin (mg), ascorbic acid (mg).

No.	Food, approximate measure	Measure	Grams	Water	Food energy	Protein	Fat	Saturated	Oleic	Linoleic	Carbohydrate	Calcium	Iron	Vitamin A	Thiamine	Riboflavin	Niacin	Ascorbic acid
	Olives, pickled:																	
572	Green	4 medium or 3 extra large or 2 giant.	16	78	15	Trace	2	Trace	2	Trace	Trace	8	.2	40	Trace	Trace	---	---
573	Ripe: Mission	3 small or 2 large.	10	73	15	Trace	2	Trace	2	Trace	Trace	9	.1	10	Trace	.01	---	---
	Pickles, cucumber:																	
574	Dill, medium, whole, 3¾ in. long, 1¼ in. diam.	1 pickle	65	93	10	1	Trace	---	---	---	1	17	.7	70	Trace	Trace	Trace	4
575	Fresh, sliced, 1½ in. diam., ¼ in. thick.	2 slices	15	79	10	Trace	Trace	---	---	---	3	5	.3	20	Trace	Trace	Trace	1
576	Sweet, gherkin, small, whole, approx. 2½ in. long, ¾ in. diam.	1 pickle	15	61	20	Trace	Trace	---	---	---	6	2	.2	10	Trace	Trace	Trace	1
577	Relish, finely chopped, sweet.	1 tbsp.	15	63	20	Trace	Trace	---	---	---	5	3	.1	---	---	---	---	---
578	Popcorn. See Grain Products. Popsicle, 3 fl. oz. size	1 popsicle	95	80	70	0	0	0	0	0	18	0	Trace	0	0	0	0	0
	Pudding, home recipe with starch base:																	
579	Chocolate	1 cup	260	66	385	8	12	7	4	Trace	67	250	1.3	390	.05	.36	.3	1
580	Vanilla (blanc mange)	1 cup	255	76	285	9	10	5	3	Trace	41	298	Trace	410	.08	.41	.3	2
581	Pudding mix, dry form, 4-oz. package.	1 pkg.	113	2	410	3	2	1	1	Trace	103	23	1.8	Trace	.02	.08	.5	0
582	Sherbet	1 cup	193	67	260	2	2	---	---	---	59	31	Trace	120	.02	.06	Trace	4
	Soups:																	
	Canned, condensed, ready-to-serve:																	
	Prepared with an equal volume of milk:																	
583	Cream of chicken	1 cup	245	85	180	7	10	3	4	3	15	172	.5	610	.05	.27	.7	2
584	Cream of mushroom	1 cup	245	83	215	7	14	4	4	5	16	191	.5	250	.05	.34	.7	1
585	Tomato	1 cup	250	84	175	7	7	3	2	1	23	168	.8	1,200	.10	.25	1.3	15
	Prepared with an equal volume of water:																	
586	Bean with pork	1 cup	250	84	170	8	6	1	2	2	22	63	2.3	650	.13	.08	1.0	3
587	Beef broth, bouillon consomme.	1 cup	240	96	30	5	0	0	0	0	3	Trace	.5	Trace	Trace	.02	1.2	---
588	Beef noodle	1 cup	240	93	70	4	3	1	1	1	7	7	1.0	50	.05	.07	1.0	Trace
589	Clam chowder, Manhattan type (with tomatoes, without milk).	1 cup	245	92	80	2	3	---	---	---	12	34	1.0	880	.02	.02	1.0	---
590	Cream of chicken	1 cup	240	92	95	3	6	1	2	3	8	24	.5	410	.02	.05	.5	Trace
591	Cream of mushroom	1 cup	240	90	135	2	10	1	3	5	10	41	.5	70	.02	.12	.7	Trace
592	Minestrone	1 cup	245	90	105	5	3	---	---	---	14	37	1.0	2,350	.07	.05	1.0	---

Table of Food Composition (continued)

[Dashes in the columns for nutrients show that no suitable value could be found although there is reason to believe that a measurable amount of the nutrient may be present]

	Food, approximate measure, and weight (in grams)	Water	Food energy	Protein	Fat	Fatty acids Saturated (total)	Fatty acids Unsaturated Oleic	Fatty acids Unsaturated Linoleic	Carbohydrate	Calcium	Iron	Vitamin A value	Thiamin	Riboflavin	Niacin	Ascorbic acid
		Per cent	Calories	Grams	Grams	Grams	Grams	Grams	Grams	Milligrams	Milligrams	International units	Milligrams	Milligrams	Milligrams	Milligrams
	MISCELLANEOUS ITEMS—Continued															
	Soups—Continued															
	Canned, condensed, ready-to-serve—Con.															
	Prepared with an equal volume of water—Con.															
593	Split pea. 1 cup, 245 Grams	85	145	9	3	1	2	Trace	21	29	1.5	440	0.25	0.15	1.5	1
594	Tomato. 1 cup, 245	90	90	2	3	Trace	1	1	16	15	.7	1,000	.05	.05	1.2	12
595	Vegetable beef. 1 cup, 245	92	80	5	2	-----	-----	-----	10	12	.7	2,700	.05	.05	1.0	-----
596	Vegetarian. 1 cup, 245	92	80	2	2	-----	-----	-----	13	20	1.0	2,940	.05	.05	1.0	-----
	Dehydrated, dry form:															
597	Chicken noodle (2-oz. package). 1 pkg., 57	6	220	8	6	2	3	1	33	34	1.4	190	.30	.15	2.4	3
598	Onion mix (1½-oz. package). 1 pkg., 43	3	150	6	5	1	2	1	23	42	.6	30	.05	.03	.3	6
599	Tomato vegetable with noodles (2½-oz. pkg.). 1 pkg., 71	4	245	6	6	2	3	1	45	33	1.4	1,700	.21	.13	1.8	18
	Frozen, condensed:															
	Clam chowder, New England type (with milk, without tomatoes):															
600	Prepared with equal volume of milk. 1 cup, 245	83	210	9	12				16	240	1.0	250	.07	.29	.5	Trace
601	Prepared with equal volume of water. 1 cup, 240	89	130	4	8				11	91	1.0	50	.05	.10	.5	-----
	Cream of potato:															
602	Prepared with equal volume of milk. 1 cup, 245	83	185	8	10	5	3	Trace	18	208	1.0	590	.10	.27	.5	Trace
603	Prepared with equal volume of water. 1 cup, 240	90	105	3	5	3	2	Trace	12	58	1.0	410	.05	.05	.5	-----

No.	Food	Measure	Grams	Water (%)	Food energy (cal.)	Protein (g)	Fat (g)	Saturated fatty acids (g)	Unsaturated oleic (g)	Unsaturated linoleic (g)	Carbohydrate (g)	Calcium (mg)	Iron (mg)	Vitamin A (I.U.)	Thiamine (mg)	Riboflavin (mg)	Niacin (mg)	Ascorbic acid (mg)
	Cream of shrimp:																	
604	Prepared with equal volume of milk.	1 cup	245	82	245	9	16	----	----	----	15	189	.5	290	.07	.27	.5	Trace
605	Prepared with equal volume of water.	1 cup	240	88	160	5	12	----	----	----	8	38	.5	120	.05	.05	.5	----
	Oyster stew:																	
606	Prepared with equal volume of milk.	1 cup	240	83	200	10	12	----	----	----	14	305	1.4	410	.12	.41	.5	Trace
607	Prepared with equal volume of water.	1 cup	240	90	120	6	8	----	----	----	8	158	1.4	240	.07	.19	.5	----
608	Tapioca, dry, quick-cooking.	1 cup	152	13	535	1	Trace	----	----	----	131	15	.6	0	0	0	0	0
	Tapioca desserts:																	
609	Apple.	1 cup	250	70	295	1	Trace	----	----	----	74	8	.5	30	Trace	Trace	Trace	Trace
610	Cream pudding.	1 cup	165	72	220	8	8	4	3	Trace	28	173	.7	480	.07	.30	.2	2
611	Tartar sauce.	1 tbsp.	14	34	75	Trace	8	1	1	4	1	3	.1	30	Trace	Trace	Trace	Trace
612	Vinegar.	1 tbsp.	15	94	Trace	Trace	0	----	----	----	1	1	.1	----	----	----	----	----
613	White sauce, medium.	1 cup	250	73	405	10	31	16	10	1	22	288	.5	1,150	.10	.43	.5	2
	Yeast:																	
614	Baker's, dry, active.	1 pkg.	7	5	20	3	Trace	----	----	----	3	3	1.1	Trace	.16	.38	2.6	Trace
615	Brewer's, dry.	1 tbsp.	8	5	25	3	Trace	----	----	----	3	17	1.4	Trace	1.25	.34	3.0	Trace
	Yoghurt. See Milk, Cheese, Cream, Imitation Cream.																	

Appendix I
Recommended Daily Dietary Allowances[1]

Revised 1973 by the Food and Nutrition Board, National Academy of Sciences-National Research Council. Designed for the maintenance of good nutrition of practically all healthy people in the United States.

	Age years	Weight (kg)	Weight (lbs)	Height (cm)	Height (in)	Energy (kcal)	Protein (g)	Vitamin A Activity (RE)	Vitamin A Activity (IU)	Vitamin D (IU)	Vitamin E Activity (IU)	Ascorbic Acid (mg)	Folacin (mcg)	Niacin (mg)	Riboflavin (mg)	Thiamin (mg)	Vitamin B₆ (mg)	Vitamin B₁₂ (mcg)	Calcium (mg)	Phosphorus (mg)	Iodine (mcg)	Iron (mg)	Magnesium (mg)	Zinc (mg)
INFANTS	0.0-0.5	6	14	60	24	kg x 117	kg x 2.2	420	1400	400	4	35	50	5	0.4	0.3	0.3	0.3	360	240	35	10	60	3
	0.5-1.0	9	20	71	28	kg x 108	kg x 2.0	400	2000	400	5	35	50	8	0.6	0.5	0.4	0.3	540	400	45	15	70	5
CHILDREN	1-3	13	28	86	34	1300	23	400	2000	400	7	40	100	9	0.8	0.7	0.6	1.0	800	800	60	15	150	10
	4-6	20	44	110	44	1800	30	500	2500	400	9	40	200	12	1.1	0.9	0.9	1.5	800	800	80	10	200	10
	7-10	30	66	135	54	2400	36	700	3300	400	10	40	300	16	1.2	1.2	1.2	2.0	800	800	110	10	250	10
MALES	11-14	44	97	158	63	2800	44	1000	5000	400	12	45	400	18	1.5	1.4	1.6	3.0	1200	1200	130	18	350	15
	15-18	61	134	172	69	3000	54	1000	5000	400	15	45	400	20	1.8	1.5	2.0	3.0	1200	1200	150	18	400	15
	19-22	67	147	172	69	3000	54	1000	5000	400	15	45	400	20	1.8	1.5	2.0	3.0	800	800	140	10	350	15
	23-50	70	154	172	69	2700	56	1000	5000		15	45	400	18	1.6	1.4	2.0	3.0	800	800	130	10	350	15
	51+	70	154	172	69	2400	56	1000	5000		15	45	400	16	1.5	1.2	2.0	3.0	800	800	110	10	350	15
FEMALES	11-14	44	97	155	62	2400	44	800	4000	400	12	45	400	16	1.3	1.2	1.6	3.0	1200	1200	115	18	300	15
	15-18	54	119	162	65	2100	48	800	4000	400	12	45	400	14	1.4	1.1	2.0	3.0	1200	1200	115	18	300	15
	19-22	58	128	162	65	2100	46	800	4000	400	12	45	400	14	1.4	1.1	2.0	3.0	800	800	100	18	300	15
	23-50	58	128	162	65	2000	46	800	4000		12	45	400	13	1.2	1.0	2.0	3.0	800	800	100	18	300	15
	51+	58	128	162	65	1800	46	800	4000		12	45	400	12	1.1	1.0	2.0	3.0	800	800	80	10	300	15
PREGNANT						+300	+30	1000	5000	400	15	60	800	+2	+0.3	+0.3	2.5	4.0	1200	1200	125	18	450	20
LACTATING						+500	+20	1200	6000	400	15	80	600	+4	+0.5	+0.3	2.5	4.0	1200	1200	150	18+	450	25

[1]The allowances are intended to provide for individual variations among most normal persons as they live in the United States under usual environmental stresses. Diets should be based on a variety of common foods in order to provide other nutrients for which human requirements have been less well defined. See text for more-detailed discussion of allowances and of nutrients not tabulated.

Index

†